Uveitis: A Clinical Guide

Uveitis: A Clinical Guide

Editor: Slade Decker

AMERICAN
MEDICAL PUBLISHERS
www.americanmedicalpublishers.com

AMERICAN MEDICAL PUBLISHERS
www.americanmedicalpublishers.com

Cataloging-in-Publication Data

Uveitis : a clinical guide / edited by Slade Decker.
p. cm.
Includes bibliographical references and index.
ISBN 979-8-88740-550-6
1. Uveitis. 2. Uveitis--Diagnosis. 3. Uveitis--Treatment. 4. Uvea--Diseases.
5. Eye--Inflammation. 6. Ophthalmology. I. Decker, Slade.
RE351 .U94 2023
617.72--dc23

American Medical Publishers,
41 Flatbush Avenue,
1st Floor, New York,
NY 11217, USA

ISBN 979-8-88740-550-6 (Hardback)

Contents

Preface

This book has been an outcome of determined endeavour from a group of educationists in the field. The primary objective was to involve a broad spectrum of professionals from diverse cultural background involved in the field for developing new researches. The book not only targets students but also scholars pursuing higher research for further enhancement of the theoretical and practical applications of the subject.

Uveitis is an inflammation of the uvea, the middle layer of tissue surrounding the eye, that consists of the iris, ciliary body and choroid. The anatomical forms of uveitis are anterior, intermediate, posterior, or diffuse. Anterior uveitis is defined as inflammation of the iris and the anterior chamber. Intermediate uveitis is defined as inflammation of the ciliary body and vitreous humor. Posterior uveitis is defined as the inflammation of the retina, choroid, or optic disc. The major cause includes an infection (viral, fungal, bacterial, or parasitic), systemic disease (typically an autoimmune disorder), or injury to the eye. The symptoms of uveitis consist of eye redness, eye pain, blurred vision, light sensitivity, floating spots and decreased vision. Treatment consists of glucocorticoid steroids, either as topical eye drops or as oral therapy that relieves pain caused by spasms of the pupil-constriction muscle. The objective of this book is to give a general view of the different causes, symptoms, and treatment methodologies of uveitis. It will serve as a valuable source of reference for graduate and postgraduate students.

It was an honour to edit such a profound book and also a challenging task to compile and examine all the relevant data for accuracy and originality. I wish to acknowledge the efforts of the contributors for submitting such brilliant and diverse chapters in the field and for endlessly working for the completion of the book. Last, but not the least; I thank my family for being a constant source of support in all my research endeavours.

Editor

1

Interrelationship of Stress, Environment and Herpes Simplex Virus Type-1 on Behçet's Disease: Using a Mouse Model

S. M. Shamsul Islam[1], *Hye-Myung Ryu*[2], *Hasan M. Sayeed*[1] *and Seonghyang Sohn*[1,2*]

[1] *Department of Biomedical Science, School of Medicine, Ajou University, Suwon, South Korea,* [2] *Department of Microbiology, Ajou University School of Medicine, Suwon, South Korea*

Correspondence:
Seonghyang Sohn
sohnsh@ajou.ac.kr

The purpose of this study was to investigate effects of stress and environment factors on the induction of Behçet's disease (BD) using HSV-1 infected mouse model. BD is a chronic multisystemic inflammatory disease of unknown etiology. Environmental factors, immune dysfunction, and herpes simplex virus type-1 (HSV) infection might be triggers of BD. To investigate effects of environmental factors on the incidence of BD, HSV was inoculated into mice. Mice were then maintained in conventional facility or SPF facility to compare BD incidence rates. The incidence of BD was also tracked by adding stressors such as substance P (anxiety stress), 4°C (cold stress), xanthine sodium salt (oxidative stress), or 77 dB noise (noise stress). To clarify immune mechanisms involved in the difference in BD incidence caused by various stresses, dendritic cell activation markers were analyzed using flow cytometry. The combination of conventional environment, noise stress, and HSV had the highest rate of BD (38.1%) among all groups. However, HSV inoculated group in a SPF environment had the lowest incidence (2.2%). Frequencies of dendritic cell activation markers such as CD40, CD83, CD80, and CD86 were expressed differently under various stresses. Noise stress increased frequencies of CD83 positive cells. Noise stress also upregulated transcription factors T-bet and ROR-γt. Different gut microbiota compositions were observed between SPF and conventional environment by 16S rRNA sequence analysis. Environment and stress influenced the incidence of HSV-induced BD. Microbial diversity due to environmental differences might be one explanation for regional differences in the incidence of BD.

Keywords: Behçet's disease, stress, environment, herpes simplex virus, gut microbiota, mouse model

INTRODUCTION

Behçet's disease (BD) is a chronic, recurrent, multisystemic variable vessel vasculitis inflammatory disorder that can cause oral and genital ulcers, papulopustular and nodular skin lesions, arthritis, uveitis, venous and arterial thrombosis, arterial aneurysms, central nervous system lesions, and gastrointestinal ulcers (1). Several studies have addressed the epidemiological complex of BD. However, the exact etiology of BD remains inconclusive. Several factors are involved in the development of BD, including environmental pollutants, viral or bacterial infections, genetic polymorphism, and immune dysregulations (2). Herpes Simplex Virus (HSV) has been isolated from patients' ocular fluids (3), saliva (4), skin lesions (5), and peripheral blood (6). It is considered a triggering factor of BD. HSV-1 inoculated ICR mice had BD-like symptoms such as oral ulcers, genital ulcers, skin ulcers, eye symptoms, intestinal ulcers, arthritis, and skin crust (7). Therefore, it has been used as a potential animal model for BD.

Stresses such as psychological, environmental, and physiological stressors are known to threaten bodies' homeostasis and nonspecific responses (8). Stress has diverse adverse health effects, many of which are mediated by stressful actions on immune system (9). It has been reported that stress can induce pro-inflammatory or type 1-type 2 cytokine-mediated immune responses, leading to inability to modulate innate and adaptive immune responses (9). Interaction between physical and psychological factors and low quality of life are associated with BD progression (10). Stress is also recognized as a modulator of gut microbiota (11). Gut microbiota is a key component of immune homeostasis (12). Dysbiosis, an imbalance of gut microbiota, has been observed in many inflammatory autoimmune diseases such as multiple sclerosis (13), rheumatoid arthritis (14), and inflammatory bowel disease (15). It has been also found that BD is associated with significant gut microbiota changes, suggesting alterations in gut microbiota might play a role in the pathogenesis of BD (16). During psychological stress, the migration of dendritic cells (DCs) is enhanced, resulting in increased T cell responses (17). DCs are known as the forefront initiator of immune signals and the most potent antigen presenting cells with the ability to activate and differentiate T lymphocytes. They can effectively connect innate and adaptive immune systems. Antigen-capturing DCs go through a maturation process. Mature DCs can differentiate naïve T cells, B cells, and NK cells (18). DCs are involved in several autoimmune diseases such as inflammatory bowel disease (IBD) (19), rheumatoid arthritis (RA) (20), uveitis (21), and Crohn's disease (CD) (22). During the maturation process of DCs, DCs accumulate peptides, major histocompatibility complex class II molecules, and costimulatory molecules. CD40, CD80, CD83, and CD86 are DC costimulatory molecules (23). Among them, CD83 is known to play a pathogenic role in BD mice (24). It has been reported that inhibition of CD83 by GC7 can affect the ability of DCs to induce T cell proliferation (25).

In the present study, an HSV-1 induced BD symptomatic mice model was used to investigate the mechanism by which stress could increase the incidence of BD. DCs and gut microbiota compositions were also studied to understand their involvement in BD. Findings of this study revealed that DC and gut microbiota were regulated under stress conditions that caused BD.

MATERIALS AND METHODS

Animal Experiment

Animals used in this study were handled according to animal protocols and guidelines established by the Ethics Review Board of Ajou University School of Medicine. All animal experiments were approved by the Institutional Animal Care and Use Committee (IACUC) of Ajou University (IACUC-2018-0017). Institute of Cancer Research (ICR) mice at 4 to 5 weeks old were used as previously described (7). Virus inoculation was performed and then observed for 16 weeks. Mice were bred in a specific pathogen free (SPF) room or a conventional room with temperature and light control (20-22°C, 12 h light/dark cycle). These mice had free access to food and water. Animals were closely monitored and photographed during experiments.

HSV-1 Induced BD Symptomatic Mice

Virus inoculation was performed using published procedures (7). Briefly, the earlobes of mice were scratched with a needle and inoculated with 20 μL of 1 x 10^6 pfu/mL of HSV-1 (F strain) grown in Vero cells. Virus inoculation was performed twice with an interval of 10 days. Mice were anesthetized by intraperitoneal injection with 2,2,2-tribromo ethanol (240 mg/kg), virus was inoculated, and BD symptoms were confirmed by follow-up for 5 to 16 weeks. Several symptoms, including oral ulcers, genital ulcers, erythema, skin pustules, skin ulcers, arthritis, diarrhea, red-eye, loss of balance, and facial edema, were observed in mice after HSV inoculation. The incidence of BD was between 2% and 38% in HSV inoculated mice. Oral, genital, skin ulcers, and eye symptoms were classified as major symptoms. Arthritis, intestinal ulceration, and neurological involvement were considered as minor symptoms. Mice with at least one major symptom and at least one minor symptom were classified as having BD. Each symptom score was one point. The sum of scores of different symptoms was used to determine the severity of BD using 2006 BD Current Activity Form prepared by the International Society for Behçet's Disease (http://medhealth.leeds.ac.uk/download/910/behcetsdiseaseactivityform). All BD mice used in this study showed ocular symptoms. The disappearance of symptoms or a reduction in skin lesion size of 20% or more indicated improvement of BD. Whether ocular symptoms were improved was not confirmed. HSV-1 inoculated and asymptomatic mice were used as BD normal (BDN) mice as previously described (7).

Induction of Stress

Mice were exposed to several types of stress. For noise stress induction, mice were exposed to noise in a noise chamber. The ventilation chamber was equipped with a high-frequency driver (Electro-Voice DH-7) and a power amplifier (Ax5505, Inkel) operated with an arbitrary waveform generator (Agilent 33210A) that generated sound waves in the range of 0.1 Hz to 15 MHz. Animals were exposed to a 77 dB sound pressure level of broadband noise measured with a dual channel real-time frequency analyzer (Type 2144, Bruel & Kjaer) for 1 hour daily for 10 consecutive days. 77 dB sound pressure is a typical construction site noise level. Each animal was placed in a separate 10 cm diameter wire mesh cage to eliminate sound pressure attenuation by adjacent animals. For the induction of anxiety stress, Substance P (SP) was injected intraperitoneally. For cold stress induction, mice were kept in a cold room at 4°C for one hour daily for 10 consecutive days. And for induction of oxidative stress, xanthine sodium salt was injected intraperitoneally.

Preparation of siRNA

CD83 siRNA preparation was performed as detailed previously (24). In brief, CD83 siRNA oligonucleotides with the following sense and antisense sequences were synthesized by Integrated DNA Technology (Coralville, IA, USA): Sense, 5'-GUGCUUUUCAGUCAUCUACAAGCTA-3'; Antisense, 3'-CUCACGAAAAGUCAGUAGAUGUUCGAU-5'.

Mouse Treatment

SP (5 μg) was injected intraperitoneally five times every other day into normal mice, HSV-1 induced single symptomatic mice, and BD mice. To induce oxidative stress, 10 mg Xanthine sodium salt was injected intraperitoneally into mice once daily for five consecutive days. As a control group, mice were treated with PBS for the same period. CD83 siRNA was prepared as previously described (24). CD83 siRNA was mixed with a transfection reagent JetPEI (Polyplus-transfection, Illkirch-Graffenstaden, France) for injection into mice. To apply siRNA to mice, 0.5 μmol CD83 siRNA was dissolved in 200 μL of 5% glucose solution, mixed with jetPEI, and injected intraperitoneally twice at 5-day intervals. As a control, mice were treated with only transfection reagent during the same period.

Flow Cytometric Analysis

Mice were euthanized and peripheral blood leukocytes (PBLs) were collected by cardiac puncture and peritoneal macrophages (pMQs) were isolated from the peritoneal cavity. PBLs were washed with ammonium-chloride-potassium (ACK) lysis buffer to lyse red blood cells. pMQs and PBLs were washed with phosphate buffered saline (PBS). Then $1x10^6$ cells were stained with Percp-eFluor-labeled anti-mouse CD40, eFluor 660-labeled anti-mouse CD83, PE-Cyanine7-labeled anti-mouse CD80, and FITC-labeled anti-mouse CD86 (eBioscience, San Diego, CA, USA) at 4°C in the dark for 30 min. Stained cells were analyzed with FACS Aria III flow cytometer (Becton Dickinson, San Jose, CA, USA) with x10,000 gated cells.

Analysis of Microbiota in Mouse Feces by 16S Ribosomal RNA (rRNA) Gene Sequencing

Fresh feces were collected from mice to analyze mouse gut microbiota based on 16S rRNA gene amplicon sequence. 16S rRNA gene sequencing of V3 and V4 amplicons was performed using 16S rRNA gene PCR primer (Forward Primer 5′-TCG TCG GCA GCG TCA GAT GTG TAT AAG AGA CAG CCT ACG GGN GGC WGC AG-3′, Reverse Primer 5′-GTC TCG TGG GCT CGG AGA TGT GTA TAA GAG ACA GGA CTA CHV GGG TAT CTA ATC C-3′). The number of operational taxonomic units (OTUs) was determined by clustering the sequence from each sample with 97% sequence identities as a cut-off using quantitative insights into microbial ecology (QIIME) software (v.1.8.0). Taxonomic abundance was counted with a National Center for Biotechnology Information (NCBI) database using a confidence threshold of 0.8 derived from preprocessed reads for each sample.

Total RNA Extraction and Quantitative RT-PCR

Total RNAs were isolated from cells using TRIzol reagent (Thermo Fisher, Waltham, MA, USA) according to the manufacturer's recommendations. RNAs were quantified with a NanoDrop spectrophotometer (NanoDrop Technologies, Wilmington, NC, USA) and reverse-transcribed into cDNA using Prime Script cDNA Synthesis kit (Takara Shuzo Co., Otsu, Shiga, Japan). qRT-PCR was performed on a 7500 Real-time PCR system (Applied Biosystems) in duplicate for each target transcript using SYBER green PCR Master Mix (Applied Biosystems, Foster City, CA, USA) and gene-specific primers. For qRT-PCR, 1 μL cDNA served as template. The final reaction volume was 20 μL. Each reaction contained gene-specific primers listed in (**Table 1**). The PCR condition was as follows: 2 min at 94°C, followed by 40 cycles at 94°C for 3s, 55°C for 30s, and 72°C for 30s, and a final extension step at 72°C for 10 min. Relative gene expression level was calculated using the $2^{-\Delta\Delta Ct}$ method and expression level of each gene was normalized against the level of β-actin, a house-keeping gene. Data are presented as fold changes relative to untreated control.

Statistical Analysis

Statistical differences between experimental groups were determined using Graphpad Prism (version 8.3.1) for Windows (Graphpad Software, La Jolla, CA, USA) and MedCalc® version 9.3.0.0. (MedCalc, Ostend, Belgium). Statistical significance was assessed by performing Mann-

TABLE 1 | List of primers used in real-time PCR.

Gene Name	Primer Sequence (Forward)	Primer Sequence (Reverse)
Egr2	5′-CTCCCGTATCCGAGTAGC-3′	5′-GATGCCCGCACTCACAAT-3′
Ripk2	5′- ATCCCGTACCACAAGCTCG-3′	5′-GGATGTGTAGGTGCTTCACTG-3′
Ptpn1	5′-GGCTATTTACCAGGACATTCGAC-3′	5′- TCCGACTGTGGTCAAAAGGG-3′
Cebpb	5′- CAACCTGGAGACGCAGCACAAG-3′	5′-GCTTGAACAAGTTCCGCAGGGT-3′
T-bet	5′-ATGTTTGTGGATGTGGTCTTGGT-3′	5′-CGGTTCCCTGGCATGCT-3′
ROR-γt	5′-GACCCACACCTCACAAATTGA-3′	5′-AGTAGGCCACATTACACTGCT-3′
Gata-3	5′-CAAGCTTCATAATACCCCTGACTATG-3′	5′-GCGCGTCATGCACCTTTT-3′
Foxp3	5′-CACAATATGCGACCCCCTTTC-3′	5′-AACATGCGAGTAAACCAATGGTA -3′
β-actin	5′- TGTCCACCTTCCAGCAGATGT-3′	5′-AGCTCAGTA ACAGTCCGCCTAG-3′

Whiteny U test and Student's *t*-test. Statistical significance was considered when *p*-value was less than 0.05.

RESULTS

Effects of Stress and Environment on the Incidence of BD in Mice

To determine the effect of environment on the prevalence of BD, HSV was inoculated into mice and the prevalence of BD was compared between mice in SPF environment and a conventional facility. Under conventional conditions, HSV inoculated mice showed higher incidence of BD than those under SPF conditions (15.0% *vs.* 2.2%, $p = 0.03$). To investigate the effect of stress on the prevalence of BD, HSV inoculated mice were given several types of stress. Types of stress applied to mice included anxiety, cold, oxidative, and noise stress. SP was used to induce anxiety stress. In order to induce cold stress, mice were placed in a cold chamber at 4°C. To induce noise stress, mice were placed inside a 77-dB noise-producing device. HSV inoculated and SP treated mice under a conventional condition showed higher incidence of BD than HSV inoculated mice in an SPF condition (17.10% vs. 2.2%, $p = 0.04$). Mice inoculated with HSV and exposed to noise stress under conventional conditions had significantly higher incidence rate of BD (38.1% vs. 2.2%, $p = 0.0001$) than HSV inoculated mice under SPF conditions. Noise stress additionally treated to HSV-inoculated mice under the conventional conditions increased the incidence of BD compared to HSV inoculated mice (38.10% *vs.* 15.00%, $p = 0.04$) (**Table 2**). However, oxidative stress and cold stress failed to increase the rate of BD incidence.

Altered Gut Microbial Compositions in Normal Mice Under Conventional and SPF Conditions

To determine differences in compositions of gut microbiota according to the environment in which mice were maintained, microbiota were analyzed for fresh feces samples of mice (five weeks old). Microbiome was determined based on 16S rRNA sequence analysis. Based on a NCBI classifier comparison of microbial community, taxonomy construct distances between conventional and SPF conditions were determined using Shannon diversity index and beta diversity and visualized by Principal Coordinate Analysis (PCoA) plot (**Figures 1A–C**). Based on fecal sample microbiome analysis, the number of OTUs was increased in SPF-maintained mice compared to that in conventionally maintained mice. There was no significant difference in alpha diversity between groups (**Figures 1A, B**). For mice maintained in the conventional facility, *Firmicutes, Bacteroids*, and *Proteobacteria* were the most prevalent phyla, while *Firmicutes, Bacteroids*, and *Deferribacteres* were the most prevalent phyla in mice maintained in the SPF facility (**Figure 1D**). *Akkermansiaceae, Defluviitaleaceae, Erysipelotrichaceae*, and *Ruminococcaceae* were microbial families that were more dominant in mice under the SPF condition than in mice under the conventional condition. *Lachnospiraceae, Porphyromonadaceae*, and *Prevotellaceae* were more dominant microbial families in mice maintained in the conventional condition than in mice maintained in the SPF condition (**Figure 1E**). At genus level, *Akkermansia, Lactobacillus, Mucispirillum, Ruminiclostridium, Ruminococcus, and Vallitalea* groups had higher populations in mice maintained under the SPF condition than mice maintained in the conventional condition. At genus level, *Candidatus, Lachnoclostridium, Parabacteroidetes, Porphyromonas, Prevotela*, and *Tyzzerella* had higher populations in mice under the conventional condition than in mice under the SPF condition, although such differences were not statistically significant (**Figure 1F**). For bacterial species, *Clostridium cellobioparum, Akkermansia muciniphila, Anaerobacterium chartisolvens, Bacteroides caccae, Lactobacillus intestinalis, Lactobacillus reuteri, Mucispirillum schaedleri*, and *Parabacteroides goldsteinii* were more dominant in mice maintained under the SPF condition, whereas *Candidatus arthromitus* and *Lactobacillus johnsonii* were more dominant in mice maintained under the conventional condition, although differences between the two groups were not statistically significant (**Figure 1G**). Differences in fecal microbiota between conventional and SPF conditions and *p*-values are shown in **Supplementary Table ST1**.

TABLE 2 | Differences in incidence of Behçet's disease between mice maintained in a conventional facility and those maintained in a specific pathogen free (SPF) facility.

Mouse Environments	Application	BD/Total Number of Mice (%)
SPF	HSV	1/45 (2.2%)
Conventional	HSV	6/40 (15.0%)*
	HSV + Substance P (Anxiety stress)	7/41 (17.1%)*
	HSV + Noise stress	8/21 (38.1%)**#

#p < 0.05 vs. HSV (Conventional).
**p < 0.05 vs. HSV (SPF).*
***p < 0.001 vs. HSV (SPF).*

Frequencies of Dendritic Cell Activation Markers CD40, CD83, CD80, and CD86-Expressing Cells in BD Mice

To determine whether there was a correlation between DC activation marker expression and BD mice with ocular symptoms, frequencies of cells expressing DC activation markers were analyzed in mice PBLs. Frequencies of activated DC molecules CD40+, CD83+, CD80+, and CD86+ cells in normal, HSV-1 inoculated, BDN, and BD mice were determined by flow cytometric analysis (FACS). Frequencies of CD83+ cells were significantly increased in BD symptomatic mice (40.00 ± 11.51%) than in BDN (28.12 ± 7.14%, $p = 0.04$), HSV inoculated (28.17 ± 3.92%, $p = 0.04$), and normal mice (28.87 ± 7.12%, $p = 0.04$) (**Figure 2B**). Frequencies of CD80+ cells were significantly higher in BD mice than in BDN mice (56.50 ± 8.98% *vs.* 46.94 ± 4.28%, $p = 0.05$) (**Figure 2C**). Frequencies of CD86+ cells were reduced in BD (4.42 ± 2.6%,

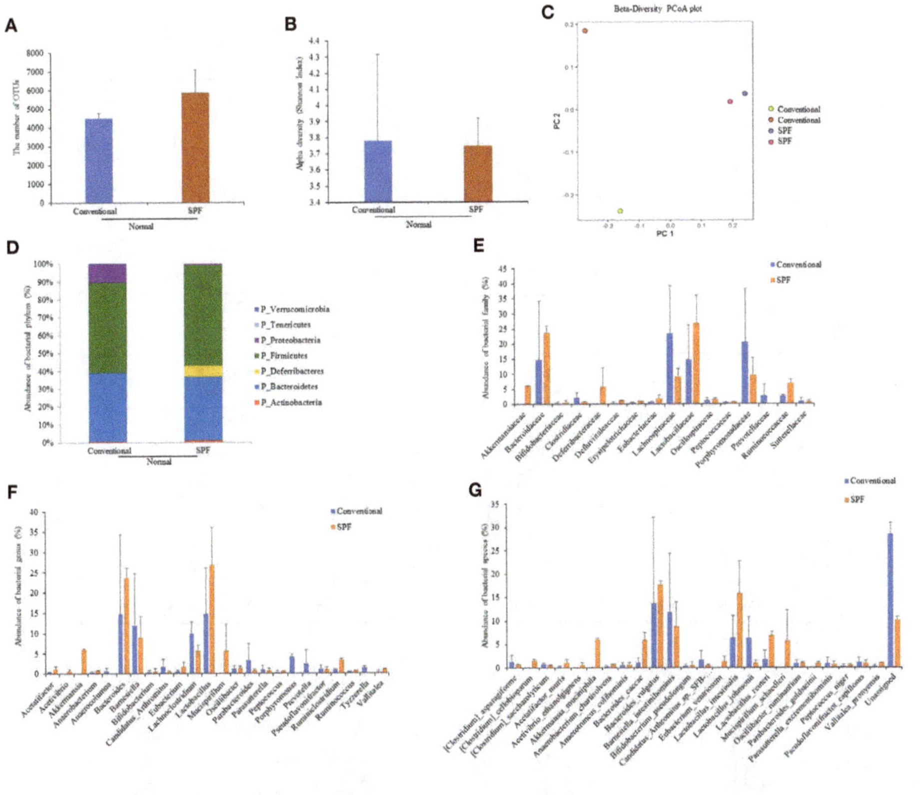

FIGURE 1 | Fecal samples were collected from normal mice maintained under conventional or SPF condition and 16S rRNA amplicons were sequenced for analysis. Microbiome analysis was performed using sequencing data of 16S rRNA V3 and V4 amplicons. The number of OTUs **(A)** and Alpha diversity (Shannon index) **(B)**, and Principal component analysis (PCA) plot **(C)** were calculated. Phylum **(D)**, family **(E)**, genus **(F)**, and species **(G)** showed significant differences in fecal 16S rRNA sequence analysis between groups. Two mice were used in each group.

p = 0.006) and BDN (4.98 ± 2.07%, p = 0.006) mice than in normal mice (12.97 ± 3.20%) (**Figure 2D**). There were no significant differences in frequencies of CD40+ cells among groups (**Figure 2A**). A representative histogram of CD83 is shown in (**Figure 2E**)

Identification of Several Genes Expressed in Eye Symptomatic BD Mice by Real-Time PCR

To determine expression levels of several genes expressed in BD mice with ocular symptoms, real-time PCR was performed using mouse PBLs. Results revealed that mRNA expression levels of Egr2 were higher in BD mice with eye symptoms than in mice with eye symptoms only (13.50 ± 0.14 *vs.* 0.6 ± 0.70, p = 0.001) and in normal mice (13.50 ± 0.14 *vs.* 1.0 ± 0.73, p = 0.001) (**Figure 3A**). Ripk2 mRNA expression levels were also higher in BD mice with eye symptoms than in mice with eye symptoms only (4.39 ± 0.30 *vs.* 0.78 ± 0.35, p = 0.008) and in normal mice (4.39 ± 0.30 *vs.* 1.0 ± 1.36, p = 0.07) (**Figure 3B**). Cebpb mRNA expression levels in PBLs of BD mice with ocular symptoms were also higher than in normal mice, although the difference between the two groups was not statistically significant (2.79 ± 0.34 *vs.* 1.00 ± 0.69, p = 0.08) (**Figure 3D**). Ptpn1 mRNA expression levels did not differ significantly among the groups (**Figure 3C**). The mice used in this experiment were 2 for each group.

Identification of Several Stressors That Influence the Activation of Dendritic Cells

To determine whether stress might affect the activation of dendritic cells, several types of stress were used to treat normal mice. Frequencies of cells expressing DC activation markers were measured by FACS. DC markers analyzed in PBLs of mice were CD40, CD83, CD80, and CD86. To induce anxiety stress, substance P was administered to mice by intraperitoneal injection. Frequencies of CD40 positive (+) and CD83+ cells were significantly increased in mice under anxiety stress than in control mice (41.80 ± 7.19% *vs.* 25.94 ± 4.16%, p = 0.008; 27.78 ± 5.45% *vs.* 11.20 ± 3.88%, p = 0.008, respectively) (**Figures 4A, B**). In mice treated with cold stress, frequencies of CD83+ and CD80+ cells were significantly increased than in control mice (27.94 ± 9.90% *vs.* 11.20 ± 3.88%, p = 0.003; 58.10 ± 8.05% *vs.* 39.90 ± 3.13%, p = 0.003, respectively) (**Figures 4B, C**), no significant differences were observed for the frequencies of CD40+ and CD86+ cells (**Figures 4A, D**). In mice treated with xanthine sodium salt for oxidative stress, frequencies of CD40+, CD83+, and CD80+ cells were significantly increased than in control mice (37.68 ± 3.04% *vs.* 25.94 ± 4.16%, p = 0.008; 37.68 ± 7.63% *vs.* 11.20 ± 3.88%, p = 0.008; 66.16 ± 6.11% *vs.* 39.90 ± 3.13%, p = 0.008, respectively) (**Figures 4A–C**). In mice treated with noise stress, frequencies of CD40+, CD83+, CD80+, and CD86+ cells were significantly

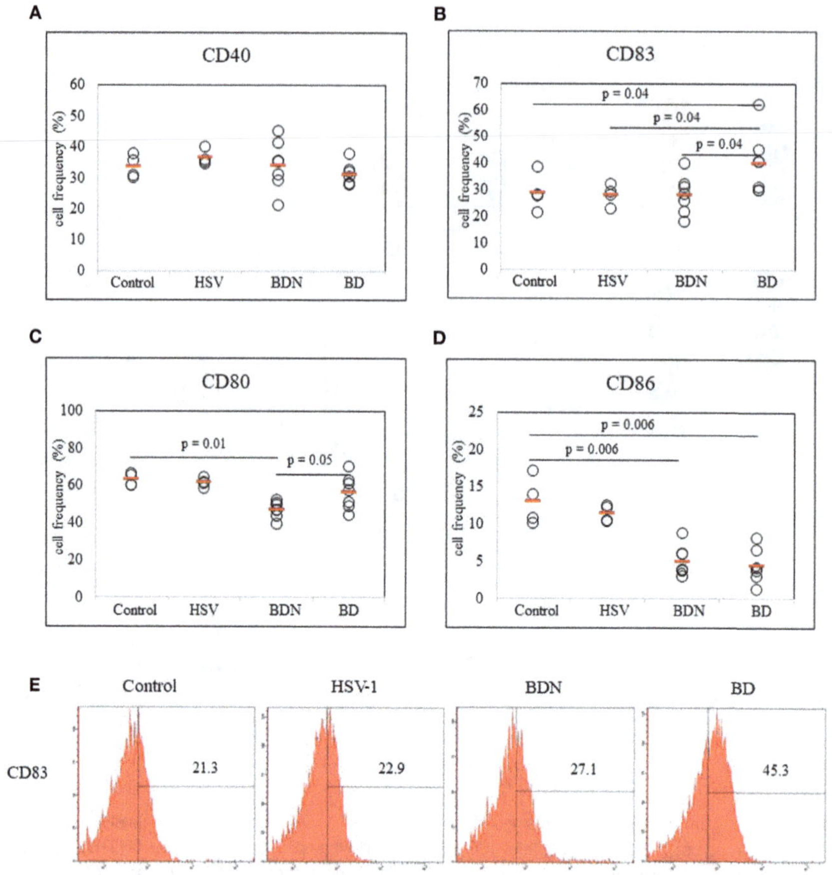

FIGURE 2 | Frequencies of DC costimulatory molecules CD40, CD83, CD80, and CD86 in peripheral blood leukocytes (PBLs) were evaluated in normal, HSV-1 inoculated, BDN, and BD mice. Isolated PBLs were analyzed by flow cytometry after surface staining **(A–D)**. Representative histogram of CD83+ cells is shown in **(E)**. For statistical analysis, the Mann-Whitney U test was performed with GraphPad. Experiments were performed independently at least three times.

increased than in control mice (39.53 ± 4.06% *vs.* 25.94 ± 4.16%, p = 0.02; 27.60 ± 2.40% *vs.* 11.20 ± 3.88%, p = 0.02; 71.57 ± 2.67% *vs.* 39.90 ± 3.13%, p = 0.02; 20.72 ± 2.00% *vs.* 5.70 ± 2.46%, p = 0.02, respectively) (**Figures 4A–D**). Noise stress treatment also regulated transcription factors in PBLs of normal mice. T-bet and ROR-γt mRNA expression levels were increased in mice treated with noise stress than in control mice (3.5 ± 0.6 *vs.* 1.0 ± 0.4, p = 0.004; 6.4 ± 3.4 *vs.* 1.0 ± 0.9, p = 0.05, respectively) (**Figures 4E, H**). There were no significant differences in Gata-3 or Foxp3 mRNA expression between the two groups (**Figures 4F, G**). The mice used in (**Figures 4E–H**) were 3 for each group. Results of each stress dose are shown in supplementary Figures (**Supplementary Figures S1–S3**).

Stress Activates Dendritic Cells in HSV-Infected State

To determine whether stress could promote dendritic cell activation in HSV-infected state, noise stress was applied to HSV inoculated mice and DC activation markers in PBLs were analyzed by FACS. Noise stress increased frequencies of CD80+ and CD83+ cells in HSV inoculated mice than in control mice (69.68 ± 3.02% *vs.* 61.42 ± 2.30%, p = 0.02; 36.62 ± 2.41% *vs.* 28.17 ± 3.92%, p = 0.02, respectively) (**Figures 5B, C**). HSV infection itself also increased frequencies of CD40+, CD83+, and CD80+ cells than in healthy, uninfected mice (36.40 ± 2.52% *vs.* 25.94 ± 4.16%, p = 0.02; 28.17 ± 3.90% *vs.* 11.20 ± 3.88%, p = 0.02; 61.42 ± 2.30% *vs.* 39.90 ± 3.13%, p = 0.02, respectively) (**Figures 5A–C**). On the other hand, HSV infection itself or with noise stress down-regulated frequencies of CD86+ cells than in uninfected noise stress induced mice (11.42 ± 1.12% *vs.* 20.72 ± 2.00%, p = 0.03; 13.82 ± 2.78% *vs.* 20.72 ± 2.00%, p = 0.03, respectively) (**Figure 5D**).

Stress Modulates Dendritic Cell Activation in BD Mice

To determine whether stress could affect additional activation of dendritic cells, noise stress was applied to BD mice. As a control group, asymptomatic mice (BD Normal, BDN) after HSV administration were used. Results revealed that noise stress decreased frequencies of CD40+ cells in BD mice (31.00 ± 3.50% *vs.* 27.30 ± 6.39%, p = 0.04) (**Figure 6A**). Noise stress did not significantly affect frequencies of CD83+ cells in BD mice (**Figure 6B**), although it increased frequencies of CD80+ cells in

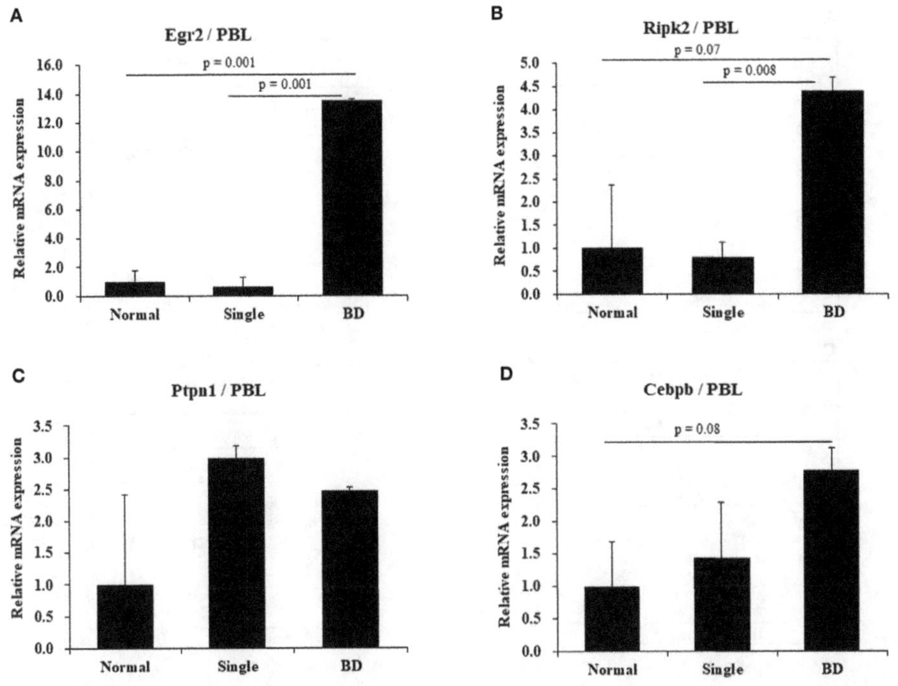

FIGURE 3 | Expression levels of several mRNAs in BD mice by real-time PCR. Expression levels of several mRNAs in peripheral blood leukocytes (PBLs) of BD mice with ocular symptoms were analyzed by real time-PCR **(A–D)**. Selected genes were Egr2, Ripk2, Rtpn1, and Cebpb. After normalization against β-actin, relative expression levels were analyzed for each sample. The experiment was conducted in duplicate.

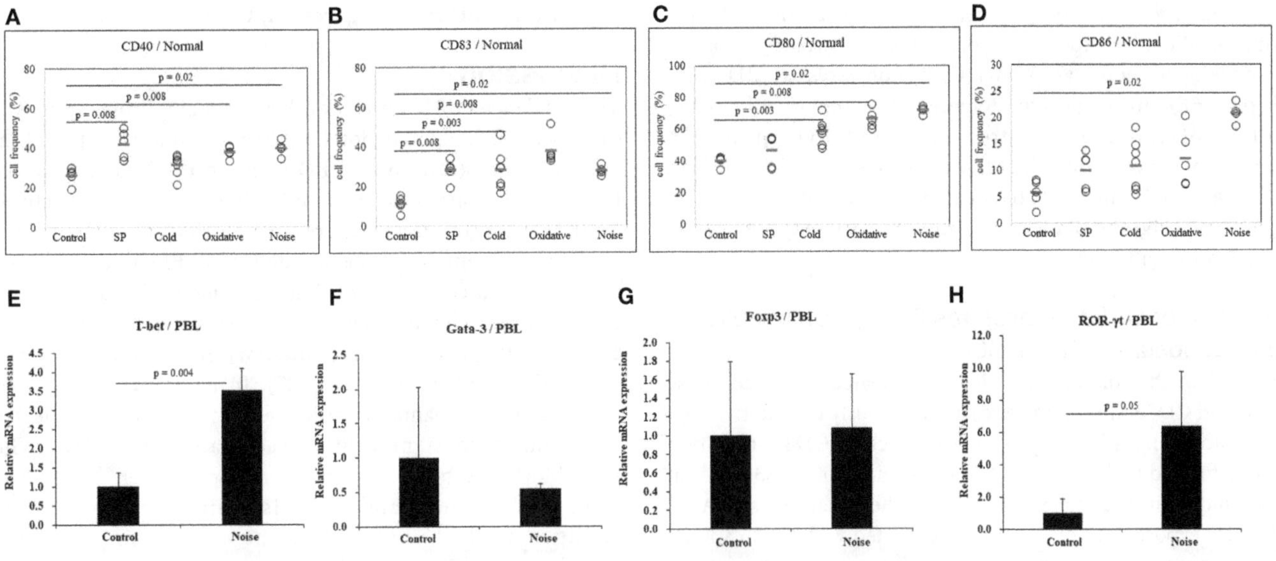

FIGURE 4 | Expression levels of dendritic cell activation markers in normal mice after stress treatment. Frequencies of DC activation molecules CD40+, CD83+, CD80+, and CD86+ cells in normal mice after stress treatment were analyzed by FACS analysis **(A–D)**. Substance P (SP) was used for anxiety stress, 4°C temperature was used for cold stress, xanthine sodium salt was used for oxidative stress, and 77dB sound was used for noise stress induction. For statistical analysis, Mann-Whitney U test was performed. Cellular transcription factor mRNA expression levels in PBLs of normal mice exposed to noise stress were analyzed by real time-PCR **(E–H)**.

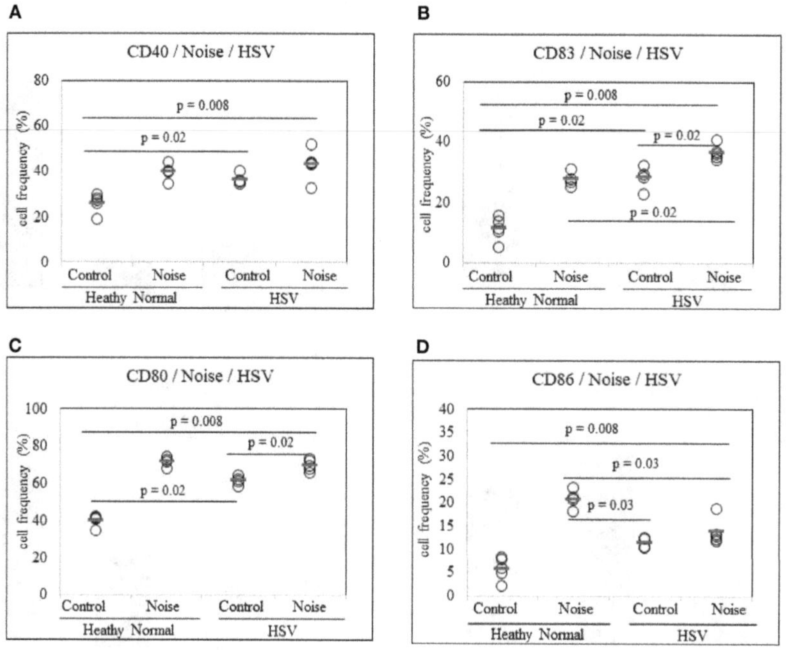

FIGURE 5 | Frequency analysis of DC-stimulating molecules CD40, CD83, CD80 and CD86-expressing cells in normal mice and HSV-1 inoculated mice with or without noise stress. Mice were exposed to noise stress for 10 days after the first HSV-1 inoculation. One day after second inoculation of HSV-1, peripheral blood leukocytes were applied to flow cytometry **(A–D)**. Experiments were conducted independently at least three times.

BD mice (56.50 ± 8.98% *vs.* 68.36 ± 7.23%, p = 0.04) and BDN mice (46.94 ± 4.28% *vs.* 67.51 ± 6.99%, p = 0.001) (**Figure 6C**). Noise stress also increased frequencies of CD86+ cells in BD mice (4.42 ± 2.26% *vs.* 8.86 ± 2.00%, p = 0.004) and BDN mice (4.98 ± 2.07% *vs.* 10.10 ± 1.94%, p = 0.008) (**Figure 6D**). BD symptomatic mice exposed to noise stress had worse symptoms or developed new symptoms than non-stressed BD mice (**Figure 6E**). In single-symptomatic mice (before BD stage) and in BD mice, noise stress increased ROR-γt mRNA expression levels but decreased GATA-3 mRNA levels, although such increase or decrease was not statistically significant (**Figures 6F, G**). The mice used in **Figures 6F, G** were 3 for each group.

Inhibition of CD83 Ameliorates BD Symptoms Even After Exposure to Noise Stress

To confirm the role of CD83 in stress-treated BD mice, noise stress and CD83 inhibition were simultaneously used to treat BD mice and changes in symptoms were tracked. CD83 inhibition was performed with CD83 siRNA. Frequencies of CD83+ cells in PBLs and peritoneal macrophages were then analyzed by FACS. BD mice exposed to noise stress were treated with CD83 siRNA and compared to BD mice exposed to noise stress only. Frequencies of CD83+ cells were significantly downregulated in mice treated with both CD83 siRNA and noise stress than in mice treated with noise stress only (39.38 ± 3.53% *vs.* 26.66 ± 10.96%, p = 0.01; 22.42 ± 4.55% *vs.* 12.18 ± 6.42%, p = 0.03, respectively) (**Figure 7B**). Treatment of BD mice exposed to noise stress with CD83 siRNA improved BD symptoms (**Figure 7E**). There were no differences of CD40+, CD80+, or CD86+ cells with or without CD83 siRNA treatment in noise stress-treated BD mice (**Figures 7A, C, D**).

Discussion

The incidence of BD varies worldwide, ranging from 3.3 to 31.8 cases per 100,000 population (26). Even in countries around the Silk Road, the prevalence of BD varies in the Middle East, Far East, and Europe. Currently, microbiota research is actively underway. Many researchers expect that microbiota can explain differences in the incidence of BD under various environmental conditions of different regions. Dysbiosis of the gut microbiome may trigger or exacerbate the inflammatory process in BD, and a reduced intestinal microbial diversity was observed in patients with BD (27). In an animal study, fecal microbiota transplantation using feces from BD patients has been shown to significantly exacerbate uveitis (16). Gut microbiota has been reported to differ between laboratory-controlled animals and animals maintained in outdoor facilities (28). To determine the relationship between microbiota and BD outbreak, BD prevalence experiments were conducted in mice maintained in different environmental facilities. We demonstrated the higher incidence of BD in mice maintained in conventional facilities than in mice maintained in SPF facilities, suggesting normal microflora can influence BD

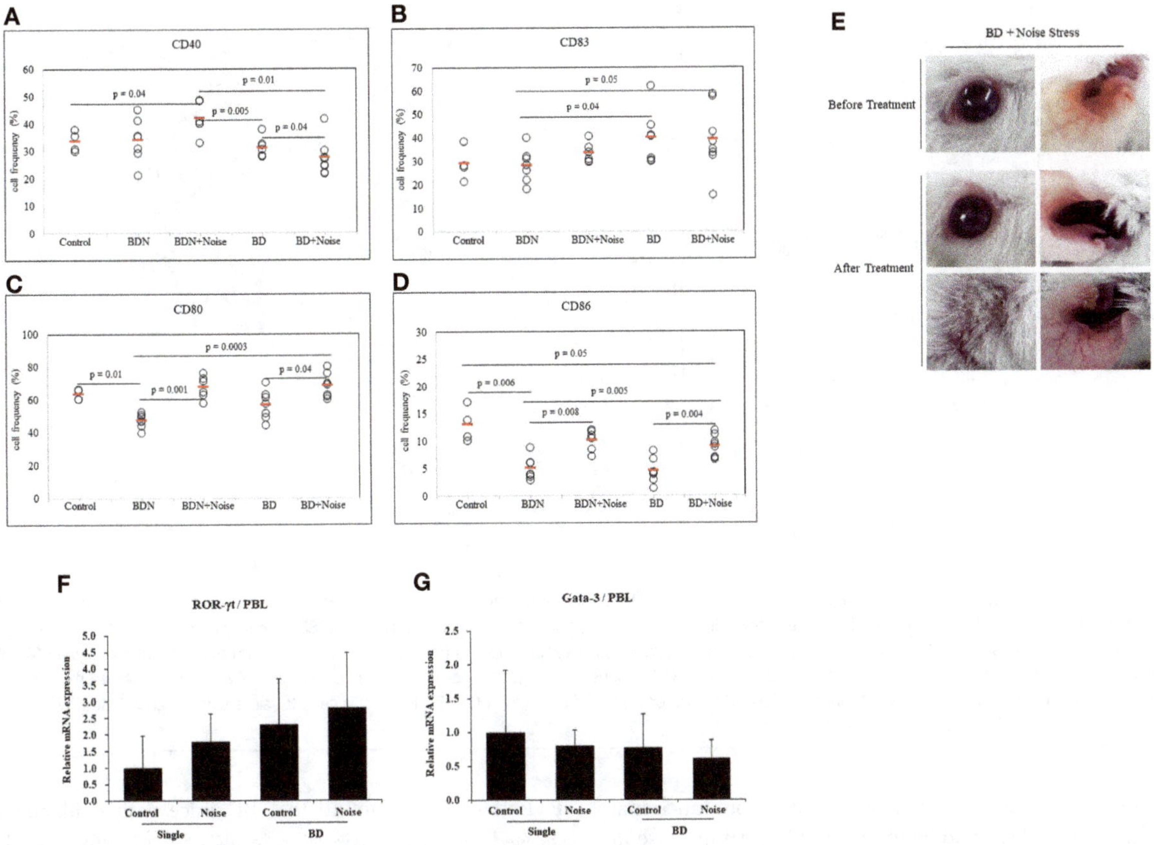

FIGURE 6 | Noise stress affects DC activation in BD mice. To investigate the correlation between noise stress and DC activation in BD, frequencies of DC activation markers CD40, CD83, CD80, and CD83 positive cells in peripheral blood leukocytes of noise-treated BD mice and BDN mouse were measured by flow cytometry **(A–D)**. BD mice under noise stress showed deteriorated or new symptoms **(E)**. Experiments were conducted independently at least three times. mRNA expression levels of cell transcription factors ROR-γt and Gata-3 in mice with only ocular symptoms and BD mice with ocular symptoms were analyzed by real time PCR. Both groups of mice were compared with mice in noise stress treated groups **(F, G)**. Statistical analysis was performed with Student's *t*-test. The experiment was conducted in duplicate.

induction. Mice maintained in the SPF facility displayed a greater number of OTUs and more bacterial phyla than mice maintained in the conventional facility. This suggests bacterial phylum diversity is associated with inhibition of BD development. Mice maintained in SPF facilities showed a greater number of *Akkermansia muciniphilia, Bacteroides caccae, Lactobacillus reuteri*, and *Parabacteroides goldsteinii* than in mice maintained in conventional facilities. *Akkermansia muciniphilia* is known to reduce IFN-γ production (29). *Bacteroides caccae* decreased IL-8 levels (30). IL-8 was upregulated in patients with active BD (31). *Lactobacillus reuteri* increased butyrate production, which alleviated airway inflammation (32), and *Parabacteroides goldsteinii* has been suggested for use as a novel probiotic in obesity and type 2 diabetes (33). This suggests environment plays a crucial role in alteration of gut microbiota.

It has been reported stress-induced vascular disease and inflammatory symptoms are associated with microbiota changes (34, 35). Stress has a variety of adverse health effects, some of which are mediated by its action on the immune system (9). In the present study, various stresses were applied to HSV-1 inoculated mice for induction of BD to determine what stresses might play an important role in BD induction. Of various stresses, noise stress was the most effective in increasing the incidence of BD in mice. Mice are sound sensitive animals (36). Although noise stress has a significant effect on the induction of BD in mice, there is still no evidence as to whether it could have the same effect on BD development in human patients. Therefore, more research is needed to determine types of stress that can affect the prevalence of BD in humans. In BD patients, stress has been defined as the most common self-reporting trigger for oral ulcer development (37).

Repeated social defeat stress can activate DC and enhance cytokine secretion (38). DC plays an important role in a variety of human and murine autoimmune diseases (39). Mature DCs express co-stimulatory molecules CD40, CD80, CD83, and CD86 on cell surfaces. These molecules can regulate inflammation (40, 41). Among DC co-stimulatory molecules, CD83 is one of the

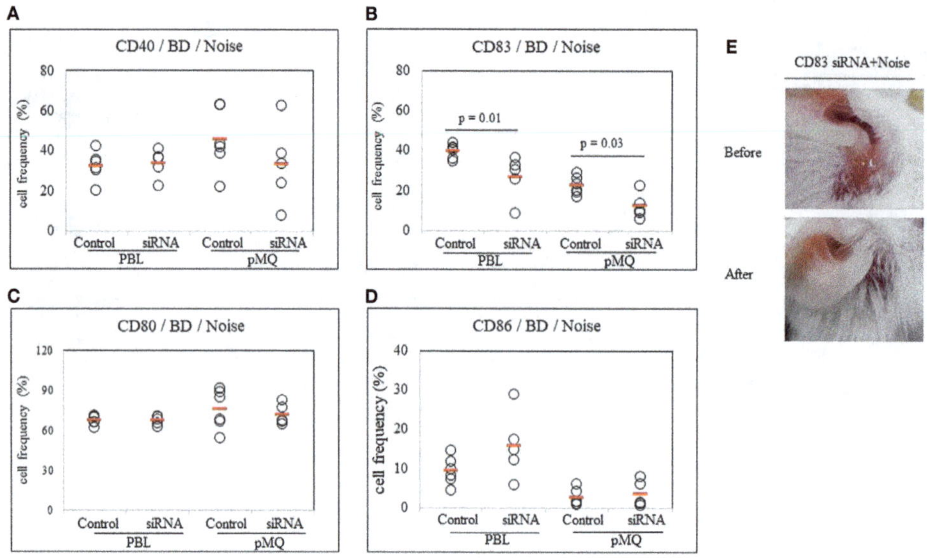

FIGURE 7 | CD83 siRNA reduces frequencies of CD83+ cells in BD mice. Both noise stress and CD83 inhibition were used to treat BD mice at the same time. Symptoms were improved and frequencies of CD83+ cells were decreased in the group that showed inhibition of CD83 after treatment with CD83 siRNA. BD mice were treated with noise stress and CD83 inhibition at the same time and changes in symptoms and frequencies of DC activation markers were analyzed **(A–D)**. In the group that showed inhibition of CD83 after treatment with CD83 siRNA, frequencies of CD83+ cells were decreased **(B)**. CD83 siRNA inhibited the increase in frequencies of CD83+ cells induced by noise stress and inhibited the deterioration of BD symptoms **(E)**. For statistical analysis, Mann-Whitney U test was performed. Experiments were conducted independently at least three times.

markers of DC maturation or activation. It carries out functional interactions between DCs and lymphocytes (42). An increase in CD83 expressing DC has been observed in patients with Crohn's disease (43) and in patients with rheumatoid arthritis (44). In the present study, frequencies of CD83 expressing cells were significantly increased in BD mice, suggesting CD83 plays an important role in BD inflammation.

Stress can suppress immune functions in some conditions, while provoking immune functions in other conditions (45). Acute stress increases blood levels of proinflammatory cytokines (46). Stressful life events are also provoking factors of BD (47). Stress can increase DC maturation by enhancing activation markers. Increased DC trafficking from skin to lymph nodes under stress has been observed (45). In uveitis, DC promotes the activation of different subsets of Th cells (48). Excessive Th1/Th17 responses in ocular BD patients can be suppressed by modulating DC function through immunomodulatory therapy (49). Oxidative stress enhances DC maturation and increases frequencies of CD86+ and CD40+ cells in mouse bone marrow-derived DC cultures (50). Substance P, a marker of pain and anxiety stress, increases DC maturation in mice skin by regulating MHCII, ICAM-1, CD11c, and langerin (51). However, there have been no reports about regulation of CD40, CD80, CD83, and CD86 by substance P. Temperature stress can also influence CD86+ DC frequencies in laboratory mice (52).

In Chinese Han BD patients, uveitis is correlated with expression levels of EGR2, RIPK2, CEBPB, LACC1, and PTPN1 (53). We found that BD mice with ocular symptoms showed increased expression levels of Egr2, Ripk2, and Cebpb mRNAs than normal mice. BD mice with ocular symptoms had similar expression patterns to those with BD patients with uveitis.

Elevated levels of Th1 and Th17 cytokines may play an important role in the pathogenesis of BD (54). Expression levels of T-bet (T-box expression in T cells) mRNA supporting the Th1 subset of T cells are increased in BD patients with uveitis (55). ROR-γt mRNA levels and frequencies of IL-17A+ Th17 cells are elevated in BD patients with uveitis (56). Results of the present mouse study shows noise stress increased T-bet and RORγt mRNA expression levels. Stress-induced Th1 and Th17 immune responses might contribute to BD inflammation response.

Proinflammatory cytokines promoted DC maturation (57). Inhibition of CD83 could significantly prevent DC-mediated T cell activation (25, 58). In our previous reports, inhibition of CD83, with CD83 siRNA, was able to improve BD symptoms in mice (24). In the current study, noise stress treated BD mice improved when CD83 was suppressed. This means that CD83 expression may be a more potent modulator than the stress in BD. This suggests CD83 is a potential molecule that can control BD symptoms.

In conclusion, we observed environmental conditions and noise stress may play important roles in BD and that it may exacerbate BD symptoms by modulating DC activating markers.

Among the DC activating markers, CD83 is a powerful molecule that regulates BD symptoms. The composition of the gut microbiota was regulated according to environmental conditions. Stress management and gut microbiota control may be complementary approaches to BD management.

ETHICS STATEMENT

The animal study was reviewed and approved by Institutional Animal Care and Use Committee (IACUC) of Ajou University (IACUC-2018-0017).

AUTHOR CONTRIBUTIONS

All authors contributed to the article and approved the submitted version. SS contributed to the concept and design of this study, data analysis, and data interpretation. SI, H-MR, and HS contributed to data acquisition, data analysis, and data interpretation. SS and SI wrote the manuscript.

SUPPLEMENTARY MATERIAL

Supplementary Figure 1 | Frequencies of DC co-stimulatory molecules CD83, CD80, and CD86 in peripheral blood leukocytes (PBLs) of normal mice were elevated after noise stress induction. Isolated PBLs were analyzed by flow cytometric after surface staining **(A–D)**. For statistical analysis, one-way analysis of variance (ANOVA) was performed using GraphPad. Experiments were conducted independently at least three times.

Supplementary Figure 2 | Substance P (SP) for anxiety stress increased frequencies of DC co-stimulatory molecules CD40 and CD83 in peripheral blood leukocytes (PBLs) of normal mice. Isolated PBLs were analyzed by flow cytometry after surface staining **(A–D)**. For statistical analysis, one-way ANOVA was performed using GraphPad. Experiments were conducted independently at least three times.

Supplementary Figure 3 | Frequencies of DC co-stimulatory molecules CD40, CD83, and CD80 in peripheral blood leukocytes (PBLs) of normal mice are elevated after inducing oxidation using xanthine sodium salt. Isolated PBLs were analyzed by flow cytometry after surface staining **(A–D)**. For statistical analysis, one-way ANOVA was performed using GraphPad. Experiments were conducted independently at least three times.

REFERENCES

1. Hatemi G, Seyahi E, Fresko I, Talarico R, Hamuryudan V. One year in review 2019: Behcet's syndrome. *Clin Exp Rheumatol* (2019) 37Suppl 121(6):3–17.
2. Islam SMS, Sohn S. HSV-Induced Systemic Inflammation as an Animal Model for Behcet's Disease and Therapeutic Applications. *Viruses* (2018) 10 (9):511. doi: 10.3390/v10090511
3. Sezer FN. The isolation of a virus as the cause of Behcet's diseases. *Am J Ophthalmol* (1953) 36(3):301–15. doi: 10.1016/0002-9394(53)91372-5
4. Lee S, Bang D, Cho YH, Lee ES, Sohn S. Polymerase chain reaction reveals herpes simplex virus DNA in saliva of patients with Behcet's disease. *Arch Dermatol Res* (1996) 288(4):179–83. doi: 10.1007/bf02505221
5. Tojo M, Zheng X, Yanagihori H, Oyama N, Takahashi K, Nakamura K, et al. Detection of herpes virus genomes in skin lesions from patients with Behcet's disease and other related inflammatory diseases. *Acta Derm Venereol* (2003) 83(2):124–7. doi: 10.1080/00015550310007472
6. Eglin RP, Lehner T, Subak-Sharpe JH. Detection of RNA complementary to herpes-simplex virus in mononuclear cells from patients with Behcet's syndrome and recurrent oral ulcers. *Lancet* (1982) 2(8312):1356–61. doi: 10.1016/s0140-6736(82)91268-5
7. Sohn S, Lee ES, Bang D, Lee S. Behcet's disease-like symptoms induced by the Herpes simplex virus in ICR mice. *Eur J Dermatol* (1998) 8(1):21–3.
8. Liu Y-Z, Wang Y-X, Jiang C-L. Inflammation: The Common Pathway of Stress-Related Diseases. *Front Hum Neurosci* (2017) 11:316. doi: 10.3389/fnhum.2017.00316
9. Dhabhar FS. Effects of stress on immune function: the good, the bad, and the beautiful. *Immunol Res* (2014) 58(2-3):193–210. doi: 10.1007/s12026-014-8517-0
10. Uğuz F, Dursun R, Kaya N, Savas Cilli A. Quality of life in patients with Behçet's disease: the impact of major depression. *Gen Hosp Psychiatry* (2007) 29(1):21–4. doi: 10.1016/j.genhosppsych.2006.10.001
11. Karl JP, Hatch AM, Arcidiacono SM, Pearce SC, Pantoja-Feliciano IG, Doherty LA, et al. Effects of Psychological, Environmental and Physical Stressors on the Gut Microbiota. *Front Microbiol* (2018) 9:2013. doi: 10.3389/fmicb.2018.02013
12. Consolandi C, Turroni S, Emmi G, Severgnini M, Fiori J, Peano C, et al. Behçet's syndrome patients exhibit specific microbiome signature. *Autoimmun Rev* (2015) 14(4):269–76. doi: 10.1016/j.autrev.2014.11.009
13. Berer K, Gerdes LA, Cekanaviciute E, Jia X, Xiao L, Xia Z, et al. Gut microbiota from multiple sclerosis patients enables spontaneous autoimmune encephalomyelitis in mice. *Proc Natl Acad Sci U S A* (2017) 114(40):10719–24. doi: 10.1073/pnas.1711233114
14. Zhang X, Zhang D, Jia H, Feng Q, Wang D, Liang D, et al. The oral and gut microbiomes are perturbed in rheumatoid arthritis and partly normalized after treatment. *Nat Med* (2015) 21(8):895–905. doi: 10.1038/nm.3914
15. Morgan XC, Tickle TL, Sokol H, Gevers D, Devaney KL, Ward DV, et al. Dysfunction of the intestinal microbiome in inflammatory bowel disease and treatment. *Genome Biol* (2012) 13(9):R79. doi: 10.1186/gb-2012-13-9-r79
16. Ye Z, Zhang N, Wu C, Zhang X, Wang Q, Huang X, et al. A metagenomic study of the gut microbiome in Behcet's disease. *Microbiome* (2018) 6(1):135–. doi: 10.1186/s40168-018-0520-6
17. Saint-Mezard P, Chavagnac C, Bosset S, Ionescu M, Peyron E, Kaiserlian D, et al. Psychological Stress Exerts an Adjuvant Effect on Skin Dendritic Cell Functions In Vivo. *J Immunol* (2003) 171(8):4073. doi: 10.4049/jimmunol.171.8.4073
18. Tanne A, Bhardwaj N. Chapter 9 - Dendritic Cells: General Overview and Role in Autoimmunity. In: GS Firestein, RC Budd, SE Gabriel, IB McInnes, JR O'Dell, editors. *Kelley and Firestein"s Textbook of Rheumatology, Tenth Edition*. Canada: Elsevier (2017). p. 126–44.e6.
19. Hart AL, Al-Hassi HO, Rigby RJ, Bell SJ, Emmanuel AV, Knight SC, et al. Characteristics of Intestinal Dendritic Cells in Inflammatory Bowel Diseases. *Gastroenterology* (2005) 129(1):50–65. doi: 10.1053/j.gastro.2005.05.013
20. Khan S, Greenberg JD, Bhardwaj N. Dendritic cells as targets for therapy in rheumatoid arthritis. *Nat Rev Rheumatol* (2009) 5(10):566–71. doi: 10.1038/nrrheum.2009.185
21. O'Rourke M, Fearon U, Sweeney CM, Basdeo SA, Fletcher JM, Murphy CC, et al. The pathogenic role of dendritic cells in non-infectious anterior uveitis. *Exp Eye Res* (2018) 173:121–8. doi: 10.1016/j.exer.2018.05.008
22. Silva MA. Intestinal Dendritic Cells and Epithelial Barrier Dysfunction in Crohn's Disease. *Inflamm Bowel Dis* (2008) 15(3):436–53. doi: 10.1002/ibd.20660
23. Kawamura K, Iyonaga K, Ichiyasu H, Nagano J, Suga M, Sasaki Y. Differentiation, Maturation, and Survival of Dendritic Cells by Osteopontin Regulation. *Clin Diagn Lab Immunol* (2005) 12(1):206. doi: 10.1128/CDLI.12.1.206-212.2005
24. Islam SMS, Byun HO, Choi B, Sohn S. Inhibition of CD83 Alleviates Systemic Inflammation in Herpes Simplex Virus Type 1-Induced Behcet's Disease Model Mouse. *Mediators Inflamm* (2019) 2019:5761392. doi: 10.1155/2019/5761392
25. Kruse M, Rosorius O, Krätzer F, Bevec D, Kuhnt C, Steinkasserer A, et al. Inhibition of Cd83 Cell Surface Expression during Dendritic Cell Maturation by Interference with Nuclear Export of Cd83 mRNA. *J Exp Med* (2000) 191 (9):1581–90. doi: 10.1084/jem.191.9.1581
26. Maldini C, Druce K, Basu N, LaValley MP, Mahr A. Exploring the variability in Behçet's disease prevalence: a meta-analytical approach. *Rheumatology* (2017) 57(1):185–95. doi: 10.1093/rheumatology/kew486
27. van der Houwen TB, van Laar JAM, Kappen JH, van Hagen PM, de Zoete MR, van Muijlwijk GH, et al. Behçet's Disease Under Microbiotic Surveillance? A

Combined Analysis of Two Cohorts of Behçet's Disease Patients. *Front Immunol* (2020) 11:1192. doi: 10.3389/fimmu.2020.01192
28. Bär J, Leung JM, Hansen C, Loke PN, Hall AR, Conour L, et al. Strong effects of lab-to-field environmental transitions on the bacterial intestinal microbiota of Mus musculus are modulated by Trichuris muris infection. *FEMS Microbiol Ecol* (2020) 96:167. doi: 10.1093/femsec/fiaa167
29. Greer RL, Dong X, Moraes ACF, Zielke RA, Fernandes GR, Peremyslova E, et al. Akkermansia muciniphila mediates negative effects of IFNγ on glucose metabolism. *Nat Commun* (2016) 7(1):13329. doi: 10.1038/ncomms13329
30. Hiippala K, Kainulainen V, Suutarinen M, Heini T, Bowers JR, Jasso-Selles D, et al. Isolation of Anti-Inflammatory and Epithelium Reinforcing Bacteroides and Parabacteroides Spp. from A Healthy Fecal Donor. *Nutrients* (2020) 12 (4):935. doi: 10.3390/nu12040935
31. Durmazlar SP, Ulkar GB, Eskioglu F, Tatlican S, Mert A, Akgul A. Significance of serum interleukin-8 levels in patients with Behcet's disease: high levels may indicate vascular involvement. *Int J Dermatol* (2009) 48(3):259–64. doi: 10.1111/j.1365-4632.2009.03905.x
32. Li L, Fang Z, Liu X, Hu W, Lu W, Lee Y-K, et al. Lactobacillus reuteri attenuated allergic inflammation induced by HDM in the mouse and modulated gut microbes. *PloS One* (2020) 15(4):e0231865. doi: 10.1371/journal.pone.0231865
33. Wu TR, Lin CS, Chang CJ, Lin TL, Martel J, Ko YF, et al. Gut commensal Parabacteroides goldsteinii plays a predominant role in the anti-obesity effects of polysaccharides isolated from Hirsutella sinensis. *Gut* (2019) 68(2):248–62. doi: 10.1136/gutjnl-2017-315458
34. He XY, Ng D, Egeblad M. Gut Feelings Block the Flow: Microbiota Links Stress to Vascular Disease. *Immunity* (2020) 53(2):238–40. doi: 10.1016/j.immuni.2020.07.013
35. Xu C, Lee SK, Zhang D, Frenette PS. The Gut Microbiome Regulates Psychological-Stress-Induced Inflammation. *Immunity* (2020) 53(2):417–28.e4. doi: 10.1016/j.immuni.2020.06.025
36. Alexander GJ, Gray R. Induction of convulsive seizures in sound sensitive albino mice: response to various signal frequencies. 1. *Proc Soc Exp Biol Med* (1972) 140(4):1284–8. doi: 10.3181/00379727-140-36659
37. İris M, Özçıkmak E, Aksoy A, Alibaz-Öner F, İnanç N, Ergun T, et al. The assessment of contributing factors to oral ulcer presence in Behçet's disease: Dietary and non-dietary factors. *Eur J Rheumatol* (2018) 5(4):240–3. doi: 10.5152/eurjrheum.2018.18094
38. Powell ND, Bailey MT, Mays JW, Stiner-Jones LM, Hanke ML, Padgett DA, et al. Repeated social defeat activates dendritic cells and enhances Toll-like receptor dependent cytokine secretion. *Brain Behav Immun* (2009) 23(2):225–31. doi: 10.1016/j.bbi.2008.09.010
39. Mehling A, Beissert S. Dendritic cells under investigation in autoimmune disease. *Crit Rev Biochem Mol Biol* (2003) 38(1):1–21. doi: 10.1080/713609208
40. Ouaaz F, Arron J, Zheng Y, Choi Y, Beg AA. Dendritic cell development and survival require distinct NF-kappaB subunits. *Immunity* (2002) 16(2):257–70. doi: 10.1016/s1074-7613(02)00272-8
41. Nolan A, Kobayashi H, Naveed B, Kelly A, Hoshino Y, Hoshino S, et al. Differential role for CD80 and CD86 in the regulation of the innate immune response in murine polymicrobial sepsis. *PloS One* (2009) 4(8):e6600. doi: 10.1371/journal.pone.0006600
42. Zhou LJ, Tedder TF. Human blood dendritic cells selectively express CD83, a member of the immunoglobulin superfamily. *J Immunol* (1995) 154 (8):3821–35.
43. Middel P, Raddatz D, Gunawan B, Haller F, Radzun HJ. Increased number of mature dendritic cells in Crohn's disease: evidence for a chemokine mediated retention mechanism. *Gut* (2006) 55(2):220–7. doi: 10.1136/gut.2004.063008
44. Prado C, Iruretagoyena M, Burgos PI, Pacheco R. Smoking promotes exacerbated inflammatory features in dendritic cells of Chilean rheumatoid arthritis patients. *Rev Med Chil* (2018) 146(2):150–9. doi: 10.4067/s0034-98872018000200150
45. Dhabhar FS. Enhancing versus Suppressive Effects of Stress on Immune Function: Implications for Immunoprotection and Immunopathology. *Neuroimmunomodulation* (2009) 16(5):300–17. doi: 10.1159/000216188
46. Marsland AL, Walsh C, Lockwood K, John-Henderson NA. The effects of acute psychological stress on circulating and stimulated inflammatory markers: A systematic review and meta-analysis. *Brain Behav Immun* (2017) 64:208–19. doi: 10.1016/j.bbi.2017.01.011
47. Karlidag R, Unal S, Evereklioglu C, Sipahi B, Er H, Yologlu S. Stressful life events, anxiety, depression and coping mechanisms in patients with Behçet's disease. *J Eur Acad Dermatol Venereol* (2003) 17(6):670–5. doi: 10.1046/j.1468-3083.2003.00760.x
48. Banchereau J, Steinman RM. Dendritic cells and the control of immunity. *Nature* (1998) 392(6673):245–52. doi: 10.1038/32588
49. Ye Z, Deng B, Wang C, Zhang D, Kijlstra A, Yang P. Decreased B and T lymphocyte attenuator in Behcet's disease may trigger abnormal Th17 and Th1 immune responses. *Sci Rep* (2016) 6:20401. doi: 10.1038/srep20401
50. Batal I, Azzi J, Mounayar M, Abdoli R, Moore R, Lee JY, et al. The mechanisms of up-regulation of dendritic cell activity by oxidative stress. *J Leukoc Biol* (2014) 96(2):283–93. doi: 10.1189/jlb.3A0113-033RR
51. Joachim RA, Handjiski B, Blois SM, Hagen E, Paus R, Arck PC. Stress-induced neurogenic inflammation in murine skin skews dendritic cells towards maturation and migration: key role of intercellular adhesion molecule-1/leukocyte function-associated antigen interactions. *Am J Pathol* (2008) 173 (5):1379–88. doi: 10.2353/ajpath.2008.080105
52. Kokolus K, Spangler H, Povinelli B, Farren M, Lee K, Repasky E. Stressful Presentations: Mild Cold Stress in Laboratory Mice Influences Phenotype of Dendritic Cells in Naïve and Tumor-Bearing Mice. *Front Immunol* (2014) 5:23. doi: 10.3389/fimmu.2014.00023
53. Wu P, Du L, Hou S, Su G, Yang L, Hu J, et al. Association of LACC1, CEBPB-PTPN1, RIPK2 and ADO-EGR2 with ocular Behcet's disease in a Chinese Han population. *Br J Ophthalmol* (2018) 102(9):1308–14. doi: 10.1136/bjophthalmol-2017-311753
54. Nanke Y, Yago T, Kotake S. The Role of Th17 Cells in the Pathogenesis of Behcet's Disease. *J Clin Med* (2017) 6(7):74. doi: 10.3390/jcm6070074
55. Li B, Yang P, Zhou H, Zhang Z, Xie C, Lin X, et al. T-bet expression is upregulated in active Behçet's disease. *Br J Ophthalmol* (2003) 87(10):1264–7. doi: 10.1136/bjo.87.10.1264
56. Albayrak O, Oray M, Can F, Uludag Kirimli G, Gul A, Tugal-Tutkun I, et al. Effect of Interferon alfa-2a Treatment on Adaptive and Innate Immune Systems in Patients With Behçet Disease Uveitis. *Invest Ophthalmol Vis Sci* (2019) 60(1):52–63. doi: 10.1167/iovs.18-25548
57. Wang C, Ye Z, Kijlstra A, Zhou Y, Yang P. Activation of the aryl hydrocarbon receptor affects activation and function of human monocyte-derived dendritic cells. *Clin Exp Immunol* (2014) 177(2):521–30. doi: 10.1111/cei.12352
58. Fujimoto Y, Tedder TF. CD83: a regulatory molecule of the immune system with great potential for therapeutic application. *J Med Dent Sci* (2006) 53(2):85–91.

2

Uveitis: Molecular Pathogenesis and Emerging Therapies

Charles E. Egwuagu[1*], *Sahar A. Alhakeem*[1,2] *and Evaristus C. Mbanefo*[1]

[1] Molecular Immunology Section, Laboratory of Immunology, National Eye Institute (NEI), National Institutes of Health, Bethesda, MD, United States, [2] Department of Biomedical Sciences, College of Health Sciences, University of Wisconsin-Milwaukee, Milwaukee, WI, United States

***Correspondence:**
Charles E. Egwuagu
egwuaguc@nei.nih.gov

The profound impact that vision loss has on human activities and quality of life necessitates understanding the etiology of potentially blinding diseases and their clinical management. The unique anatomic features of the eye and its sequestration from peripheral immune system also provides a framework for studying other diseases in immune privileged sites and validating basic immunological principles. Thus, early studies of intraocular inflammatory diseases (uveitis) were at the forefront of research on organ transplantation. These studies laid the groundwork for foundational discoveries on how immune system distinguishes self from non-self and established current concepts of acquired immune tolerance and autoimmunity. Our charge in this review is to examine how advances in molecular cell biology and immunology over the past 3 decades have contributed to the understanding of mechanisms that underlie immunopathogenesis of uveitis. Particular emphasis is on how advances in biotechnology have been leveraged in developing biologics and cell-based immunotherapies for uveitis and other neuroinflammatory diseases.

Keywords: molecular therapies, cellular therapies, autoimmunity, immunobiology, EAU, uveitis

INTRODUCTION

The vertebrate immune system is comprised of the adaptive and innate immune systems and the two limbs have unique as well as overlapping functions that are seamlessly integrated (1). During antigen priming in secondary lymphoid or peripheral tissues, innate immune cells such as dendritic cells (DC) secrete cytokines that instruct the naïve lymphocyte to differentiate and generate effector lymphocyte subsets that orchestrate humoral or cell-mediated immunity to pathogens (2). The immense capacity of lymphocyte response to diverse antigens derives from diversity of their cell surface antigen receptors and a critical function of the immune system is to establish tolerance against self-antigens while allowing selective immunity to pathogens (3, 4). Thus, exuberant effector immune responses that cause pathogenic autoimmunity are restrained or prevented by specialized regulatory cells that secrete immune-suppressive cytokines (5). Defects in central and/or peripheral tolerance mechanisms can result in autoimmune diseases such as uveitis, the focus of this review. Uveitis is a group of potentially blinding intraocular inflammatory diseases of infectious or autoimmune etiology and accounts for more than 10% of severe visual handicaps in the United States (6, 7). Although steroids and other anti-inflammatory drugs are effective therapies, renal toxicity and other adverse effects preclude their prolonged usage. Development of effective and safe therapies thus requires a better understanding of molecular and cellular mechanisms that maintain ocular immunity and how dysregulation of these pathways contribute to pathogenesis of uveitis. In this review, we highlight recent advances in understanding of mechanisms that underlie susceptibility to uveitis and summarize emerging therapeutic approaches that show promise in suppressing ocular inflammation and uveitis.

THE VERTEBRATE EYE

The eye is segregated from the peripheral immune system and is arguably one of the most anatomically complex organs in mammals (**Figure 1**). It is composed of: (i) the outer coat of the eye comprised of the opaque sclera (outer white layer of the eyeball) and the transparent cornea which is a continuation of the sclera; (ii) The retinal pigment epithelium (RPE) is a single layer of hexagonal pigmented cells overlying the retina and attached to the underlying choroid. It functions in phagocytosis of photoreceptor outer segment membranes, light absorption, epithelial transport and nourishment of visual cells of the neuroretina. (iii) The Mueller/Glia cell is a specialized glial cell type that supports and supplies nutrients and oxygen to retinal neurons and serves in maintaining the functional stability of retinal cells. The Mueller cell also insulates neurons from each other, uptakes neurotransmitters and regulates the extracellular environment. (iv) The uvea is the pigmented middle layer of the eye beneath the cornea and sclera and is comprised of the vascularized choroid, iris and ciliary body. It performs most visual functions of the eye including focusing on objects at various distances to the retina and changing the pupil size in response to light intensity. (v) The neural retina is the innermost, light-sensitive layer consisting of five types of neurons that receive photons transmitted through the cornea and lens. It consists of the photosensitive ganglion cells, amacrine cells, bipolar cells, horizontal cells and photoreceptors (rods and cones). They generate two-dimensional image of an object and converts it to electrical signals that are then transduced to the brain to create visual perception. The embryonic vertebrate retina and optic nerve derive from the diencephalon of the developing brain and are considered part of the CNS. Similar to brain, the retina is an immune privileged tissue.

THE EYE AS AN IMMUNE PRIVILEGED SITE

Developments in ocular immunology led to appreciation of the special relationship between the eye and the immune system and this foundational research led to our current concept of immune privilege. Sir Peter Medawar who shared the 1960 Nobel Prize in physiology and medicine with Sir Frank Macfarlane Burnet coined the term "Immune Privilege" based on studies showing that tumor or skin allograft when placed in the anterior chamber of the eye is not rejected (8). Immune privilege was then viewed as a unique feature of the eye and failure to reject an allograft or alloantigen was attributed to the lack of blood vessels in retina (9). A modern explanation of immune privilege is that proteins in immune privileged tissues of the CNS are sequestrated from the peripheral immune system by the blood-retina barrier (BRB), blood-brain-barrier (BBB) and the neurovascular unit (NVU) comprised of pericytes, perivascular macrophages, neuronal dendrites, glia limitans of the Müler/microglia and tightly bound endothelial cells that surround the NVU (10, 11). The avascular immunosuppressive environment of the retina lacks lymphatic drainage, contains resident regulatory cells that secrete neuropeptides and anti-inflammatory cytokines and also contributes to immunological sequestration of the retina (10). In addition, the RPE and resident retinal cells that express inhibitory cell surface associated proteins (TGF-β, FAS/FAS ligand, CD46 and CD59) limit inflammation in the retina by inactivating lymphocytes (12–14). Normal development of the gut microbiome during early infancy is now recognized to play

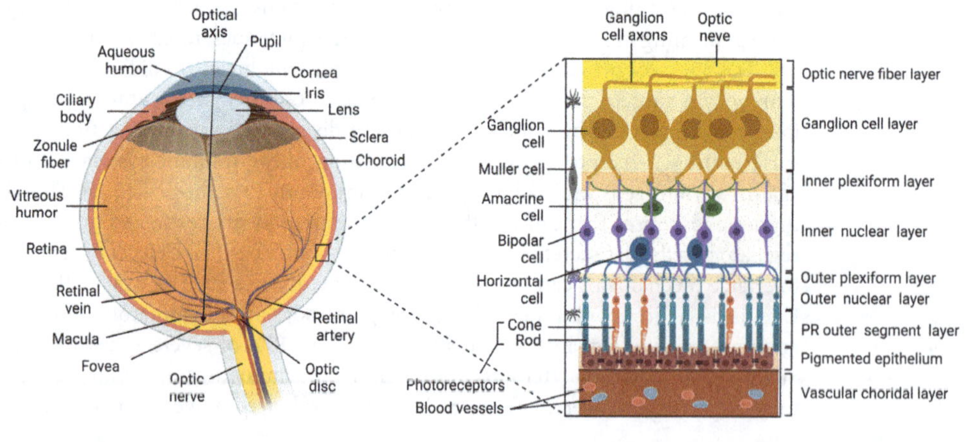

FIGURE 1 | Structure of the Vertebrate Eye. The eye is composed of: (i) the outer tunic of the eye comprised of the sclera and cornea (ii) the uvea comprised of the choroid, the iris and the ciliary body; (iii) the neural retina comprised of five types of neurons (ganglion cell, amacrine cells, bipolar cells, horizontal cells and photoreceptors (rods and cones); (iv) Muller cell; (v) RPE.

important roles in establishing the BBB or BRB (15) and studies in mice with defective gut microbiome have established a link between dysbiosis and susceptibility to inflammatory diseases including, acute anterior uveitis (AAU) (16, 17). Despite these safeguards, intense and persistent inflammation can still overwhelm the multilayered barriers and peripheral tolerance mechanisms that maintain immune privilege. Th17 cells play important roles of in early events that initiate pathogenesis of inflammatory diseases (18–20). They produce granzyme B that promotes disruption of the BBB and initiate CNS autoimmune diseases including multiple sclerosis and experimental autoimmune encephalomyelitis (EAE) (21). Similar to other CNS autoimmune diseases, adoptive transfer studies have shown that as few as $1x10^7$ uveitogenic Th1 and Th17 cells also promote breakdown of the BRB and the retinal NVU, resulting in the recruitment of bystander lymphocytes and myeloid cells that exacerbate uveitis (20). However, individuals with intact immune system eventually re-establish immune privilege *via* induction of regulatory T cells (Tregs, Tr1, Tr3) and B cells (Bregs) that secrete immune-suppressive cytokines in the retina and lymphoid tissues.

HUMAN UVEITIS

CNS inflammatory diseases present unique challenges because the need to eliminate a pathogen is as important as avoiding exuberant inflammatory response associated with photoreceptor cell deficit and development of severe uveitis. A cross-sectional study in California documented an incidence rate of 25.6 /100,000 person-years and prevalence rate of 69 cases/100,000 persons (22). However, infectious uveitis accounts for less than 20% of uveitis/scleritis, with incidence rate of 18.9/100,000 and prevalence of 60.6/100,000 persons (23). Uveitis is classified as anterior, intermediate, posterior or pan uveitis depending on the anatomic location (24). Anterior segment uveitis is the most common form and manifests as iritis or iridocyclitis while Intermediate uveitis is characterized by vitritis and peripheral retinal vasculitis. Posterior uveitis is a disease of the posterior segment (retina, choroid and vitreous) and symptoms include blurred vision, photophobia, retinal neovascularization, retinal detachment and macular edema. Although the precise etiology of most uveitis is difficult to ascertain, Fuchs' heterochromic iridocyclitis, birdshot retinochoroidopathy, multifocal choroiditis, pars planitis and sympathetic ophthalmia are thought to be of autoimmune etiology (24). Uveitis can also be associated with systemic diseases such as sarcoidosis, psoriatic arthritis, ankylosing spondylitis, juvenile rheumatoid arthritis (JRA), MS, Vogt-Koyanagi-Harada's disease, Behçet's disease, systemic lupus erythematosus (SLE) and collagen vascular diseases (24).

ANIMAL MODELS OF UVEITIS

Animal models of human uveitis have contributed to understanding of immunopathogenic mechanisms of uveitis. Two of the best characterized models of anterior uveitis are endotoxin-induced uveitis (EIU) (25) and experimental autoimmune anterior uveitis (EAAU), also called experimental melanin-induced uveitis (EMIU) (26, 27). Posterior uveitis poses the greatest risk of blindness and the best characterized model of posterior uveitis is experimental autoimmune uveitis (EAU) (28–30). Study of EAU using a variety of genetically modified mouse strains have identified critical pathways that mediate posterior uveitis. These studies have identified transcription factors (STAT3, IRF4, IRF8), regulatory proteins (SOCS1, SOCS3) or cytokine signaling pathways that regulate EAU and can serve as potential therapeutic targets for ameliorating uveitis (20, 31–35). Of particular interest is a transgenic mouse strain expressing a TCR specific for $IRBP_{161-180}$ that develops spontaneous ocular autoimmunity. Analysis of EAU in these mice has revealed that gut commensals might be a source of signals that prime autoreactive retina-specific T cells to trigger uveitis (36).

Experimental Models of Anterior Uveitis

Endotoxin-induced uveitis (EIU) is a rodent model of acute anterior segment inflammation induced by subcutaneous or intraperitoneal injection of lipopolysaccharide (LPS) and is characterized by infiltration of inflammatory cells into the anterior segment (37). Although EIU exhibits immunohistopathologic features of human anterior uveitis, duration of the inflammatory response is relatively short (< 72h) and does not cause lasting tissue damage (37). On the other hand, EAAU is induced by peripheral administration of proteins bound to melanin granules and the inflammatory response is more representative of human anterior uveitis (26, 27, 38). EAAU is characterized by massive infiltration of mononuclear and polymorphonuclear cells into the anterior chamber, iris and ciliary body vessels, with limited posterior segment involvement. Although none of these models manifest full spectrum of clinical and histopathological features of human uveitis, each contributes to understanding of particular aspects of the disease process.

Experimental Autoimmune Uveitis: Model of Posterior Uveitis

Experimental autoimmune uveitis (EAU) is a T-cell-mediated intraocular inflammatory disease induced in susceptible species by active immunization with ocular-specific proteins or peptides in an emulsion containing Complete Freund's Adjuvant (CFA). Full-blown disease requires coadministration of pertussis toxin and heat-killed tuberculosis bacteria, which activate bacterial pattern recognition receptors on innate immune cells (28). Commonly used retinal protein for inducing EAU in mice and rats are S-Antigen (S-Ag or arrestin) and interphotoreceptor retinoid-binding protein (IRBP) (39, 40). EAU is considered a useful model of posterior uveitis because of its immunopathologic features that include iritis, choroiditis, vitritis, retinal vasculitis, destruction of photoreceptor cells and retinal edema (20). The disease is transferable to naive syngeneic animals by injection of *in vitro* activated $CD4^+$ T cells specific to retinal antigens (28–30).

CELLULAR AND MOLECULAR MECHANISMS THAT DETERMINE SUSCEPTIBILITY OR RESISTANCE TO UVEITIS

Although lymphocytes from uveitis patients respond to retinal S-Ag *in vitro* and a number of retinal antigens induce disease in rodents and non-human primates, the putative retinal antigens involved in human uveitis have not been defined. On the other hand, it has been suggested that the response to S-Ag might be secondary to retinal tissue damage induced by inflammation. Nevertheless, animal models of uveitis exhibit essential immunopathogenic features of human uveitis. In this section of the review, we summarize what we know of the molecular pathogenesis of uveitis with particular focus on: molecular basis of susceptibility to autoimmune uveitis and source of the autoreactive memory T cells that mediate relapsing-remitting inflammation that characterize potentially blinding chronic uveitis.

Defects in Central Tolerance Mechanism and Susceptibility to Uveitis

The mature T lymphocyte derives from bone marrow hematopoietic stem cells (HSC) and acquires capacity to mediate immunological responses following maturation in the thymus. At very early stages of its development, bone marrow-derived lymphoid-primed multipotent progenitor (LMPP) and common lymphoid progenitor (CLP) enter the thymic cortex and undergo positive and negative selection processes (central tolerance) that endows the developing T cell with the capacity to discriminate between self and non-self-antigens (41, 42). T cells that express a functional TCR and develop tolerance for self-antigens encountered in the thymus exit the thymus to enter secondary lymphoid organs and the peripheral circulation (**Figure 2**). The AIRE transcription factor (autoimmune regulator) plays a critical role in central tolerance mechanism by promoting the expression of self-proteins on medullary thymic epithelial cells (mTEC) at levels detectable by the

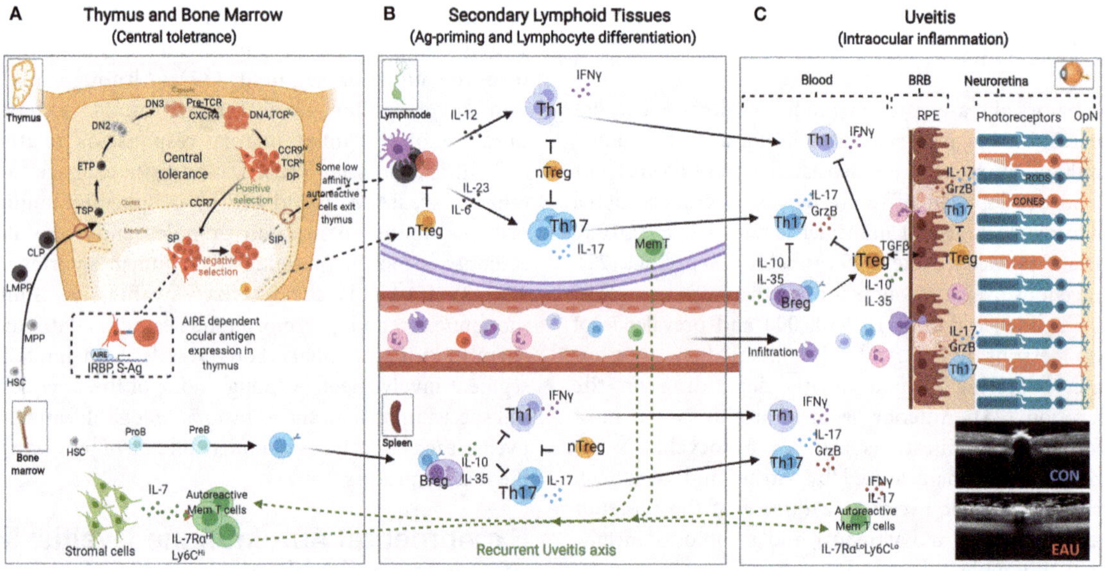

FIGURE 2 | Immunopathogenic Mechanisms of experimental autoimmune uveitis (EAU). **(A)** Central tolerance mechanism: Bone marrow derived lymphoid-primed multipotent progenitors (LMPPs) and common lymphoid progenitors (CLPs) enter the thymus near the cortico-medullary junction. Thymus-settling progenitors cells give rise to early T cell progenitors (ETPs), double negative 1 (DN1), DN2 and DN3 thymocytes that then migrate to the subcapsular zone for further development (42). DN3 thymocytes that express functional pre-T cell receptor and CXCR4 receive survival signals that promote proliferation and eventual differentiate to DN4 and then double positive (DP) thymocytes. The DP thymocytes (CCR9^{Hi}) undergoing positive selection interact with self-peptide/MHC complexes on cortical thymic epithelial cells, upregulate CCR7 and mature into single positive (SP) mature T cells that migrate to the thymic medulla (42). The medullary thymic epithelial cells (mTEC) in collaboration with the AIRE transcription factor (autoimmune regulator) in the medulla, promiscuously express tissue-restrictive antigens of major proteins in peripheral tissues. AIRE also contributes to mechanism of negative selection, which eliminates self-reactive T cells that would cause autoimmune diseases. T cells with normal low affinity/avidity recognition of self-antigens are induced to upregulate sphingosine-1-phosphate receptor 1 (S1P1), exit the thymus and enter the blood and peripheral lymphoid tissues. **(B)** Peripheral tolerance mechanisms mediated by nTregs render potentially autoreactive T cells anergic or "ignorant". Naïve T cells that enter the circular or peripheral tissues differentiate to various T-helper subsets in response to PAMPs (pathogen associated molecular patterns) or molecular mimicry mechanism. During EAU, active immunization with ocular antigens (e.g. IRBP or S-Ag) in CFA emulsion induces clonal expansion of Th1 and Th17 resulting in disease by day 14-20 followed by Treg and Breg-mediated resolution of the acute inflammatory response between days 25-32 after disease induction. However, few autoreactive memory T cells expressing IL-7Rα persist and they eventually migrate to the bone marrow (BM) where they reside and can be reactivated to mediate recurrent uveitis. **(C)** Schematic representation of early events associated with loss of immune privilege of the eye and induction of retinal protective mechanism in rodent model of uveitis. Effector molecules such as Granzyme B and proinflammatory cytokines secreted by Th17 cells facilitate breakdown of blood retina barrier (BRB), resulting in the influx of other inflammatory cells such as Th1, Th2, and monocytes. The inflammatory cells entering the eye encounter hostile environment of the neuroretina consisting of anti-inflammatory molecules as well as regulatory T and B cells secreting IL-10 and/or IL-35. RPE, retinal pigment epithelium; OPN, optic nerve; CON, control retina; EAU, OCT image of mouse with uveitis.

maturing T cells. T cells with very high affinity for cognate self-protein are eliminated because they pose danger of pathogenic autoimmunity (1, 43). However, some T cells that detect cognate antigens just below the threshold required for tolerance induction are not eliminated and these renegade autoreactive T cells are thought to be the cause of organ-specific autoimmune diseases (44). In immune-competent hosts, these potentially autoreactive T cells are maintained at low levels by an immune-suppressive T cell subset that also develops in the thymus (45). These specialized Foxp3$^+$ T cells are called natural regulatory T cells (nTregs) and they constitutively secrete IL-10, an immune-suppressive cytokine that suppresses autoreactive T cells and inflammation (5). These nTregs also migrate from the thymus into peripheral tissues and play critical roles in peripheral tolerance.

A major contribution of ocular immunology and uveitis to our current understanding of the molecular basis of resistance or susceptibility to organ-specific autoimmune diseases derived from a series of EAU studies performed in the late nineties. Genetic and molecular studies of the thymus of mouse strains (B10RIII, B10A, C57BL/6 and BALB/c) and rat strains (Lewis and Brown-Norway) that vary in their relative susceptibility to EAU provided direct evidence that ocular proteins are not sequestered from the peripheral immune system and are accessible for tolerance induction in the thymus (43). These studies showed that ocular proteins are expressed in the thymus, but the level of expression varied even among animals of the same species including mice, rats and non-human primates (43, 46, 47). High level expression of ocular proteins (IRBP or S-Antigen) in the thymus correlated with resistance to EAU development while low levels correlated with susceptibility to uveitis. This observation was subsequently validated in a mouse model of PLP-induced EAE (48) and in human studies showing that transcription levels of the insulin gene in the thymus correlated with susceptibility to type 1 diabetes (49). This seminal discovery from EAU studies thus provided mechanistic explanation for differential susceptibility to autoimmune uveitis and suggested that resistance to uveitis is regulated at least in part by capacity to establish central tolerance to retinal autoantigens (43).

Pro-inflammatory T-Helper Cells Mediate Acute and Chronic Relapsing-Remitting Uveitis

Uveitis correlates with HLA class I or class II genes, with HLA-DR4 strongly associated with sympathetic ophthalmia or VKH while HLA-A29 is strongly associated with birdshot retinochoroidopathy (50, 51). On the other hand, HLA-B27 is strongly associated with anterior uveitis and patients with acute anterior uveitis and ankylosing spondylitis (52). Similar to humans, susceptibility of mice to uveitis is linked to certain genetic loci, with strong correlations to certain MHC class II haplotypes (53). Among mouse strains the most susceptible is B10.RIII with decreasing susceptibility: B10.RIII (H-2r)> B10.BR (H-2k) >C57BL/6 (H-2b) (53). However, the genetic influences of the MHC molecules are not the only predisposing factors.

The heterodimeric IL-12 family of cytokines play critical roles during Ag-presentation in developmental decisions of differentiating naïve lymphocytes and in determining the intensity, duration and nature of the inflammatory response (54). The family is comprised of IL-12 (IL-12p35/IL-12p40), IL-23 (IL-23p19/IL-12p40), IL-27 (IL-27p28/Ebi3), IL-35 (IL-12p35/Ebi3), and IL-39 (IL-23p19/Ebi3) (54, 55). Studies in the late nineties demonstrated that IL-12 skewed the uveitogenic T cell response towards the Th1 developmental pathway while IL-12p40-deficient mice were found to be resistant to EAU, leading to the suggestion that Th1 cells mediated EAU (56). Subsequent discovery of IL-23 that shares the IL-12p40 subunit with IL-12 led to appreciation of the role of IL-23 in several autoimmune diseases and eventual identification of the Th17 as the lymphocyte subset that mediated these diseases (19). IL-12 was subsequently shown to confer protection against EAU (57), leading to the revised conclusion that IL-23 rather than IL-12 is critical for the development of EAU induced by immunization with IRBP in CFA (58). Soon after the discovery of Th17, its role in EAU was established (59). This was confirmed by studies showing that mutant mice with targeted deletion of STAT3 in the CD4 T cell compartment do not develop EAU because their T cells cannot differentiate into Th17 cells (31). The EAU-resistant CD4-STAT3KO mice exhibited exaggerated increase of Th1 cells and elevated levels of IFN-γ, providing suggestive evidence that increase in Th1 cells does not cause EAU (31). Subsequent studies revealed that Th1 expansion during EAU antagonized Th17 responses through IFN-γ/STAT1-dependent expression of IL-27 cytokine, an immune-suppressive member of the IL-12 family (59). It is notable that involvement of Th17 cells in a human autoimmune disease was first demonstrated in study of uveitis and scleritis patients. Blood of patients with active uveitis or scleritis contained elevated levels of Th17 which correlated with increase in IL-2 (59).

Organ-specific CNS autoimmune diseases such as uveitis and multiple sclerosis are characterized by repeated cycles of remission and recurrent inflammation and it is not known where the auto-reactive memory T cells that initiate recurrent uveitis or MS reside during periods of disease remission. This age-old question was addressed in a chronic uveitis model by monitoring IRBP-specific autoreactive memory T cells (IL-7Rα^{High}Ly6C^{High}CD4$^+$) for 6 months and showing that the uveitogenic T cells relocated from the retina and peripheral lymphoid tissues into the bone marrow (BM) (20) (**Figure 2**). The autoreactive memory T cells resided in a resting state in the BM and upon restimulation converted to Th17 effector cells (IL-7Rα^{Low}Ly6C^{Low}CD4$^+$). It is notable that while BM cells from WT EAU mice transferred uveitis to naive mice, IRBP-specific autoreactive memory T cells of CD4-STAT3KO mice could not traffic to the BM and BM cells from the IRBP-immunized CD4-STAT3KO mice could not transfer EAU upon reactivation (20). These studies identified BM as a niche for IRBP-specific memory T cells that caused recurrent uveitis and suggested that BM stromal cells provide survival signals to autoreactive memory T cells through STAT3-dependent mechanisms (20). Taken together, analysis of mouse uveitis model and the blood of human uveitis patients identified roles of Th17 cells and STAT3 pathway in uveitis and that STAT3 pathway is a potential target for treatment of uveitis.

TREATMENT OF UVEITIS

Topical or systemic steroids are effective therapies for uveitis. While topical corticosteroid is effective for anterior uveitis, severe intermediate or posterior uveitis might require periocular corticosteroid injections. On the other hand, standard of care for vision-threatening uveitis, especially if accompanied by cystoid macular edema is systemic immunosuppression with oral corticosteroid (prednisone). If ineffective, low dose prednisone in combination with cyclosporin A, antimetabolites (methotrexate, azathioprine) or anti-inflammatory (colchicine) is indicated. When combination of corticosteroid with these second line drugs are ineffective, alkylating agents such as cyclophosphamide or chlorambucil which are associated with significant adverse effects are employed as a last resort. Nonetheless, prolonged use of systemic corticosteroids increases risk of infections, malignancy and decreased lifespan. Thus, the adverse effects of prolonged use of corticosteroids, alkylating agents and immunosuppressive drugs such as cyclosporin A, FK-506 or rapamycin are impetus to develop less toxic and more specific therapies for uveitis.

POSTERIOR UVEITIS THERAPY

Targeting Cytokines and Cytokine Receptors

Commonly used therapies for posterior uveitis are steroids and although they are effective in suppressing ocular inflammation, they do not directly target memory autoreactive T cells that perpetuate cycles of recurrence and remission that characterize blinding posterior uveitis.

Besides steroids, biologics that target T cell receptors or effector functions are gaining acceptance although Adalimumab (Humira) is the only FDA approved biologic for uveitis. Other biologics include: (i) Blockage of T cell signaling pathways (cyclosporine, FK-506 and rapamycin); (ii) Anti-CD4 T cell function (anti-IL-2R, anti-IFN-γ Abs; (iii) Targeting TNF-α (Etanercept (Enbrel®), Infliximab (Remicade®), Thalidomide); (iv) Biologics that target immune modulatory molecules (adhesion, co-stimulatory molecules) (60–63). This section of the review will focus on new therapeutic strategies that target signal transduction pathways utilized by pathogenic lymphocytes.

Targeting Janus Kinases

The JAK/STAT pathway regulates growth and survival of mammalian cells and signal transduction through this evolutionarily conserved pathway is mediated by Janus kinases (Jak1, Jak2, Jak3 and Tyk2) and Signal Transducers and Activators of Transcription (STAT1, STAT2, STAT3, STAT4, STAT5a, STAT5b, and STAT6), a 7-member family of latent cytoplasmic transcription factors (64). Immunoregulatory cytokines secreted by innate cells (IL-12, IL-23, IL-27) or lymphocytes (IFN-γ, IL-2, IL-4, IL-6, IL-10, IL-21) mediate their biological activities through receptor-associated Janus kinases (Jaks) and Stat proteins (65). Cytokine-binding to its cognate receptor selectively activates Jaks by transphosphorylation of specific tyrosine residues, followed by recruitment of cytokine-specific Stats to the receptor complex (66). Tyrosine-phosphorylated Stats form homo- or hetero-dimers, translocate into the nucleus and mediate transcription of cognate genes. Thus, cytokine-mediated activation of Jak/Stat pathway provides a rapid membrane to nucleus mechanism for regulating gene expression and altering behavior of the cell (66). Because persistent activation of Jak/Stat signals dysregulate the immune system and cause many autoimmune diseases and cancer, cytokine responses are under stringent regulation. Thus, pharmacological regulation of Jak kinase activities has been exploited for treatment of autoimmune and neoplastic diseases (67–71). Of note, Jak inhibitors have been found to be effective in treating anterior uveitis and associated macular edema (72).

Targeting Stat3 Pathway Utilized by Th17 Cells

Most cytokines that regulate lymphocyte growth, development, survival or effector functions activate STAT3 pathway (73, 74). CD4-STAT3KO mice do not develop EAU because of defect in generating Th17 cells (31), suggesting that STAT3 is a potential therapeutic target for modulating uveitis. Surprisingly, mice with loss of STAT3 in the CD19 B cell compartment (CD19-STAT3KO) have exacerbate EAU (32), suggesting that intrinsic functions of STAT3 are diametrically opposite in T and B cells. Another target of Stat3 that promotes ocular inflammation is miR-155-5p (miR-155). Stat3 activates miR-155 and the Stat3/miR-155 axis mediate severe uveitis by promoting the expansion of pathogenic Th17 cells (75). Inflammatory cytokines have also been shown to induce expression of miR-155 in human RPE cells (76), further suggesting that Stat3 is a potential therapeutic target for treating uveitis. We describe here strategies that have been successful in targeting Stat pathway and suppressing uveitis in mice.

Synthetic STAT3 Inhibitors

ORLL-NIH001 is a synthetic 406-kDa small chemical compound that targets STAT3 (**Figure 3**) by antagonizing Th17 cells, down-regulating α4;β1, α4β7, CCR6 and CXCR3 and inhibiting trafficking of lymphocytes into the retina (77). However, a drawback to therapeutic use of ORLL-NIH001 is its relatively poor bioavailability and frequent administration of the drug is required. Although delivery of the drug by intravenous injection is effective, oral administration or subcutaneous injection may be attractive alternatives.

Suppressor of Cytokine Signaling and SOCS Mimetic Peptide Therapy

Suppressor of cytokine signaling (SOCS) are an 8-member family of intracellular proteins that are rapidly induced in many cell types in response to cytokines (IFN-γ, IL-2, IL-4, IL-6, IL-10, IL-12, IL-21, IL-23, IL-27) or growth factors (CNTF, LIF, FGF, IGF-

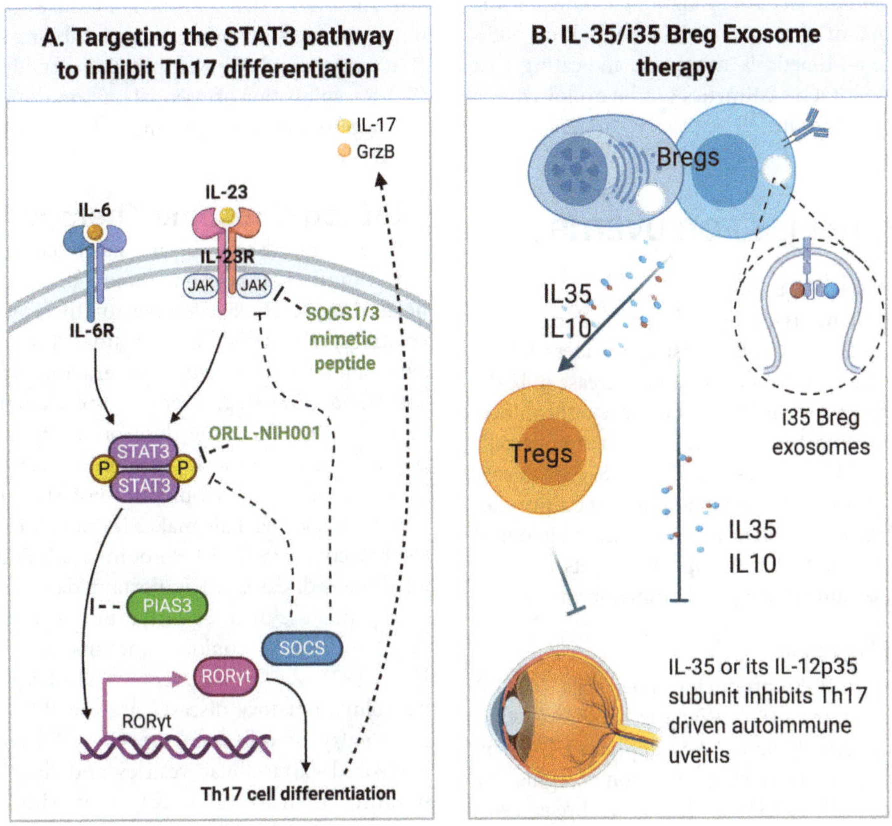

FIGURE 3 | Emerging Therapies for Uveitis. **(A)** Regulation of STAT3 pathway. Cytokines such as IL-6 or IL-23 bind their cognate receptor on lymphocytes and activate receptor-associated JAK kinases. Following the recruitment of latent STAT3 proteins to the activated receptor complex, the STAT3 protein is Tyrosine-phosphorylated, forms pSTAT3:pSTAT3 homodimers that translocate to the nucleus and activate STAT3-responsive genes. SOCS (SOCS1, SOCS3) proteins are immediate early genes activated by pSTAT3 and they are negative feedback regulators of JAK/STAT pathway. They inhibit or terminate JAK/STAT signals by binding to Tyrosine-phosphorylated JAKs or cytokine receptors, targeting them for degradation in the proteosome. PIAS3 protein also inhibits STAT3 transcriptional activities by binding STAT3 DNA binding domain and physically preventing STAT3 binding to target genes. **(B)** Other emerging therapies for the treatment of uveitis include: (i) Immunotherapy with IL-35-producing Breg cells (i35-Breg) (ii) Administration of biologics (IL-35, IL12p35); (iii) Exosome treatment with IL-35-containing exosomes (i35-Exosomes).

1, insulin). However, unabated stimulation of Stat signaling pathway during chronic inflammation or cellular stress induces SOCS proteins, particularly SOCS1 and SOCS3 that function as components of a negative feedback loop that regulate the initiation, intensity and duration of inflammatory cytokine responses (78). Their inhibitory effects derive from direct interaction with cytokine/growth-factor receptors, STAT proteins and Jak kinases, leading to proteasomal degradation of target proteins or receptor complex and termination of the signal (79, 80). SOCS1 and SOCS3 are well established as important regulators of inflammatory diseases including allergy, autoimmune diseases, diabetes, metabolic syndrome and cancer (79, 80). In context of potential involvement of SOCS proteins in uveitis, transgenic rats and mice with targeted overexpression of SOCS1 in the retina are protected from severe uveitis and scleritis patients exhibit a defect in SOCS1 expression as their lymphocytes could not induce SOCS1 in response to IL-2 (81). These observations suggest that enhancing SOC1 levels in the retina can be used to suppress uveitis. However, a major impediment to use of SOCS1 or SOCS3 for therapy is that they are intracellular proteins and the lack of efficient means to deliver these proteins into cells. A promising new approach is the development of SOCS1 and SOCS3 mimetic peptides that incorporate an N-terminal or carboxy-terminal lipid moiety, which then allows SOCS mimetic peptides to be delivered directly into cells.

Topical SOCS1 Mimetic Peptide Therapy

The SOCS1 protein possesses a kinase inhibitory region (KIR) and binding of the KIR to activated Jak1 or Jak2 suppresses their kinase activities (82). SOCS1 mimetic peptide of varying length have been shown to be effective in inhibiting Stat1/Stat3 signaling (83, 84). Topical administration of a formulation consisting of membrane-penetrating 16 amino acid SOCS1 peptide, with a lipophilic palmitoyl-lysine group attached to its NH2-terminus (SOCS1-KIR), was effective in suppressing uveitis in mice EAU (**Figure 3**) (85). The SOCS1-Mimetic ameliorated uveitis by suppressing the expansion of pathogenic Th17 cells and trafficking of inflammatory cells into the neuroretina during EAU. Photopic and scotopic electroretinograms confirmed the neuroprotective effects of the SOCS1-KIR in uveitis (85). Importantly, the SOCS1-Mimetic is non-toxic, indicating that topical administration of SOCS1-Mimetics can be exploited as a non-invasive treatment for uveitis.

EMERGING THERAPIES FOR UVEITIS

Therapeutic Cytokines

The IL-12 family of cytokines is comprised of proinflammatory (IL-12, IL-23, IL-39) and immunosuppressive members (IL-27 and IL-35) (54). In mouse models of uveitis, the increase of IL-12 or IL-23 during antigen priming in LN or the eye promotes uveitis (86) while increased secretion of IL-27 by microglial cells or lymphocytes during EAU suppressed EAU (59, 87, 88). These reports suggest that identifying factors that induce the immune-suppressive IL-27 and IL-35 cytokines or enhance their biological activities *in vivo* might be potential therapeutic targets that can be exploited to suppress human ocular inflammatory diseases.

Interleukin 35 Therapy

Following discovery that IL-35-producing Treg cells (iT_R35) suppressed colitis in the mouse (89), Wang et al. showed that treatment of mice with recombinant IL-35 suppressed EAU by inhibiting Th-17 responses and inducing expansion of regulatory B cells (Breg) that produce IL-10 (B10) or IL-35 (i35-Bregs) (90). Adoptive transfer of *ex-vivo* generated i35-Bregs cells was also shown to suppress EAU, providing evidence that i35-Breg immunotherapy may also be efficacious in uveitis (90) (**Figure 3**). Mechanistically, the i35-Bregs also suppressed EAU by inhibiting expansion of pathogenic Th17 cells and converting conventional lymphocytes to B10, iTR35 or i35-Breg. These observations have led to significant interest in using IL-35 or i35-Bregs as treatment for uveitis. However, before i35-Breg immunotherapy can be brought to the clinic, additional preclinical investigations are needed to establish IL-35 pharmacokinetics and detailed characterization of human i35-Breg to demonstrate that it is a stable Breg phenotype with immune-suppressive activity and functions.

IL-35 Subunit Therapy

Despite significant interest in IL-35 as a potential biologic or use of i35-Breg immunotherapy for autoimmune diseases, less is known about mechanisms by which IL-35 mediates its immune suppressive functions. It is still not clear whether immune-suppressive activities of IL-35 derive exclusively by the pairing of IL-12p35 and Ebi3 subunits to form the heterodimeric IL-35 or if IL-12p35 or Ebi3 also possesses intrinsic functions independent of IL-35. Recent reports revealed that recombinant IL-12p35 (rIL-12p35) has immunoregulatory activities that regulated immunity and suppressed neuroinflammation in the EAE mouse model (91). Similar to IL-35, the rIL-12p35 subunit suppressed EAU and EAE by inducing expansion of B10 and i35-Bregs while inhibiting Th17 responses (91, 92). However, a major difference is that while IL-35 upregulates inhibitory receptor proteins (Lag3, PD-1) that induce T cell exhaustion, rIL-12p35 did not induce these inhibitory receptors but suppressed inflammation by inhibiting signals downstream of IL-6 receptor and cell-cycle proteins that inhibit T cell proliferation (91). Recapitulation of essential immunosuppressive activities of IL-35 suggests that IL-12p35 may also be used as immunotherapy for uveitis.

i35-Breg-Exosome Therapy

Although IL-35 shows promise as biologics for the treatment of autoimmune diseases, a major disadvantage of using the heterodimeric IL-35 cytokine for therapy is its instability and relatively short-half-life. Besides the technical challenges associated with *ex-vivo* generation of large amounts of functional i35-Breg, there is the difficulty of reproducibly administering the same dose of IL-35 each time. It is a very unstable heterodimeric cytokine because association of its IL-12p35 and Ebi3 subunits is not strong (non-covalent) and readily dissociate. This makes it difficult to ascertain the dose of the bioactive p35:Ebi3 heterodimer administered or required to ameliorate disease. An important development relating to the therapeutic use of IL-35 or i35-Breg is the recent discovery that i35-Bregs secrete copious amounts of exosomes that contain IL-35 (93). An impediment to i35-Breg immunotherapy for neuroinflammatory diseases are the BBB, BRB and NVU that limit entry of cells into the CNS. Exosomes are 30-150 nm nanosized extracellular vesicles and their relatively small size, making them suitable for delivering immunoregulatory molecules to the CNS. Mice treated with IL-35 containing exosomes (i35-Exosomes) were protected from developing severe uveitis and disease protection correlated with expansion of IL-10 and IL-35 secreting Treg cells with concomitant suppression of Th17 responses (93) (**Figure 3**). i35-Exosome therapy thus overcomes the technically difficult and labor-intensive effort required to produce sufficient amounts of IL-35-producing i35-Bregs for immunotherapy: as much as 32×10^{10} exosomes can be isolated from a mouse and 2×10^{10} i35-exosomes contain ~15ng IL-35. Another advantage of i35-Exosomes therapy is that IL-12p35/Ebi3 heterodimers are confined in the same vesicle which obviates the dosing issue of determining the precise amount of bioactive IL-35 administered to the subject (93). Taken together, i35-Exosomes are an attractive therapeutic option for delivering IL-35 to the retina.

PERSPECTIVES

The remarkable advances in ocular immunology over the past 3 decades have led to a better understanding of the molecular mechanisms that underlie etiology and susceptibility to uveitis. Genetically modified mouse strains with targeted deletion or overexpression of transcription factors, regulatory proteins or cytokines that control lymphocyte development or functions have led to identification of critical pathways that regulate uveitis. Results from these studies have ushered in a new era of targeted therapies for these family of potentially blinding diseases that are a major cause of morbidity. In conclusion, we highlight three promising and effective treatment modalities without the adverse effects associated with steroids, which are the commonly used drugs for uveitis. (i) Regulatory B cell (Breg) therapy: Breg immunotherapy with as few as $5x10^6$ cells is sufficient to suppress uveitis by inhibiting Th17/Th1 lymphocytes and converting conventional lymphocytes into IL-10 and/or IL-35-producing regulatory cells. Because the Bregs proliferate *in vivo* they are able to sustain secretion of anti-inflammatory cytokines in target tissues. (ii) i35-Exosome therapy: i35-Exosomes suppress uveitis by upregulating inhibitory receptors (PD1, LAG3), propagating infectious-tolerance signals which induced conventional lymphocytes to acquire capacity for producing immunosuppressive cytokines. (iii) Topical SOCS1-Mimetic therapy: The SOCS1-Mimetic inhibits Jak kinases and is an effective non-invasive treatment for uveitis in mice. Although therapy for uveitis will continue to depend in part upon the location, underlying cause and any associated complications, availability of alternative therapeutic options for patients is clearly a major dividend.

AUTHOR CONTRIBUTIONS

CE, SA, and EM wrote and reviewed manuscript. All authors contributed to the article and approved the submitted version.

REFERENCES

1. Gery I, Egwuagu CE. Central Tolerance Mechanisms in Control of Susceptibility to Autoimmune Uveitic Disease. *Int Rev Immunol* (2002) 21 (2-3):89–100. doi: 10.1080/08830180212061
2. Takenaka MC, Quintana FJ. Tolerogenic Dendritic Cells. *Semin Immunopathol* (2017) 39(2):113–20. doi: 10.1007/s00281-016-0587-8
3. Theofilopoulos AN, Kono DH, Baccala R. The Multiple Pathways to Autoimmunity. *Nat Immunol* (2017) 18(7):716–24. doi: 10.1038/ni.3731
4. Amaya-Uribe L, Rojas M, Azizi G, Anaya JM, Gershwin ME. Primary Immunodeficiency and Autoimmunity: A Comprehensive Review. *J Autoimmun* (2019) 99:52–72. doi: 10.1016/j.jaut.2019.01.011
5. Sakaguchi S, Mikami N, Wing JB, Tanaka A, Ichiyama K, Ohkura N. Regulatory T Cells and Human Disease. *Annu Rev Immunol* (2020) 38:541–66. doi: 10.1146/annurev-immunol-042718-041717
6. Gritz DC, Wong IG. Incidence and Prevalence of Uveitis in Northern California; the Northern California Epidemiology of Uveitis Study. *Ophthalmology* (2004) 111(3):491–500; discussion 500. doi: 10.1016/j.ophtha.2003.06.014
7. Caspi RR. A Look At Autoimmunity and Inflammation in the Eye. *J Clin Invest* (2010) 120(9):3073–83. doi: 10.1172/JCI42440
8. Medawar PB. Immunity to Homologous Grafted Skin; the Fate of Skin Homografts Transplanted to the Brain, to Subcutaneous Tissue, and to the Anterior Chamber of the Eye. *Br J Exp Pathol* (1948) 29(1):58–69.
9. Medawar PB. Immunological Tolerance. *Science* (1961) 133(3449):303–6. doi: 10.1126/science.133.3449.303
10. Molzer C, Heissigerova J, Wilson HM, Kuffova L, Forrester JV. Immune Privilege: The Microbiome and Uveitis. *Front Immunol* (2020) 11:608377. doi: 10.3389/fimmu.2020.608377
11. Forrester JV, McMenamin PG, Dando SJ. CNS Infection and Immune Privilege. *Nat Rev Neurosci* (2018) 19(11):655–71. doi: 10.1038/s41583-018-0070-8
12. Kawazoe Y, Sugita S, Keino H, Yamada Y, Imai A, Horie S, et al. Retinoic Acid From Retinal Pigment Epithelium Induces T Regulatory Cells. *Exp Eye Res* (2012) 94(1):32–40. doi: 10.1016/j.exer.2011.11.002
13. Zamiri P, Masli S, Streilein JW, Taylor AW. Pigment Epithelial Growth Factor Suppresses Inflammation by Modulating Macrophage Activation. *Invest Ophthalmol Vis Sci* (2006) 47(9):3912–8. doi: 10.1167/iovs.05-1267
14. Zamiri P, Masli S, Kitaichi N, Taylor AW, Streilein JW. Thrombospondin Plays a Vital Role in the Immune Privilege of the Eye. *Invest Ophthalmol Vis Sci* (2005) 46(3):908–19. doi: 10.1167/iovs.04-0362
15. Braniste V, Al-Asmakh M, Kowal C, Anuar F, Abbaspour A, Toth M, et al. The Gut Microbiota Influences Blood-Brain Barrier Permeability in Mice. *Sci Transl Med* (2014) 6(263):263ra158. doi: 10.1126/scitranslmed.3009759
16. Rosenbaum JT. New Developments in Uveitis Associated With HLA B27. *Curr Opin Rheumatol* (2017) 29(4):298–303. doi: 10.1097/BOR.0000000000000403
17. Rosenbaum JT, Asquith M. The Microbiome and HLA-B27-associated Acute Anterior Uveitis. *Nat Rev Rheumatol* (2018) 14(12):704–13. doi: 10.1038/s41584-018-0097-2
18. Boivin WA, Cooper DM, Hiebert PR, Granville DJ. Intracellular Versus Extracellular Granzyme B in Immunity and Disease: Challenging the Dogma. *Lab Invest* (2009) 89(11):1195–220. doi: 10.1038/labinvest.2009.91
19. Cua DJ, Sherlock J, Chen Y, Murphy CA, Joyce B, Seymour B, et al. Interleukin-23 Rather Than interleukin-12 is the Critical Cytokine for Autoimmune Inflammation of the Brain. *Nature* (2003) 421(6924):744–8. doi: 10.1038/nature01355
20. Oh HM, Yu CR, Lee Y, Chan CC, Maminishkis A, Egwuagu CE. Autoreactive Memory CD4+ T Lymphocytes That Mediate Chronic Uveitis Reside in the Bone Marrow Through STAT3-dependent Mechanisms. *J Immunol* (2011) 187(6):3338–46. doi: 10.4049/jimmunol.1004019
21. Kebir H, Kreymborg K, Ifergan I, Dodelet-Devillers A, Cayrol R, Bernard M, et al. Human TH17 Lymphocytes Promote Blood-Brain Barrier Disruption and Central Nervous System Inflammation. *Nat Med* (2007) 13(10):1173–5. doi: 10.1038/nm1651
22. Suhler EB, Lloyd MJ, Choi D, Rosenbaum JT, Austin DF. Incidence and Prevalence of Uveitis in Veterans Affairs Medical Centers of the Pacific Northwest. *Am J Ophthalmol* (2008) 146(6):890–896 e898. doi: 10.1016/j.ajo.2008.09.014
23. Zhang Y, Amin S, Lung KI, Seabury S, Rao N, Toy BC. Incidence, Prevalence, and Risk Factors of Infectious Uveitis and Scleritis in the United States: A Claims-Based Analysis. *PloS One* (2020) 15(8):e0237995. doi: 10.1371/journal.pone.0237995
24. Nussenblatt RB. The Natural History of Uveitis. *Int Ophthalmol* (1990) 14(5-6):303–8. doi: 10.1007/BF00163549
25. Rosenbaum JT, McDevitt HO, Guss RB, Egbert PR. Endotoxin-Induced Uveitis in Rats as a Model for Human Disease. *Nature* (1980) 286 (5773):611–3. doi: 10.1038/286611a0
26. Broekhuyse RM, Kuhlmann ED, Winkens HJ, Van Vugt AH. Experimental Autoimmune Anterior Uveitis (EAAU), a New Form of Experimental Uveitis. I. Induction by a Detergent-Insoluble, Intrinsic Protein Fraction of the Retinal Pigment Epithelium. *Exp Eye Res* (1991) 52(4):465–74. doi: 10.1016/0014-4835(91)90044-f
27. Broekhuyse RM, Kuhlmann ED, Winkens HJ. Experimental Autoimmune Anterior Uveitis (EAAU). III. Induction by Immunization With Purified Uveal and Skin Melanins. *Exp Eye Res* (1993) 56(5):575–83. doi: 10.1006/exer.1993.1071
28. Wacker WB, Donoso LA, Kalsow CM , Yankeelov JA Jr., Organisciak DT. Experimental Allergic Uveitis. Isolation, Characterization, and Localization of a Soluble Uveitopathogenic Antigen From Bovine Retina. *J Immunol (Baltimore Md.* (1977) 119(6):1949–58.
29. Caspi RR, Roberge FG, Chan CC, Wiggert B, Chader GJ, Rozenszajn LA, et al. A New Model of Autoimmune Disease. Experimental Autoimmune Uveoretinitis Induced in Mice With Two Different Retinal Antigens. *J Immunol (Baltimore Md.* (1988) 140(5):1490–5.
30. McAllister CG, Wiggert B, Chader GJ, Kuwabara T, Gery I. Uveitogenic Potential of Lymphocytes Sensitized to Interphotoreceptor Retinoid-Binding Protein. *J Immunol* (1987) 138(5):1416–20.

31. Liu X, Lee YS, Yu CR, Egwuagu CE. Loss of STAT3 in CD4+ T Cells Prevents Development of Experimental Autoimmune Diseases. *J Immunol* (2008) 180 (9):6070–6. doi: 10.4049/jimmunol.180.9.6070
32. Oladipupo FO, Yu CR, Olumuyide E, Jittaysothorn Y, Choi JK, Egwuagu CE. STAT3 Deficiency in B Cells Exacerbates Uveitis by Promoting Expansion of Pathogenic Lymphocytes and Suppressing Regulatory B Cells (Bregs) and Tregs. *Sci Rep* (2020) 10(1):16188. doi: 10.1038/s41598-020-73093-1
33. Kim SH, Burton J, Yu CR, Sun L, He C, Wang H, et al. Dual Function of the IRF8 Transcription Factor in Autoimmune Uveitis: Loss of IRF8 in T Cells Exacerbates Uveitis, Whereas Irf8 Deletion in the Retina Confers Protection. *J Immunol* (2015) 195(4):1480–8. doi: 10.4049/jimmunol.1500653
34. Yu CR, Hayashi K, Lee YS, Mahdi RM, Shen de F, Chan CC, et al. Suppressor of Cytokine Signaling 1 (SOCS1) Mitigates Anterior Uveitis and Confers Protection Against Ocular HSV-1 Infection. *Inflammation* (2015) 38(2):555–65. doi: 10.1007/s10753-014-9962-6
35. Egwuagu CE, Sztein J, Mahdi RM, Li W, Chao-Chan C, Smith JA, et al. IFN-Gamma Increases the Severity and Accelerates the Onset of Experimental Autoimmune Uveitis in Transgenic Rats. *J Immunol* (1999) 162(1):510–7.
36. Horai R, Caspi RR. Microbiome and Autoimmune Uveitis. *Front Immunol* (2019) 10:232. doi: 10.3389/fimmu.2019.00232
37. McMenamin PG, Crewe J. Endotoxin-Induced Uveitis. Kinetics and Phenotype of the Inflammatory Cell Infiltrate and the Response of the Resident Tissue Macrophages and Dendritic Cells in the Iris and Ciliary Body. *Invest Ophthalmol Vis Sci* (1995) 36(10):1949–59.
38. Jha P, Sohn JH, Xu Q, Nishihori H, Wang Y, Nishihori S, et al. The Complement System Plays a Critical Role in the Development of Experimental Autoimmune Anterior Uveitis. *Invest Ophthalmol Vis Sci* (2006) 47(3):1030–8. doi: 10.1167/iovs.05-1062
39. Zigler JS Jr., Mochizuki M, Kuwabara T, Gery I. Purification of Retinal S-antigen to Homogeneity by the Criterion of Gel Electrophoresis Silver Staining. *Invest Ophthalmol Vis Sci* (1984) 25(8):977–80.
40. Gery I, Wiggert B, Redmond TM, Kuwabara T, Crawford MA, Vistica BP, et al. Uveoretinitis and Pinealitis Induced by Immunization With Interphotoreceptor Retinoid-Binding Protein. *Invest Ophthalmol Vis Sci* (1986) 27(8):1296–300.
41. Hogquist KA, Baldwin TA, Jameson SC. Central Tolerance: Learning Self-Control in the Thymus. *Nat Rev Immunol* (2005) 5(10):772–82. doi: 10.1038/nri1707
42. Love PE, Bhandoola A. Signal Integration and Crosstalk During Thymocyte Migration and Emigration. *Nat Rev Immunol* (2011) 11(7):469–77. doi: 10.1038/nri2989
43. Egwuagu CE, Charukamnoetkanok P, Gery I. Thymic Expression of Autoantigens Correlates With Resistance to Autoimmune Disease. *J Immunol* (1997) 159(7):3109–12.
44. Roep BO. Autoreactive T Cells in Endocrine/Organ-Specific Autoimmunity: Why has Progress Been So Slow? *Springer Semin Immunopathol* (2002) 24 (3):261–71. doi: 10.1007/s00281-002-0109-8
45. Kronenberg M, Rudensky A. Regulation of Immunity by Self-Reactive T Cells. *Nature* (2005) 435(7042):598–604. doi: 10.1038/nature03725
46. Ham DI, Fujimoto C, Gentleman S, Chan CC, Yu CR, Yu S, et al. The Level of Thymic Expression of RPE65 Inversely Correlates With its Capacity to Induce Experimental Autoimmune Uveitis (EAU) in Different Rodent Strains. *Exp Eye Res* (2006) 83:897–902. doi: 10.1016/j.exer.2006.04.013
47. Takase H, Yu CR, Mahdi RM, Douek DC, Dirusso GB, Midgley FM, et al. Thymic Expression of Peripheral Tissue Antigens in Humans: A Remarkable Variability Among Individuals. *Int Immunol* (2005) 17(8):1131–40. doi: 10.1093/intimm/dxh275
48. Klein L, Klugmann M, Nave KA, Tuohy VK, Kyewski B. Shaping of the Autoreactive T-cell Repertoire by a Splice Variant of Self Protein Expressed in Thymic Epithelial Cells. *Nat Med* (2000) 6(1):56–61. doi: 10.1038/71540
49. Pugliese A, Zeller M, Fernandez A Jr., Zalcberg LJ, Bartlett RJ, Ricordi C, et al. The Insulin Gene is Transcribed in the Human Thymus and Transcription Levels Correlated With Allelic Variation At the INS Vntr-IDDM2 Susceptibility Locus for Type 1 Diabetes. *Nat Genet* (1997) 15(3):293–7. doi: 10.1038/ng0397-293
50. Nussenblatt RB, Mittal KK, Ryan S, Green WR, Maumenee AE. Birdshot Retinochoroidopathy Associated With HLA-A29 Antigen and Immune Responsiveness to Retinal s-Antigen. *Am J Ophthalmol* (1982) 94(2):147–58. doi: 10.1016/0002-9394(82)90069-1
51. Gocho K, Kondo I, Yamaki K. Identification of Autoreactive T Cells in Vogt-Koyanagi-Harada Disease. *Invest Ophthalmol Vis Sci* (2001) 42(9):2004–9.
52. Yang P, Wan W, Du L, Zhou Q, Qi J, Liang L, et al. Clinical Features of HLA-B27-positive Acute Anterior Uveitis With or Without Ankylosing Spondylitis in a Chinese Cohort. *Br J Ophthalmol* (2018) 102(2):215–9. doi: 10.1136/bjophthalmol-2016-309499
53. Caspi RR, Grubbs BG, Chan CC, Chader GJ, Wiggert B. Genetic Control of Susceptibility to Experimental Autoimmune Uveoretinitis in the Mouse Model. Concomitant Regulation by MHC and non-MHC Genes. *J Immunol* (1992) 148(8):2384–9.
54. Vignali DA, Kuchroo VK. Il-12 Family Cytokines: Immunological Playmakers. *Nat Immunol* (2012) 13(8):722–8. doi: 10.1038/ni.2366
55. Wang X, Wei Y, Xiao H, Liu X, Zhang Y, Han G, et al. A Novel IL-23p19/Ebi3 (Il-39) Cytokine Mediates Inflammation in Lupus-like Mice. *Eur J Immunol* (2016) 46(6):1343–50. doi: 10.1002/eji.201546095
56. Tarrant TK, Silver PB, Chan CC, Wiggert B, Caspi RR. Endogenous IL-12 is Required for Induction and Expression of Experimental Autoimmune Uveitis. *J Immunol (Baltimore Md.* (1998) 161(1):122–7.
57. Tarrant TK, Silver PB, Wahlsten JL, Rizzo LV, Chan CC, Wiggert B, et al. Interleukin 12 Protects From a T Helper Type 1-Mediated Autoimmune Disease, Experimental Autoimmune Uveitis, Through a Mechanism Involving Interferon Gamma, Nitric Oxide, and Apoptosis. *J Exp Med* (1999) 189 (2):219–30. doi: 10.1084/jem.189.2.219
58. Luger D, Caspi RR. New Perspectives on Effector Mechanisms in Uveitis. *Semin Immunopathol* (2008) 30:135–43. doi: 10.1007/s00281-008-0108-5
59. Amadi-Obi A, Yu CR, Liu X, Mahdi RM, Clarke GL, Nussenblatt RB, et al. T (H)17 Cells Contribute to Uveitis and Scleritis and are Expanded by IL-2 and Inhibited by IL-27/STAT1. *Nat Med* (2007) 13(6):711–8. doi: 10.1038/nm1585
60. Takeuchi M. A Systematic Review of Biologics for the Treatment of Noninfectious Uveitis. *Immunotherapy* (2013) 5(1):91–102. doi: 10.2217/imt.12.134
61. Podojil JR, Miller SD. Targeting the B7 Family of Co-Stimulatory Molecules: Successes and Challenges. *BioDrugs* (2013) 27(1):1–13. doi: 10.1007/s40259-012-0001-6
62. Lechner MG, Russell SM, Bass RS, Epstein AL. Chemokines, Costimulatory Molecules and Fusion Proteins for the Immunotherapy of Solid Tumors. *Immunotherapy* (2011) 3(11):1317–40. doi: 10.2217/imt.11.115
63. Ford ML, Adams AB, Pearson TC. Targeting Co-Stimulatory Pathways: Transplantation and Autoimmunity. *Nat Rev Nephrol* (2014) 10(1):14–24. doi: 10.1038/nrneph.2013.183
64. Darnell JE Jr. Stats and Gene Regulation. *Science* (1997) 277(5332):1630–5. doi: 10.1126/science.277.5332.1630
65. Egwuagu CE, Larkin Iii J. Therapeutic Targeting of STAT Pathways in CNS Autoimmune Diseases. *Jakstat* (2013) 2(1):e24134. doi: 10.4161/jkst.24134
66. Levy DE , Darnell JE Jr. Stats: Transcriptional Control and Biological Impact. *Nat Rev Mol Cell Biol* (2002) 3(9):651–62. doi: 10.1038/nrm909
67. Leonard WJ, Lin JX, O'Shea JJ. The Gammac Family of Cytokines: Basic Biology to Therapeutic Ramifications. *Immunity* (2019) 50(4):832–50. doi: 10.1016/j.immuni.2019.03.028
68. Kontzias A, Kotlyar A, Laurence A, Changelian P, O'Shea JJ. Jakinibs: A New Class of Kinase Inhibitors in Cancer and Autoimmune Disease. *Curr Opin Pharmacol* (2012) 12(4):464–70. doi: 10.1016/j.coph.2012.06.008
69. Laurence A, Pesu M, Silvennoinen O, O'Shea J. Jak Kinases in Health and Disease: An Update. *Open Rheumatol J* (2012) 6:232–44. doi: 10.2174/1874312901206010232
70. O'Shea JJ, Kontzias A, Yamaoka K, Tanaka Y, Laurence A. Janus Kinase Inhibitors in Autoimmune Diseases. *Ann Rheum Dis* (2013) 72 Suppl 2:ii111–115. doi: 10.1136/annrheumdis-2012-202576
71. O'Shea JJ, Schwartz DM, Villarino AV, Gadina M, McInnes IB, Laurence A. The JAK-STAT Pathway: Impact on Human Disease and Therapeutic Intervention. *Annu Rev Med* (2015) 66:311–28. doi: 10.1146/annurev-med-051113-024537
72. Bauermann P, Heiligenhaus A, Heinz C. Effect of Janus Kinase Inhibitor Treatment on Anterior Uveitis and Associated Macular Edema in an Adult

Patient With Juvenile Idiopathic Arthritis. *Ocul Immunol Inflammation* (2019) 27(8):1232–4. doi: 10.1080/09273948.2019.1605453

73. Egwuagu CE. STAT3 in CD4+ T Helper Cell Differentiation and Inflammatory Diseases. *Cytokine* (2009) 47(3):149–56. doi: 10.1016/j.cyto.2009.07.003
74. Liu X, Nurieva RI, Dong C. Transcriptional Regulation of Follicular T-helper (Tfh) Cells. *Immunol Rev* (2013) 252(1):139–45. doi: 10.1111/imr.12040
75. Escobar T, Yu CR, Muljo SA, Egwuagu CE. STAT3 Activates miR-155 in Th17 Cells and Acts in Concert to Promote Experimental Autoimmune Uveitis. *Invest Ophthalmol Vis Sci* (2013) 54(6):4017–25. doi: 10.1167/iovs.13-11937
76. Kutty RK, Nagineni CN, Samuel W, Vijayasarathy C, Hooks JJ, Redmond TM. Inflammatory Cytokines Regulate microRNA-155 Expression in Human Retinal Pigment Epithelial Cells by Activating JAK/STAT Pathway. *Biochem Biophys Res Commun* (2010) 402(2):390–5. doi: 10.1016/j.bbrc.2010.10.042
77. Yu CR, Lee YS, Mahdi RM, Surendran N, Egwuagu CE. Therapeutic Targeting of STAT3 (Signal Transducers and Activators of Transcription 3) Pathway Inhibits Experimental Autoimmune Uveitis. *PloS One* (2012) 7(1):e29742. doi: 10.1371/journal.pone.0029742
78. Hilton DJ. Negative Regulators of Cytokine Signal Transduction. *Cell Mol Life Sci* (1999) 55(12):1568–77. doi: 10.1007/s000180050396
79. Alexander WS. Suppressors of Cytokine Signalling (SOCS) in the Immune System. *Nat Rev Immunol* (2002) 2(6):410–6. doi: 10.1038/nri818
80. Alexander WS, Hilton DJ. The Role of Suppressors of Cytokine Signaling (SOCS) Proteins in Regulation of the Immune Response. *Annu Rev Immunol* (2004) 22:503–29. doi: 10.1146/annurev.immunol.22.091003.090312
81. Yu CR, Mahdi RR, Oh HM, Amadi-Obi A, Levy-Clarke G, Burton J, et al. Suppressor of Cytokine Signaling-1 (SOCS1) Inhibits Lymphocyte Recruitment Into the Retina and Protects SOCS1 Transgenic Rats and Mice From Ocular Inflammation. *Invest Ophthalmol Vis Sci* (2011) 52(9):6978–86. doi: 10.1167/iovs.11-7688
82. Starr R, Willson TA, Viney EM, Murray LJ, Rayner JR, Jenkins BJ, et al. A Family of Cytokine-Inducible Inhibitors of Signalling. *Nature* (1997) 387 (6636):917–21. doi: 10.1038/43206
83. Flowers LO, Johnson HM, Mujtaba MG, Ellis MR, Haider SM, Subramaniam PS. Characterization of a Peptide Inhibitor of Janus Kinase 2 That Mimics Suppressor of Cytokine Signaling 1 Function. *J Immunol* (2004) 172 (12):7510–8. doi: 10.4049/jimmunol.172.12.7510
84. Waiboci LW, Ahmed CM, Mujtaba MG, Flowers LO, Martin JP, Haider MI, et al. Both the Suppressor of Cytokine Signaling 1 (SOCS-1) Kinase Inhibitory Region and SOCS-1 Mimetic Bind to JAK2 Autophosphorylation Site: Implications for the Development of a SOCS-1 Antagonist. *J Immunol* (2007) 178(8):5058–68. doi: 10.4049/jimmunol.178.8.5058
85. He C, Yu CR, Sun L, Mahdi RM, Larkin J,3, Egwuagu CE. Topical Administration of a Suppressor of Cytokine Signaling-1 (SOCS1) Mimetic Peptide Inhibits Ocular Inflammation and Mitigates Ocular Pathology During Mouse Uveitis. *J Autoimmun* (2015). doi: 10.1016/j.jaut.2015.05.011
86. Luger D, Silver PB, Tang J, Cua D, Chen Z, Iwakura Y, et al. Either a Th17 or a Th1 Effector Response can Drive Autoimmunity: Conditions of Disease Induction Affect Dominant Effector Category. *J Exp Med* (2008) 205:799–810. doi: 10.1084/jem.20071258
87. Amadi-Obi A, Yu CR, Dambuza I, Kim SH, Marrero B, Egwuagu CE. Interleukin 27 Induces the Expression of Complement Factor H (CFH) in the Retina. *PloS One* (2012) 7(9):e45801. doi: 10.1371/journal.pone.0045801
88. Lee YS, Amadi-Obi A, Yu CR, Egwuagu CE. Retinal Cells Suppress Intraocular Inflammation (Uveitis) Through Production of interleukin-27 and Interleukin-10. *Immunology* (2011) 132(4):492–502. doi: 10.1111/j.1365-2567.2010.03379.x
89. Collison LW, Chaturvedi V, Henderson AL, Giacomin PR, Guy C, Bankoti J, et al. Il-35-mediated Induction of a Potent Regulatory T Cell Population. *Nat Immunol* (2010) 11(12):1093–101. doi: 10.1038/ni.1952
90. Wang RX, Yu CR, Dambuza IM, Mahdi RM, Dolinska MB, Sergeev YV, et al. Interleukin-35 Induces Regulatory B Cells That Suppress Autoimmune Disease. *Nat Med* (2014) 20(6):633–41. doi: 10.1038/nm.3554
91. Choi JK, Dambuza IM, He C, Yu CR, Uche AN, Mattapallil MJ, et al. IL-12p35 Inhibits Neuroinflammation and Ameliorates Autoimmune Encephalomyelitis. *Front Immunol* (2017) 8:1258. doi: 10.3389/fimmu.2017.01258
92. Dambuza IM, He C, Choi JK, Yu CR, Wang R, Mattapallil MJ, et al. Il-12p35 Induces Expansion of IL-10 and IL-35-expressing Regulatory B Cells and Ameliorates Autoimmune Disease. *Nat Commun* (2017) 8(1):719. doi: 10.1038/s41467-017-00838-4
93. Kang M, Choi JK, Jittayasothorn Y, Egwuagu CE. Interleukin 35-Producing Exosomes Suppress Neuroinflammation and Autoimmune Uveitis. *Front Immunol* (2020) 11:1051. doi: 10.3389/fimmu.2020.01051

3

Altered Metabolic Phenotype of Immune Cells in a Spontaneous Autoimmune Uveitis Model

*Claudia Barfüßer, Carmen Wiedemann, Anne L. C. Hoffmann, Sieglinde Hirmer and Cornelia A. Deeg**

Chair of Physiology, Department of Veterinary Sciences, Ludwig-Maximilians-Universität (LMU) Munich, Martinsried, Germany

***Correspondence:**
Cornelia A. Deeg
Cornelia.Deeg@lmu.de

As one of the leading causes of blindness worldwide, uveitis is an important disease. The exact pathogenesis of autoimmune uveitis is not entirely elucidated to date. Equine recurrent uveitis (ERU) represents the only spontaneous animal model for autoimmune uveitis in humans. As the metabolism of immune cells is an emerging field in research and gains more and more significance to take part in the pathogenesis of various diseases, we conducted experiments to investigate the metabolism of immune cells of ERU cases and healthy controls. To our knowledge, the link between a deviant immunometabolism and the pathogenesis of autoimmune uveitis was not investigated so far. We showed that PBMC of ERU cases had a more active metabolic phenotype in basal state by upregulating both the oxidative phosphorylation and the glycolytic pathway. We further revealed an increased compensatory glycolytic rate of PBMC and CD4$^+$ T cells of ERU cases under mitochondrial stress conditions. These findings are in line with metabolic alterations of immune cells in other autoimmune diseases and basic research, where it was shown that activated immune cells have an increased need of energy and molecule demand for their effector function. We demonstrated a clear difference in the metabolic phenotypes of PBMC and, more specifically, CD4$^+$ T cells of ERU cases and controls. These findings are another important step in understanding the pathogenesis of ERU and figuratively, human autoimmune uveitis.

Keywords: immunometabolism, PBMC, CD4$^+$ T cell, OXPHOS, glycolysis, mitochondria, autoimmunity, equine recurrent uveitis (ERU)

INTRODUCTION

Equine recurrent uveitis (ERU) is an important disease in horses worldwide (1, 2), which, being untreated, eventually leads to loss of vision in the affected eyes (3). It is characterized by recurrent and painful episodes of inflammation, which are mainly caused by autoaggressive CD4$^+$ T cells that migrate from the peripheral blood through the blood retinal barrier into the eye to attack and destroy retinal structures (1). Few monocytes can be observed among these infiltrating CD4$^+$ T cells, but the driving force during an uveitic attack are the CD4$^+$ T cells (4, 5). Like in other autoimmune diseases, the pathogenesis of ERU is still not fully elucidated (1, 6). ERU represents the only spontaneous animal model for human autoimmune uveitis (HAU), a sight-threatening disease with a similar pathogenesis as ERU (1, 7–9). Thus, new findings concerning the underlying pathogenesis of ERU are of great value for both, veterinary and human medicine. For example, our group identified CRALBP as autoantigen in horses with ERU (10). Later on, CRALBP was also verified as important autoantigen in human autoimmune uveitis (11), autoimmune retinopathy (12) and juvenile idiopathic arthritis-associated uveitis (JIAU) (13). Patients with autoimmune uveitis receive long-term treatment with immune suppressants like high-dosed corticosteroids, cyclophosphamides or azathioprine or they are treated with antibodies against TNFα or IL-17 [reviewed in (14)]. Unlike these human patients, horses affected by ERU are only treated for a few days when they experience an acute inflammatory episode and not in the quiescent stage of the disease (5, 15, 16), therefore it is possible to examine immune reactions in the quiescent stage unaffected by long-term treatment.

The area of immune cell metabolism has gained more and more interest in the last decades. Immune cells produce ATP and other metabolites through metabolic pathways, which are closely connected with each other. The two major pathways for an immune cell to obtain ATP are oxygen-consuming oxidative phosphorylation (OXPHOS) and glycolysis, in which ATP is generated *via* oxygen independent substrate-level phosphorylation reactions [reviewed in (17, 18)]. Changes in metabolism are interdependent with oxidation-reduction (redox) reactions, for example electrons derived in glycolysis and the tricarboxylic acid (TCA) cycle are necessary to generate reducing equivalents contained in NADH. The NAD^+/FAD coenzymes can be seen as the main oxidizing agents in cellular catabolism (19, 20). They are needed to transfer electrons from glucose (glycolysis), fatty acids (β-oxidation) and activated acetic acid (TCA cycle) to the mitochondrial respiratory chain for ATP generation [reviewed in (21)]. Most cells can quickly adapt to environmental changes and varying energy sources by switching between the dominantly used energy-delivering pathways (22). The interrelation between immune cell metabolism and the cell's activation status was revealed through research in the last two decades (23). Naïve $CD4^+$ T cells primarily rely on OXPHOS to generate ATP, for which the TCA cycle delivers electrons stored in NADH and $FADH_2$ (21, 24). Upon activation, $CD4^+$ T cells raise glycolysis not only for ATP production, but also to generate metabolic intermediates such as pyruvate, which are crucial for synthesizing amino acids and fatty acids to cover the demand for proliferation and effector function [reviewed in (21)]. Furthermore, different metabolic pathways dominate in $CD4^+$ T cell subsets. For example, memory T cells rely primarily on catabolic pathways such as OXPHOS (including fatty acid oxidation as electron source) to cover their metabolic needs, while effector T cells (Th1, Th2 and Th17) exhibit a glycolysis-dominated metabolism (25, 26).

A first approach to identifying changes in metabolism of healthy and degenerated cells was taken over 60 years ago, as tumor cells were shown to shift from oxidative phosphorylation to the glycolytic pathway, more precisely to aerobic glycolysis (27–29). This showed that healthy and cancer cells, which have the same origin, can be distinguished upon their different metabolism. The microenvironment also affects cell metabolism, as it was shown in human T cell subsets in healthy and cancerous tissue (30). The $CD4^+$ T cells in tumorous environment displayed decreased mitochondrial enzyme activity and reduced aerobic glycolysis compared to $CD4^+$ T cells in an healthy microenvironment (30). Thus, cells with the same protein profile can be differentiated by their distinct metabolism in a healthy or tumorous microenvironment (30). Interestingly, the meaning behind the term "aerobic glycolysis" differs upon context. In cancerous cells, aerobic glycolysis, also known as the Warburg effect, describes their ability to convert pyruvate to lactate in the presence of oxygen (30, 31). In healthy cells, this reaction re-oxidizes NADH for continuing glycolysis under anaerobic conditions (32). Concerning biochemistry and activated immune cells, the term "aerobic glycolysis" mainly describes the conversion of pyruvate to Acetyl-CoA, which fuels the tricarboxylic acid cycle, in the presence of oxygen (27). To sum it up, cells in health and disease exert a distinct metabolic phenotype despite expressing the same protein profile.

Furthermore, metabolic aberrations of immune cells in autoimmune diseases are implicated to contribute to their autoaggressive and inflammatory phenotype (17). For example, systemic lupus erythematosus (SLE) $CD4^+$ T cells of lupus-prone mice had enriched OXPHOS and glycolytic pathways and combined treatment with 2-DG and metformin *in vivo* could normalize metabolism of these $CD4^+$ T cells and reverse biomarkers of the disease (33). This underlines the importance of not only investigating metabolic features of healthy immune cells, but to uncover possible differences in metabolism of immune cells of diseased individuals. However, over the last years, studies on spontaneous autoimmune uveitis mostly concentrated on different protein expressions in healthy and autoimmune cells. For example, our group previously demonstrated a correlation of higher integrin-linked kinase expression and a lower apoptosis rate of ERU lymphocytes, whereas necrosis rates were not significantly different, compared to cells of eye-healthy horses (6). To our knowledge, studies to distinguish autoaggressive immune cells from normal immune cells upon their metabolic phenotype were not yet performed in context of spontaneous autoimmune uveitis in humans or horses, although immunometabolism is considered to play a tremendous role in autoimmune diseases (29). Thus, the goal of the study was to characterize the metabolic features of equine PBMC and $CD4^+$ T cells in health and ERU to detect possible alterations in the uveitic phenotype. This could contribute to identify and possibly even target the autoaggressive cells therapeutically in the peripheral blood before they migrate into the eye and attack retinal tissue.

MATERIALS AND METHODS

Isolation of Primary Peripheral Blood Mononuclear Cells and Ethics Approval for Animal Research

Peripheral blood mononuclear cells (PBMC) of 25 healthy and 29 ERU cases were used in this study. Horses were regarded as eye-healthy, when no previous ocular inflammation was reported by the owner and the standard clinical routine examination did not indicate pathophysiological changes in the eye. These eye-healthy horses are referred to as controls in the following parts of the manuscript. Horses with ERU were diagnosed by experienced clinicians of the Equine Hospital of LMU Munich based on typical clinical signs of uveitis along with a documented history of multiple episodes of inflammation in the affected eye (34). All ERU blood samples were obtained in the quiescent stage of the disease. Equine whole blood samples of controls and ERU cases were taken from the *vena jugularis* in tubes with heparin sodium (50 I.U. per ml blood; Ratiopharm, Ulm, Germany). After sedimentation of blood components, the leukocyte-rich plasma was isolated by density gradient centrifugation (room temperature, 350 x g, 25 min, low acceleration, low break) using Pancoll separation solution (PanBiotech, Aidenbach, Germany). PBMC were extracted from the intermediate phase, washed in phosphate buffered saline (PBS) three times (4°C, 500 x g, 10 min) and counted with trypan blue solution (VWR Life Science, Darmstadt, Germany). Cells were either used the same day or stored in RPMI 1640 medium (PanBiotech, Aidenbach, Germany), supplemented with 1% penicillin/streptomycin and 10% heat-inactivated fetal bovine serum (both Biochrom, part of Merck, Darmstadt, Germany) overnight at 4°C, until further processing. Some horses' cells were tested in multiple assays. No experimental animals were used in this study. Collection of blood was permitted by the local authority, Regierung von Oberbayern (Permit number: ROB-55.2Vet-2532.Vet_03-17-88).

Magnetic Activated Cell Sorting (MACS) of $CD4^+$ T Cells Using LS Columns

1 x 10^8 PBMC were washed (4°C, 500 x g, 10 min) and then resuspended in 10 ml MACS buffer (phosphate-buffered saline (pH 7.2), supplemented with 2 mM EDTA (AppliChem, Darmstadt, Germany) and 0.5% bovine serum albumin (Serva, Heidelberg, Germany)). After another washing step, cells were incubated at 4°C with 1 ml mouse anti horse CD4 antibody (clone MCA 1078, Biorad, Feldkirchen, Germany, 1:2000) per 1x10^7 cells. After 20 minutes, 5 ml MACS buffer were added for washing (4°C, 500 x g, 10 min). Cells were resuspended with 80 µl buffer per 10^7 cells before adding 20 µl anti-mouse IgG1 microbeads (Miltenyi Biotec, Bergisch Gladbach, Germany) per 10^7 cells. After incubation for 15 minutes at 4°C, another washing step (4°C, 300 x g, 10 min) was performed and cells were resuspended in 500 µl MACS buffer for cell sorting. Magnetic separation was performed using LS columns (Miltenyi Biotec, Bergisch Gladbach, Germany). Magnetically labelled $CD4^+$ T cells were retained in the magnetic field, while unlabeled $CD4^-$ cells were washed through the columns by three washing steps (3 x 3 ml MACS buffer). The $CD4^+$ T cell fraction was eluted by removing the column from the magnetic field and rinsing with 5 ml MACS buffer. Purity of $CD4^+$ fraction was tested *via* flow cytometry, by staining with 30 µl mouse anti horse CD4 FITC labelled antibody (clone MCA1078F, Biorad, Feldkirchen, Germany, 1:10) and 30 µl mouse anti horse CD8 FITC labelled antibody (clone MCA1080F, Biorad, Feldkirchen, Germany, 1:10) (**Supplementary Figure 1**, ≥ 96% purity of the $CD4^+$ fraction).

Cell Proliferation Assay

PBMC, $CD4^+$ and $CD4^-$ cells of controls and ERU cases were stimulated with three different mitogens to assess their proliferative response. 1 x 10^5; cells in 200 µl RPMI 1640 medium (PanBiotech, Aidenbach, Germany) supplemented with 1% penicillin/streptomycin and 10% heat-inactivated fetal bovine serum (both Biochrom, part of Merck, Darmstadt, Germany) were seeded per well in 96-well plates. Triplicates (technical replicates) of the cells were either stimulated with pokeweed mitogen (PWM; 5 µg/mL), concanavalin A (ConA; 5 µg/mL) or phytohemagglutinin (PHA-L; 5 µg/mL) (all three Merck, Darmstadt, Germany). One triplicate of each cell type was left unstimulated as a medium control. After incubating for 32 hours (37°C, 5% CO_2), H^3-thymidine (Perkin Elmer, Germany) was added to each well (1 µCi/well) for radioactive labelling. After another 16 hours of incubation (37°C, 5% CO_2), the cells were harvested onto a glass fiber filter and the H^3-thymidine incorporation was quantified as radioactivity by liquid scintillation in a beta counter (MicroBeta, Perkin Elmer, Germany). Counts per minute were measured for each well and means of triplicates were calculated. To determine the proliferation rate, the mean value of the stimulated cells was divided by the mean value of the medium control, separately for each mitogen. No significant differences in the proliferation capacity of PBMC, $CD4^+$ T cells and $CD4^-$ cells of ERU cases compared to controls upon polyclonal stimulation were detected (**Supplementary Figures 2A–C**).

Measurement of Equine Cell Metabolism Through Seahorse XFe Analyzer

Metabolic features of equine PBMC, $CD4^+$ T cells and $CD4^-$ cells were measured by characterizing oxygen consumption rates (OCR), extracellular acidification rates (ECAR) and glycolytic rates (glycoPER) of respective cells using a Seahorse XFe Analyzer (Agilent Technologies, Waldbronn, Germany). Following the manufacturer's instructions, 24-well plates were coated with 52 µl Poly-D-Lysin (Merck, Darmstadt, Germany) one day prior to the assay. 8 x 10^5 cells were seeded per well, suspended in 200 µl XF medium (Seahorse XF RPMI Medium (pH 7.4), Agilent Technologies, Waldbronn, Germany), which was supplemented with 100 mM Pyruvate, 2.5 mM Glucose and 200 mM L-Glutamine (all three Merck, Darmstadt, Germany) prior. Experiments were performed with at least two technical replicates per horse. Four wells on each 24-well plate were filled with medium and served as background correction. To ensure an evenly distributed cell layer on the bottom of each well, the plate was centrifuged for 1 minute at 2000 rpm with low acceleration and low break. All wells of the 24-well plate were filled up with XF medium to reach a total volume of 500 µl. The plate was put into a CO_2-free incubator for 20 minutes before starting the experiment. The calibration plate was also prepared as described in the user guides of the manufacturer for each assay. OCR and ECAR rates were determined using the mito stress test (Agilent Technologies, Waldbronn, Germany). GlycoPER rates were measured with glycolytic rate assay kits (Agilent Technologies, Waldbronn, Germany). Data analysis and interpretation was done using WAVE 2.6 software according to the manufacturer's manual (both Agilent Technologies, Waldbronn, Germany). Ratios were determined after normalizing each measurement against the baseline mean. To perform statistical analysis, data from three time-points per measurement were used.

Western Blot

$CD4^+$ T cells were lysed in lysis buffer (9 M Urea, 2 M Thiourea, 65 mM Dithioerythritol, 4% CHAPS) and protein concentration was determined *via* Bradford assay. A 12% gel was loaded with 5 µg protein/slot. Three slots were functioning as blanks. Serva Triple Color Protein Standard III (Serva Electrophoresis, Heidelberg, Germany) was used as marker. Proteins were separated by SDS-PAGE and blotted semidry onto 8.5 × 6 cm PVDF membranes (GE Healthcare, Freiburg, Germany). To prevent unspecific binding, the membrane was blocked with 4% BSA for one hour at room temperature. After three washing steps with phosphate buffered saline supplemented with 0.05% Tween (PBS-T) at room temperature for 10 minutes, it was incubated with the primary antibodies mouse anti ATP5β (Santa Cruz, Heidelberg, Germany, 1:100) and anti GAPDH (Merck, Darmstadt, 1:500) overnight at 4°C. This was followed by another three washing steps in PBS-T and subsequent incubation with POD-conjugated goat anti mouse IgG (Merck, Darmstadt, Germany, 1:5000) as secondary antibody for one hour at room temperature. After 1 hour, 6 washing steps with PBS-T were performed before re-incubation with primary antibody rabbit anti β-actin (Cell Signaling, Frankfurt am Main, Germany, 1:40000) for 3 hours at room temperature. After washing the membrane 3 x 10 minutes with PBS-T, it was incubated with POD-conjugated goat anti rabbit IgG (Life Technologies, Darmstadt, Germany, 1:10000) for one hour at room temperature. Afterwards, the membrane was washed 6 x 10 minutes with PBS-T before detection of the signals by enhanced chemiluminescence (Amersham Imager680, Analysis2.0, GE Healthcare, Freiburg, Germany). The signal intensity of ATP5β was normalized to β-actin for each horse before statistical evaluation of the differences in signal intensity between controls and ERU cases.

Detection of Mitochondria *via* Immunocytochemical Staining

2×10^5 $CD4^+$ T cells of ERU cases and controls were stained with 100 µl prewarmed (37°C) MitoTracker Deep Red (ThermoFisher Scientific, Ulm, Germany, 200 nM) at 37°C and 5% CO_2 for 30 minutes. 100 µl prewarmed (37°C) PBS were added and cells were washed (room temperature, 810 x g, 1 min), resuspended with 200 µl prewarmed PBS and washed again (room temperature, 810 x g, 1 min) before fixation in prewarmed PBS supplemented with 1% paraform aldehyde (PFA; Merck, Darmstadt, Germany) for 20 min at 37°C, 5% CO_2. Cell nuclei were stained with 4', 6-Diamidin-2-phenylindol (DAPI; Invitrogen, Karlsruhe, Germany, 1:100). 1×10^5 cells were transferred to microscope slides and centrifuged (300 x g, 10 min) before coverslips were applied using fluoromount medium (Serva, Heidelberg, Germany). Visualization was performed using a Leica Dmi8 microscope with associated LAS-X-software, version 3.4.2 (both Leica, Wetzlar, Germany).

Statistical Analysis

Kolmogorov-Smirnov (KS) test was used for determination of Gaussian distribution. If KS test was significant ($p < 0.05$; no normal distribution), Mann-Whitney test was used for statistical analysis. If KS test was not significant ($p > 0.05$; normal distribution), statistics were performed using student's t-test. In both tests, statistical probabilities were considered not significant (ns) at $p > 0.05$ and significant at $p \leq 0.05$. Significances are indicated by asterisks with * $p \leq 0.05$, ** $p \leq 0.01$ and *** $p \leq 0.001$. OriginPro2020 software, version 9.7 (Additive, Friedrichsdorf, Germany) was used for statistical analysis and graph creation.

RESULTS

PBMC and $CD4^+$ T Cells Display Increased Basal Oxygen Consumption Rate (OCR) in ERU

We analyzed metabolic features of PBMC, $CD4^+$ T cells and $CD4^-$ cells of ERU cases and controls with a Seahorse XFe analyzer, which detects concentrations of oxygen and protons within the cell-surrounding medium. Therefore, higher oxygen consumption rates positively correlate to higher mitochondrial activity and respective oxidative phosphorylation (OXPHOS). By blocking mitochondrial respiration with rotenone/antimycin A (Rot/AA), the remaining OCR resembles the non-mitochondrial oxygen consumption, which is likely caused by the activity of oxidoreductases and other enzymes and which remains as background in all other measurements addressed in the following. Oligomycin and FCCP were used to access and influence only parts of the oxidative chain: Oligomycin inhibits the ATP synthase (complex V) of the respiratory chain reaction, which means that the decrease in OCR following oligomycin injection resembles the oxygen level used by ATP-linked respiration. Carbonyl cyanide-4 (trifluoromethoxy) phenylhydrazone (FCCP) is used as an uncoupling substance for mitochondrial respiration, thus the level of OCR after injection of FCCP shows the maximum respiration capacity of the cells.

PBMC and $CD4^-$ cells of ERU cases consumed significantly more oxygen (** $p \leq 0.01$) in basal state through their mitochondria, represented through a higher OCR level compared to controls. Likewise, $CD4^+$ T cells of ERU cases showed significantly increased basal oxidative phosphorylation (*** $p \leq 0.001$) compared to control $CD4^+$ T cells (**Figure 1A**). Furthermore, all three tested subsets of immune cells showed differing OCRs between ERU cases and controls after injection of the reagents oligomycin, FCCP and Rot/AA (data not shown). To ensure that these differing reactions to the injected reagents were independent of the different basal oxygen consumption rates between controls and ERU cases, we then normalized all measurements against the baseline mean and compared

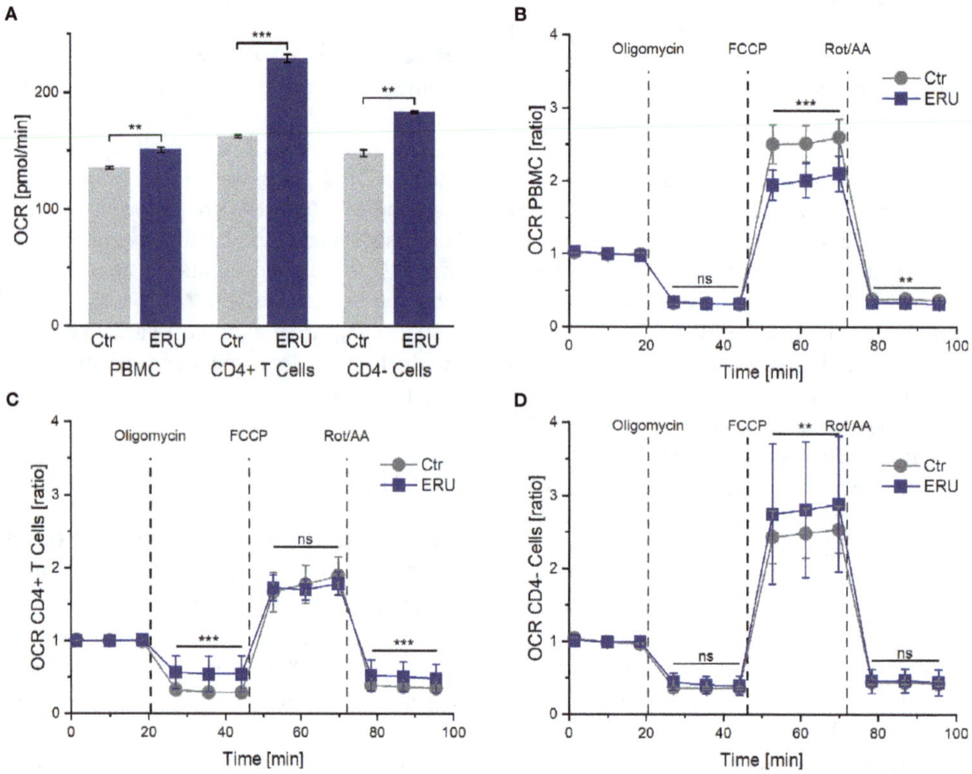

FIGURE 1 | Oxygen consumption rates (OCR) and OCR ratios by mitochondrial metabolism of PBMC, $CD4^+$ T cells and $CD4^-$ cells of healthy and ERU cases. Controls (n=16) are presented as grey lines whereas ERU cases (n=9) are illustrated as blue lines. OCR is shown by graph **(A)** and OCR ratios are illustrated by graphs **(B–D)**. First three measurements (dots) show basal respiration, followed by injections of oligomycin (after the third measurement point), FCCP (after the sixth measurement point) and Rot/AA (after the ninth measurement point). Data are shown as mean ± SEM. **(A)** Significantly higher basal oxygen consumption rates of equine PBMC (**$p \leq 0.01$), $CD4^+$ T cells (***$p \leq 0.001$) and $CD4^-$ cells (**$p \leq 0.01$) of ERU cases compared to controls. **(B)** After normalization against the baseline mean, PBMC of ERU cases showed significantly lower OCR ratio after FCCP (***$p \leq 0.001$) and Rot/AA (**$p \leq 0.01$) injection compared to controls. **(C)** $CD4^+$ T cells of ERU cases showed significantly higher OCR ratio (***$p \leq 0.001$) when injected with oligomycin and Rot/AA. **(D)** $CD4^-$ cells of horses with ERU had significantly increased OCR ratio (**$p \leq 0.01$) after FCCP injection. No significant difference is represented by ns (ns $p > 0.05$).

respective OCR ratios as reaction to the injected substances between the two tested groups.

Maximum Respiration Capacity and Non-Mitochondrial Oxygen Consumption Is Lower in PBMC of ERU Cases

After adding oligomycin, no significant difference in the ATP-linked respiration was measured between PBMC of healthy and diseased groups (ns $p > 0.05$). However, PBMC of ERU cases had significantly decreased maximum respiration capacity (*** $p \leq 0.001$) after uncoupling the mitochondria with FCCP. Non-mitochondrial oxygen consumption was also lower in PBMC of ERU cases (** $p \leq 0.01$) compared to controls (**Figure 1B**).

$CD4^+$ T Cells of ERU Horses Display Decreased ATP-Linked Respiration but Similar Maximum Respiration Capacity Compared to Controls

OCR ratios of $CD4^+$ T cells of ERU cases were significantly higher (*** $p \leq 0.001$) compared to controls after oligomycin and Rot/AA injection. These results point to a significantly decreased ATP-linked respiration and to an increased non-mitochondrial oxygen consumption in ERU $CD4^+$ T cells. $CD4^+$ T cells of controls and ERU cases had similar maximum respiration capacities (ns $p > 0.05$) after uncoupling the mitochondria with FCCP (**Figure 1C**). In contrast, the maximum respiration capacity of $CD4^-$ cells of ERU cases was significantly increased (** $p \leq 0.01$) compared to controls (**Figure 1D**).

The Extracellular Acidification Rate (ECAR) Is Basal Higher in PBMC and $CD4^-$ Cells of ERU Cases

Simultaneously to the measurement of the oxygen consumption rate in the mito stress test assay, the seahorse analyzer measures the pH change of the cell culture medium and provides this information as extracellular acidification rate (ECAR). ECAR mainly resembles the glycolytic activity of the cells, in the course of which lactate is produced and excreted. However, the extracellular acidification rate may also be influenced to a smaller amount by respiration linked acidification. This means that CO_2, produced in the cause of respiration, is forming a week acid (H_2CO_3) in the cell-surrounding medium, which then dissociates into a proton and hydrogen carbonate. PBMC of ERU cases had a significantly higher basal ECAR rates (*** $p \leq 0.001$) than control PBMC. This only applied to the CD4⁻ cells of ERU cases, whereas $CD4^+$ T cells of controls and ERU cases had no significant difference (ns $p > 0.05$) in the basal extracellular acidification rate (**Figure 2A**). To further analyze the effects of oligomycin, FCCP and Rot/AA unaffected by differing baseline values of ERU cases and controls, all following measurements were then normalized to the baseline mean value.

ECAR of Tested Cell Subsets of ERU Cases Decreases After Blocking and Uncoupling the Respiratory Chain

PBMC, $CD4^+$ T cells and $CD4^-$ cells of horses with ERU had lower extracellular acidification rates than controls after inhibiting the ATP synthase with oligomycin (PBMC * $p \leq 0.05$; **Figure 2B**. $CD4^+$ T cells ** $p \leq 0.01$; **Figure 2C**. $CD4^-$ cells *** $p \leq 0.001$; **Figure 2D**). Furthermore, all tested cell subsets of ERU cases showed lower extracellular acidification than controls after uncoupling the oxidative chain reaction with FCCP (*** $p \leq 0.001$) and after blocking the mitochondrial respiratory chain through Rot/AA (*** $p \leq 0.001$; **Figures 2B–D**).

The Basal Glycolytic Proton Efflux Rate (glycoPER) Is Increased in PBMC of ERU Cases, but Decreased in $CD4^+$ T Cells of ERU Cases

Since ECAR measurement in the mito stress test represents the proton production of glycolysis indirectly, we next analyzed PBMC and CD4 sorted cells of controls and ERU cases with the glycolytic rate assay. Our goal was to determine whether resting equine immune cells also generate energy through the glycolytic pathway and whether the rate of glycolysis varied with autoimmunity. PBMC of ERU cases had significantly increased basal glycolysis (*** $p \leq 0.001$) compared to controls, whereas $CD4^+$ T cells of ERU cases had significantly lower basal glycolysis (* $p \leq 0.05$). Furthermore, our data show that $CD4^-$ cells of ERU cases caused significantly higher basal glycolytic rates (*** $p \leq$

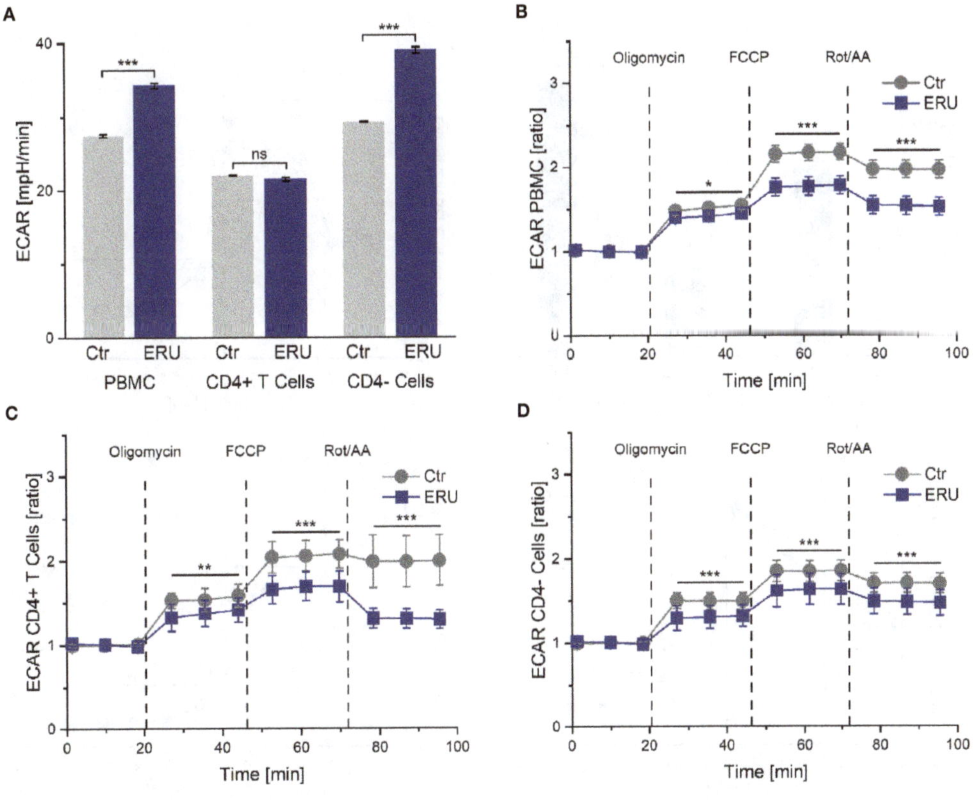

FIGURE 2 | Extracellular acidification rate (ECAR) of PBMC, $CD4^+$ T cells and $CD4^-$ cells of healthy and ERU cases. Graphs display the extracellular acidification rate (ECAR) of cells of healthy (grey, n=14) and ERU diseased cases (blue, n=8). Graph **(A)** shows extracellular acidification rates, graphs **(B–D)** show ECAR ratios of healthy and ERU cases. First three measurements (dots) show basal respiration, followed by injections of oligomycin (after the third measurement point), FCCP (after the sixth measurement point) and Rot/AA (after the ninth measurement point). Data are shown as mean ± SEM. **(A)** PBMC and more specifically $CD4^-$ cells of ERU cases showed significantly increased basal extracellular acidification (***$p \leq 0.001$) compared to controls, whereas no significant difference (ns $p > 0.05$) between the basal extracellular acidification rate of $CD4^+$ T cells of healthy and diseased horses was detectable. **(B)** ECAR ratio of PBMC of ERU cases decreased significantly after injection of the reagents of the mito stress test. **(C)** $CD4^+$ T cells had a significantly lower ECAR ratio than controls after injection of oligomycin, FCCP and Rot/AA. **(D)** ECAR ratio of $CD4^-$ cells was significantly lower in ERU cases than in controls after injection of the mito stress test reagents. Statistical significances are represented by asterisks (*$p \leq 0.05$; **$p \leq 0.01$; ***$p \leq 0.001$).

0.001) compared to controls (**Figure 3A**). As before, we normalized the measurements against the baseline mean to see whether the effects reached by injections of the two reagents of the glycolytic rate assay kit were independent of the significantly different basal glycolytic rates of ERU cases and controls.

The Compensatory Glycolysis of PBMC and CD4$^+$ T Cells Is Increased in ERU

Injection of Rot/AA inhibits the mitochondrial chain reaction and therefore mitochondrial respiration. Thus, a rise in glycoPER after Rot/AA injection resembles compensatory glycolysis. Blocking glycolysis through competitive binding of glucose hexokinase with the glucose analog 2-deoxy-D-glucose (2-DG) should lead to a decrease of glycoPER, which would confirm that the protons measured before were primarily generated through glycolysis.

Our experiments revealed a significant increase in compensatory glycolysis (* $p \leq 0.05$) of PBMC of ERU cases compared to controls (**Figure 3B**). CD4 cell sorting showed that isolated CD4$^+$ T cells of ERU cases caused the significantly increased levels of compensatory glycolysis (* $p \leq 0.05$; **Figure 3C**), whereas CD4$^-$ cells had a similar proton production as controls (ns $p > 0.05$; **Figure 3D**). Furthermore, there was no significant difference in glycoPER ratio (ns $p > 0.05$) after 2-DG injection of the tested cell subsets compared to the control group (**Figures 3B–D**). This means that the measured protons were similarly generated through glycolysis in control and ERU cases.

CD4$^+$ T Cells of ERU Cases Do Not Have Significant Difference in the Amount of Mitochondria

To elucidate if the higher basal oxygen consumption rate of CD4$^+$ T cells in ERU was due to more mitochondria per cell, we performed western blot analysis using the mitochondrial marker ATP5β (**Figure 4A**). CD4$^+$ T cells of ERU cases and controls revealed no significant differences in ATP5β abundances, thus the total amount of mitochondria (ns $p > 0.05$; **Figure 4B**). Immunocytochemical staining of CD4$^+$ T cells of a representative control and ERU case with the mitochondrial marker MitoTracker Deep Red illustrates this finding (**Figure 4C**).

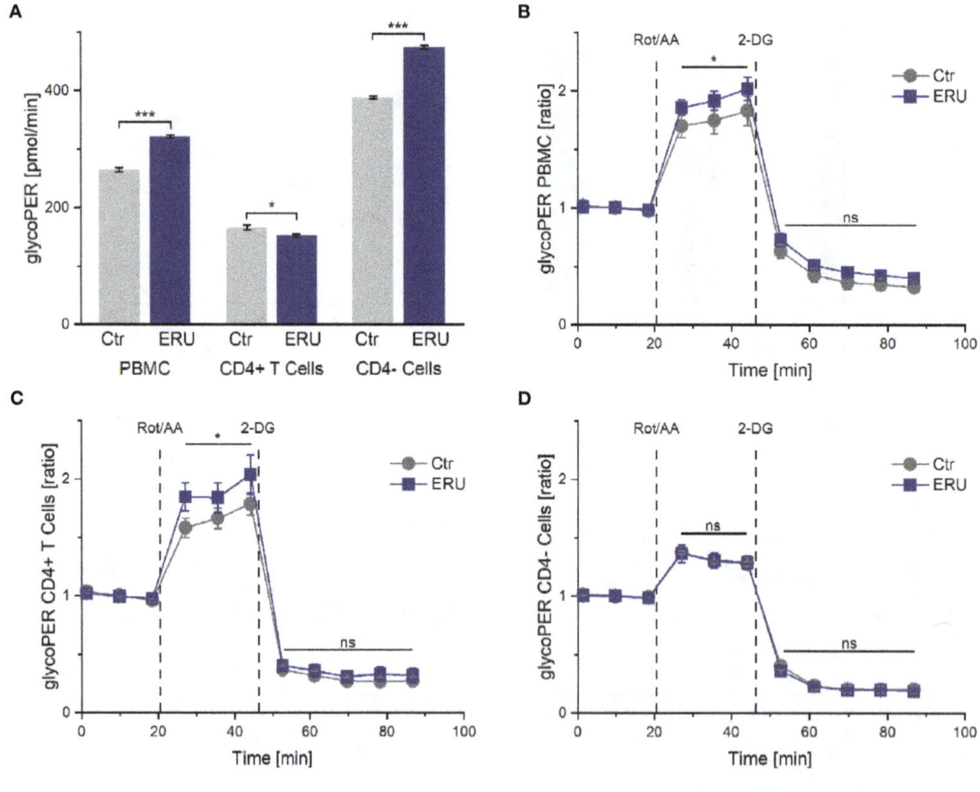

FIGURE 3 | Glycolytic proton efflux (glycoPER) of PBMC, CD4$^+$ T cells and CD4$^-$ cells of healthy and ERU cases. Graph **(A)** shows the glycolytic proton efflux rates of controls (grey, n=8) and ERU cases (blue, n=10), graphs **(B–D)** represent glycoPER ratios, normalized against the baseline mean. First three measurements (dots) show basal respiration, followed by injections of Rot/AA (after the third measurement point) and 2-DG (after the sixth measurement point). Data are shown as mean ± SEM. **(A)** Significantly increased basal glycolysis (***$p \leq 0.001$) of PBMC and more precisely CD4$^-$ cells of ERU cases, whereas CD4$^+$ T cells of horses with ERU showed significantly lower basal glycolysis (*$p \leq 0.05$). **(B)** Significantly higher glycoPER ratio (*$p \leq 0.05$) of ERU PBMC after Rot/AA injection. **(C)** Significantly increased glycoPER (*$p \leq 0.05$) of CD4$^+$ T cells of ERU cases after Rot/AA injection. **(D)** CD4$^-$ cells showed no difference in glycolysis ratios (ns $p > 0.05$) after treatment with Rot/AA and 2-DG compared to controls.

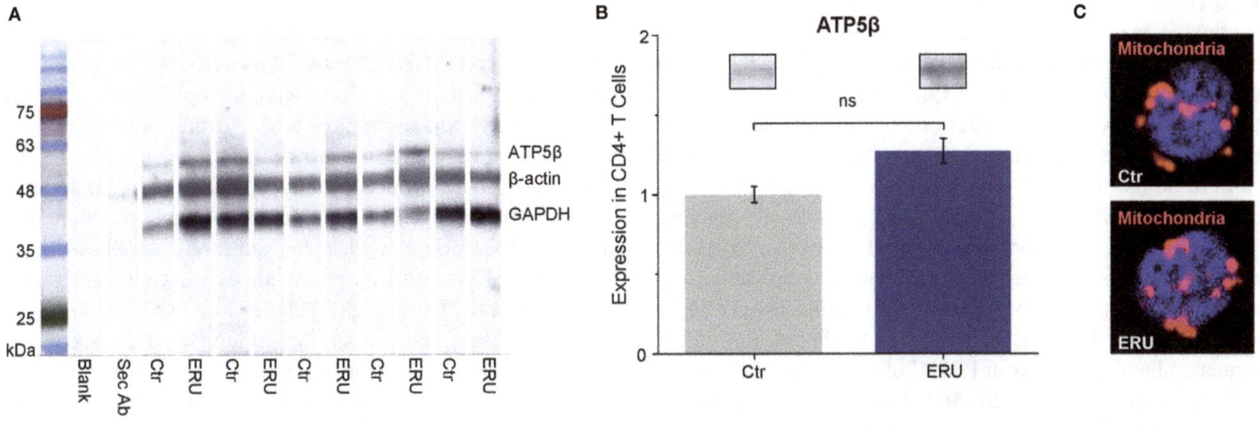

FIGURE 4 | ATP5β in CD4⁺ T cells of healthy and ERU cases. **(A)** Western blot with CD4⁺ T cells of control and ERU horses (n=5 each) stained with anti ATP5β antibody, anti GAPDH antibody and anti β-actin antibody for normalization. A molecular weight marker is shown on the left, followed by a blank lane and a lane only incubated with the secondary antibody. **(B)** Statistical analysis of the volume of ATP5β lanes of control and ERU cases after normalization to the respective β-actin lane showed no significant difference (ns $p > 0.05$). Data are represented as mean ± SEM. The ERU bar (blue) was set accordingly to the control bar (grey), which was set as 1. **(C)** Representative immunocytochemically stained CD4⁺ T cell of a control (upper picture) and an ERU case (lower picture). Mitochondria were stained with MitoTracker Deep Red (red). Cell nuclei were counterstained with DAPI (blue). x1000 magnification.

DISCUSSION

Research on immunometabolism is an emerging field and new insight can help to understand pathogenesis of diseases, including autoimmune diseases, and searching for adequate therapy (27, 29, 35). To our knowledge, the link between immunometabolism and the pathogenesis of spontaneous autoimmune uveitis was not investigated so far. In this study, we therefore aimed to elucidate the metabolic phenotype and to identify metabolic alterations of leukocytes of ERU cases, which could lead to a better understanding of the autoimmune nature of the cells, the pathogenesis of uveitis and provide a basis to identify the autoreactive cells in the periphery before they can harm the eye. We showed that the metabolic phenotype of immune cells of ERU cases significantly differed in 9 of 11 tested parameters in PBMC and in 8 of 11 tested parameters in $CD4^+$ T cells compared to controls, although the amount of mitochondria was unaffected by the disease. Peripheral lymphocytes are the most promising cell type to investigate ERU pathogenesis since every uveitic episode starts in the periphery, where autoaggressive T cells are activated in the spleen to migrate into the eye and destroy retinal tissue (1, 36). Caspi and colleagues further demonstrated in adoptive transfer experiments with Lewis rats that peripheral T cells specific to retinal proteins induce EAU in healthy recipient rats upon peripheral injection (37).

Since PBMC of horses with induced autoimmune uveitis had different protein expressions even in the quiescent stage of the disease compared to lymphocytes of eye-healthy horses (38), we were interested whether lymphocytes of uveitic horses also had a deviant metabolism than controls. Indeed, PBMC of ERU cases displayed a different energetic phenotype than PBMC of eye-healthy horses, namely higher basal OCR, ECAR and glycoPER rates (**Figures 1A, 2A, 3A**). Thus, one could conclude that the mitochondrial respiration and glycolysis pathways were both more active in PBMC of horses with ERU than in control cells. To our knowledge, this is a novel finding in the context of spontaneous uveitis, thus we do not know the functional meaning of increased basal mitochondrial respiration and glycolytic rates in uveitic pathogenesis so far. Increased basal mitochondrial respiration and glycolysis were also described in PBMC of a transgenic pig model for diabetes compared to the wild-type littermates (39). Interestingly, these findings correlate with the findings in our study concerning PBMC in recurrent autoimmune uveitis. Since the authors indicated a link between the metabolic alterations at the early stage of the disease and the inflammatory character of $CD4^+$ T cells in this diabetic pig model (39), one might conclude that the increased basal mitochondrial respiration and glycolysis of PBMC of ERU cases, revealed in the present study, might also contribute to the augmented effector functions and therefore autoimmune character of these cells. A similar metabolic phenotype was seen in autoreactive lymphocytes of KBN mice, which are a spontaneous autoimmune arthritis model and were tested at an early stage of the disease (40). More precisely, $CD4^+$ T cells of these KBN mice were shown to have increased basal mitochondrial and glycolytic rates compared to control mice and B cells also revealed a higher glycolytic rate than controls (40). The researchers linked the higher metabolism to the enhanced effector functions of $CD4^+$ T cells and B cells of KBN mice compared to controls (40). Furthermore, they strengthened their theory by inhibiting glycolysis of KBN lymphocytes with 2-DG, which stopped the development and, when treatment was carried out early and continuous, decreased the severity of joint inflammation (40). Thus, the study managed to link the high glycolytic rates of lymphocytes in an autoimmune disease model with the disease's severity.

PBMC are a heterogeneous cell population comprised of T cells, B cells, monocytes, dendritic cells and natural killer cells (41), thus it was unclear for us which cell types caused the observed changes in metabolism in the ERU group. By testing and comparing the metabolic reactions of $CD4^+$ and $CD4^-$ cells with the collective PBMC fraction, we could clarify some parameters. While discussing these results, it is important to keep in mind that the $CD4^-$ cell fraction is comprised of the cell subsets in the PBMC population remaining after density gradient centrifugation and CD4 sorting, namely $CD8^+$ T cells, γδ T cells, B cells, monocytes, dendritic cells and natural killer cells (41). Both $CD4^+$ T cells and $CD4^-$ cells caused the higher basal OCR level in PBMC of ERU cases (**Figure 1A**), whereas the highly upregulated basal glycolysis in PBMC of ERU cases was caused only by $CD4^-$ cells (**Figures 2A, 3A**). To our knowledge, we are the first to describe these differences in a direct comparison between PBMC and CD4 sorted subpopulations. Since $CD4^+$ T cells are the major players in HAU, ERU and the induced uveitis models (1, 42, 43), we subsequently focused on the metabolic phenotype of this specific cell subset. We could demonstrate that $CD4^+$ T cells of ERU cases utilized the oxidative phosphorylation pathway in basal state to a significantly higher amount than control cells (**Figure 1A**). Furthermore, $CD4^+$ T cells of horses with ERU were engaged to a lower level in the glycolytic pathway in their basal energy state than control $CD4^+$ T cells (**Figure 3A**). We therefore demonstrated that $CD4^+$ T cells of ERU cases and controls had different basal metabolic phenotypes. The higher OCR level in ERU might be caused by higher mitochondrial respiration rates. To our knowledge, we are the first to describe this altered metabolic phenotype in $CD4^+$ T cells of cases affected by spontaneous autoimmune uveitis. Still, these results are mostly in line with the findings of altered T cell metabolism in mouse models of other autoimmune diseases like rheumatoid arthritis or SLE (33, 40). In SLE, an autoimmune disease mainly driven by autoreactive $CD4^+$ T cells and B cells (44), studies revealed an increased level of glycolysis and mitochondrial activity of $CD4^+$ T cells of lupus patients and the lupus-prone mouse model (33, 44). The authors suggested that this altered T cell metabolism could cause SLE (33). With this in mind, we hypothesize that the altered T cell metabolism of ERU cases revealed in the present study might also play an important part in the pathogenesis of this disease. Functional studies are necessary to further research this interesting topic in the future, like it was recently done in a study on murine interferon regulatory factor-4 (IRF4) depleted $CD4^+$ T cells of an experimental autoimmune uveitis model (EAU) (45). Here, a connection between knockout of IRF4 and lower mitochondrial respiration in basal state in $CD4^+$ T cells and suppressed autoimmune uveitis could be shown (45). Unfortunately, this study did not include $CD4^+$ T cells of eye-healthy control mice, thus is it uncertain whether IRF4 depletion adjusted the mitochondrial respiration level of $CD4^+$ T cells of EAU cases to that of respective cells of healthy mice.

Interestingly, $CD4^+$ T cells of ERU cases were able to reach higher rates in compensatory glycolysis compared to controls, when mitochondrial activity was blocked (**Figure 3C**). We hypothesize that the ability of autoreactive $CD4^+$ T cells to achieve higher glycolytic rates when needed, might be due to higher expression levels of glucose transporters. In human $CD4^+$ effector T cells, GLUT1 was shown to be essential, as its impairment led to decreased glucose uptake, glycolysis and effector T cell differentiation (46). Furthermore, in a mouse model of inflammatory bowel disease *in vivo*, GLUT1 deficiency led to reduced ability of effector T cells to induce inflammation (46). Autoimmune phenotypes in spontaneous and induced mouse models for SLE were ameliorated upon inhibition of glucose transport with CG-5, a glucose transport inhibitor (44). Thus, higher expression levels of GLUT1 or another glucose transporter in immune cells of uveitis cases might increase their ability to induce inflammation in the immune privileged eye, which merits further investigations in the future, as soon as antibodies for equine glucose transporters are available.

Furthermore, $CD4^+$ T cells of ERU cases showed decreased ATP-linked respiration and increased non-mitochondrial oxygen consumption compared to controls, when complexes of their mitochondrial respiratory chain were blocked (**Figure 1C**). Noteworthy, these differences could not be seen when $CD4^+$ T cells were tested together with $CD4^-$ cells (**Figure 1B**). The reason for that might be that sorting out the $CD4^+$ T cells impacts the relative proportions of the remaining cell subsets in the $CD4^-$ fraction. One could speculate that subset-specific metabolic patterns could now have a stronger effect on the $CD4^-$ cell metabolic curve than on the PBMC metabolic curve. Another possible explanation for this observation might be that the diverse cell subsets in the PBMC population influence each other in their metabolism, especially when some complexes of the respiratory chain or the glycolytic pathway are blocked or uncoupled. This might result in the specific metabolic curve of the PBMC group, but does not evenly represent the metabolic curves of every cell subset within this group. Taken together, our results point to altered parts of $CD4^+$ T cell metabolism of horses affected by ERU, namely spending less oxygen on producing ATP through oxidative phosphorylation and in return using more oxygen for non-mitochondrial processes such as glycolysis. Our study is the first to describe these results for immune cells in autoimmune uveitis. In basic research however, effector T cells of C57BL/6 mice were shown to engage in aerobic glycolysis upon pro-inflammatory signals (27, 47, 48). We therefore hypothesize that $CD4^+$ T cells of ERU cases as well rather use oxygen to engage in aerobic glycolysis than trying to compensate impaired mitochondrial function with an upregulated OXPHOS. This leap between ERU $CD4^+$ T cells, obtained in the quiescent stage of the disease, and T cells in inflammatory studies is possible, because former studies demonstrated that PBMC of ERU cases are locked in an inflammatory state even in the quiescent stage of the disease. For example, PBMC of ERU cases, which were obtained in a quiescent stage of the disease, had higher lactotransferrin concentrations, which the authors linked to the presence of activated immune cells (49). ERU immune cells also demonstrated a more intense reaction to the autoantigen cellular retinaldehyde binding protein, more specifically a more directed and significantly closer movement toward this autoantigen, than control cells (1). Furthermore, the higher concentration of formin like 1 in CD4$^+$ T cells of ERU cases was also linked to the activation of those cells in the quiescent stage of equine recurrent autoimmune uveitis (50).

Concerning the increased mitochondrial activity of PBMC and CD4$^+$ T cells of ERU cases, another interesting aspect to investigate is if this enhanced activity influences the mass and formation of mitochondria within immune cells of ERU cases compared to controls. T cells of human SLE patients were shown to have higher mitochondrial mass than controls (51) and the increased mitochondrial mass of M2 macrophages of C57BL/6 mice with melanoma was suggested to be linked to the higher mitochondrial OXPHOS levels of these cells (52). Furthermore, mitochondrial remodeling is known to affect the metabolic status of a cell (29). For example, mitochondrial fission shifts the metabolism to aerobic glycolysis, whereas fusion processes shift the metabolism to OXPHOS (29). As a first step towards this research area, we investigated the amount of mitochondria in CD4$^+$ T cells of controls and ERU cases. We could show that the mitochondrial marker protein ATP5β was expressed to same amounts (**Figures 4A, B**) and that mitochondria were located in the same cellular regions (**Figure 4C**) in health and ERU. This finding is in line with former studies concerning the equine CD4$^+$ T cell proteome, where mitochondrial markers like Timm13, Tomm70, ATP5β and other ATP synthase subunits were not expressed significantly different in healthy horses and ERU cases (53). Thus, the metabolic alterations seen in ERU cases do not stem from a differing amount of mitochondria but more likely from a deviant metabolic activity. The altered metabolic phenotype of immune cells is not only investigated in diseases, but also in basic research, since the finding of functionally different cells that can be solely identified by their metabolic phenotype is intriguing. Mitochondria were shown to not only generate ATP and metabolic metabolites but also to control signaling pathways of a cell (54). By producing mitochondrial reactive oxygen species (mROS), they can influence the activation of transcription factors like HIF1α or NFAT, which ultimately resulted in functional changes of the cell, for example a differentiation into a pro-inflammatory effector T cell in mice [reviewed in (54)]. The knowledge in this field is emerging and many details of mROS generation and functioning are still not fully understood to date, whether in basic research nor in disease [reviewed in (54)]. Therefore, studies in a species like the horse and spontaneous disease models are scarce to date and build a first basis for further knowledge in this complex field.

Linking the results of the mito stress test to the amount of mitochondria and mitochondrial markers found in CD4$^+$ T cells in controls and ERU cases, an intriguing fact comes to attention: Although ERU and control CD4$^+$ T cells had the same amount of ATP5β, the ATP synthase (complex V) used less oxygen in ERU CD4$^+$ T cells compared to controls (**Figure 1C**). Future research will be necessary to elucidate the reason for this in the equine model of autoimmune uveitis. One possible explanation might be that CD4$^+$ effector T cells of ERU cases are likely to use the glycolytic pathway to a higher extend than control cells, as previously described for CD4$^+$ T cells of an EAE mouse model (55). Another possible explanation could be a functional defect in complex V of the respiratory chain of ERU cells, as it was shown in immortalized human ME/CFS lymphoblasts (56).

Taken together, our findings prove a clear difference in the metabolic phenotype of peripheral CD4$^+$ T cells of ERU cases and controls, which allows researchers to identify and possibly target the autoreactive cells in the periphery before they migrate into the eye and destroy retinal tissue. With an increased mitochondrial metabolism under basal conditions and the ability to switch to alternative pathways when the mitochondria are impaired and to engage in higher glycolysis when needed, CD4$^+$ T cells of ERU cases are metabolically suited to lead an autoimmune attack. Overall, our results provide a basis for further investigations concerning the functional implication of the altered phenotype of autoreactive lymphocytes in the pathogenesis of autoimmune uveitis.

ETHICS STATEMENT

The animal study was reviewed and approved by Regierung von Oberbayern, Permit number: ROB-55.2Vet-2532.Vet_03-17-88.

AUTHOR CONTRIBUTIONS

CD conceived, designed and analyzed the experiments and supervised the project. CB, CW, AH and SH performed the experiments. CB, AH and CD analyzed the data. CB, CW, AH and CD wrote the manuscript. All authors contributed to the article and approved the submitted version.

ACKNOWLEDGMENTS

The authors would like to thank Hartmut Gerhards, Bettina Wollanke and Lutz S. Göhring as well as the staff of the Equine Hospital at LMU Munich for providing blood samples of the animals. We also thank Tanja Witte, Kirsten Hahn, Claudia Julius-Wilhelm and Yvette Ballauf for support in blood withdrawal from the horses as well as Lydia Hoffmann, Stefanie Püls and Barbara Amann for technical assistance. We also thank Lea Lorenz, Lucia Korbonits and Roxane Degroote, as well as Joachim Manning and Herbert Kaltner for critical discussion.

REFERENCES

1. Wiedemann C, Amann B, Degroote RL, Witte T, Deeg CA. Aberrant Migratory Behavior of Immune Cells in Recurrent Autoimmune Uveitis in Horses. *Front Cell Dev Biol* (2020) 8(101):1–15. doi: 10.3389/fcell.2020.00101
2. Malalana F, Stylianides A, McGowan C. Equine Recurrent Uveitis: Human and Equine Perspectives. *Vet J* (2015) 206(1):22–9. doi: 10.1016/j.tvjl.2015.06.017
3. Gerding JC, Gilger BC. Prognosis and Impact of Equine Recurrent Uveitis. *Equine Vet J* (2016) 48(3):290–8. doi: 10.1111/evj.12451

4. Zipplies JK, Kirschfink M, Amann B, Hauck SM, Stangassinger M, Deeg CA. Complement Factor B Expression Profile in a Spontaneous Uveitis Model. *Immunobiology* (2010) 215(12):949–55. doi: 10.1016/j.imbio.2010.02.003
5. Deeg CA, Kaspers B, Gerhards H, Thurau SR, Wollanke B, Wildner G. Immune Responses to Retinal Autoantigens and Peptides in Equine Recurrent Uveitis. *Invest Ophthalmol Vis Sci* (2001) 42(2):393–8.
6. Schauer M, Kleinwort KJH, Degroote RL, Wiedemann C, Kremmer E, Hauck SM, et al. Interaction of Septin 7 and DOCK8 in Equine Lymphocytes Reveals Novel Insights Into Signaling Pathways Associated With Autoimmunity. *Sci Rep* (2018) 8(1):12332. doi: 10.1038/s41598-018-30753-7
7. Doycheva D, Preuss B, Klein R, Zierhut M. High Incidence of Antibodies to Lens Proteins in Sera From Patients With Uveitis. *Graefes Arch Clin Exp Ophthalmol* (2007) 245(5):683–8. doi: 10.1007/s00417-006-0407-2
8. Doycheva D, Preuss B, Deuter C, Zierhut M, Klein R. Identification of Immunodominant Epitopes of Alpha-Crystallins Recognized by Antibodies in Sera of Patients With Uveitis. *Graefes Arch Clin Exp Ophthalmol* (2012) 250 (2):297–305. doi: 10.1007/s00417-011-1758-x
9. Deeg CA, Hauck SM, Amann B, Pompetzki D, Altmann F, Raith A, et al. Equine Recurrent Uveitis–a Spontaneous Horse Model of Uveitis. *Ophthalmic Res* (2008) 40(3-4):151–3. doi: 10.1159/000119867
10. Deeg CA, Pompetzki D, Raith AJ, Hauck SM, Amann B, Suppmann S, et al. Identification and Functional Validation of Novel Autoantigens in Equine Uveitis. *Mol Cell Proteomics* (2006) 5(8):1462–70. doi: 10.1074/mcp.M500352-MCP200
11. Deeg CA, Raith AJ, Amann B, Crabb JW, Thurau SR, Hauck SM, et al. CRALBP is a Highly Prevalent Autoantigen for Human Autoimmune Uveitis. *Clin Dev Immunol* (2007) 2007:39245. doi: 10.1155/2007/39245
12. Neutzner RV, Jager M, Friedburg C, Deeg CA, Lorenz B. [Blind Spot Enlargement Syndrome in Acute Zonal Occult Outer Retinopathy With Detection of Autoantibodies Against the Retinal Antigens CRALBP and s-Ag]. *Ophthalmologe* (2011) 108(11):1045–9. doi: 10.1007/s00347-011-2406-x
13. Busch M, Wefelmeyer KL, Walscheid K, Rothaus K, Bauer D, Deeg CA, et al. Identification of Ocular Autoantigens Associated With Juvenile Idiopathic Arthritis-Associated Uveitis. *Front Immunol* (2019) 10:1–12. doi: 10.3389/fimmu.2019.01793
14. Prete M, Dammacco R, Fatone MC, Racanelli V. Autoimmune Uveitis: Clinical, Pathogenetic, and Therapeutic Features. *Clin Exp Med* (2016) 16 (2):125–36. doi: 10.1007/s10238-015-0345-6
15. Brandes K, Wollanke B, Niedermaier G, Brem S, Gerhards H. Recurrent Uveitis in Horses: Vitreal Examinations With Ultrastructural Detection of Leptospires. *J Vet Med* (2007) 54:270–5. doi: 10.1111/j.1439-0442.2007.00921.x
16. Voelter K, Vial Z, Pot SA, Spiess BM. Leptospiral Antibody Prevalence and Surgical Treatment Outcome in Horses With Equine Recurrent Uveitis (ERU) in Switzerland. *Vet Ophthalmol* (2020) 23(4):648–58. doi: 10.1111/vop.12767
17. Stathopoulou C, Nikoleri D, Bertsias G. Immunometabolism: An Overview and Therapeutic Prospects in Autoimmune Diseases. *Immunotherapy* (2019) 11:813–29. doi: 10.2217/imt-2019-0002
18. Brooks GA. The Science and Translation of Lactate Shuttle Theory. *Cell Metab* (2018) 27(4):757–85. doi: 10.1016/j.cmet.2018.03.008
19. Covarrubias AJ, Perrone R, Grozio A, Verdin E. NAD(+) Metabolism and its Roles in Cellular Processes During Ageing. *Nat Rev Mol Cell Biol* (2021) 22 (2):119–41. doi: 10.1038/s41580-020-00313-x
20. Clanton TL. Hypoxia-Induced Reactive Oxygen Species Formation in Skeletal Muscle. *J Appl Physiol (1985)* (2007) 102(6):2379–88. doi: 10.1152/japplphysiol.01298.2006
21. Muri J, Kopf M. Redox Regulation of Immunometabolism. *Nat Rev Immunol* (2021) 21:363–81. doi: 10.1038/s41577-020-00478-8
22. O'Neill LA, Kishton RJ, Rathmell J. A Guide to Immunometabolism for Immunologists. *Nat Rev Immunol* (2016) 16(9):553–65. doi: 10.1038/nri.2016.70
23. Teng X, Li W, Cornaby C, Morel L. Immune Cell Metabolism in Autoimmunity. *Clin Exp Immunol* (2019) 197(2):181–92. doi: 10.1111/cei.13277
24. Klein Geltink RI, Kyle RL, Pearce EL. Unraveling the Complex Interplay Between T Cell Metabolism and Function. *Annu Rev Immunol* (2018) 36:461–88. doi: 10.1146/annurev-immunol-042617-053019
25. Angiari S, Runtsch MC, Sutton CE, Palsson-McDermott EM, Kelly B, Rana N, et al. Pharmacological Activation of Pyruvate Kinase M2 Inhibits CD4(+) T Cell Pathogenicity and Suppresses Autoimmunity. *Cell Metab* (2020) 31 (2):391–405.e8. doi: 10.1016/j.cmet.2019.10.015
26. Buck MD, O'Sullivan D, Klein Geltink RI, Curtis JD, Chang CH, Sanin DE, et al. Mitochondrial Dynamics Controls T Cell Fate Through Metabolic Programming. *Cell* (2016) 166(1):63–76. doi: 10.1016/j.cell.2016.05.035
27. Pålsson-McDermott EM, O'Neill LAJ. Targeting Immunometabolism as an Anti-Inflammatory Strategy. *Cell Res* (2020) 30:300–14. doi: 10.1038/s41422-020-0291-z
28. Warburg O. On the Origin of Cancer Cells. *Science* (1956) 123:309–14. doi: 10.1126/science.123.3191.309
29. Takeshima Y, Iwasaki Y, Fujio K, Yamamoto K. Metabolism as a Key Regulator in the Pathogenesis of Systemic Lupus Erythematosus. *Semin Arthritis Rheum* (2019) 48(6):1142–5. doi: 10.1016/j.semarthrit.2019.04.006
30. Miller A, Nagy C, Knapp B, Laengle J, Ponweiser E, Groeger M, et al. Exploring Metabolic Configurations of Single Cells Within Complex Tissue Microenvironments. *Cell Metab* (2017) 26:788–0. doi: 10.1016/j.cmet.2017.08.014
31. Vander Heiden MG, Cantley LC, Thompson CB. Understanding the Warburg Effect: The Metabolic Requirements of Cell Proliferation. *Science* (2009) 324 (5930):1029–33. doi: 10.1126/science.1160809
32. Orang AV, Petersen J, McKinnon RA, Michael MZ. Micromanaging Aerobic Respiration and Glycolysis in Cancer Cells. *Mol Metab* (2019) 23:98–126. doi: 10.1016/j.molmet.2019.01.014
33. Yin Y, Choi SC, Xu Z, Perry DJ, Seay H, Croker BP, et al. Normalization of CD4+ T Cell Metabolism Reverses Lupus. *Sci Transl Med* (2015) 7 (274):274ra18. doi: 10.1126/scitranslmed.aaa0835
34. Wollanke B, Rohrbach BW, Gerhards H. Serum and Vitreous Humor Antibody Titers in and Isolation of *Leptospira Interogans* From Horses With Recurrent Uveitis. *Sci Rep* (2001) 219:795–800. doi: 10.2460/javma.2001.219.795
35. O'Sullivan D, Pearce EL. Targeting T Cell Metabolism for Therapy. *Trends Immunol* (2015) 36(2):71–80. doi: 10.1016/j.it.2014.12.004
36. Streilein JW, Niederkorn JY. Induction of Anterior Chamber-Associated Immune Deviation Requires an Intact, Functional Spleen. 1981. *Ocul Immunol Inflamm* (2007) 15(3):187–94. doi: 10.1080/09273940701382473
37. Caspi RR, Roberge FG, McAllister CG, el-Saied M, Kuwabrara T, Gery I, et al. T Cell Lines Mediating Experimental Autoimmune Uveoretinitis (EAU) in the Rat. *J Immunol* (1986) 136:928–33.
38. Hauck SM, Lepper MF, Hertl M, Sekundo W, Deeg CA. Proteome Dynamics in Biobanked Horse Peripheral Blood Derived Lymphocytes (PBL) With Induced Autoimmune Uveitis. *Proteomics* (2017) 17(19):1–5. doi: 10.1002/pmic.201700013
39. Giese IM, Schilloks MC, Degroote RL, Weigand M, Renner S, Wolf E, et al. Chronic Hyperglycemia Drives Functional Impairment of Lymphocytes in Diabetic INS (C94Y) Transgenic Pigs. *Front Immunol* (2021) 11:607473. doi: 10.3389/fimmu.2020.607473
40. Abboud G, Choi SC, Kanda N, Zeumer-Spataro L, Roopenian DC, Morel L. Inhibition of Glycolysis Reduces Disease Severity in an Autoimmune Model of Rheumatoid Arthritis. *Front Immunol* (2018) 9:1973. doi: 10.3389/fimmu.2018.01973
41. Ventura G, Calvano CD, Porcelli V, Palmieri L, De Giacomo A, Xu Y, et al. Phospholipidomics of Peripheral Blood Mononuclear Cells (PBMCs): The Tricky Case of Children With Autism Spectrum Disorder (ASD) and Their Healthy Siblings. *Anal Bioanal Chem* (2020) 412(25):6859–74. doi: 10.1007/s00216-020-02817-z
42. Radosavljevic A, Agarwal M, Bodaghi B, Smith JR, Zierhut M. Medical Therapy of Uveitic Macular Edema: Biologic Agents. *Ocul Immunol Inflamm* (2020) 28:1239–50. doi: 10.1080/09273948.2019.1709648
43. Chen YH, Eskandarpour M, Gondrand A, Zhang X, Gu R, Galatowicz G, et al. Functionally Distinct Ifngamma(+) IL-17A(+) Th Cells in Experimental Autoimmune Uveitis: T Cell Heterogeneity, Migration and Steroid Response. *Eur J Immunol* (2020) 50(12):1941–51. doi: 10.1002/eji.202048616
44. Li W, Qu G, Choi SC, Cornaby C, Titov A, Kanda N, et al. Targeting T Cell Activation and Lupus Autoimmune Phenotypes by Inhibiting Glucose Transporters. *Front Immunol* (2019) 10:833. doi: 10.3389/fimmu.2019.00833
45. Kang M, Lee HS, Choi JK, Yu CR, Egwuagu CE. Deletion of Irf4 in T Cells Suppressed Autoimmune Uveitis and Dysregulated Transcriptional Programs Linked to CD4(+) T Cell Differentiation and Metabolism. *Int J Mol Sci* (2021) 22(5):1–15. doi: 10.3390/ijms22052775
46. Macintyre AN, Gerriets VA, Nichols AG, Michalek RD, Rudolph MC, Deoliveira D, et al. The Glucose Transporter Glut1 is Selectively Essential

for CD4 T Cell Activation and Effector Function. *Cell Metab* (2014) 20(1):61–72. doi: 10.1016/j.cmet.2014.05.004

47. Pearce EL, Poffenberger MC, Chang CH, Jones RG. Fueling Immunity: Insights Into Metabolism and Lymphocyte Function. *Science* (2013) 342 (6155):1242454. doi: 10.1126/science.1242454
48. Chang CH, Curtis JD, Maggi LBJr., Faubert B, Villarino AV, O'Sullivan D, et al. Posttranscriptional Control of T Cell Effector Function by Aerobic Glycolysis. *Cell* (2013) 153(6):1239–51. doi: 10.1016/j.cell.2013.05.016
49. Degroote RL, Hauck SM, Amann B, Hirmer S, Ueffing M, Deeg CA. Unraveling the Equine Lymphocyte Proteome: Differential Septin 7 Expression Associates With Immune Cells in Equine Recurrent Uveitis. *PLoS One* (2014) 9(3):e91684. doi: 10.1371/journal.pone.0091684
50. Degroote RL, Uhl PB, Amann B, Krackhardt AM, Ueffing M, Hauck SM, et al. Formin Like 1 Expression Is Increased on CD4+ T Lymphocytes in Spontaneous Autoimmune Uveitis. *J Proteomics* (2017) 154:102–8. doi: 10.1016/j.jprot.2016.12.015
51. Lai ZW, Marchena-Mendez I, Perl A. Oxidative Stress and Treg Depletion in Lupus Patients With Anti-Phospholipid Syndrome. *Clin Immunol* (2015) 158 (2):148–52. doi: 10.1016/j.clim.2015.03.024
52. Yu Q, Wang Y, Dong L, He Y, Liu R, Yang Q, et al. Regulations of Glycolytic Activities on Macrophages Functions in Tumor and Infectious Inflammation. *Front Cell Infect Microbiol* (2020) 10:287. doi: 10.3389/fcimb.2020.00287
53. Degroote RL, Helm S, Klein U, Schmitt R, Ueffing M, Hauck SM, et al. The Equine CD4+ Lymphocyte Proteome. *Hindawi* (2014) 2014:1–4. doi: 10.1155/2014/105312
54. Mehta MM, Weinberg SE, Chandel NS. Mitochondrial Control of Immunity: Beyond ATP. *Nat Rev Immunol* (2017) 17(10):608–20. doi: 10.1038/nri.2017.66
55. Wu L, Hollinshead KER, Hao Y, Au C, Kroehling L, Ng C, et al. Niche-Selective Inhibition of Pathogenic Th17 Cells by Targeting Metabolic Redundancy. *Cell* (2020) 182(3):641–54. doi: 10.1016/j.cell.2020.06.014
56. Missailidis D, Annesley SJ, Allan CY, Sanislav O, Lidbury BA, Lewis DP, et al. An Isolated Complex V Inefficiency and Dysregulated Mitochondrial Function in Immortalized Lymphocytes From ME/CFS Patients. *Int J Mol Sci* (2020) 21(3):1–26. doi: 10.3390/ijms21031074

4

Metabolomic Analysis of Aqueous Humor Identifies Aberrant Amino Acid and Fatty Acid Metabolism in Vogt-Koyanagi-Harada and Behcet's Disease

*Jing Xu [1], Guannan Su [1], Xinyue Huang [1], Rui Chang [1], Zhijun Chen [1], Zi Ye [1], Qingfeng Cao [1], Aize Kijlstra [2] and Peizeng Yang [1]**

[1] The First Affiliated Hospital of Chongqing Medical University, Chongqing Branch of National Clinical Research Center for Ocular Diseases, Chongqing, China, [2] University Eye Clinic Maastricht, Maastricht, Netherlands

***Correspondence:**
Peizeng Yang
peizengycmu@126.com

To investigate aqueous metabolic profiles in Vogt-Koyanagi-Harada (VKH) and Behcet's disease (BD), we applied ultra-high-performance liquid chromatography equipped with quadrupole time-of flight mass spectrometry in aqueous humor samples collected from these patients and controls. Metabolite levels in these three groups were analyzed by univariate logistic regression. The differential metabolites were subjected to subsequent pathway analysis by MetaboAnalyst. The results showed that both partial-least squares discrimination analysis and hierarchical clustering analysis showed specific aqueous metabolite profiles when comparing VKH, BD, and controls. There were 28 differential metabolites in VKH compared to controls and 29 differential metabolites in BD compared to controls. Amino acids and fatty acids were the two most abundant categories of differential metabolites. Furthermore, pathway enrichment analysis identified several perturbed pathways, including pantothenate and CoA biosynthesis when comparing VKH with the control group, and D-arginine and D-ornithine metabolism and phenylalanine metabolism when comparing BD with the control group. Aminoacyl-tRNA biosynthesis was altered in both VKH and BD when compared to controls. Our findings suggest that amino acids metabolism as well as two fatty acids, palmitic acid and oleic acid, may be involved in the pathogenesis of BD and VKH.

Keywords: Vogt-Koyanagi-Harada disease, Behcet's disease, metabolomics, pathway, amino acids, fatty acids

INTRODUCTION

Uveitis known as intraocular inflammation is one of the leading causes of visual impairment and blindness in the world (1, 2). Vogt-Koyanagi-Harada (VKH) disease and Behcet's disease (BD) are two of the most commonly seen uveitis entities in China (3, 4). The incidence rate of uveitis in China is 111.3 persons per 100,000 person-years (5) and a frequency of 12.7% and 8.7% has been reported for VKH and BD in Chinese uveitis patients, respectively (4). VKH disease is a multisystemic autoimmune disease characterized by recurrent bilateral granulomatous panuveitis accompanied with systemic involvements including poliosis, alopecia, vitiligo, central nervous system, and auditory abnormalities (6). BD is recognized as an autoinflammatory disorder accompanied with recurrent uveitis, oral aphthae, genital ulcers, and typical skin lesions (7). The exact pathogenesis of both VKH disease and BD remains unclear and omics analysis may advance the understanding of these diseases.

Metabolomics is a rapidly expanding field in life science which leads to the growing interest in metabolism (8). Metabolites, serving as downstream products of transcription, translation, and post-translational protein modification, can reflect and be influenced by local physiological events (9). Therefore, a study of metabolomics could contribute to a better understanding of the pathophysiology of intraocular inflammation. Recent metabolomic studies in VKH disease or BD, using sweat or urine samples have revealed a specific metabolite profile (10, 11). Aqueous humor fills the anterior chamber of the eye and contributes to a normal intraocular homeostatic environment (12). Its composition may probably be a better reflection of local physiological changes associated with intraocular diseases than the analysis of samples obtained from peripheral sites. As far as we know, no aqueous metabolomic study has been reported for VKH or BD and this was therefore the subject of the study described here.

Liquid chromatography/mass spectrometry (LC/MS) is a commonly applied technique for untargeted metabolomics detection with robust reliability and reproducibility (13–15). In view of these features, we performed an untargeted metabolomic analysis of aqueous humor samples from VKH disease and BD patients taken during cataract surgery and compared it with samples from senile cataract controls, applying ultra-high-performance liquid chromatography equipped with quadrupole time-of-flight mass spectrometry (UPLC-Q-TOF/MS).

MATERIALS AND METHODS

Participants

Individuals selected for this study included 15 VKH patients, 15 BD patients, and 15 senile cataract controls. The VKH and BD patients included, had developed cataract as a complication of their uveitis. The demographic data of the cohorts were collected (16) and shown in **Table 1**. Criteria of an international committee and those developed by our group were used to make the diagnosis of VKH disease (17, 18). Diagnosis of BD was based on the International Study Group's criteria (19). Patients with any unclear diagnosis were excluded from the study. We also excluded patients with other ocular condition such as optic nerve disease, macular abnormalities or diabetic retinopathy. As for controls, the exclusion criteria were subjects with uveitis and a history of any other autoimmune disease.

All participants underwent cataract surgery at the First Affiliated Hospital of Chongqing Medical University (Chongqing, China) from August, 2017 to May, 2019. Our method for cataract removal in uveitis patients has been reported elsewhere (20). Signed informed consents were obtained from all enrolled participants. The study received the approval of the Ethics Committee of the First Affiliated Hospital of Chongqing Medical University and followed the tenets of the Declaration of Helsinki.

Sample Collection and Preparation

Anterior chamber paracentesis was performed to collect approximately 200 µl of aqueous humor samples at the beginning of the cataract surgery under the sterile condition. Care was taken to avoid contamination of samples with blood or touching intraocular tissues. The specimens were stored at −80°C until UPLC-Q-TOF/MS analysis. All specimens were thawed at 4°C. To remove protein, 80 µl aqueous humor aliquots were mixed with 320 µl of cold methanol/acetonitrile (1:1, v/v) which was then centrifuged for 20 min (14,000 g, 4°C). The supernatant was dried in a vacuum centrifuge. Quality control (QC) specimens consisting of mixing with 10 µl of each sample were analyzed with other samples to monitor the repeatability and stability of instrument. The QC specimens were inserted regularly in the cohort of tested samples, which could monitor the reliability of the whole procedure.

UPLC-Q-TOF/MS Analysis

Aqueous metabolomic analyses were applied using an Agilent 1290 Infinity LC system (Agilent Technologies, Santa-Clara, California, USA) coupled with an AB SCIEX Triple TOF 6600 System (AB SCIEX, Framingham, MA, USA). For chromatographic separation, ACQUITY HSS T3 1.8 mm (2.1 mm × 100 mm) columns were used for sample analyses in both positive and negative modes. The column temperature was

TABLE 1 | Demographic and clinical characteristics of participants.

Characteristics	VKH	BD	Controls	*p* value
Number (n)	15	15	15	–
Laterality (OD/OS)	7/8	5/10	8/7	–
Age (years)	45.8 ± 9.79	35.93 ± 10.72	60.6 ± 7.44	<0.001[a]
Gender (Male/Female)	8/7	9/6	6/9	0.54[b]
IOP (mmHg)	13.5 ± 2.8	15.7 ± 3.5	15.1 ± 2.6	0.13[a]
Systemic corticosteroids, (n, %)	15 (100%)	15 (100%)	n.a.	–
Immunosuppressant, (n, %)	15 (100%)	13 (86.67%)	n.a.	0.48[b]
Biological agents, (n, %)	0	0	n.a.	–

VKH, Vogt-Koyanagi-Harada disease; BD, Behcet's disease; IOP, intraocular pressure; n.a., not applicable.
Continuous variables are expressed as mean ± standard deviation.
[a]Analyzed by ANOVA; [b]Analyzed by Pearson chi-square test/Fischer's exact test.

set at 25°C. The mobile phase was set as follows: A = 25 mM ammonium acetate and 25 mM ammonium hydroxide in water, and B = acetonitrile. The elution procedure was set as follows. After keeping for 0.5 min, the gradient of 95% B was linearly reduced to 65% in 6.5 min. Then it was decreased to 40% in 1 min. After keeping 40% B for 1 min, it was increased to 95% in 10 s. A 3-min re-equilibration period was employed in the procedure. The delivery flow rate was set at 300 μl/min, and 2 μl aqueous specimen was injected into the column.

UPLC-Q-TOF/MS was conducted in both positive and negative ion modes. Electrospray ionization source conditions were set as Ion Source Gas1 = 60 psi, Ion Source Gas2 = 60 psi, curtain gas = 30 psi, source temperature = 600°C, and IonSpray Voltage Floating = 5500 V (+) and −5500 V (−). The MS/MS spectra were obtained by using information dependent acquisition (IDA) coupled with the selected high sensitivity mode. The parameters were set as the collision energy = 50 eV (+) and −20 eV (−), declustering potential = 60 V (+), and −60 V (−), excluding isotopes within 4 Da, and candidate ions to monitor per cycle = 6.

Metabolomics Data Processing

The raw UPLC-Q-TOF/MS data were converted to MzXML files using Proteo Wizard MSconverter, and then imported with XCMS online software for data processing (https://xcmsonline.scripps.edu/landing_page.php?pgcontent=mainPage). The parameters including peak picking, retention time, and peak grouping were aligned by XCMS. We completed compound identification of metabolites by comparing the accuracy m/z value (<25 ppm) and MS/MS spectra. After being normalized, the processed data were uploaded into SIMCA-P (version 14.1, Umetrics, Umea, Sweden) for multivariate data analysis. Then we conducted principal component analysis (PCA) and partial least square discriminant analysis (PLS-DA) to acquire an overview of the metabolomics data in both positive and negative models. The contribution of each metabolite was calculated from the PLS-DA model and expressed as variable importance in the projection (VIP) score. To evaluate the significance of metabolites, those metabolites with a VIP score >1 were analyzed statistically with Student's t-test. We performed the Benjamini–Hochberg procedure for multiple testing adjustments, whereby the critical false discovery rate (FDR) was set to 0.05. The Human Metabolome Database (HMDB) (https://hmdb.ca/) was used to define the classes of metabolites.

Bioinformatics Analysis

Venny software version 2.1.0 (https://bioinfogp.cnb.csic.es/tools/venny/) was used to generate a Venn diagram which could directly show the common and unique differential metabolites among the three groups. Multi Experiment Viewer (MeV) software version 4.9.0 was applied for the heat plot and hierarchical cluster analysis of metabolites. A Volcano plot was made with Graphpad Prism 7.0. MetaboAnalyst (https://www.metaboanalyst.ca/), an open database source, was used to identify metabolic pathways and to perform pathway enrichment analysis.

Statistical Analysis

Statistical analysis of the data was performed using SPSS 22.0. Results are presented as the mean ± standard deviation (SD) for continuous variables. Normality was assessed by the Shapiro-Wilk test and $p > 0.05$ referred to normally distributed data. Student's t-test, Variance (ANOVA), Fisher's exact test and the Pearson chi-square test were used where appropriate. Age was adjusted by univariate logistic regression analysis to reduce bias. A p value less than 0.05 was considered as statistically significant.

RESULTS

Characteristics of Study Participants

A total of 45 participants were enrolled in the study, including 15 VKH subjects (male/female: 8/7), 15 BD subjects (male/female: 9/6), and 15 senile cataract controls (male/female: 6/9) (**Table 1**). No significant differences were present with regards to sex and IOP among the groups ($p = 0.54$ and $p = 0.13$, respectively). All the 30 uveitis patients were on treatment with systemic corticosteroids, without additional biologic agents. The number of VKH patients receiving immunosuppressants (15/15, 100%) was similar to that in the BD group (13/15, 86.57%). Overall, the treatment regimens did not vary between the BD and VKH groups.

Aqueous Metabolomics in VKH, BD, and Controls

To identify the aqueous metabolic profiles among the three groups tested, aqueous humor specimens were applied for untargeted metabolomics analysis. The total ion chromatograms are shown in **Figure S1**. Only slight changes of the spectral peaks of the QC samples were found, indicating that the method showed a satisfactory reproducibility. A total of 14,592 positive-model signals and 10,985 negative-model signals were detected in this study after signal filtering and peak alignment. After pareto scaling of the data, PCA models showed that the QC samples were tightly clustered in both positive and negative modes (**Figure S2**), which also suggests the high reproducibility of the method and credibility of the data. PLS-DA plots were performed to characterize the metabolic profiles for both positive and negative modes, and revealed clear differences when comparing VKH vs. control, BD vs. control, and VKH vs. BD (**Figure 1**).

Differentially Expressed Metabolites Were Identified Between Groups

Metabolites with a VIP > 1 were filtered to perform Student's t-test. The results were adjusted with FDR < 0.05 for multiple comparisons. To identify differentially expressed metabolites for subsequent analysis, we further raised the criteria to a VIP > 1.5. In total, 84 metabolites with a VIP > 1.5 and $p < 0.05$ (FDR corrected) were considered as differentially expressed between the groups (**Table S1**). HMDB was used to gain the classes of the 84 metabolites. It was found that amino acids and fatty acids were the two categories with the most abundant differential metabolites. As shown in **Figure S3**, 64 metabolites for VKH

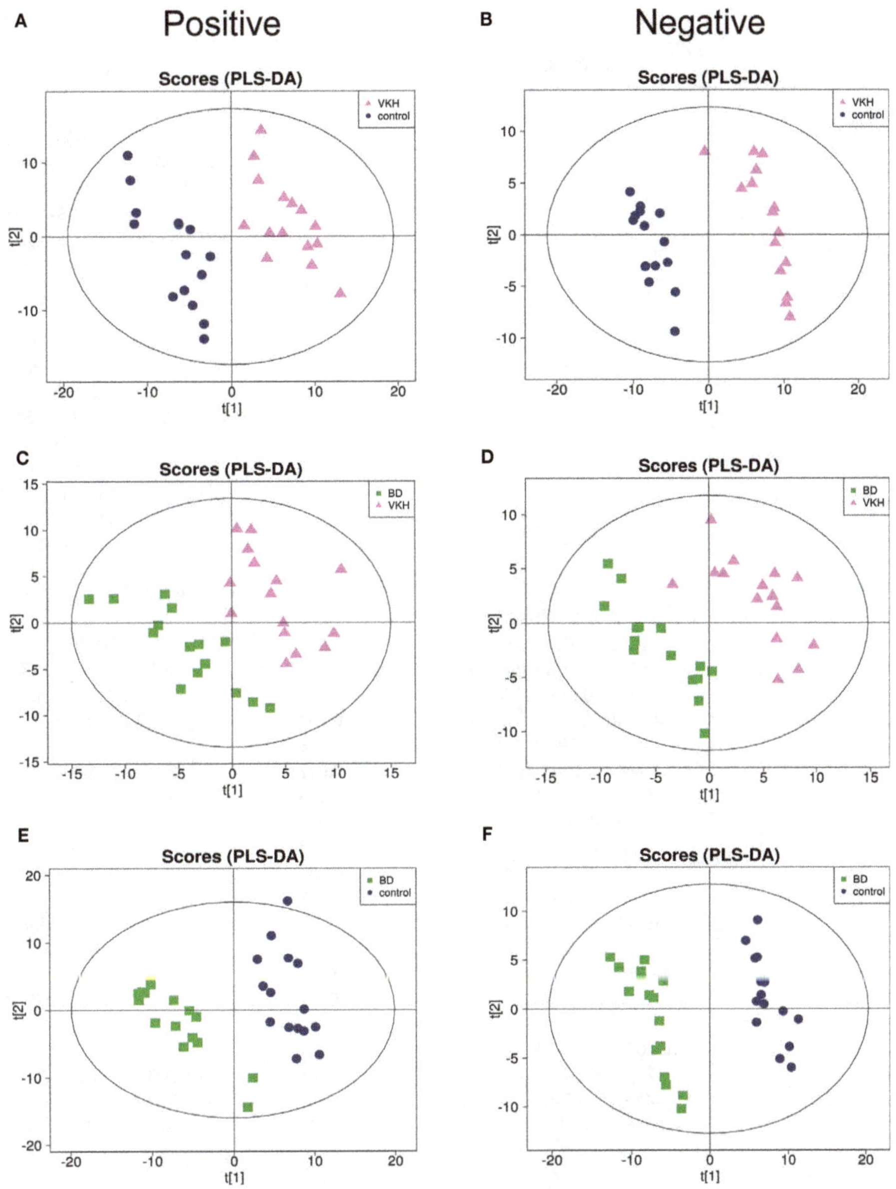

FIGURE 1 | Partial least square discriminant analysis (PLS-DA) for any two of the three groups. PLS-DA plots for Vogt-Koyanagi-Harada disease (VKH) versus senile cataract controls separation in positive mode **(A)** and negative mode **(B)**; PLS-DA plots for VKH disease and Behcet's disease (BD) separation in positive mode **(C)** and negative mode **(D)**; PLS-DA plots for BD and senile cataract controls separation in positive mode **(E)** and negative mode **(F)**.

vs. control and 65 metabolites for BD vs. control showed significant differences. We found 27 differentially expressed metabolites between VKH and BD (data not shown). However, the significance was lost after FDR correction. The volcano plots were made to describe the variation tendencies of metabolites for VKH vs. control and BD vs. control (**Figure S4**).

To further investigate metabolites that could differentiate a group of patients from the other participants, we conducted univariate logistic regression analysis (**Table 2**). There were 41 differential metabolites between the groups after adjustment (**Figure 2**). There were 28 and 29 significantly differential metabolites for VKH vs. control and BD vs. control, respectively (**Figure 3**). Among them, nine amino acids and two fatty acids were overlapping differential metabolites. Palmitic acid and oleic acid levels, the two long-chain fatty acids, were significantly elevated in both VKH and BD compared to controls. Except for N-acetylhistidine, the other eight amino acids were significantly increased in both VKH and BD compared to controls, including asymmetric dimethylarginine, L-lysine, D-ornithine, D-pipecolic acid, L-methionine, creatinine, L-pipecolic acid, and gamma-Glutamyllysine. L-histidine, ornithine, and L-valine were differential amino acids

TABLE 2 | Results of univariate logistic regression analysis comparing the differential metabolites levels of patients to those of controls.

Metabolites	VKH		BD	
	OR (95% CI)	*p* value	OR (95% CI)	*p* value
Pyroglutamic acid	–	–	–	–
L-Phenylalanine	–	–	13.054 (1.589–107.249)	**0.017**
Cyclohexylamine	–	–	63.537 (1.657–2,435.857)	**0.026**
Citramalic acid	–	–	5.975E+9 (0.334–1.068E+20)	0.062
L-Tyrosine	–	–	3.165 (0.728–13.761)	0.124
L-Tryptophan	–	–	14.504 (1.951–107.815)	**0.009**
gamma-Glutamylalanine	–	–	2.814 (0.42–18.854)	0.286
L-Glutamine	–	–	8.622 (0.891–83.397)	0.063
Arachidonic Acid	–	–	–	–
Uracil mustard	–	–	55.004 (0.216–14,034.571)	0.156
Pseudouridine	–	–	17.51 (1.043–293.893)	**0.047**
Phenylacetic acid	–	–	0.098 (0.015–0.652)	**0.016**
N-Alpha-acetyllysine	–	–	37.793 (0.81–1,764.335)	0.064
Heptadecanoic acid	–	–	5.641 (1.217–26.149)	**0.027**
D-Arginine	–	–	26.544 (2.55–276.276)	**0.006**
D-Lactic acid	–	–	0.366 (0.101–1.334)	0.128
Ribothymidine	–	–	9.92 (1.402–70.182)	**0.022**
Cytosine	–	–	0.198 (0.045–0.865)	**0.031**
N-Acetyl-L-aspartic acid	–	–	0.11 (0.019–0.644)	**0.014**
Androsterone sulfate	–	–	661.353 (0.142–3.087E+06)	0.132
Acetylcarnitine	218.881 (0.558–85,932.722)	0.077	–	–
Palmitic acid	5.908 (1.403–24.874)	**0.015**	5.137 (1.101–23.956)	**0.037**
Linoleic acid	1.096E+18 (0–3.648E+39)	0.1	3.69E+17 (0–1.223E+39)	0.11
Sorbitol	0.095 (0.011–0.843)	**0.035**	0.126 (0.014–1.146)	0.66
Asymmetric dimethylarginine	84.921 (1.512–4,769.689)	**0.031**	162.346 (2.59–10,176.585)	**0.016**
Betaine	2.906 (0.896–9.431)	0.076	–	–
Oleic acid	51.746 (2.053–1,304.351)	**0.017**	56.921 (2.086–1,553.162)	**0.017**
2-Methylbutyroylcarnitine	16.964 (1.481–194.372)	**0.023**	–	–
L-Histidine	0.121 (0.015–0.995)	**0.049**	–	–
D-Mannitol	0.425 (0.112–1.611)	0.208	–	–
Malonic acid	0.264 (0.067–1.041)	0.057	0.269 (0.055–1.303)	0.103
Glyceric acid	7.073 (1.128–44.344)	**0.037**	–	–
Uric acid	19.491 (0.552–687.894)	0.102	13.981 (0.385–507.987)	0.15
myo-Inositol	0.173 (0.036–0.824)	**0.028**	0.181 (0.034–0.948)	**0.043**
2-Hydroxy-3-methylbutyric acid	82.362 (1.693–4,007.462)	**0.026**	41.241 (0.851–1,997.65)	0.06
Threonic acid	0.02 (0.001–0.391)	**0.01**	0.028 (0.001–0.59)	**0.021**
Myristic acid	–	–	–	–
Trimethylamine N-oxide	182.074 (1.236–26,828.903)	**0.041**	–	–
N6-N6-N6-Trimethyl-L-lysine	1,706.774 (0.047–6.198E+07)	0.165	1,346.868 (0.037–4.916E+07)	0.179
Gamma-Linolenic acid	1.0042E+16 (0.046–2.349E+33)	0.07	3.922E+15 (0.018–8.718E+32)	0.078
Dehydroascorbic acid	4.264E–5 (4.047E–9–0.449)	**0.033**	0.001 (6.958E–7–1.951)	0.074
Urea	2.666 (0.802–8.861)	0.11	–	–
Coniferyl aldehyde	0.369 (0.108–1.266)	0.113	–	–
Hydroxyisocaproic acid	–	–	–	–
Palmitoleic acid	12.937 (0.581–288.155)	0.106	8.423 (0.37–191.537)	0.181
N-Acetylhistidine	0.147 (0.022–0.961)	**0.045**	0.038 (0.004–0.361)	**0.004**
L-Carnitine	1,067.081 (0.272–4.189E+06)	0.099	875.146 (0.222–3.443E+06)	0.109
L-Alanine	4.092 (0.823–20.35)	0.085	6.525 (1.095–38.886)	**0.039**
N-a-Acetyl-L-arginine	8.079 (0.677–96.481)	0.099	9.484 (0.748–120.32)	0.083
Melamine	0.349 (0.111–1.101)	0.072	–	–
L-Lysine	24.662 (1.365–445.649)	**0.03**	64.749 (3.039–1,379.643)	**0.008**
Oxalate	0.083 (0.01–0.708)	**0.023**	0.091 (0.01–0.854)	**0.036**
D-Proline	49,040.59 (0.371–6.479E+09)	0.073	22,919.578 (0.173–3.031E+09)	0.095
D-Galactarate	–	–	–	–
Citraconic acid	–	–	–	–
Xanthine	–	–	–	–
Allantoin	4.834 (0.652–35.834)	0.123	3.476 (0.44–27.484)	0.238
D-Ornithine	3.764 (1.026–13.807)	**0.046**	5.059 (1.182–21.652)	**0.029**
D-Pipecolic acid	13.908 (1.11–174.212)	**0.041**	28.391 (1.909–422.144)	**0.015**
L-Methionine	654.271 (1.167–366,750.445)	**0.045**	995.407 (1.702–582,209.079)	**0.034**
cis-Aconitic acid	–	–	–	–

(Continued)

TABLE 2 | Continued

Metabolites	VKH		BD	
	OR (95% CI)	*p* value	OR (95% CI)	*p* value
Adenosine	0.097 (0.017–0.568)	**0.01**	–	–
3-Hydroxybutyric acid	0.4 (0.122–1.313)	0.131	0.379 (0.074–1.952)	0.246
Arginyl-Cysteine	245.905 (0.69–87,593.484)	0.066	538.096 (1.4–206,887.842)	**0.038**
L-Arginine	21.832 (0.923–516.491)	0.056	77.246 (2.72–2,193.341)	**0.011**
L-Cystine	–	–	–	–
Ornithine	225.963 (1.195–42,724.551)	**0.043**	–	–
Creatinine	273.817 (1.073–69,863.673)	**0.047**	357.107 (1.324–96,291.296)	**0.04**
3-Methoxy-4-Hydroxyphenylglycol Sulfate	56.764 (0.917–3,514.634)	0.055	31.913 (0.502–2,026.769)	0.102
Diethanolamine	0.049 (0.001–2.441)	0.13	0.026 (0–1.825)	0.093
L-Pipecolic acid	17.021 (1.272–227.676)	**0.032**	35.008 (2.225–550.864)	**0.011**
Gluconic acid	2,563.115 (2.053–3.2E+06)	**0.031**	6561.35 (4.931–8.731E+06)	**0.017**
Decanoylcarnitine	9,139.504 (0.401–2.084E+08)	0.075	–	–
Galacturonic acid	–	–	–	–
m-Chlorohippuric acid	2.328 (0.665–8.151)	0.186	2.558 (0.627–10.447)	0.191
Stearidonic acid	48083.35 (0.451–5.124E+09)	0.068	–	–
Uracil	56.065 (1.229–2557.482)	**0.039**	–	–
7-Methylxanthine	0.24 (0.059–0.984)	**0.047**	–	–
L-Valine	0.118 (0.022–0.643)	**0.013**	–	–
Methylmalonic acid	0.014 (2.655E–5–6.897)	0.176	0.017 (1.92E–05–14.773)	0.238
L-Malic acid	42,033.685 (0.085–2.076E+10)	0.111	–	–
Stavudine	162.849 (1.062–24,967.269)	**0.047**	272.228 (1.645–45,052.551)	**0.031**
gamma-Glutamyllysine	36.475 (1.135–1,171.916)	**0.042**	38.583 (1.147–1,297.405)	**0.042**
L-Kynurenine	24,202.338 (0.025–2.307E+10)	0.151	–	–

VKH, Vogt-Koyanagi-Harada disease; BD, Behcet's disease; OR, odds ratio; CI, confidence interval.
P value in bold was less than 0.05 which was regarded as statistically significant.

when VKH patients were compared with controls. L-phenylalanine, D-arginine, N-acetyl-L-aspartic acid, L-alanine, arginyl-cysteine, and L-arginine were differential amino acids for BD vs. controls.

Pathway Analysis of Differential Aqueous Metabolites

Subsequently, MetaboAnalyst was used to compare metabolic disturbances between VKH, BD, and the control groups (**Figure 4**). There were two metabolic pathways that were significantly perturbed when comparing VKH patients with controls, and three pathways when comparing BD patients with controls (**Table 3**). The aminoacyl-tRNA biosynthesis pathway was significantly altered in both VKH and BD as compared to controls. In addition, we found significant differences in pantothenate and coenzyme A (CoA) biosynthesis for VKH vs. control, and in D-arginine and D-ornithine metabolism and phenylalanine metabolism for BD vs. control.

DISCUSSION

In the present study, we found that aqueous humor from VKH and BD patients showed distinct metabolic profiles compared to senile cataract controls. After correction, 28 and 29 metabolites were differentially expressed for VKH vs. control and BD vs. control, respectively. Amino acids and fatty acids were the two most abundant differential metabolite categories. Also, significant alterations were found in several metabolic pathways, including aminoacyl-tRNA biosynthesis, pantothenate and CoA biosynthesis, D-arginine and D-ornithine metabolism and phenylalanine metabolism. Experimental verification is needed to validate the role of the pathways identified in this clinical study in the pathogenesis of uveitis. There are very good animal models of autoimmune uveitis (21–23) and further studies are planned to confirm our clinical findings in these models.

Fatty acids are of great importance for immune regulation and may contribute to the development of some autoimmune diseases (24–27). Previous studies have shown that serum oleic acid level and urine palmitic acid and oleic acid levels were significantly higher in BD (11, 28). Moreover, our recent studies in VKH disease identified that sweat palmitic acid level (10) and serum oleic acid level (unpublished data) were increased in VKH. In the current study aqueous palmitic acid and oleic acid levels were significantly higher in VKH and BD compared to controls. The elevated intraocular and peripheral levels of both palmitic acid and oleic acid levels observed in VKH and BD indicates that they may play an important role in the pathophysiology of uveitis. Further studies are needed to investigate the functions of these two fatty acids and their association in the pathogenesis of uveitis.

Amino acids are important protein building stones but can also play a role in the functioning of the immune system (29). It was reported that glutamine metabolism had a distinct role to promote Th17 cells but constrained Th1 cell differentiation (30). Moreover, alanine was recently found to be essential for early T cell activation and deprivation of it might impair T cell effector functions (31). Previous metabolic profiling of aqueous humor obtained from acute anterior uveitis and Posner–Schlossman syndrome patients showed differences concerning amino acid metabolism (32, 33). Our previous metabolomics study of sweat

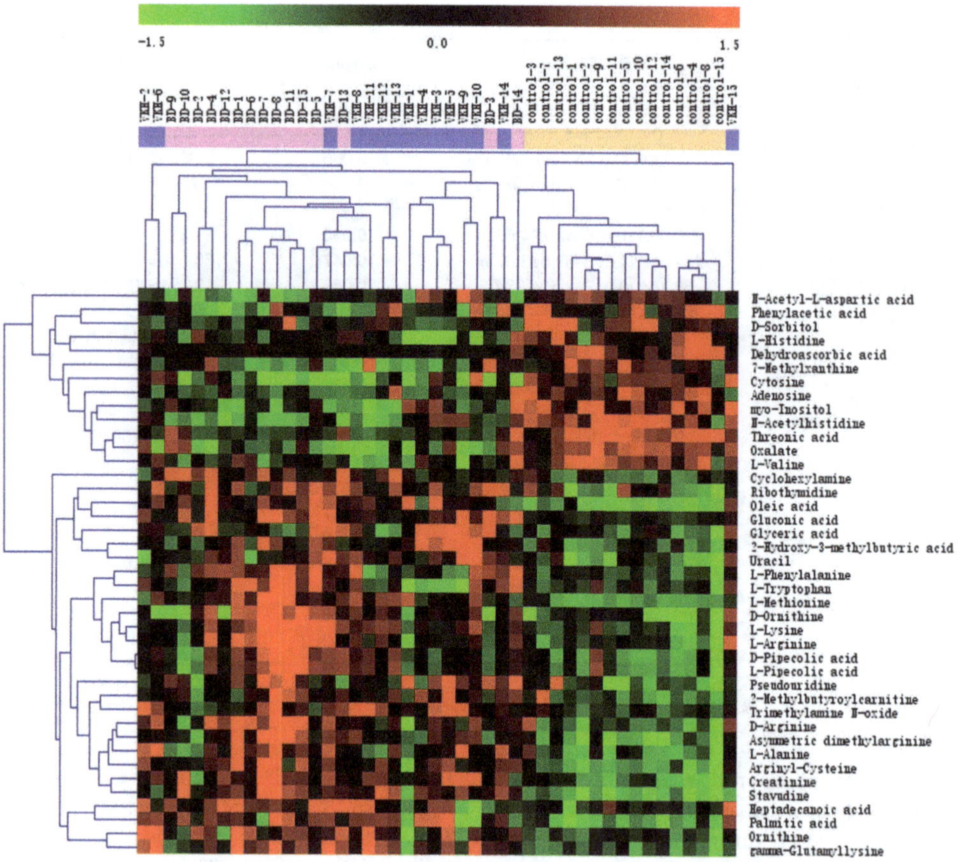

FIGURE 2 | Heat plot of the significantly differential metabolites among three groups. VKH, Vogt-Koyanagi-Harada disease; BD, Behcet's disease.

also revealed an important role for amino acid metabolism in the pathogenesis of VKH disease (10). In our present study, we found 12 and 15 amino acids were differentially expressed in VKH vs. control and BD vs. control, respectively. When compared to controls, D-arginine, D-ornithine, and L-phenylalanine, as well as its catabolite phenylacetic acid were significantly increased in BD patients, suggesting a possible role for the pathways regulating these specific amino acids in the pathogenesis of BD. Several studies have reported that the pantothenate and CoA biosynthesis pathway is associated with amino acid metabolism, whereby branched-chain amino acids provide CoA derivatives to enter the tricarboxylic acid cycle (29, 34, 35). The involvement of pantothenate and CoA biosynthesis was evident from a decrease in L-valine and increase in uracil that we observed in VKH compared to controls.

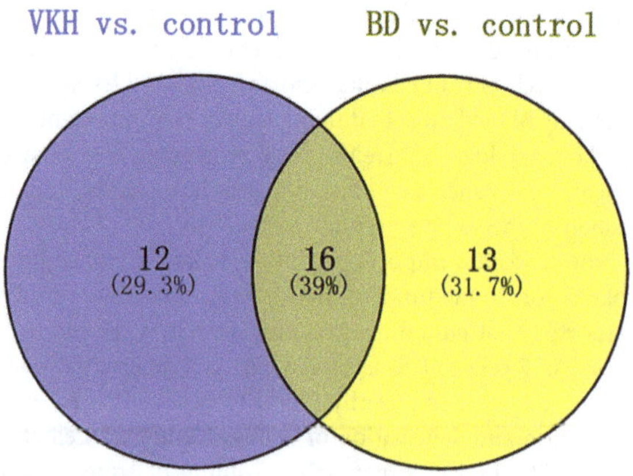

FIGURE 3 | Venn diagram of metabolites after logistic regression analyses adjusting which significantly differed in comparisons between VKH disease, BD, and control groups. VKH, Vogt-Koyanagi-Harada disease; BD, Behcet's disease.

Another interesting finding from our current study came from the analysis of Aminoacyl-tRNAs, which are the essential substrates that transport specific amino acids to incorporate them into the polypeptide chain produced during translation (36, 37). The aminoacyl-tRNA biosynthesis pathway is associated with various diseases, including several autoimmune diseases (38–40). Of interest is our finding that the most significant pathway in our study was aminoacyl-tRNA biosynthesis which involved L-Histidine, L-Methionine, L-Lysine and L-Valine for VKH, and L-Phenylalanine, L-Arginine, L-Methionine, L-Alanine, L-Lysine and L-Tryptophan for BD. Both VKH disease and BD showed an increase of L-Methionine and L-Lysine and the involvement of the associated

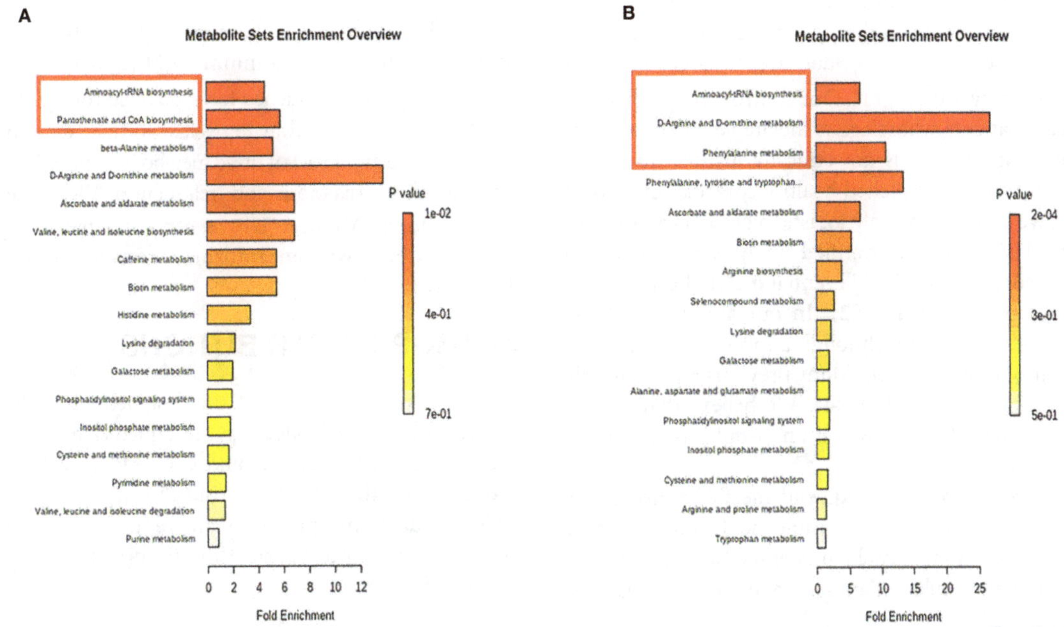

FIGURE 4 | Pathway analysis of the differential metabolites in Vogt-Koyanagi-Harada disease group **(A)** and Behcet's disease group **(B)**. The significantly perturbed pathways were in red rectangle.

aminoacyl-tRNA biosynthesis pathway (**Figure 3**). Therefore, we speculated that these two uveitis entities might share metabolic regulation pathways. Although these two uveitis entities show very specific features, they could be driven by common immunopathological mechanisms (41, 42).

There are several limitations in the current study. First, for ethical reasons, we used aqueous humor samples obtained during cataract surgery. Prior to cataract surgery for uveitis, the inflammation in these eyes has to be controlled and patients enrolled in our study are therefore in an inactive state. Despite this limitation, we do believe that the data are interesting because the composition of the aqueous humor can reflect the status of the basic intraocular environment in a uveitis patient. Second, the sample size used in our study may seem small, but aqueous humor is not easily accessible like serum or urine. In view of ethical considerations and current practice in our hospital, we only collected aqueous humor when the patient was undergoing an operation to remove a cataract from their eyes. These operations are not very frequently done and it therefore took us quite some time to collect the desired number of samples from these two well-defined uveitis entities. Most aqueous metabolomics studies in the field of ophthalmology consist of less than 30 samples in each group (32, 33). The relatively small sample size might limit the finding of other differentially expressed metabolites. This may explain why the significance of differential metabolites was lost when comparing VKH with BD. Both entities are very different from each other, both from a clinical and a pathological perspective (6). A larger population is therefore needed to validate the results in future. Third, patients enrolled in our study were still on treatment with a low dose of systemic corticosteroids and immunosuppressants and we cannot exclude an effect of treatment on our findings. It is not

TABLE 3 | The significantly altered pathways in Vogt-Koyanagi-Harada disease and Behcet's disease.

Pathways	VKH			BD		
	p value	Hit	Metabolites	*p* value	Hit	Metabolites
Aminoacyl-tRNA biosynthesis	0.01	4	L-Histidine, L-Methionine, L-Lysine, L-Valine	<0.001	6	L-Phenylalanine, L-Arginine, L-Methionine, L-Alanine, L-Lysine, L-Tryptophan
D-Arginine and D-ornithine metabolism	–	–	–	0.002	2	D-Arginine, D-Ornithine
Phenylalanine metabolism	–	–	–	0.014	2	L-Phenylalanine, Phenylacetic acid
Pantothenate and CoA biosynthesis	0.045	2	L-Valine, Uracil	–	–	–

VKH, Vogt-Koyanagi-Harada disease; BD, Behcet's disease.

ethical to terminate therapy in these patients for the mere purpose of research. On the other hand our data are different from those reported in an earlier study on glucocorticoid-induced metabolome changes (43), and are in agreement with metabolic studies in uveitis (10, 11). Our control group consisted of senile cataract patients whose age is inevitable older than our uveitis patients, but again, it is not ethically justified to collect aqueous samples from age matched healthy controls. In view of this limitation, we used a univariate logistic regression analysis to adjust for age. Using an age-stratified analysis we found no significant differences for the 41 differential metabolites between the different age groups (**Table S2**). In our study we set the accuracy m/z value at 25 ppm, although a more strict setting of 10 ppm might also have been used. Many previous reports in this field use a setting of 25 ppm (10, 44). We believe that several metabolites might have been missed if one would use a smaller accuracy m/z value.

In summary, we found specific aqueous metabolic profiles for VKH disease and BD. Differential amino acid and fatty acid expression in aqueous humor could play important roles in the pathogenesis of the intraocular inflammation in these two diseases.

ETHICS STATEMENT

The studies involving human participants were reviewed and approved by the Ethics Committee of the First Affiliated Hospital We further provide evidence for a possible role of the aminoacyl-tRNA biosynthesis pathway in uveitis. Further research is needed to investigate the exact role of these metabolites and relevant metabolic pathways in the diagnosis and treatment of VKH disease and BD. of Chongqing Medical University. The patients/participants provided their written informed consent to participate in this study.

AUTHOR CONTRIBUTIONS

PY and JX conceived the idea and designed the study. PY, JX, and QC contributed to collecting the aqueous humor and clinical data. JX, XH, RC, ZC, ZY, and GS performed the experiments and analyzed the data. JX wrote the manuscript. PY and AK reviewed data interpretation and edited the manuscript. All authors contributed to the article and approved the submitted version.

REFERENCES

1. Rothova A, Suttorp-van Schulten MS, Frits Treffers W, Kijlstra A. Causes and frequency of blindness in patients with intraocular inflammatory disease. *Br J Ophthalmol* (1996) 80:332–6. doi: 10.1136/bjo.80.4.332
2. McCluskey PJ, Towler HM, Lightman S. Management of chronic uveitis. *BMJ* (2000) 320:555–8. doi: 10.1136/bmj.320.7234.555
3. Yang P, Zhang Z, Zhou H, Li B, Huang X, Gao Y, et al. Clinical patterns and characteristics of uveitis in a tertiary center for uveitis in China. *Curr Eye Res* (2005) 30:943–8. doi: 10.1080/02713680500263606
4. Yang P, Zhong Z, Du L, Li F, Chen Z, Zhu Y, et al. Prevalence and clinical features of systemic diseases in Chinese patients with uveitis. *Br J Ophthalmol* (2021) 105:75–82. doi: 10.1136/bjophthalmol-2020-315960
5. Hwang DK, Chou YJ, Pu CY, Chou P. Epidemiology of uveitis among the Chinese population in Taiwan: a population-based study. *Ophthalmology* (2012) 119:2371–6. doi: 10.1016/j.ophtha.2012.05.026
6. Yang P, Ren Y, Li B, Fang W, Meng Q, Kijlstra A. Clinical characteristics of Vogt-Koyanagi-Harada syndrome in Chinese patients. *Ophthalmology* (2007) 114:606–14. doi: 10.1016/j.ophtha.2006.07.040
7. Yang P, Fang W, Meng Q, Ren Y, Xing L, Kijlstra A. Clinical features of chinese patients with Behçet's disease. *Ophthalmology* (2008) 115:312–8.e4. doi: 10.1016/j.ophtha.2007.04.056
8. Wishart DS. Metabolomics for Investigating Physiological and Pathophysiological Processes. *Physiol Rev* (2019) 99:1819–75. doi: 10.1152/physrev.00035.2018
9. Oldiges M, Lütz S, Pflug S, Schroer K, Stein N, Wiendahl C. Metabolomics: current state and evolving methodologies and tools. *Appl Microbiol Biotechnol* (2007) 76:495–511. doi: 10.1007/s00253-007-1029-2
10. Cui X, Su G, Zhang L, Yi S, Cao Q, Zhou C, et al. Integrated omics analysis of sweat reveals an aberrant amino acid metabolism pathway in Vogt-Koyanagi-Harada disease. *Clin Exp Immunol* (2020) 200:250–9. doi: 10.1111/cei.13435
11. Ahn JK, Kim J, Hwang J, Song J, Kim KH, Cha HS. Urinary Metabolomic Profiling to Identify Potential Biomarkers for the Diagnosis of Behcet's Disease by Gas Chromatography/Time-of-Flight-Mass Spectrometry. *Int J Mol Sci* (2017) 18:2039. doi: 10.3390/ijms18112309
12. Streilein JW. Ocular immune privilege: therapeutic opportunities from an experiment of nature. *Nat Rev Immunol* (2003) 3:879–89. doi: 10.1038/nri1224
13. Sindelar M, Patti GJ. Chemical Discovery in the Era of Metabolomics. *J Am Chem Soc* (2020) 142:9097–105. doi: 10.1021/jacs.9b13198
14. Fan Y, Li Y, Chen Y, Zhao YJ, Liu LW, Li J, et al. Comprehensive Metabolomic Characterization of Coronary Artery Diseases. *J Am Coll Cardiol* (2016) 68:1281–93. doi: 10.1016/j.jacc.2016.06.044
15. Gika HG, Theodoridis GA, Wingate JE, Wilson ID. Within-day reproducibility of an HPLC-MS-based method for metabonomic analysis: application to human urine. *J Proteome Res* (2007) 6:3291–303. doi: 10.1021/pr070183p
16. Yang P, Du L, Ye Z. How To Deal With Uveitis Patients? *Curr Mol Med* (2018) 17:468–70. doi: 10.2174/1566524018666180207153342
17. Read RW, Holland GN, Rao NA, Tabbara KF, Ohno S, Arellanes-Garcia L, et al. Revised diagnostic criteria for Vogt-Koyanagi-Harada disease: report of an international committee on nomenclature. *Am J Ophthalmol* (2001) 131:647–52. doi: 10.1016/s0002-9394(01)00925-4
18. Yang P, Zhong Y, Du L, Chi W, Chen L, Zhang R, et al. Development and Evaluation of Diagnostic Criteria for Vogt-Koyanagi-Harada Disease. *JAMA Ophthalmol* (2018) 136:1025–31. doi: 10.1001/jamaophthalmol.2018.2664
19. Criteria for diagnosis of Behçet's disease. International Study Group for Behçet's Disease. *Lancet* (1990) 335:1078–80.
20. Ji Y, Hu K, Li C, Li P, Kijlstra A, Eghrari AO, et al. Outcome and Prognostic Factors of Phacoemulsification Cataract Surgery in Vogt-Koyanagi-Harada Uveitis. *Am J Ophthalmol* (2018) 196:121–8. doi: 10.1016/j.ajo.2018.08.041
21. Luger D, Caspi RR. New perspectives on effector mechanisms in uveitis. *Semin Immunopathol* (2008) 30:135–43. doi: 10.1007/s00281-008-0108-5
22. Bing SJ, Shemesh I, Chong WP, Horai R, Jittayasothorn Y, Silver PB, et al. AS101 ameliorates experimental autoimmune uveitis by regulating Th1 and Th17 responses and inducing Treg cells. *J Autoimmun* (2019) 100:52–61. doi: 10.1016/j.jaut.2019.02.006
23. Qiu Y, Zhu Y, Yu H, Zhou C, Kijlstra A, Yang P. Dynamic DNA Methylation Changes of Tbx21 and Rorc during Experimental Autoimmune Uveitis in Mice. *Mediators Inflamm* (2018) 2018:9129163. doi: 10.1155/2018/9129163
24. Yaqoob P. Fatty acids as gatekeepers of immune cell regulation. *Trends Immunol* (2003) 24:639–45. doi: 10.1016/j.it.2003.10.002
25. Batista-Gonzalez A, Vidal R, Criollo A, Carreño LJ. New Insights on the Role of Lipid Metabolism in the Metabolic Reprogramming of Macrophages. *Front Immunol* (2019) 10:2993. doi: 10.3389/fimmu.2019.02993
26. Frommer KW, Schäffler A, Rehart S, Lehr A, Müller-Ladner U, Neumann E. Free fatty acids: potential proinflammatory mediators in rheumatic diseases. *Ann Rheum Dis* (2015) 74:303–10. doi: 10.1136/annrheumdis-2013-203755
27. Tsoukalas D, Fragoulakis V, Sarandi E, Docea AO, Papakonstaninou E, Tsilimidos G, et al. Targeted Metabolomic Analysis of Serum Fatty Acids for the Prediction of Autoimmune Diseases. *Front Mol Biosci* (2019) 6:120. doi: 10.3389/fmolb.2019.00120
28. Ahn JK, Kim J, Hwang J, Song J, Kim KH, Cha HS. Potential metabolomic biomarkers for reliable diagnosis of Behcet's disease using gas chromatography/ time-of-flight-mass spectrometry. *Joint Bone Spine* (2018) 85:337–43. doi: 10.1016/j.jbspin.2017.05.019

29. Kelly B, Pearce EL. Amino Assets: How Amino Acids Support Immunity. *Cell Metab* (2020) 32:154–75. doi: 10.1016/j.cmet.2020.06.010
30. Johnson MO, Wolf MM, Madden MZ, Andrejeva G, Sugiura A, Contreras DC, et al. Distinct Regulation of Th17 and Th1 Cell Differentiation by Glutaminase-Dependent Metabolism. *Cell* (2018) 175:1780–95.e19. doi: 10.1016/j.cell.2018.10.001
31. Ron-Harel N, Ghergurovich JM, Notarangelo G, LaFleur MW, Tsubosaka Y, Sharpe AH, et al. T Cell Activation Depends on Extracellular Alanine. *Cell Rep* (2019) 28:3011–21.e4. doi: 10.1016/j.celrep.2019.08.034
32. Verhagen FH, Stigter ECA, Pras-Raves ML, Burgering BMT, Imhof SM, Radstake T, et al. Aqueous Humor Analysis Identifies Higher Branched Chain Amino Acid Metabolism as a Marker for Human Leukocyte Antigen-B27 Acute Anterior Uveitis and Disease Activity. *Am J Ophthalmol* (2019) 198:97–110. doi: 10.1016/j.ajo.2018.10.004
33. Wang H, Zhai R, Sun Q, Wu Y, Wang Z, Fang J, et al. Metabolomic Profile of Posner-Schlossman Syndrome: A Gas Chromatography Time-of-Flight Mass Spectrometry-Based Approach Using Aqueous Humor. *Front Pharmacol* (2019) 10:1322. doi: 10.3389/fphar.2019.01322
34. Neinast MD, Jang C, Hui S, Murashige DS, Chu Q, Morscher RJ, et al. Quantitative Analysis of the Whole-Body Metabolic Fate of Branched-Chain Amino Acids. *Cell Metab* (2019) 29:417–29.e4. doi: 10.1016/j.cmet.2018.10.013
35. Zhou J, Tang L, Wang JS. Assessment of the adverse impacts of aflatoxin B(1) on gut-microbiota dependent metabolism in F344 rats. *Chemosphere* (2019) 217:618–28. doi: 10.1016/j.chemosphere.2018.11.044
36. Sheppard K, Yuan J, Hohn MJ, Jester B, Devine KM, Söll D. From one amino acid to another: tRNA-dependent amino acid biosynthesis. *Nucleic Acids Res* (2008) 36:1813–25. doi: 10.1093/nar/gkn015
37. Yao P, Fox PL. Aminoacyl-tRNA synthetases in medicine and disease. *EMBO Mol Med* (2013) 5:332–43. doi: 10.1002/emmm.201100626
38. Santos ALM, Vitório JG, de Paiva MJN, Porto BLS, Guimarães HC, Canuto GAB, et al. Frontotemporal dementia: Plasma metabolomic signature using gas chromatography-mass spectrometry. *J Pharm BioMed Anal* (2020) 189:113424. doi: 10.1016/j.jpba.2020.113424
39. Zhang Q, Yin X, Wang H, Wu X, Li X, Li Y, et al. Fecal Metabolomics and Potential Biomarkers for Systemic Lupus Erythematosus. *Front Immunol* (2019) 10:976. doi: 10.3389/fimmu.2019.00976
40. Koch MW, Ilnytskyy Y, Golubov A, Metz LM, Yong VW, Kovalchuk O. Global transcriptome profiling of mild relapsing-remitting versus primary progressive multiple sclerosis. *Eur J Neurol* (2018) 25:651–8. doi: 10.1111/ene.13565
41. Geri G, Terrier B, Rosenzwajg M, Wechsler B, Touzot M, Seilhean D, et al. Critical role of IL-21 in modulating TH17 and regulatory T cells in Behçet disease. *J Allergy Clin Immunol* (2011) 128:655–64. doi: 10.1016/j.jaci.2011.05.029
42. Li F, Yang P, Liu X, Wang C, Hou S, Kijlstra A. Upregulation of interleukin 21 and promotion of interleukin 17 production in chronic or recurrent Vogt-Koyanagi-Harada disease. *Arch Ophthalmol* (2010) 128:1449–54. doi: 10.1001/archophthalmol.2010.265
43. Bordag N, Klie S, Jürchott K, Vierheller J, Schiewe H, Albrecht V, et al. Glucocorticoid (dexamethasone)-induced metabolome changes in healthy males suggest prediction of response and side effects. *Sci Rep* (2015) 5:15954. doi: 10.1038/srep15954
44. Zhou X, Liu L, Lan X, Cohen D, Zhang Y, Ravindran AV, et al. Polyunsaturated fatty acids metabolism, purine metabolism and inosine as potential independent diagnostic biomarkers for major depressive disorder in children and adolescents. *Mol Psychiatry* (2019) 24:1478–88. doi: 10.1038/s41380-018-0047-z

5

Immunological Insights in Equine Recurrent Uveitis

Roxane L. Degroote and Cornelia A. Deeg*

Chair of Physiology, Department of Veterinary Sciences, LMU Munich, Munich, Germany

Correspondence:
Roxane L. Degroote
r.degroote@lmu.de

Horses worldwide suffer from equine recurrent uveitis (ERU), an organ-specific, immune-mediated disease with painful, remitting-relapsing inflammatory attacks alternating with periods of quiescence, which ultimately leads to blindness. In course of disease, both eyes can eventually be affected and since blind horses pose a threat to themselves and their surroundings, these animals have to be killed. Therefore, this disease is highly relevant for veterinary medicine. Additionally, ERU shows strong clinical and pathological resemblance to autoimmune uveitis in man. The exact cause for the onset of ERU is unclear to date. T cells are believed to be the main effector cells in this disease, as they overcome the blood retinal barrier to invade the eye, an organ physiologically devoid of peripheral immune cells. These cells cause severe intraocular inflammation, especially in their primary target, the retina. With every inflammatory episode, retinal degeneration increases until eyesight is completely lost. In ERU, T cells show an activated phenotype, with enhanced deformability and migration ability, which is reflected in the composition of their proteome and downstream interaction pathways even in quiescent stage of disease. Besides the dysregulation of adaptive immune cells, emerging evidence suggests that cells of the innate immune system may also directly contribute to ERU pathogenesis. As investigations in both the target organ and the periphery have rapidly evolved in recent years, giving new insights on pathogenesis-associated processes on cellular and molecular level, this review summarizes latest developments in ERU research.

Keywords: retina, Mueller glia, vitreous, serum, lymphocyte, granulocyte, complement system, cytokines

INTRODUCTION

Insights in the pathogenesis of equine recurrent uveitis (ERU) have grown in recent years, especially on cellular and molecular level in periphery and in the eye itself. ERU is an organ-specific, immune-mediated disease, which is predominantly driven by CD4+ T cells (1–3). These are somehow activated in periphery and then manage to overcome the blood retinal barrier (BRB), entering the eye and causing intraocular inflammation (4). Since ERU has a remitting-relapsing character (2), increasing numbers of immune cells invade and accumulate in the eye with every inflammatory attack, gradually destroying their main target, the retina. These acute phases alternate with periods of quiescence and increase in severity as the disease progresses (5). Factors associating to ERU onset are still discussed and an exact cause is elusive to date. A genome-wide association study suggested a correlation of genetic variants influencing the expression of IL-17A and IL-17F with the development of ERU (6). This study also substantiated previous reports linking ERU to MHC class I haplotype ELA-A9 in warmblood horses (7). Direct evidence for a genetic component in ERU of warmblood horses, however, is still lacking. Disease prevalence among the horse population is high, ranging from 2%–25% in the US and 8%–10% in Europe (5, 8). ERU often affects both eyes and eventually leads to blindness if left untreated (9). These two factors, high prevalence and loss of sight, explain its importance for veterinary medicine, since blind horses have to be killed due to the threat they pose to their surroundings and themselves, which has a great personal but also economic impact on horse owners. Moreover, ERU has great potential to serve as a valuable spontaneous model for autoimmune uveitis in man, due to strong clinical and pathological similarities (3, 4, 10, 11).

In the past, several studies could show that the dysregulated immune response in ERU is directed against retinal autoantigens such as interphotoreceptor retinoid-binding protein (IRBP) and cellular retinaldehyde-binding protein (CRALBP) (4, 12), which, along with other factors, suggests presence of autoimmune reactions in ERU. These autoantigens not only remain stably expressed in advanced stages of ERU, when retinal architecture is drastically destructed (13), IRBP can also induce experimental uveitis in the horse itself, which shows close similarity to the spontaneous disease on clinical, cellular and molecular level (4, 14). Moreover, studies on ERU horses firstly provided CRALBP as novel autoantigen (12), which was subsequently proven to also have high prevalence in human patients with autoimmune uveitis (15). As shown in previous studies, the recognition of these autoantigens and the subsequent spreading of epitope recognition to a new determinant may be the cause for the relapsing character of ERU (12, 16). This process known as epitope spreading describes the reaction of immune cells against the initial epitope of an ERU autoantigen, which then redirects against a different, but structurally similar epitope, re-initializing an inflammatory response after the initial inflammation has subsided (17, 18).

In addition to the retinal-autoantigen specific T cells driving ERU from periphery, further studies suggested that the retina itself promotes the intraocular inflammatory processes through active abundance downscaling of proteins which protect the maintenance of the blood-retina-barrier (19) and through secretion of the pro inflammatory cytokine interferon gamma (IFNγ) by retinal Mueller glial cells (20). Since then, research has advanced on the target organ of ERU as well as the cellular and molecular components in periphery. This review summarizes the latest immunological insights in ERU pathogenesis.

PERIPHERY

Adaptive Immune System

Although the concept of immune privilege is increasingly discussed since its initial description (21, 22), the eye is considered to be an immune privileged organ (23, 24), and is therefore usually devoid of immune cells form peripheral blood stream. In ERU, however, we find major cell infiltrates in the eye (2, 3, 25–27), which mainly consist of CD4+ lymphocytes (2, 27). To date, the exact mechanisms enabling these autoreactive cells to overcome the BRB in ERU are still elusive. Experimental autoimmune uveitis (EAU) is a valuable tool to investigate these mechanisms, not only in common rodent models (28–31), but to a certain extent also in the horse (4). Immunization of healthy horses with the retinal autoantigen IRBP mimics the spontaneous disease through the formation of auto-aggressive, IRBP specific T cells, which leave the peripheral blood stream to invade the eye directly prior to a uveitic attack (4). These cells show distinct protein changes before immunization, during the inflammatory phase and in quiescent episodes (14), which points to a highly dynamic functional phenotype depending on the stage of disease. During quiescence of this IRBP induced equine EAU, protein abundance changes in immune cells show many similarities to those observed in freshly obtained cells from horses in quiescent stage of ERU (14), underlining the close resemblance of the spontaneous and the induced disease in the horse. Although this type of induced horse model may allow more in depth investigations on ERU pathomechanisms, which is especially interesting for assessment of protein and cellular dynamics throughout the different stages of ERU, it is less suitable for large-scale experiments comparable to those performed on the several existing rodent models for autoimmune uveitis.

Analysis of primary T cells from horses with spontaneously occurring ERU revealed distinct proteome changes, mainly of proteins with a role in cell adhesion, cell migration and regulation of cell shape (32–34). In transmigration experiments, CD4+ T cells from ERU horses showed increased migration rates, which was linked to increased expression of the protein formin-like 1 (FMNL1) in the membranes of these cells (33). As shown in a new FMNL1 knock-out mouse model, FMNL1 deficiency impedes extravasation and trafficking of T cells to sites of inflammation (35), further undermining the importance of this protein and its functional effects in ERU pathogenesis. Furthermore, lymphocytes from ERU horses displayed significantly higher cell motility, cell speed and directness toward selected chemoattractants, especially IFNγ, and toward the ERU autoantigen CRALBP, in live-cell imaging experiments (36), which was associated to lower abundance of the protein septin 7 in these cells (32, 36). Previous studies on septin 7-depleted murine CD4+ T cells (clone D10.G4, as well as primary T cells from DO11.10 TCR transgenic mice), showed less rigidity and aberrant cell morphology in these depleted cells, resulting in the ability to migrate through narrow pores (37), which was also hypothesized for ERU (32), but never directly proven. Identification of interactors of septin 7, most importantly dedicator of cytokinesis 8 (DOCK8), which was decreased in ERU (34), pointed to impaired immunity and increased risk for recurrent inflammation, as suggested in studies on human cells from patients with DOCK8 deficiency (38). Furthermore, increased expression of DOCK8 interacting protein integrin-linked kinase (ILK) was functionally associated to a decreased apoptosis rate in ERU cells (34). Combined results from these *in vitro* experiments - increased life span, increased migratory reactivity toward chemokines and autoantigens and enhanced migration ability of

ERU lymphocytes - underlines the dysregulated nature of these cells in ERU. Although the transfer of these interpretations from *in vitro* experiments to *in vivo* mechanisms needs to be assessed with care, these insights further support the role of CD4+ T cells as key players in ERU pathogenesis.

Recent studies showed that, although percentage of CD3+, CD8+, and CD4+ lymphocytes does not differ between healthy horses and those with ERU, only the disease-driving CD4+ T cells have an activated phenotype in ERU horses (39). These cells show significantly increased expression levels of IFNγ and decreased expression of IL-10, indicating Th1 immune response (39). This supports previous findings of increased levels of IFNγ as well as cytokine Interferon gamma-induced protein 10 (IP-10) in serum of ERU horses (40). A further known immune response in autoimmune uveitis in man as well as EAU in rodents is mediated through Th17 cells (41). In ERU, the exact role of Th17 cells has not been established to date, however, detection of cytokines IL-6, IL-17, and IL-23 *via* crossreactive anti-human antibodies in histological sections of the iris and the ciliary body of ERU horses provide first indications pointing toward a contribution of these cells to ERU pathogenesis (42). Similar conclusions could be drawn from *M. tuberculosis* (strain H37Ra) induced experimental uveitis in horses, where high levels of IL-17 were detected in aqueous humor and vitreous *via* Enzyme-linked Immunosorbent Assay (ELISA) (43).

Contrary to the Th1 and/or Th17 immune response inducing and maintaining inflammation in the uveitic eye, remission of each inflammatory bout in autoimmune uveitis and EAU can be associated to T regulatory cells (Treg) (44–46). During an acute inflammatory uveitic attack, these cells show decreased abundance in peripheral blood as opposed to phases of quiescence, suggesting a crucial role in the remitting-relapsing character of autoimmune uveitis (47, 48). These differences, however, could not be detected in peripheral blood of ERU horses compared to healthy controls (39). To date, no direct evidence for Tregs in the equine eye could be found. Nevertheless, the role of Treg in periodic remission of ERU is highly probable and thus merits further investigations.

Although an autoreactive Th1 response against retinal antigens is widely supported as the key process in ERU pathogenesis, one pivotal question remains: how can peripheral T cells be primed against tissue specific self-antigens which are "hidden" in an immune privileged organ? Emerging investigations on autoimmune uveitis suggest that commensal microbiota, if dysregulated (dysbiosis), may show sequence similarities with self-antigens (49, 50). This in turn may induce T cell cross-activation and priming against retina-specific antigens, triggering autoimmune reactions (49, 50). Other studies suggest, that a healthy gut microbiome is needed for prevention of autoimmunity through Treg homeostasis and that dysbiosis leads to changed or insufficiently effective Treg populations (51, 52). In ERU, the involvement of commensal microbiota has not been proven to date, however it is highly likely to play a possible role.

Equine T cell activation can be markedly reduced by co-incubation with adipose-derived equine mesenchymal stem cells (MSC) *in vitro*, resulting in downscaling of CD25 as well as intracellular IFNγ, IL-10, and FoxP3 (39). This feature of MSC might be useful for the development of new therapeutic approaches in ERU (53), as suggested by in equine immune-mediated keratitis, where subconjunctival injection of autologous MSCs improved clinical signs of disease (54). Although clinical application of this therapeutic strategy needs more in-depth validation, it might have the potential of broadening the currently applied methods of medical and surgical therapy, which classically comprise the systemical and topical application of immunosuppressive and anti-inflammatory medication, placement of a suprachoroidal cyclosporine sustainded-release device or pars plana vitrectomy (9, 55, 56).

Innate Immune System

The role of innate immune cells in autoimmune uveitis has been intensely investigated in the eyes of rodent EAU models (57–60) and infiltration of these cells in eyes of ERU horses, although to a lesser extent, has also been observed (3). The involvement of monocytes, which might promote pro-inflammatory behavior, as well as destruction of the targeted retinal cells in ERU could be shown by expression of CD68 on infiltrating peripheral immune cells in the diseased retina (61). Monocytes are major mediators of tissue damage in EAU (62, 63) and are potent antigen-presenting cells (64), which makes their role in ERU especially interesting, particularly in regard to their interaction with specific retinal cells (65). Further indication of participation of innate immune cells in ERU was proven by identification of decreased talin 1 abundance, a key integrin regulator in leukocytes, and its interacting proteins in low-density-neutrophils which were obtained as byproduct of lymphocyte isolation (25, 66). Targeted investigations of pure granulocyte fractions of healthy and ERU horses revealed significant proteome changes in diseased state, which associated to MHC-I-mediated antigen presentation, RAF/MAP kinase cascade, and neutrophil degranulation (67). Interestingly, increased neutrophil degranulation was also described in other T-cell driven autoimmune diseases, such as multiple sclerosis, where it is linked to a generally pre-activated state of these cells (68). Moreover, neutrophil degranulation relates to deviant equine granulocyte proteome after *in vitro* stimulation (69), underlining a latent state of activation of granulocytes in ERU, even in quiescent stage of disease (67). The fact that neutrophils from ERU horses more readily perform NETosis supports these findings (70). The exact role of innate immune cells and their timing in and impact on ERU pathogenesis, however, is still not completely understood to date and needs more in-depth investigation.

Implication of a role of the complement system was shown by the identification of several complement factors and split factors and their increased expression in ERU sera and eyes (19, 61, 71). Namely complement factor B, as well as C3 derived split products C3d and iC3b showed highly increased abundance, indicating strong activation of the complement system not only in the peripheral blood stream but also locally in the eye itself (61, 71). Although the exact source of these complement components in ERU eyes is still unclear, they might be macrophage-derived, as suggested by studies on human retinas from patients with age-related macular degeneration (AMD) and *in vivo* retina analyses of rodent models for AMD (72). Other studies on C57BL/6 mice showed that complement factor B is constitutively expressed by RPE cells and this expression is positively regulated by inflammatory cytokines in the human RPE cell line ARPE19 (73), a process which might also apply to the increased occurrence in ERU eyes. Deviant regulation of the complement system is involved in the pathogenesis of various ocular diseases, including autoimmune uveitis (74, 75) and the severity of experimental autoimmune uveitis drastically decreases in complement-receptor deficient rodent models (76–78). Moreover, EAU can be effectively suppressed in C57BL/6 mice when activation of complement *via* the alternative pathway is blocked through complement receptor CRIg-Fc. Since complement factor B is exclusive to the alternative pathway, increased intraocular levels in EAU suggest a role of this pathway in disease pathogenesis (79). Despite the high abundance of complement factor B in uveitic horse eyes, indicating a possible contribution of the alternative pathway to ERU pathogenesis, this correlation has not yet been assessed.

Serum Proteins

In the last decade, proteomic studies on sera of ERU diseased horses revealed substantial differences compared to sera of healthy horses (80). Due to breakdown of the BRB in course of multiple uveitic attacks, several of these proteins can also be detected inside the eye (3, 71, 81, 82).

Among these differentially expressed proteins, kininogen was identified with decreased abundance in sera of ERU horses (71). Contrary to this, kininogen showed increased levels in vitreous and retina in ERU, whereas it was not detectable in healthy eyes (71). Kininogen promotes angiogenesis and neovascularization (83), a process that plays a significant role in the pathogenesis of autoimmune uveitis (71). It is also a part of the kallikrein-kinin system, which promotes integrity loss of barrier systems, such as the blood-brain-barrier in a mouse model of multiple sclerosis (84). Increased vitreal and retinal kininogen levels combined with a decrease in serum of ERU horses therefore points to disruption of the BRB in course of disease. IgM levels were also increased in ERU sera compared to healthy horses, suggesting a recent immune response pattern prior to blood sampling (71).

Decreased levels of pigment epithelium derived factor (PEDF) could be shown in sera of ERU horses (82), which was also observed in the retina and the vitreous of these animals in earlier studies (19, 20). PEDF was also decreased in plasma and retina from rats with endotoxin-induced uveitis, describing PEDF as a negative acute-phase protein (85). Furthermore, PEDF plays an important role in the viability of rat and mouse retinal cells (86, 87), the protection of human retinal pigment epithelium cells (ARPE-19 cell line) against oxidative stress (88) and the protection of tight junction proteins in rat eyes (85). Therefore, the decrease of PEDF in periphery as well as the target organ suggests increased permeability of the blood retinal-barrier.

TARGET ORGAN

Retinal Pigment Epithelium

Increased BRB permeability in ERU is supported by studies on the outer BRB, which physiologically maintains ocular immune privilege through disconnection of the inner eye from peripheral blood-derived immune cells (24). The outer BRB is formed by retinal pigment epithelium (RPE) cells, which play a crucial role in the mainly avascular retina of the horse, since they maintain homeostasis of retinal cells (89). This is also reflected in the RPE surface proteome, which strongly associates to transport processes (90). Furthermore, horses with ERU display a distinctly changed RPE membrane protein repertoire in ERU (91). A significant decrease of peripherin 2, a protein that is associated with membrane fusion processes, in RPE cells of ERU horses is thought to provoke disruption of the cell-to-cell junctions which are physiolocically maintained through these cells (92), which in turn points to increased permeability of the outer BRB. As also hypothesized for PEDF (19, 20, 82), this might promote integrity loss of the BRB. Although loss of barrier function of the BRB and leukocyte infiltration in course of ERU is evident (4, 27, 91, 92), the exact chronological order of these events is still not completely clear. Integrity loss of the BRB may occur either as an initial process which subsequently facilitates migration of peripheral immune cells into the eye, or as a secondary effect in response to leukocyte recruitment. The latter could be shown in an IRBP-induced B10.RIII mouse EAU model, where Evans blue dye, which was injected shortly before killing of the mice, could be observed leaking into the retinal parenchyma only after intravascular sticking and extravasation of blood-derived leukocytes from retinal venules took place (93). Further studies on murine EAU models implied that BRB breakdown might be a result of several consecutive steps, actively triggered by intravascular adherence of primed lymphocytes, followed by changed expression of adhesion molecules and chemokine receptors in the vascular epithelium and reduced shear stress in retinal veins prior to infiltration (93–97). Interestingly, adoptive transfer of EAU in lewis rats could show that antigen specificity for retinal antigens is not a prerequisite for migration of activated T cells through the BRB, however, for the induction of actual intraocular inflammation, it is indispensable (98).

Retina and Vitreous

After infiltrating the eye, peripheral immune cells accumulate in the iris, ciliary body and retina of horses with ERU (4, 27). Although the vast majority of the infiltrating cells were identified as CD4+ T cells (2, 27), pure granulocyte infiltrates can be observed in few spontaneous ERU and IRBP induced cases (3, 4). This is in stark contrast to the composition of the cellular infiltrate in IRBP-induced murine EAU models, where a more heterogeneous cell infiltrate can be observed, containing around 30% CD4+ T cells and a high percentage of macrophages (99, 100). This points to different molecular pathways and cellular processes in EAU and ERU, underlining the great variability of disease pathogenesis between species, which needs to be kept in mind while interpreting associated data. In the base of the ciliary body and the iris of ERU horses, the infiltrated cells organize into lymphoid follicle nodules, which predominantly comprise CD3+ T cells (26, 27). In the retina, we mostly see scattered areas of T cell infiltration, especially near the ora ciliaris retinae and the optic disc, but occasional lymphoid follicle formation is also observed (27). Interestingly, the majority of infiltrated CD4+ lymphocytes in the ERU retina also show surface expression of CD166, a molecule associated with activation and transmigration of T cells into inflamed tissues (26). Presence of phosphorylated signal transducer and activator of transcription (STAT) proteins 1 and 5 in these cells underline the role of activated Th1 cells in ERU but also indirectly point toward inhibition of the Th17 pathway (26). Detection of IL-6, IL-17, and IL-23 in cell infiltrates of the ciliary body and iris, on the other hand, indirectly suggests that a Th17 mediated immune reaction might also present in ERU eyes (42). In rodent models, EAU can develop either as a Th1 or a Th17 response depending on the model and the antigen used for induction, showing the importance of both T cell subpopulations in disease pathogenesis (41, 101–104). In ERU, on the other hand, the important role of Th1 lymphocytes as effector cells is well known (2, 3, 36), the exact impact of Th17 cells on disease pathogenesis, however, merits further investigations.

Through membrane proteome analyses of equine retinae, numerous differentially expressed proteins were identified in ERU, several of which were associated to retinal Mueller glia cell derived proteins (105). Retinal Mueller glia cells, the main macroglial cells of the retina, are indispensable for the maintenance of retinal function and integrity (106). Apart from their proinflammatory role in ERU (20) and in murine EAU (65), these cells display a gliotic phenotype, which presents with morphological changes and impaired functionality in diseased retinae (12, 20, 105, 107). One of the important functions of these cells is the regulation of potassium and water homeostasis in the retina (108, 109), which shows severe misbalance in ERU (105, 107). This is mirrored in changed abundance and distribution pattern of potassium channels Kir4.1 and Kir2.1 as well as water channels AQP4, AQP5, and AQP11 which is hypothesized to contribute to impaired Mueller cell function and intracellular fluid regulation and, subsequently, retinal edema (105, 107, 110), a severe complication of ERU (27). Furthermore, in ERU, dysfunctional RMG are connected to decreased secretion of Wnt signaling inhibitors DKK3 and SFRP2, which point to a regulatory role of Wnt signaling in ERU (111), similar to other autoimmune diseases (112, 113). These insights on RMG support the role of these cells as prime responders to autoimmune triggers in ERU, promoting inflammatory processes and increasing severity of disease pathogenesis.

Additionally, severe extracellular matrix (ECM) remodeling in ERU was suggested through the identification of the proteins fibronectin and osteopontin (OPN) (105, 114). Fibronectin is an important constituent of the vertebrate ECM, mediates cell-ECM interactions (115) and also plays a role in adhesion and migration of cultured rat Mueller cells (116). Since fibronectin expression in Mueller cell endfeet might contribute to the attachment of the retina to the vitreous body, the changed distribution of fibronectin in ERU retinae points to impaired Mueller cell adhesion (114). OPN is a multifunctional protein with pro-inflammatory as well as neuroprotective properties (117, 118). In EAU mice, an increased abundance of OPN correlates with severity of inflammation (119), whereas Mueller glia-derived OPN promotes photoreceptor survival in the Pde6brd1 mouse model of retinal degeneration (120). OPN also shows neuroprotective properties in porcine Mueller glia cells *in vitro* (121). Decreased expression of OPN in vitreous and retina might therefore point to reduced neuroprotection in ERU retinae (114). ERU-associated lack of neuroprotection in the retina was underlined by the identification of decreased levels and decreased activity of tissue inhibitor of metalloproteinases (TIMP)-2 in retina and vitreous (122). TIMP2 influences the activity of metalloproteinases (MMP) (123), which modulate cell-cell and cell-ECM interactions (124). It also has neuroprotective properties (125) and can inhibit migration of cells over physiological barriers (126). Hence, decrease in TIMP2 activity might promote the inflammatory responses in ERU. It has been shown that migrating immune cells, especially Th1 cells, increase their MMP2 and MMP9 expression to overcome blood-tissue barriers (127) and that inhibition of these MMPs ameliorates experimental autoimmune uveitis in rodent models (128, 129). Interestingly, infiltrating cells in ERU retinae stained highly positive for MMP9 (122).

Apart from high levels of IgG in eyes of ERU horses (3), ERU vitreous also contains various immunoglobulins of the subclass M (IgM), which show a broad reaction pattern against retinal proteins (81), whereas healthy eyes contain no IgM (or IgG). Since IgM is an activator of the complement system and complement has been proven to be highly present in the inner eye of ERU horses (61, 111), the presence of IgM in the ERU vitreous further implies involvement of innate immune system components in this T cell driven autoimmune disease. Further screening of retinal protein with vitreous from ERU horses provided potential retinal autoantigens which are targeted by IgM autoantibodies (81). One of these IgM targets was identified as neurofilament medium (NF-M) (81, 130). Interestingly, IgG response to NF-M was merely detectable, supporting the presence of a thymus-independent immune reaction with prolonged persistence of IgM response toward NF-M and lack of IgM/IgG switch (130). In the retina, on the other hand, NF-M showed decreased expression (130). The combination of active downscaling in damaged RMG and release of NF-M fragments into the adjacent vitreous might cause this combination of high vitreal occurrence and low retinal levels of NF-M (130). A further novel membrane-bound autoantigen, synaptotagmin-1, was identified with decreased expression in ERU (131), which might be a result of active downscaling of this protein in the retina through impaired neurotransmitter release in ERU. Since Synaptotagmin-1 is also expressed in the pineal gland, and pinealitis is known to concurrently develop in ERU horses (132), synaptotagmin-1 might play a role in pineal immunopathology in ERU (131). Whether these IgM-targeted retinal antigens qualify as autoantigen targets for ERU, however, remains to be proven in further studies.

CONCLUSIONS

Overall, these novel immunological insights in ERU pathogenesis point to a complex interplay of several dysregulated mechanisms, which, on the one hand, can be linked to changes in cellular and humoral components of the immune system, such as a deviant functional phenotype of T cells with increased migratory ability and a decreased apoptosis rate, latently activated granulocytes and involvement of the alternative pathway of the complement system. On the other hand, this dysregulation points to a pivotal pro-inflammatory role of retinal cells with critically impaired function in the target organ itself. Although these findings shed more light on disease mechanisms, the interaction of these dysfunctional molecular mechanisms driving ERU as well as their exact individual role and timing in ERU pathogenesis needs further assessment. Establishment of a Mueller glia cell line (133) and characterization of cultured RPE cells (90) provide valuable tools for more in depth functional examinations of ERU pathology. Additionally, the possibility of commensal microbiota involvement in ERU onset needs to be addressed.

AUTHOR CONTRIBUTIONS

CD conceived the outline of the manuscript. CD and RD wrote the manuscript. All authors contributed to the article and approved the submitted version.

REFERENCES

1. Romeike A, Brugmann M, Drommer W. Immunohistochemical studies in equine recurrent uveitis (ERU). *Vet Pathol* (1998) 35(6):515–26. doi: 10.1177/030098589803500606
2. Gilger BC, Malok E, Cutter KV, Stewart T, Horohov DW, Allen JB. Characterization of T-lymphocytes in the anterior uvea of eyes with chronic equine recurrent uveitis. *Vet Immunol Immunopathol* (1999) 71 (1):17–28. doi: 10.1016/S0165-2427(99)00082-3
3. Deeg CA, Kaspers B, Gerhards H, Thurau SR, Wollanke B, Wildner G. Immune responses to retinal autoantigens and peptides in equine recurrent uveitis. *Invest Ophthalmol Vis Sci* (2001) 42(2):393–8.
4. Deeg CA, Thurau SR, Gerhards H, Ehrenhofer M, Wildner G, Kaspers B. Uveitis in horses induced by interphotoreceptor retinoid-binding protein is similar to the spontaneous disease. *Eur J Immunol* (2002) 32(9):2598–606. doi: 10.1002/1521-4141(200209)32:9<2598::AID-IMMU2598>3.0.CO;2-#
5. Gerding JC, Gilger BC. Prognosis and impact of equine recurrent uveitis. *Equine Vet J* (2016) 48(3):290–8. doi: 10.1111/evj.12451
6. Kulbrock M, Lehner S, Metzger J, Ohnesorge B, Distl O. A genome-wide association study identifies risk loci to equine recurrent uveitis in German warmblood horses. *PloS One* (2013) 8(8):e71619. doi: 10.1371/journal.pone.0071619
7. Deeg CA, Marti E, Gaillard C, Kaspers B. Equine recurrent uveitis is strongly associated with the MHC class I haplotype ELA-A9. *Equine Vet J* (2004) 36 (1):73–5. doi: 10.2746/0425164044864651
8. Spiess BM. Equine recurrent uveitis: the European viewpoint. *Equine Vet J Suppl* (2010) 37:50–6. doi: 10.1111/j.2042-3306.2010.tb05635.x
9. McMullen RJJr., Fischer BM. Medical and Surgical Management of Equine Recurrent Uveitis. *Vet Clin North Am Equine Pract* (2017) 33(3):465–81. doi: 10.1016/j.cveq.2017.07.003
10. Deeg CA, Hauck SM, Amann B, Pompetzki D, Altmann F, Raith A, et al. Equine recurrent uveitis–a spontaneous horse model of uveitis. *Ophthalmic Res* (2008) 40(3-4):151–3. doi: 10.1159/000119867
11. Neutzner RV, Jager M, Friedburg C, Deeg CA, Lorenz B. [Blind spot enlargement syndrome in acute zonal occult outer retinopathy with detection of autoantibodies against the retinal antigens CRALBP and S-Ag]. *Ophthalmologe* (2011) 108(11):1045–9. doi: 10.1007/s00347-011-2406-x
12. Deeg CA, Pompetzki D, Raith AJ, Hauck SM, Amann B, Suppmann S, et al. Identification and functional validation of novel autoantigens in equine uveitis. *Mol Cell Proteomics* (2006) 5(8):1462–70. doi: 10.1074/mcp.M500352-MCP200 doi: M500352-MCP200 [pii].
13. Deeg CA, Hauck SM, Amann B, Kremmer E, Stangassinger M, Ueffing M. Major retinal autoantigens remain stably expressed during all stages of spontaneous uveitis. *Mol Immunol* (2007) 44(13):3291–6. doi: 10.1016/j.molimm.2007.02.027 doi: S0161-5890(07)00096-X [pii].
14. Hauck SM, Lepper MF, Hertl M, Sekundo W, Deeg CA. Proteome Dynamics in Biobanked Horse Peripheral Blood Derived Lymphocytes (PBL) with Induced Autoimmune Uveitis. *Proteomics* (2017) 17(19):1–5. doi: 10.1002/pmic.201700013
15. Deeg CA, Raith AJ, Amann B, Crabb JW, Thurau SR, Hauck SM, et al. CRALBP is a highly prevalent autoantigen for human autoimmune uveitis. *Clin Dev Immunol* (2007) 2007:39245. doi: 10.1155/2007/39245
16. Deeg CA, Amann B, Raith AJ, Kaspers B. Inter- and intramolecular epitope spreading in equine recurrent uveitis. *Invest Ophthalmol Vis Sci* (2006) 47 (2):652–6. doi: 10.1167/iovs.05-0789 doi: 47/2/652 [pii].
17. Vanderlugt CJ, Miller SD. Epitope spreading. *Curr Opin Immunol* (1996) 8 (6):831–6. doi: 10.1016/s0952-7915(96)80012-4
18. Ujiie H, Yoshimoto N, Natsuga K, Muramatsu K, Iwata H, Nishie W, et al. Immune Reaction to Type XVII Collagen Induces Intramolecular and Intermolecular Epitope Spreading in Experimental Bullous Pemphigoid Models. *Front Immunol* (2019) 10:1410. doi: 10.3389/fimmu.2019.01410
19. Deeg CA, Altmann F, Hauck SM, Schoeffmann S, Amann B, Stangassinger M, et al. Down-regulation of pigment epithelium-derived factor in uveitic lesion associates with focal vascular endothelial growth factor expression and breakdown of the blood-retinal barrier. *Proteomics* (2007) 7(9):1540–8. doi: 10.1002/pmic.200600795
20. Hauck SM, Schoeffmann S, Amann B, Stangassinger M, Gerhards H, Ueffing M, et al. Retinal Mueller glial cells trigger the hallmark inflammatory process in autoimmune uveitis. *J Proteome Res* (2007) 6(6):2121–31. doi: 10.1021/pr060668y
21. Forrester JV, Xu H. Good news-bad news: the Yin and Yang of immune privilege in the eye. *Front Immunol* (2012) 3:338. doi: 10.3389/fimmu.2012.00338
22. Forrester JV, McMenamin PG, Dando SJ. CNS infection and immune privilege. *Nat Rev Neurosci* (2018) 19(11):655–71. doi: 10.1038/s41583-018-0070-8
23. Streilein JW, Takeuchi M, Taylor AW. Immune privilege, T-cell tolerance, and tissue-restricted autoimmunity. *Hum Immunol* (1997) 52(2):138–43. doi: 10.1016/S0198-8859(96)00288-1 doi: S0198-8859(96)00288-1 [pii].
24. Taylor AW, Ng TF. Negative regulators that mediate ocular immune privilege. *J Leukoc Biol* (2018) 103(6)1179–87. doi: 10.1002/JLB.3MIR0817-337R
25. Degroote RL, Hauck SM, Treutlein G, Amann B, Frohlich KJ, Kremmer E, et al. Expression Changes and Novel Interaction Partners of Talin 1 in Effector Cells of Autoimmune Uveitis. *J Proteome Res* (2013) 12(12):5812–9. doi: 10.1021/pr400837f
26. Kleinwort KJ, Amann B, Hauck SM, Feederle R, Sekundo W, Deeg CA. Immunological Characterization of Intraocular Lymphoid Follicles in a Spontaneous Recurrent Uveitis Model. *Invest Ophthalmol Vis Sci* (2016) 57(10):4504–11. doi: 10.1167/iovs.16-19787

27. Deeg CA, Ehrenhofer M, Thurau SR, Reese S, Wildner G, Kaspers B. Immunopathology of recurrent uveitis in spontaneously diseased horses. *Exp Eye Res* (2002) 75(2):127–33. doi: 10.1006/exer.2002.2011
28. Caspi RR, Roberge FG, McAllister CG, el-Saied M, Kuwabara T, Gery I, et al. T cell lines mediating experimental autoimmune uveoretinitis (EAU) in the rat. *J Immunol* (1986) 136(3):928–33.
29. Palestine AG, Mc Allister C, Carter C, Keenan AM, Vistica B, Gery I, et al. Lymphocyte migration in the adoptive transfer of EAU. *Invest Ophthalmol Vis Sci* (1986) 27(4):611–5.
30. Caspi RR. Th1 and Th2 responses in pathogenesis and regulation of experimental autoimmune uveoretinitis. *Int Rev Immunol* (2002) 21(2-3):197–208. doi: 10.1080/08830180212063
31. Caspi RR, Chan CC, Fujino Y, Najafian F, Grover S, Hansen CT, et al. Recruitment of antigen-nonspecific cells plays a pivotal role in the pathogenesis of a T cell-mediated organ-specific autoimmune disease, experimental autoimmune uveoretinitis. *J Neuroimmunol* (1993) 47 (2):177–88. doi: 10.1016/0165-5728(93)90028-w
32. Degroote RL, Hauck SM, Amann B, Hirmer S, Ueffing M, Deeg CA. Unraveling the equine lymphocyte proteome: differential septin 7 expression associates with immune cells in equine recurrent uveitis. *PloS One* (2014) 9(3):e91684. doi: 10.1371/journal.pone.0091684
33. Degroote RL, Uhl PB, Amann B, Krackhardt AM, Ueffing M, Hauck SM, et al. Formin like 1 expression is increased on CD4+ T lymphocytes in spontaneous autoimmune uveitis. *J Proteomics* (2017) 154:102–8. doi: 10.1016/j.jprot.2016.12.015
34. Schauer M, Kleinwort KJH, Degroote RL, Wiedemann C, Kremmer E, Hauck SM, et al. Interaction of septin 7 and DOCK8 in equine lymphocytes reveals novel insights into signaling pathways associated with autoimmunity. *Sci Rep* (2018) 8(1):12332. doi: 10.1038/s41598-018-30753-7
35. Thompson SB, Sandor AM, Lui V, Chung JW, Waldman MM, Long RA, et al. Formin-like 1 mediates effector T cell trafficking to inflammatory sites to enable T cell-mediated autoimmunity. *Elife* (2020) 9:1–27. doi: 10.7554/eLife.58046
36. Wiedemann C, Amann B, Degroote RL, Witte T, Deeg CA. Aberrant Migratory Behavior of Immune Cells in Recurrent Autoimmune Uveitis in Horses. *Front Cell Dev Biol* (2020) 8:101. doi: 10.3389/fcell.2020.00101
37. Tooley AJ, Gilden J, Jacobelli J, Beemiller P, Trimble WS, Kinoshita M, et al. Amoeboid T lymphocytes require the septin cytoskeleton for cortical integrity and persistent motility. *Nat Cell Biol* (2009) 11(1):17–26. doi: 10.1038/ncb1808 doi: ncb1808 [pii].
38. Aydin SE, Kilic SS, Aytekin C, Kumar A, Porras O, Kainulainen L, et al. DOCK8 deficiency: clinical and immunological phenotype and treatment options - a review of 136 patients. *J Clin Immunol* (2015) 35(2):189–98. doi: 10.1007/s10875-014-0126-0
39. Saldinger LK, Nelson SG, Bellone RR, Lassaline M, Mack M, Walker NJ, et al. Horses with equine recurrent uveitis have an activated CD4+ T-cell phenotype that can be modulated by mesenchymal stem cells in vitro. *Vet Ophthalmol* (2020) 23(1):160–70. doi: 10.1111/vop.12704
40. Curto E, Messenger KM, Salmon JH, Gilger BC. Cytokine and chemokine profiles of aqueous humor and serum in horses with uveitis measured using multiplex bead immunoassay analysis. *Vet Immunol Immunopathol* (2016) 182:43–51. doi: 10.1016/j.vetimm.2016.09.008
41. Luger D, Silver PB, Tang J, Cua D, Chen Z, Iwakura Y, et al. Either a Th17 or a Th1 effector response can drive autoimmunity: conditions of disease induction affect dominant effector category. *J Exp Med* (2008) 205(4):799–810. doi: 10.1084/jem.20071258 doi: jem.20071258 [pii].
42. Regan DP, Aarnio MC, Davis WS, Carmichael KP, Vandenplas ML, Lauderdale JD, et al. Characterization of cytokines associated with Th17 cells in the eyes of horses with recurrent uveitis. *Vet Ophthalmol* (2012) 15 (3):145–52. doi: 10.1111/j.1463-5224.2011.00951.x
43. Simeonova GP, Krastev SZ, Simeonov RS. Immunological and pathological investigations in equine experimental uveitis. *Vet Res Commun* (2016) 40(3-4):107–15. doi: 10.1007/s11259-016-9659-4
44. Sharma A, Rudra D. Emerging Functions of Regulatory T Cells in Tissue Homeostasis. *Front Immunol* (2018) 9:883. doi: 10.3389/fimmu.2018.00883
45. Silver PB, Horai R, Chen J, Jittayasothorn Y, Chan CC, Villasmil R, et al. Retina-specific T regulatory cells bring about resolution and maintain remission of autoimmune uveitis. *J Immunol* (2015) 194(7):3011–9. doi: 10.4049/jimmunol.1402650
46. Gilbert RM, Zhang X, Sampson RD, Ehrenstein MR, Nguyen DX, Chaudhry M, et al. Clinical Remission of Sight-Threatening Non-Infectious Uveitis Is Characterized by an Upregulation of Peripheral T-Regulatory Cell Polarized Towards T-bet and TIGIT. *Front Immunol* (2018) 9:907. doi: 10.3389/fimmu.2018.00907
47. Ruggieri S, Frassanito MA, Dammacco R, Guerriero S. Treg lymphocytes in autoimmune uveitis. *Ocul Immunol Inflammation* (2012) 20(4):255–61. doi: 10.3109/09273948.2012.681830
48. Yeh S, Li Z, Forooghian F, Hwang FS, Cunningham MA, Pantanelli S, et al. CD4+Foxp3+ T-regulatory cells in noninfectious uveitis. *Arch Ophthalmol* (2009) 127(4):407–13. doi: 10.1001/archophthalmol.2009.32
49. Horai R, Zarate-Blades CR, Dillenburg-Pilla P, Chen J, Kielczewski JL, Silver PB, et al. Microbiota-Dependent Activation of an Autoreactive T Cell Receptor Provokes Autoimmunity in an Immunologically Privileged Site. *Immunity* (2015) 43(2):343–53. doi: 10.1016/j.immuni.2015.07.014
50. Horai R, Caspi RR. Microbiome and Autoimmune Uveitis. *Front Immunol* (2019) 10:232. doi: 10.3389/fimmu.2019.00232
51. Ye Z, Wu C, Zhang N, Du L, Cao Q, Huang X, et al. Altered gut microbiome composition in patients with Vogt-Koyanagi-Harada disease. *Gut Microbes* (2020) 11(3):539–55. doi: 10.1080/19490976.2019.1700754
52. Shimizu J, Kubota T, Takada E, Takai K, Fujiwara N, Arimitsu N, et al. Bifidobacteria Abundance-Featured Gut Microbiota Compositional Change in Patients with Behcet's Disease. *PloS One* (2016) 11(4):e0153746. doi: 10.1371/journal.pone.0153746
53. MacDonald ES, Barrett JG. The Potential of Mesenchymal Stem Cells to Treat Systemic Inflammation in Horses. *Front Vet Sci* (2019) 6:507. doi: 10.3389/fvets.2019.00507
54. Davis AB, Schnabel LV, Gilger BC. Subconjunctival bone marrow-derived mesenchymal stem cell therapy as a novel treatment alternative for equine immune-mediated keratitis: A case series. *Vet Ophthalmol* (2019) 22(5):674–82. doi: 10.1111/vop.12641
55. Werry H, Gerhards H. [The surgical therapy of equine recurrent uveitis]. *Tierarztl Prax* (1992) 20(2):178–86.
56. Gilger BC, Salmon JH, Wilkie DA, Cruysberg LP, Kim J, Hayat M, et al. A novel bioerodible deep scleral lamellar cyclosporine implant for uveitis. *Invest Ophthalmol Vis Sci* (2006) 47(6):2596–605. doi: 10.1167/iovs.05-1540 doi: 47/6/2596 [pii].
57. Pepple KL, Wilson L, Van Gelder RN. Comparison of Aqueous and Vitreous Lymphocyte Populations From Two Rat Models of Experimental Uveitis. *Invest Ophthalmol Vis Sci* (2018) 59(6):2504–11. doi: 10.1167/iovs.18-24192
58. Kerr EC, Raveney BJ, Copland DA, Dick AD, Nicholson LB. Analysis of retinal cellular infiltrate in experimental autoimmune uveoretinitis reveals multiple regulatory cell populations. *J Autoimmun* (2008) 31(4):354–61. doi: 10.1016/j.jaut.2008.08.006
59. Jones LS, Rizzo LV, Agarwal RK, Tarrant TK, Chan CC, Wiggert B, et al. IFN-gamma-deficient mice develop experimental autoimmune uveitis in the context of a deviant effector response. *J Immunol* (1997) 158(12):5997–6005.
60. Kim SJ, Zhang M, Vistica BP, Chan CC, Shen DF, Wawrousek EF, et al. Induction of ocular inflammation by T-helper lymphocytes type 2. *Invest Ophthalmol Vis Sci* (2002) 43(3):758–65.
61. Zipplies JK, Kirschfink M, Amann B, Hauck SM, Stangassinger M, Deeg CA. Complement factor B expression profile in a spontaneous uveitis model. *Immunobiology* (2010) 215(12):949–55. doi: 10.1016/j.imbio.2010.02.003
62. Robertson MJ, Erwig LP, Liversidge J, Forrester JV, Rees AJ, Dick AD. Retinal microenvironment controls resident and infiltrating macrophage function during uveoretinitis. *Invest Ophthalmol Vis Sci* (2002) 43(7):2250–7.
63. Khera TK, Copland DA, Boldison J, Lait PJ, Szymkowski DE, Dick AD, et al. Tumour necrosis factor-mediated macrophage activation in the target organ is critical for clinical manifestation of uveitis. *Clin Exp Immunol* (2012) 168 (2):165–77. doi: 10.1111/j.1365-2249.2012.04567.x
64. Chinnery HR, McMenamin PG, Dando SJ. Macrophage physiology in the eye. *Pflugers Arch* (2017) 469(3-4):501–15. doi: 10.1007/s00424-017-1947-5
65. Okunuki Y, Mukai R, Nakao T, Tabor SJ, Butovsky O, Dana R, et al. Retinal microglia initiate neuroinflammation in ocular autoimmunity. *Proc Natl Acad Sci U.S.A.* (2019) 116(20):9989–98. doi: 10.1073/pnas.1820387116
66. Degroote RL, Hauck SM, Kremmer E, Amann B, Ueffing M, Deeg CA. Altered expression of talin 1 in peripheral immune cells points to a significant role of the innate immune system in spontaneous autoimmune uveitis. *J Proteomics* (2012) 75(14):4536–44. doi: 10.1016/j.jprot.2012.01.023

67. Weigand M, Hauck SM, Deeg CA, Degroote RL. Deviant proteome profile of equine granulocytes associates to latent activation status in organ specific autoimmune disease. *J Proteomics* (2020) 230:1–9. doi: 10.1016/j.jprot.2020.103989
68. Naegele M, Tillack K, Reinhardt S, Schippling S, Martin R, Sospedra M. Neutrophils in multiple sclerosis are characterized by a primed phenotype. *J Neuroimmunol* (2012) 242(1-2):60–71. doi: 10.1016/j.jneuroim.2011.11.009
69. Degroote RL, Weigand M, Hauck SM, Deeg CA. IL8 and PMA Trigger the Regulation of Different Biological Processes in Granulocyte Activation. *Front Immunol* (2019) 10:3064. doi: 10.3389/fimmu.2019.03064
70. Fingerhut L, Ohnesorge B, von Borstel M, Schumski A, Strutzberg-Minder K, Morgelin M, et al. Neutrophil Extracellular Traps in the Pathogenesis of Equine Recurrent Uveitis (ERU). *Cells* (2019) 8(12):1–22. doi: 10.3390/cells8121528
71. Zipplies JK, Hauck SM, Schoeffmann S, Amann B, van der Meijden CH, Stangassinger M, et al. Kininogen in autoimmune uveitis: decrease in peripheral blood stream versus increase in target tissue. *Invest Ophthalmol Vis Sci* (2010) 51(1):375–82. doi: 10.1167/iovs.09-4094
72. Natoli R, Fernando N, Jiao H, Racic T, Madigan M, Barnett NL, et al. Retinal Macrophages Synthesize C3 and Activate Complement in AMD and in Models of Focal Retinal Degeneration. *Invest Ophthalmol Vis Sci* (2017) 58 (7):2977–90. doi: 10.1167/iovs.17-21672
73. Chen M, Muckersie E, Robertson M, Forrester JV, Xu H. Up-regulation of complement factor B in retinal pigment epithelial cells is accompanied by complement activation in the aged retina. *Exp Eye Res* (2008) 87(6):543–50. doi: 10.1016/j.exer.2008.09.005
74. Mohlin C, Sandholm K, Ekdahl KN, Nilsson B. The link between morphology and complement in ocular disease. *Mol Immunol* (2017) 89:84–99. doi: 10.1016/j.molimm.2017.05.028
75. Bora NS, Jha P, Bora PS. The role of complement in ocular pathology. *Semin Immunopathol* (2008) 30(2):85–95. doi: 10.1007/s00281-008-0110-y
76. Zhang L, Bell BA, Yu M, Chan CC, Peachey NS, Fung J, et al. Complement anaphylatoxin receptors C3aR and C5aR are required in the pathogenesis of experimental autoimmune uveitis. *J Leukoc Biol* (2016) 99(3):447–54. doi: 10.1189/jlb.3A0415-157R
77. Jha P, Sohn JH, Xu Q, Wang Y, Kaplan HJ, Bora PS, et al. Suppression of complement regulatory proteins (CRPs) exacerbates experimental autoimmune anterior uveitis (EAAU). *J Immunol* (2006) 176(12):7221–31. doi: 10.4049/jimmunol.176.12.7221
78. Jha P, Sohn JH, Xu Q, Nishihori H, Wang Y, Nishihori S, et al. The complement system plays a critical role in the development of experimental autoimmune anterior uveitis. *Invest Ophthalmol Vis Sci* (2006) 47(3):1030–8. doi: 10.1167/iovs.05-1062
79. Chen M, Muckersie E, Luo C, Forrester JV, Xu H. Inhibition of the alternative pathway of complement activation reduces inflammation in experimental autoimmune uveoretinitis. *Eur J Immunol* (2010) 40(10):2870–81. doi: 10.1002/eji.201040323
80. Chiaradia E, Miller I. In slow pace towards the proteome of equine body fluids. *J Proteomics* (2020) 225:103880. doi: 10.1016/j.jprot.2020.103880
81. Zipplies JK, Hauck SM, Eberhardt C, Hirmer S, Amann B, Stangassinger M, et al. Miscellaneous vitreous-derived IgM antibodies target numerous retinal proteins in equine recurrent uveitis. *Vet Ophthalmol* (2012) 15 Suppl;2:57–64. doi: 10.1111/j.1463-5224.2012.01010.x
82. Zipplies JK, Hauck SM, Schoeffmann S, Amann B, Stangassinger M, Ueffing M, et al. Serum PEDF levels are decreased in a spontaneous animal model for human autoimmune uveitis. *J Proteome Res* (2009) 8(2):992–8. doi: 10.1021/pr800694y 10.1021/pr800694y [pii].
83. Guo YL, Colman RW. Two faces of high-molecular-weight kininogen (HK) in angiogenesis: bradykinin turns it on and cleaved HK (HKa) turns it off. *J Thromb Haemost* (2005) 3(4):670–6. doi: 10.1111/j.1538-7836.2005.01218.x
84. Gobel K, Asaridou CM, Merker M, Eichler S, Herrmann AM, Geuss E, et al. Plasma kallikrein modulates immune cell trafficking during neuroinflammation via PAR2 and bradykinin release. *Proc Natl Acad Sci USA* (2019) 116(1):271–6. doi: 10.1073/pnas.1810020116
85. Zhang SX, Wang JJ, Gao G, Shao C, Mott R, Ma JX. Pigment epithelium-derived factor (PEDF) is an endogenous antiinflammatory factor. *FASEB J* (2006) 20(2):323–5. doi: 10.1096/fj.05-4313fje doi: 05-4313fje [pii].
86. Comitato A, Subramanian P, Turchiano G, Montanari M, Becerra SP, Marigo V. Pigment epithelium-derived factor hinders photoreceptor cell death by reducing intracellular calcium in the degenerating retina. *Cell Death Dis* (2018) 9(5):560. doi: 10.1038/s41419-018-0613-y
87. Eichler W, Savkovic-Cvijic H, Burger S, Beck M, Schmidt M, Wiedemann P, et al. Muller Cell-Derived PEDF Mediates Neuroprotection via STAT3 Activation. *Cell Physiol Biochem* (2017) 44(4):1411–24. doi: 10.1159/000485537
88. Wang X, Liu X, Ren Y, Liu Y, Han S, Zhao J, et al. PEDF protects human retinal pigment epithelial cells against oxidative stress via upregulation of UCP2 expression. *Mol Med Rep* (2019) 19(1):59–74. doi: 10.3892/mmr.2018.9645
89. Strauss O. The retinal pigment epithelium in visual function. *Physiol Rev* (2005) 85(3):845–81. doi: 10.1152/physrev.00021.2004
90. Szober CM, Hauck SM, Euler KN, Frohlich KJ, Alge-Priglinger C, Ueffing M, et al. Profound re-organization of cell surface proteome in equine retinal pigment epithelial cells in response to in vitro culturing. *Int J Mol Sci* (2012) 13(11):14053–72. doi: 10.3390/ijms131114053
91. Uhl PB, Szober CM, Amann B, Alge-Priglinger C, Ueffing M, Hauck SM, et al. In situ cell surface proteomics reveals differentially expressed membrane proteins in retinal pigment epithelial cells during autoimmune uveitis. *J Proteomics* (2014) 109:50–62. doi: 10.1016/j.jprot.2014.06.020
92. Uhl PB, Amann B, Hauck SM, Deeg CA. Novel localization of peripherin 2, the photoreceptor-specific retinal degeneration slow protein, in retinal pigment epithelium. *Int J Mol Sci* (2015) 16(2):2678–92. doi: 10.3390/ijms16022678
93. Xu H, Forrester JV, Liversidge J, Crane IJ. Leukocyte trafficking in experimental autoimmune uveitis: breakdown of blood-retinal barrier and upregulation of cellular adhesion molecules. *Invest Ophthalmol Vis Sci* (2003) 44(1):226–34. doi: 10.1167/iovs.01-1202
94. Xu H, Manivannan A, Liversidge J, Sharp PF, Forrester JV, Crane IJ. Involvement of CD44 in leukocyte trafficking at the blood-retinal barrier. *J Leukoc Biol* (2002) 72:1133–41, 72(6).
95. Xu H, Manivannan A, Goatman KA, Jiang HR, Liversidge J, Sharp PF, et al. Reduction in shear stress, activation of the endothelium, and leukocyte priming are all required for leukocyte passage across the blood–retina barrier. *J Leukoc Biol* (2004) 75(2):224–32. doi: 10.1189/jlb.1002479
96. Xu H, Manivannan A, Jiang HR, Liversidge J, Sharp PF, Forrester JV, et al. Recruitment of IFN-gamma-producing (Th1-like) cells into the inflamed retina in vivo is preferentially regulated by P-selectin glycoprotein ligand 1: P/E-selectin interactions. *J Immunol* (2004) 172(5):3215–24. doi: 10.4049/jimmunol.172.5.3215
97. Crane IJ, Xu H, Wallace C, Manivannan A, Mack M, Liversidge J, et al. Involvement of CCR5 in the passage of Th1-type cells across the blood-retina barrier in experimental autoimmune uveitis. *J Leukoc Biol* (2006) 79 (3):435–43. doi: 10.1189/jlb.0305130
98. Thurau SR, Mempel TR, Flugel A, Diedrichs-Mohring M, Krombach F, Kawakami N, et al. The fate of autoreactive, GFP+ T cells in rat models of uveitis analyzed by intravital fluorescence microscopy and FACS. *Int Immunol* (2004) 16(11):1573–82. doi: 10.1093/intimm/dxh158
99. Zhao J, Chen M, Xu H. Experimental autoimmune uveoretinitis (EAU)-related tissue damage and angiogenesis is reduced in CCL2(-)/(-)CX(3) CR1gfp/gfp mice. *Invest Ophthalmol Vis Sci* (2014) 55(11):7572–82. doi: 10.1167/iovs.14-15495
100. Chen M, Zhao J, Ali IHA, Marry S, Augustine J, Bhuckory M, et al. Cytokine Signaling Protein 3 Deficiency in Myeloid Cells Promotes Retinal Degeneration and Angiogenesis through Arginase-1 Up-Regulation in Experimental Autoimmune Uveoretinitis. *Am J Pathol* (2018) 188 (4):1007–20. doi: 10.1016/j.ajpath.2017.12.021
101. Amadi-Obi A, Yu CR, Liu X, Mahdi RM, Clarke GL, Nussenblatt RB, et al. TH17 cells contribute to uveitis and scleritis and are expanded by IL-2 and inhibited by IL-27/STAT1. *Nat Med* (2007) 13(6):711–8. doi: 10.1038/nm1585 doi: nm1585 [pii].
102. Bing SJ, Shemesh I, Chong WP, Horai R, Jittayasothorn Y, Silver PB, et al. AS101 ameliorates experimental autoimmune uveitis by regulating Th1 and Th17 responses and inducing Treg cells. *J Autoimmun* (2019) 100:52–61. doi: 10.1016/j.jaut.2019.02.006
103. Horai R, Caspi RR. Cytokines in autoimmune uveitis. *J Interferon Cytokine Res* (2011) 31(10):733–44. doi: 10.1089/jir.2011.0042
104. Weinstein JE, Pepple KL. Cytokines in uveitis. *Curr Opin Ophthalmol* (2018) 29(3):267–74. doi: 10.1097/ICU.0000000000000466

105. Hauck SM, Dietter J, Kramer RL, Hofmaier F, Zipplies JK, Amann B, et al. Deciphering membrane-associated molecular processes in target tissue of autoimmune uveitis by label-free quantitative mass spectrometry. *Mol Cell Proteomics* (2010) 9(10):2292–305. doi: 10.1074/mcp.M110.001073
106. Newman E, Reichenbach A. The Muller cell: a functional element of the retina. *Trends Neurosci* (1996) 19(8):307–12. doi: 10.1016/0166-2236(96)10040-0
107. Eberhardt C, Amann B, Feuchtinger A, Hauck SM, Deeg CA. Differential expression of inwardly rectifying K+ channels and aquaporins 4 and 5 in autoimmune uveitis indicates misbalance in Muller glial cell-dependent ion and water homeostasis. *Glia* (2011) 59(5):697–707. doi: 10.1002/glia.21139
108. Bringmann A, Pannicke T, Grosche J, Francke M, Wiedemann P, Skatchkov SN, et al. Muller cells in the healthy and diseased retina. *Prog Retin Eye Res* (2006) 25(4):397–424. doi: 10.1016/j.preteyeres.2006.05.003
109. Bringmann A, Iandiev I, Pannicke T, Wurm A, Hollborn M, Wiedemann P, et al. Cellular signaling and factors involved in Muller cell gliosis: neuroprotective and detrimental effects. *Prog Retin Eye Res* (2009) 28(6):423–51. doi: 10.1016/j.preteyeres.2009.07.001
110. Deeg CA, Amann B, Lutz K, Hirmer S, Lutterberg K, Kremmer E, et al. Aquaporin 11, a regulator of water efflux at retinal Muller glial cell surface decreases concomitant with immune-mediated gliosis. *J Neuroinflammation* (2016) 13(1):89. doi: 10.1186/s12974-016-0554-2
111. Hauck SM, Hofmaier F, Dietter J, Swadzba ME, Blindert M, Amann B, et al. Label-free LC-MSMS analysis of vitreous from autoimmune uveitis reveals a significant decrease in secreted Wnt signalling inhibitors DKK3 and SFRP2. *J Proteomics* (2012) 75(14):4545–54. doi: 10.1016/j.jprot.2012.04.052
112. Shi J, Chi S, Xue J, Yang J, Li F, Liu X. Emerging Role and Therapeutic Implication of Wnt Signaling Pathways in Autoimmune Diseases. *J Immunol Res* (2016) 2016:9392132. doi: 10.1155/2016/9392132
113. Cici D, Corrado A, Rotondo C, Cantatore FP. Wnt Signaling and Biological Therapy in Rheumatoid Arthritis and Spondyloarthritis. *Int J Mol Sci* (2019) 20(22):1–15. doi: 10.3390/ijms20225552
114. Deeg CA, Eberhardt C, Hofmaier F, Amann B, Hauck SM. Osteopontin and fibronectin levels are decreased in vitreous of autoimmune uveitis and retinal expression of both proteins indicates ECM re-modeling. *PloS One* (2011) 6(12):e27674. doi: 10.1371/journal.pone.0027674
115. Pankov R, Yamada KM. Fibronectin at a glance. *J Cell Sci* (2002) 115(Pt 20):3861–3. doi: 10.1242/jcs.00059
116. Wang XL, Yu T, Zhang JS, Yan QC, Luo YH. Fibronectin and focal adhesion kinase small interfering RNA modulate rat retinal Muller cells adhesion and migration. *Cell Mol Neurobiol* (2009) 29(4):549–56. doi: 10.1007/s10571-009-9346-x
117. Braitch M, Constantinescu CS. The role of osteopontin in experimental autoimmune encephalomyelitis (EAE) and multiple sclerosis (MS). *Inflammation Allergy Drug Targets* (2010) 9(4):249–56. doi: 10.2174/187152810793358778
118. Hikita ST, Vistica BP, Jones HR, Keswani JR, Watson MM, Ericson VR, et al. Osteopontin is proinflammatory in experimental autoimmune uveitis. *Invest Ophthalmol Vis Sci* (2006) 47(10):4435–43. doi: 10.1167/iovs.06-0064
119. Kitamura M, Iwabuchi K, Kitaichi N, Kon S, Kitamei H, Namba K, et al. Osteopontin aggravates experimental autoimmune uveoretinitis in mice. *J Immunol* (2007) 178(10):6567–72. doi: 10.4049/jimmunol.178.10.6567
120. Del Rio P, Irmler M, Arango-Gonzalez B, Favor J, Bobe C, Bartsch U, et al. GDNF-induced osteopontin from Muller glial cells promotes photoreceptor survival in the Pde6brd1 mouse model of retinal degeneration. *Glia* (2011) 59(5):821–32. doi: 10.1002/glia.21155
121. Ruzafa N, Pereiro X, Lepper MF, Hauck SM, Vecino E. A Proteomics Approach to Identify Candidate Proteins Secreted by Muller Glia that Protect Ganglion Cells in the Retina. *Proteomics* (2018) 18(11):e1700321. doi: 10.1002/pmic.201700321
122. Hofmaier F, Hauck SM, Amann B, Degroote RL, Deeg CA. Changes in matrix metalloproteinase network in a spontaneous autoimmune uveitis model. *Invest Ophthalmol Vis Sci* (2011) 52(5):2314–20. doi: 10.1167/iovs.10-6475
123. Brew K, Dinakarpandian D, Nagase H. Tissue inhibitors of metalloproteinases: evolution, structure and function. *Biochim Biophys Acta* (2000) 1477(1-2):267–83. doi: 10.1016/s0167-4838(99)00279-4
124. Murphy G, Nagase H. Progress in matrix metalloproteinase research. *Mol Aspects Med* (2008) 29(5):290–308. doi: 10.1016/j.mam.2008.05.002
125. Magnoni S, Baker A, Thomson S, Jordan G, George SJ, McColl BW, et al. Neuroprotective effect of adenoviral-mediated gene transfer of TIMP-1 and -2 in ischemic brain injury. *Gene Ther* (2007) 14(7):621–5. doi: 10.1038/sj.gt.3302894
126. Woods CC, Sundar K, Tessler C, Lebsack TW, Grainger L, Nielsen A, et al. Tissue inhibitor of metalloproteinase-2 inhibits T-cell infiltration and preserves pancreatic beta-cell function in an in vitro type 1 diabetes mellitus model. *J Autoimmun* (2006) 27(1):28–37. doi: 10.1016/j.jaut.2006.04.004
127. Abraham M, Shapiro S, Karni A, Weiner HL, Miller A. Gelatinases (MMP-2 and MMP-9) are preferentially expressed by Th1 vs. Th2 cells. *Cells J Neuroimmunol* (2005) 163(1-2):157–64. doi: 10.1016/j.jneuroim.2005.02.001
128. Wu B, Crampton SP, Hughes CC. Wnt signaling induces matrix metalloproteinase expression and regulates T cell transmigration. *Immunity* (2007) 26(2):227–39. doi: 10.1016/j.immuni.2006.12.007
129. El-Shabrawi Y, Walch A, Hermann J, Egger G, Foster CS. Inhibition of MMP-dependent chemotaxis and amelioration of experimental autoimmune uveitis with a selective metalloproteinase-2 and -9 inhibitor. *J Neuroimmunol* (2004) 155(1-2):13–20. doi: 10.1016/j.jneuroim.2004.05.010
130. Swadzba ME, Hirmer S, Amann B, Hauck SM, Deeg CA. Vitreal IgM autoantibodies target neurofilament medium in a spontaneous model of autoimmune uveitis. *Invest Ophthalmol Vis Sci* (2012) 53(1):294–300. doi: 10.1167/iovs.11-8734
131. Swadzba ME, Hauck SM, Naim HY, Amann B, Deeg CA. Retinal glycoprotein enrichment by concanavalin a enabled identification of novel membrane autoantigen synaptotagmin-1 in equine recurrent uveitis. *PloS One* (2012) 7(12):e50929. doi: 10.1371/journal.pone.0050929
132. Kalsow CM, Dubielzig RR, Dwyer AE. Immunopathology of pineal glands from horses with uveitis. *Invest Ophthalmol Vis Sci* (1999) 40(7):1611–5.
133. Eberhardt C, Amann B, Stangassinger M, Hauck SM, Deeg CA. Isolation, characterization and establishment of an equine retinal glial cell line: a prerequisite to investigate the physiological function of Muller cells in the retina. *J Anim Physiol Anim Nutr (Berl)* (2012) 96(2):260–9. doi: 10.1111/j.1439-0396.2011.01147.x

6

CD73+ Dendritic Cells in Cascading Th17 Responses of Experimental Autoimmune Uveitis-Induced Mice

*MinHee K. Ko [1], Hui Shao [2], Henry J. Kaplan [3] and Deming Sun [1]**

[1] Doheny Eye Institute and Department of Ophthalmology, David Geffen School of Medicine at UCLA, Los Angeles, CA, United States, [2] Department of Ophthalmology and Visual Sciences, Kentucky Lions Eye Center, University of Louisville, Louisville, KY, United States, [3] Department of Ophthalmology, Saint Louis University (SLU) Eye Institute, SLU School of Medicine, Saint Louis, MO, United States

***Correspondence:**
Deming Sun
dsun@doheny.org

Previous studies have shown that CD73 is pivotal in the conversion of pro-inflammatory adenosine triphosphate into anti-inflammatory adenosine and that immune cells of the same type that express different levels of CD73 are functionally distinct. In this study we show that adenosine enhances the Th17 promoting effect of dendritic cells (DCs), and DCs expressing CD73 critically augment Th17 responses. Bone marrow dendritic cells (BMDCs) do not constantly express CD73; however, a significant portion of the BMDCs expressed CD73 after exposure to Toll-like receptor ligand, leading to stronger Th17 responses by converting adenosine monophosphate to adenosine. We show that the CD73$^+$ BMDCs play a critical role in cascading Th17 responses, and CD73$^+$ BMDCs are functionally augmented after treatment with Toll-like receptor ligand. Splenic antigen presenting cells (DCs) of CD73$^{-/-}$ mouse have a poor Th17-stimulating effect, even after exposure to lipopolysaccharide (LPS) or γδ T cells, indicating that induction of CD73$^+$ DCs is critically involved in augmented Th17 responses. We conclude that CD73$^+$ DCs critically trigger cascading Th17 responses, and the activated Th17 cells that express CD73 further augment Th17 responses, leading to cascading exacerbation. Hence, disabling the CD73 function of DCs should block this cascading response and mitigate Th17 responses.

Keywords: autoimmunity, adenosine receptors, bone marrow dendritic cells, bone marrow culture dendritic cells, CD73, experimental autoimmune uveitis, γδ T cells, uveitis

INTRODUCTION

Under pathologic conditions, a large amount of adenosine triphosphate (ATP) is released into the extracellular compartment by injured and dying cells (1–4). The released ATP acts as an endogenous Toll-like receptor (TLR) ligand to enhance immune responses and inflammation (5–9). A combination of the ectoenzymes CD39 and CD73 degrades ATP, adenosine diphosphate (ADP), and adenosine monophosphate (AMP) to adenosine, thereby quenching the ATP-driven proinflammatory processes (10). Consequently, generated adenosine counteracts ATP-mediated immune stimulation, preventing uncontrolled inflammation and lessening the collateral damage to healthy tissues (1, 2, 11). Hence, the metabolic process of ATP conversion to adenosine has been viewed as an 'immunological switch' that shifts ATP-driven proinflammatory immune cell activity toward an anti-inflammatory state (12–14).

The glycosylphosphatidylinositol-linked membrane protein CD73 is the main enzyme responsible for the conversion of AMP into immunosuppressive adenosine (12, 13, 15–17). Studies have shown that CD73-deficient mice have altered inflammatory reactions (18–20). Expression of CD73 is functionally important for Foxp3$^+$ regulatory T cells (10, 21), Myeloid-derived suppressor cells (22), and M2 macrophages (23–25), as well as for γδ T cells (26, 27); and immune cells of the same type that express different levels of CD73 are functionally distinct (24, 25). To determine whether dendritic cells (DCs) express CD73 and whether CD73 is functionally important for DCs, we examined CD73$^+$ cells among cultured bone marrow dendritic cells (BMDCs) and splenic CD11c$^+$ cells.

DCs are the principal antigen-presenting (AP) cells for initiating immune responses. Previous studies showed that DC differentiation and function is profoundly affected by TLR ligand (28) and adenosine (23, 29, 30). Since levels of extracellular adenosine increase greatly during inflammation (31–33), and since our previous studies showed that adenosine has an opposite effect on Th1 and Th17 pathogenic responses in experimental autoimmune uveitis, we examined whether adenosine and adenosine metabolism of DCs contribute to a biased effect of adenosine on Th1 and Th17 responses: particularly, whether CD73-expressing DCs differ in supporting Th1 vs Th17 responses. Our results show that BMDCs cultured with granulocyte–macrophage colony-stimulating factor (GM-CSF) do not express detectable levels of CD73; however, a significant portion of the BMDCs become CD73$^+$ after exposure to TLR ligand or γδ T cells, suggesting that CD73 is not constantly expressed by BMDCs but is inducible. Functional comparison between induced CD73$^+$ and CD73$^-$ BMDCs and between BMDCs from CD73$^{+/+}$ (wt-B6 mouse) and CD73$^{-/-}$ (CD73$^{-/-}$ mouse) showed that CD73$^+$ BMDCs are stronger stimulators for IL-17$^+$ T cells whereas CD73$^-$ BMDCs preferentially stimulate Th1 responses. The CD73$^+$ BMDCs produce unique patterns and amounts of cytokines as compared to CD73$^-$ DCs. Our results demonstrated that the induction of CD73$^+$ DCs is crucially involved in cascading Th17 responses and that disabling CD73 function on DCs effectively mitigates the Th17 pathogenic responses in autoimmune diseases.

MATERIALS AND METHODS

Animals and Reagents

Female C57BL/6 (B6) mice and CD73$^{-/-}$ and TCR-δ$^{-/-}$ mice were purchased from Jackson Laboratory (Bar Harbor, ME); 12- to 16-week-old mice were used in all studies. All mice were housed and maintained in the animal facilities of the University of California Los Angeles. Institutional approval (Protocol number: ARC#2014-029-03A) was obtained from the Institutional Animal Care and Use Committee of the Doheny Eye Institute, University of California Los Angeles, and institutional guidelines regarding animal experimentation were followed. Veterinary care was provided by IACUC faculty. Immunized animals that displayed swelling joints were either humanely euthanatized or administered an analgesic (buprenorphine, 0.1 mg/kg sc. twice daily or ketoprofen, 2 mg/kg sc. daily) until the swelling resolved. By the end of the study, mice were euthanized by cervical dislocation after a lethal injection of ketamine and xylazine prior to tissue collection. Recombinant murine IL-1β, IL-7, IL-12 and IL-23 were purchased from R & D (Minneapolis, MN). Fluorescein isothiocyanate (FITC)-, phycoerythrin (PE)-, or allophycocyanin (APC)-conjugated antibodies (Abs) against mouse CD4 (GK1.5), αβ T cell receptor (TCR) (H57-597), or γδ TCR (GL3) and their isotype control antibodies were purchased from Biolegend (San Diego, CA). (PE)-conjugated anti-mouse IFN-γ (XMG1.2) and IL-17 (TC11-18H10.1) monoclonal antibody was purchased from Santa Cruz Biotechnology (Dallas, Texas). The non-selective AR agonist 5'-N-ethylcarboxamidoadenosine (NECA) (34) and AMP were purchased from Sigma-Aldrich (St. Louis, MO, USA). Toll-like receptors ligand LPS was purchased from Invivogen (San Diego, CA).

Immunization and EAU Induction

EAU was induced in B6 mice by subcutaneous injection of 200 µl of emulsion containing 200 µg of human IRBP$_{1-20}$ (Sigma-Aldrich, St. Louis, MO) in complete Freund's adjuvant (CFA; Difco, Detroit) at six spots at the tail base and on the flank and intraperitoneal (i.p.) injection with 300 ng of pertussis toxin.

T Cell Preparation

All αβ T cells used were purified from the spleen or draining lymph nodes of IRBP$_{1-20}$-immunized mice at day 13 post-immunization using an auto-MACS separator system, as described previously [29]. The purity of the purified cells was >95%, as determined by flow cytometric analysis using phycoerythrin-conjugated antibodies against αβ T cells. The cells were then cultured in RPMI 1640 medium containing 10% fetal calf serum (Corning).

Prepare γδ T Cells

Non-activated and activated γδ T cells were separated from either naïve B6 mice or IRBP$_{1-20}$-immunized B6 mice, respectively, by positive selection using a combination of FITC-conjugated anti-TCR-δ antibody and anti-FITC antibody-coated Microbeads, followed by separation using an auto-MACS.

Generation of Bone Marrow Dendritic Cells

Bone marrow dendritic cells were generated by incubating bone marrow cells for 5 days in the presence of 10 ng/ml of recombinant murine GM-CSF and IL-4 (R&D Systems), as described previously (35). Cytokine (IL-1β, IL-6, L-12 and IL-23) levels in the culture medium were measured by ELISA.

To determine the antigen-presenting function, BMDCs were incubated in a 24-well plate with responder T cells isolated from immunized B6 mice under Th1- or Th17-polarizing conditions. Forty-eight hours after stimulation, IFN-γ and IL-17 in the culture medium were measured by ELISA. The percentage of IFN-γ$^+$ and IL-17$^+$ T cells among the responder T cells was determined by intracellular staining after 5 days of culture as described above.

Adenosine Assay

Adenosine in the medium of cultured cells was measured by an Adenosine Assay Kit (Fluorometric) from Biovision (CA).

Briefly, 25 μl of cultured cell supernatant were mixed with assay buffer, adenosine convertor, adenosine detector, adenosine developer and adenosine probe from the kits to compose a 100 μl reaction system. Kept in room temperature for 15 min and protected from the light. Fluorescence was read in a SpectraMax iD5 multi-mode microplate reader (Molecular Devices, LLC. USA) at Ex/Em = 535/587 nm.

CFSE Assay

Purified $CD3^+$ T cells from $IRBP_{1-20}$-immunized TCR-$\delta^{-/-}$ mice were stained with CFSE (Sigma-Aldrich) as described previously (36). Briefly, the cells were washed and suspended at 5×10^6 cells/ml in serum-free RPMI 1640 medium; cells were then incubated at 37°C for 10 min with gentle shaking with a final concentration of 5 μM CFSE before being washed twice with, and suspended in, complete medium, stimulated with anti-CD3 antibodies which were pre-coated on 24 well plate. Some 48 h later, the T cells were harvested and analyzed by flow cytometry.

Experimental Setting for Interaction of T Cells and Dendritic Cells and Measurement of Th1 and Th17 Responses

In a 6-well plate, 2×10^6/well BMDCs were co-cultured with 1×10^5/well γδ or αβ T cells for 24 h. After DCs were separated from T cells, the BMDCs were irradiated (5,000 Rad) and seeded in a 24-well plate at 3×10^4/well with $CD3^+$ cells isolated from immunized B6 mice. Five days later, the percentage of IFN-γ^+ and IL-17^+ T cells among the responder T cells was determined by intracellular staining, followed by FACS analysis, as described previously (37).

αβ T cells (1.8×10^6) were collected from $IRBP_{1-20}$-immunized B6 mice on day 13 post-immunization. To obtain enough cells, the cells obtained from all six mice in the same group are routinely pooled before the T cells are further enriched. The cells were co-cultured for 48 h with irradiated spleen cells (1.5×10^6/well) as APCs and $IRBP_{1-20}$ (10 μg/ml) in a 24-well plate under either Th1 (culture medium supplemented with 10 ng/ml of IL-12) or Th17 polarized conditions (culture medium supplemented with 10 ng/ml of IL-23) (37, 38). Cytokine (IFN-γ and IL-17) levels in the serum and 48 h of culture supernatants were measured by ELISA (R & D Systems).

ELISA Measurement of Cytokine

ELISA kits (E-Bioscience) were used to measure serum IFN-γ and IL-17 levels on day 13 post-immunization and in the 48 h culture supernatants of responder T cells isolated on day 13 post-immunization from $IRBP_{1-20}$-immunized B6 or TCR-$\delta^{-/-}$ mice.

Statistical Analysis

The results in the figures are from a representative experiment, which was repeated 3–5 times. We used 2-way Students t-tests unless otherwise specified. Data were presented as the means with error bars for standard error of mean (SEM). Statistical analysis and graphing were performed in Excel software (Microsoft Corp). Asterisks (**) in graphs indicated $p \leq 0.05$ representing statistical significance.

RESULTS

Adenosine Augments DCs' Th17 Promoting Activity

Our recent studies showed that adenosine has a distinct effect on Th17 versus Th1 responses; it tips the balance between Th1 and Th17 responses towards the latter (38, 39). To determine the contribution of DCs to such contradictory effects of adenosine on antigen-specific Th1 and Th17 responses, we examined the antigen presenting (AP) function of BMDCs, before and after exposure to NECA—a non-selective adenosine receptor agonist (34). The $\alpha\beta TCR^+$ responder T cells obtained from immunized B6 mice were stimulated *in vitro* with the immunizing antigen and the treated BMDCs at ratio of DC:T = 1:20 under Th1 (culture medium added with IL-12) or Th-17 (culture medium added with IL-23) polarizing conditions (39, 40). Th17 responses were assessed by evaluating numbers of IL-17^+ T cells activated after a 5-day *in vitro* stimulation under Th17 polarizing conditions. After a 5-day *in vitro* stimulation by the immunizing antigen, under Th1 or Th17 polarizing conditions (27, 38), a significantly increased number of the $CD3^+$ responder T cells became IFN-γ and IL-17 positive after stimulation by lipopolysaccharide (LPS)-treated BMDCs (**Figure 1A**, upper panel). The IL-17^+, but not the IFN-γ^+, cells further increased if BMDCs were dually treated with LPS and NECA (**Figure 1A**, lower panel). Cytokine tests (**Figure 1B**) showed that IL-17 production by responder T cells was also enhanced after stimulation by BMDCs dually treated with LPS and NECA, whereas the IFN-γ production was inhibited.

LPS Treatment Triggers BMDCs' Response to AMP

To determine whether AMP has a similar effect on BMDCs or whether BMDCs can convert AMP to adenosine and thus augment Th17 responses, the AP function of BMDCs was examined, before and after treatment with AMP, with or without a prior LPS treatment. Results in **Figure 2A** (upper panels) showed that AMP enhances Th17 promoting activity in LPS-treated, but not untreated, BMDCs. The number of IL-17^+ T cells among the responder T cells was higher when BMDCs were pretreated with LPS. The number was further increased when the LPS-treated BMDCs were additionally treated with AMP (**Figure 2B**). However, BMDCs that were not treated with LPS did not respond to AMP, suggesting that LPS-treatment enabled BMDCs to respond to AMP. The effective doses of AMP range are from 1 to 8 μM and dose dependent effect was not apparent. Therefore, in subsequent studies we used the concentration of 1 μM.

AMP Augmented Th17 Response but Only in the Presence of $CD73^{+/+}$, but Not $CD73^{-/-}$ BMDCs

CD73 is the main ecto-enzyme converting AMP to adenosine (12, 15). To test the prediction that LPS treatment enables BMDCs to express CD73, which allows BMDCs to convert AMP to adenosine, leading to augmented Th17 responses, we prepared $CD73^{+/+}$ (isolated from $CD73^{+/+}$ B6 mouse) and $CD73^{-/-}$ BMDCs (isolated from $CD73^{-/-}$ mouse) and compared the AP function

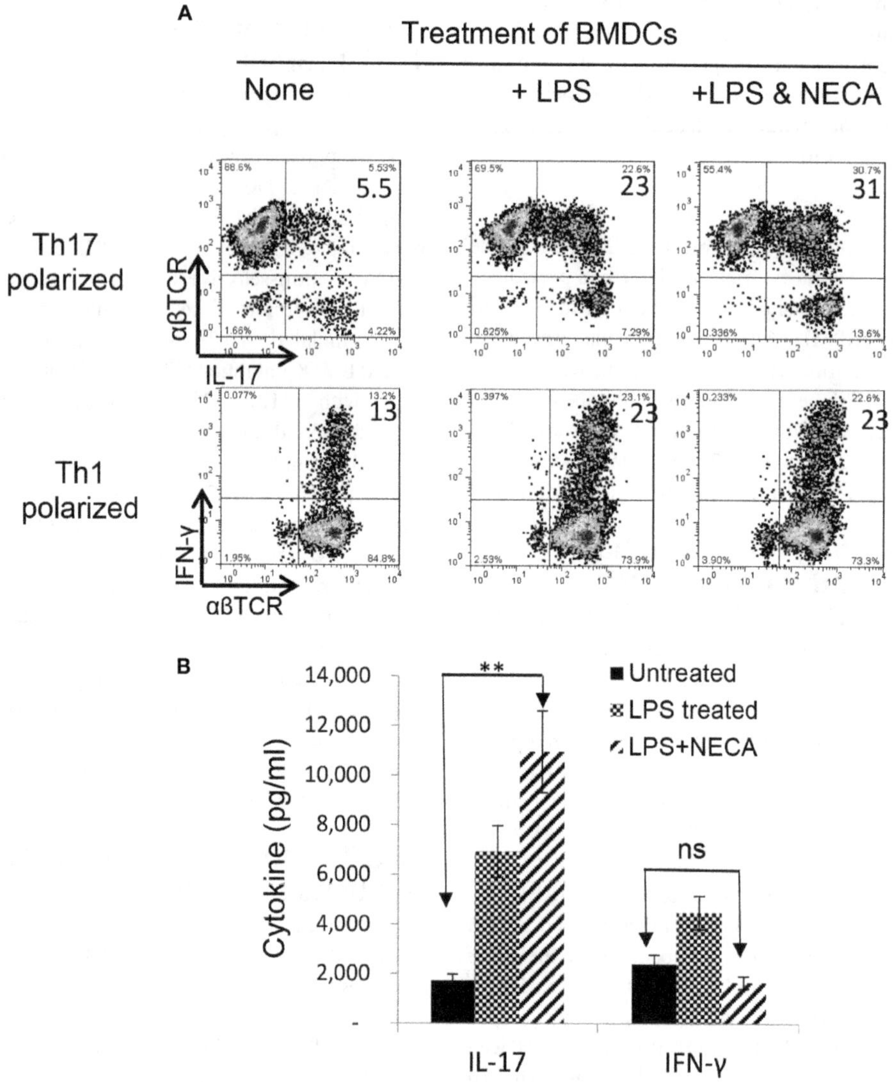

FIGURE 1 | Adenosine augments DCs' Th17 promoting activity **(A)**. Exposure of bone marrow dendritic cells (BMDCs) to a non-selective adenosine receptor agonist NECA enhanced DCs' Th17-promoting activity. BMDCs were generated by incubation of bone marrow cells in the presence of granulocyte-macrophage colony-stimulating factor and IL-4 (35). They were treated or untreated with lipopolysaccharide (LPS, 100 ng/ml)) or LPS + NECA (100 nM). In 24 well plated, the αβ responder T cells obtained from immunized B6 mice were stimulated *in vitro* with the immunizing antigen and the treated BMDCs at ratio of DC:T = 1:20. The numbers of IL-17$^+$ T cells activated after a 5-day *in vitro* stimulation under Th17 polarizing conditions were examined **(B)**. ELISA assay measuring IFN-γ and IL-17 production of αβTCR$^+$ responder T cells. IL-17 production by responder T cells were also enhanced by NECA treatment, whereas the IFN-γ production was inhibited. The data are from one single experiment and are representative of those obtained in three independent experiments. Values are expressed as mean ± SEM (n = 6). **$p < 0.05$. ns, not significant.

between CD73$^{+/+}$ and CD73$^{-/-}$ BMDCs, before and after treatment with LPS (100 ng/ml) and/or AMP (1 μM) (**Figure 2A**). The results show that treatment with LPS enhanced the Th17-promoting effect of both CD73$^{+/+}$ and CD73$^{-/-}$ BMDCs; however, additional treatment of BMDCs with AMP augmented the Th17 responses presented by CD73$^{+/+}$, but not by CD73$^{-/-}$, BMDCs (**Figure 2A**, lower panels). These results indicate that CD73$^{-/-}$ BMDCs were unresponsive to AMP and that CD73 expressed by BMDCs may convert AMP to adenosine, which augments Th17 responses (41). We also measured IL-12/IL-23 production of BMDCs, after treatment with LPS and/or AMP. As demonstrated in **Figures 3A, B**, LPS exposure induced both CD73$^{+/+}$ and CD73$^{-/-}$ BMDCs to produce increased amounts of IL-12 and IL-23. However, double exposure to LPS plus AMP enabled CD73$^{+/+}$, but not CD73$^{-/-}$, BMDCs to further increase IL-23 production and decrease IL-12 production.

Testing of AMP function by assessing cytokine production of responder T cells showed that AMP treatment further enhanced Th17 responses presented by CD73$^{+/+}$ but not CD73$^{-/-}$ BMDCs (**Figure 3C**). Phenotypic examination of BMDCs, before and after LPS treatment, showed (**Figure 3D**). LPS-treated BMDCs expressed significant levels of CD73, whereas the CD73 level had

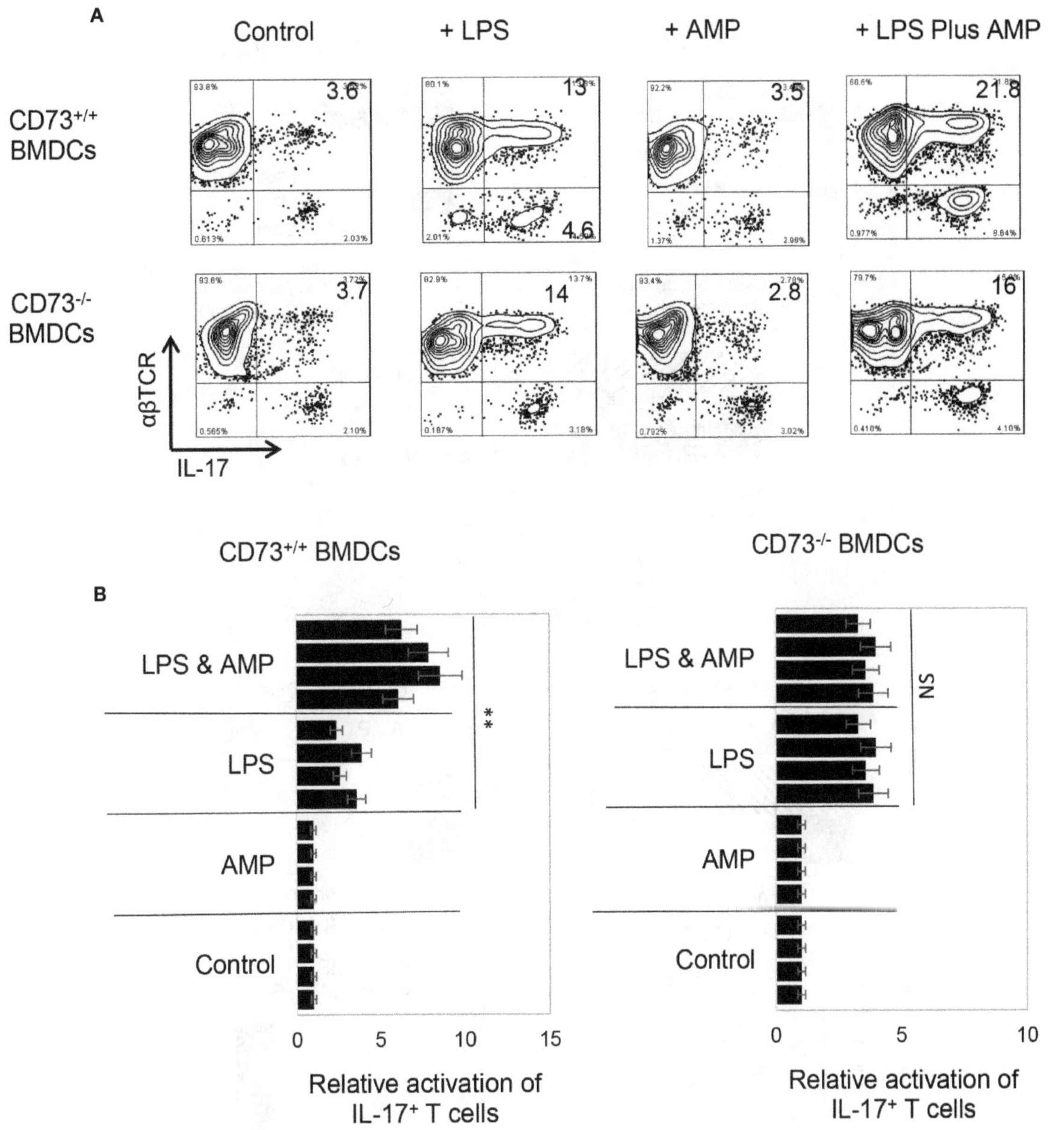

FIGURE 2 | Bone marrow dendritic cells acquire response to adenosine monophosphate after lipopolysaccharide treatment **(A)**. Synergistic effect between lipopolysaccharide (LPS) and adenosine monophosphate (AMP) in enhancing bone marrow dendritic cells' (BMDCs') Th17 promoting activity. BMDCs from B6 (CD73$^{+/+}$) (upper panels) or CD73$^{-/-}$ (lower panels) mouse were examined for antigen presenting function, after exposure to LPS (100 ng/ml) or LPS plus AMP (1 μM). Responder T cells obtained from immunized B6 mice. The numbers of IL-17^{+} T cells among responder T cells were examined after staining with anti-IL-17 and anti-αβTCR mABs, after a 5-day *in vitro* stimulation under Th17 polarizing conditions. The data are from one single experiment and are representative of those obtained in three independent experiments **(B)**. Summarized data of four separate experiments showing that AMP enhanced BMDCs' Th17 stimulating effect only after LPS treatment (left panels) and that the CD73$^{-/-}$ BMDCs remained unresponsive to AMP even LPS treatment (right panels). Values of relative activation of Th17^{+} T cells were calculated by number of IL-17^{+} T cells in testing group divided by number of IL-17^{+} T cells in the control group (in the absence of LPS and AMP) and are expressed as mean ± SEM (n = 4). **$p < 0.05$. ns, not significant.

been undetectable before treatment. We also measured adenosine amounts in the cultured supernatants of CD73$^{+/+}$ and CD73$^{-/-}$ BMDCs after stimulation with LPS with or without AMP treatment. The results show that the adenosine concentration was significantly increased in AMP-treated CD73$^{+/+}$ but not CD73$^{-/-}$ BMDCs (**Figure 3E**).

AMP Enhances Th17 Responses Supported by CD73$^{+/+}$, but Not CD73$^{-/-}$, Splenic DCs

To determine whether CD73 expressed on splenic DCs is also functionally important, we examined the AP function of CD73$^{+/+}$ (isolated from B6 mouse) and CD73$^{-/-}$ (isolated from CD73$^{-/-}$

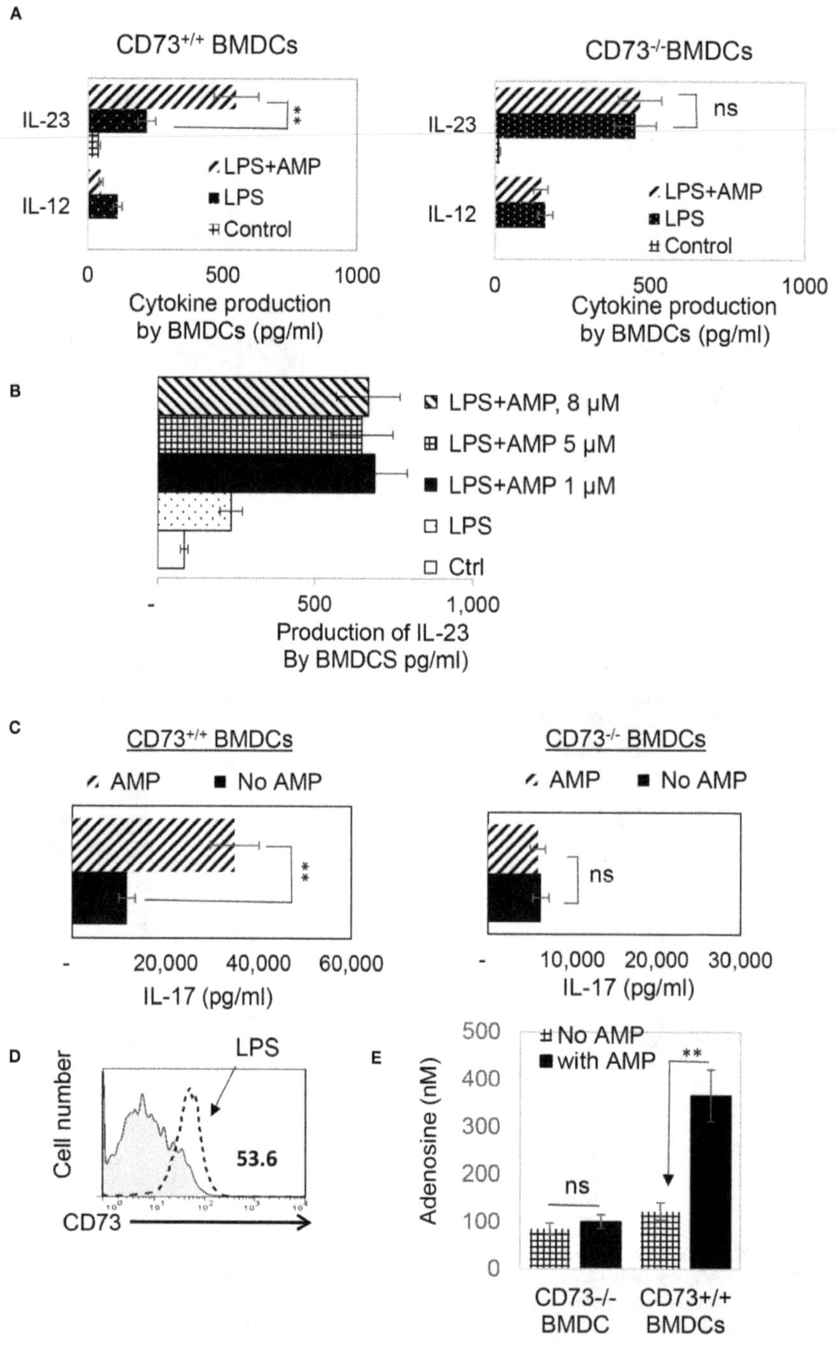

FIGURE 3 | In response to AMP LPS-treated CD73$^{+/+}$, but not CD73$^{-/-}$, BMDCs produced greater amounts of IL-23 and acquired greater Th17 stimulating activity **(A)**. ELISA assays for IL-12 and IL-23 production by CD73$^{+/+}$ and CD73$^{-/-}$ BMDCs. 48h stimulated culture supernatants of CD73$^{+/+}$ and CD73$^{-/-}$ BMDCs were assessed for IL-12 and IL-23, after being stimulated with LPS or LPS plus AMP. The control BMDCs remained untreated. The data are from one single experiment and are representative of those obtained in three independent experiments. Values are expressed as mean ± SEM (n = 6). **p <0.05. ns, not significant **(B)**. ELISA assay test AMP doses ranging from 1 to 8 µM showed no apparent dose dependent effect. The experimental setting was the same as **Figure 3A (C)**. ELISA assays for IL-17 production by responder T cells after 48h stimulation by the immunizing antigen and CD73$^{+/+}$ or CD73$^{-/-}$ BMDCs. The data are from one single experiment and are representative of those obtained in three independent experiments **(D)**. LPS exposed BMDCs expressed increased amount of CD73. BMDCs were treated (dotted line) or untreated with a small dose of LPS (50 ng/ml) before stained with anti-CD73 mAB followed by FACS analysis **(E)**. Adenosine assay. Adenosine in the supernatants of cultured BMDCs was measured by an Adenosine Assay Kit (Fluorometric) after the CD73$^{+/+}$ or CD73$^{-/-}$ BMDCs were treated with LPS (100 ng/ml) with or with additional treatment of AMP (1 µM). ns, not significant.

mouse) splenic DCs. As demonstrated in **Figure 4A**, approximately one third of the splenic CD11c$^+$ cells in wt-B6, but not the CD73$^{-/-}$ mouse are CD73$^+$. αβTCR$^+$ responder T cells separated from immunized B6 mice were stimulated for 5 days *in vitro* with the immunizing antigen and irradiated splenic DCs, under Th1- or Th17-polarizing conditions. Evaluating numbers of IFN-γ$^+$ and IL-17$^+$ T cells among responder T cells shows that AMP enhances Th17 responses (**Figure 4B**, left panels) stimulated by CD73$^{+/+}$, but not CD73$^{-/-}$, splenic DCs and it inhibits Th1 responses (**Figure 4B**, right panels) stimulated by CD73$^{+/+}$, but not CD73$^{-/-}$ as well. Cytokine test (**Figure 4C**) showed that responder T cells produced comparable amounts of IFN-γ and IL-17 when stimulated by either CD73$^{+/+}$ or CD73$^{-/-}$, splenic DCs in the absence of AMP. In the presence of AMP, however, increased IL-17 production was seen in stimulation of responder T cells by CD73$^{+/+}$, but not CD73$^{-/-}$, splenic DCs. Also, AMP inhibits IFN-γ production of responder T cells stimulated by CD73$^{+/+}$, but not CD73$^{-/-}$, splenic DCs.

CD73 Expressed by αβ T Cells Does Not Contribute to the AMP Enhancing Effect

CD73 is constantly expressed in ~80% of αβ T cells (**Figure 5A**). To determine whether CD73 molecules expressed on αβ T cells contribute to AMP-mediated enhancement of Th17 responses, αβTCR$^+$ responder T cells enriched by MACS column were CFSE labeled before stimulating with plated bound anti-CD3 antibodies, in the absence or presence of AMP (1 μM), under Th17 polarizing conditions. The results show that AMP treatment does not significantly affect the Th17 responses (**Figure 5B**), which agreed with our previous finding that CD73 expressing αβ T cells are incapable of degrading AMP to adenosine (26). To further exclude the possibility that CD73 expressed on BMDCs but not on αβ T cells accounted for the augmented Th17 responses, we conducted a crisscross test in which responder T cells isolated from immunized CD73$^{+/+}$ (B6) and CD73$^{-/-}$ (CD73$^{-/-}$ mouse) mice were stimulated by CD73$^{+/+}$ and CD73$^{-/-}$ splenic DCs. The results showed that AMP enhancement of Th17 responses is seen only in the presence of CD73$^{+/+}$ splenic DCs (**Figure 5C**). AMP suppressed Th1 responses, which is also seen only in the presence of CD73$^{+/+}$, but not CD73$^{-/-}$, splenic DCs, suggesting that CD73 expressing DCs are required in degradation of AMP to adenosine leading to inhibited Th1 and enhanced Th17 responses.

Requirement of CD73$^{+/+}$ BMDCs in DC γδ T Cell Interaction

We have observed that mouse BMDCs acquired an increased ability to enhance Th17 responses after exposure to γδ T cells, and a significant portion of the BMDCs expressed CD73 after exposure to γδ T cells. To determine whether CD73 expression by BMDCs is required for DC-γδ interaction, we compared Th17 responses presented by CD73$^{+/+}$ and CD73$^{-/-}$ BMDCs, after exposure to γδ T cells. Three BMDC preparations were compared for their interactive ability with γδ T cells—the CD73$^{+/+}$ BMDCs with (**Figure 6A**, mid panels) or without (**Figure 6A** top panels) prior exposure to LPS and the CD73$^{-/-}$ BMDCs treated with LPS (**Figure 6A**, lower panels). The γδ T cells were separated from immunized B6 mice using a MACS column (38). BMDCs were exposed to γδ T cells at a pre-determined optimal ratio of T: DC = 1:20 for 24 h. Then, the γδ T cells were removed and the BMDCs were collected, irradiated, and seeded onto 24-well plates (5×10^5/well), followed by co-culture with responder T cells. The AP function of BMDCs was assessed by measuring IFN-γ$^+$ and IL-17$^+$ T cells among responder T cells and cytokine production, under Th1-, or Th17-polarizing conditions (27, 38). Results show that the LPS-treated (**Figure 6A**, mid panels), but not the untreated (**Figure 6A**, Top panels), CD73$^{+/+}$ BMDCs stimulated a significantly greater number of IL-17$^+$ cells among responder T cells, after exposure to γδ T cells. However, the CD73$^{-/-}$ BMDCs were unable to augment Th17 response by exposure to γδ T cells (**Figure 6A**, lower panels). Cytokine tests showed that the LPS-treated, but not the untreated, CD73$^{+/+}$ BMDCs induced greater amounts of IL-17 production of responder T cells after interacting with γδ T cells (**Figure 6B**). IFN-γ production of responder T cells remained unchanged after the BMDCs were exposed to γδ T cells, further supporting the prediction that expression of CD73 by DCs crucially triggers a strong Th17 response; whereas disabling CD73 function on DCs prevents higher Th17 responses.

DISCUSSION

Under pathologic conditions, a large amount of ATP is released into the extracellular compartment by injured and stressed cells (3, 4). Extracellular ATP acts on many immune cells to promote inflammation (5–9). Due to the potent immune stimulatory actions of ATP, the extracellular concentrations are kept in check by enzymatic digestion of ATP. The ecto-enzyme CD73 (ecto-5'-nucleotidase), a molecule pivotally involved in converting non-immunosuppressive AMP into immunosuppressive adenosine (12, 16), is expressed by many cell types, including Treg cells (17, 21, 42, 43), B cells (44) and endothelial cells (45). Previous studies showed that myeloid cells express altered levels of CD73 depending on their activation state (46), which is closely associated with pro- and anti-inflammatory functions of myeloid cells (47–50). In addition, the function of regulatory cells relies on expression of CD39 and CD73, and generation of adenosine mediates the immunosuppressive ability of regulatory T cells (Tregs) (21).

Adenosine is an important regulatory molecule which modulates a wide range of physiological functions (51), including the immune response (51–54), by acting on T cells (16, 55), macrophages/DCs (24, 56), NK cells (57), neutrophils (58), platelets (59), and regulatory T cells (25, 60). Previous studies showed that adenosine diminishes the capacity of DCs to initiate and amplify Th1 immune responses and that CD73 expressed on DC/macrophages is anti-inflammatory. For example, M2 macrophages generate an adenosine-rich environment, which in turn can augment the anti-inflammatory and tissue remodeling activities of these cells (11, 23). Here we show that BMDCs preferentially activate Th1 responses; after treatment with TLR ligands, both Th1 and Th17 stimulating effects of BMDCs were enhanced. However, dual treatment with LPS and adenosine enabled BMDCs to acquire greatly increased Th17 promoting activity. Both Th1 and Th17 pathogenic T cells contribute to the pathogenesis of

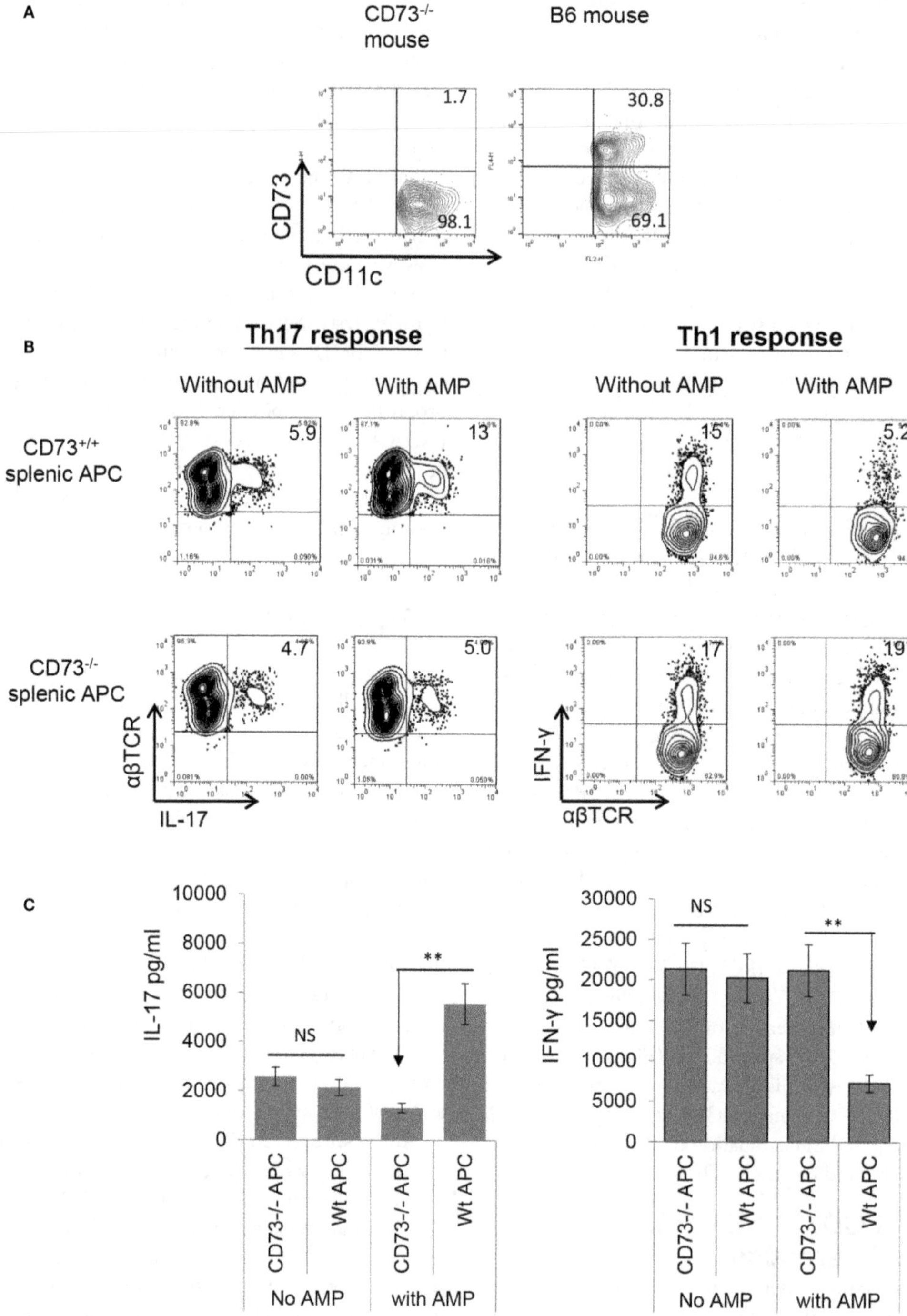

FIGURE 4 | Adenosine monophosphate enhanced Th17 responses and inhibited Th1 responses in the presence of CD73^{+} splenic APCs **(A)**. Approximated one third of the splenic CD11c^{+} cells of B6, but not CD73$^{-/-}$ mouse expressed CD73. Splenic cells of B6 and CD73$^{-/-}$ mouse were double stained by FITC-anti-CD11c and PE-anti-mouse CD73. The staining profile of gated CD11c^{+} cells is shown **(B)**. MACS column separated αβ T cells from immunized B6 mice were stimulated for 5 days with the immunizing peptide and antigen presenting cells under either Th17 (left panels) or Th1 (right panels) polarizing conditions; then the numbers of IL-17^{+} and IFN-γ^{+} cells among the TCRαβ^{+} responder T cells was assessed after intracellular staining with anti-IL-17 and anti-αβTCR mAbs. Upper panels are the responses stimulated by CD73$^{+/+}$ splenic APCs and lower panels are responses stimulated by CD73$^{-/-}$ splenic APCs **(C)**. ELISA assays for IL-17 and IFN-γ production by responder αβ T cells after 48 h stimulation by the immunizing antigen and CD73$^{+/+}$ or CD73$^{-/-}$ splenic APCs. CD73$^{+/+}$ and CD73$^{-/-}$ BMDCs, with or without a prior treatment of splenic APCs with adenosine monophosphate. The data are from one single experiment and are representative of those obtained in three independent experiments. ns, not significant.

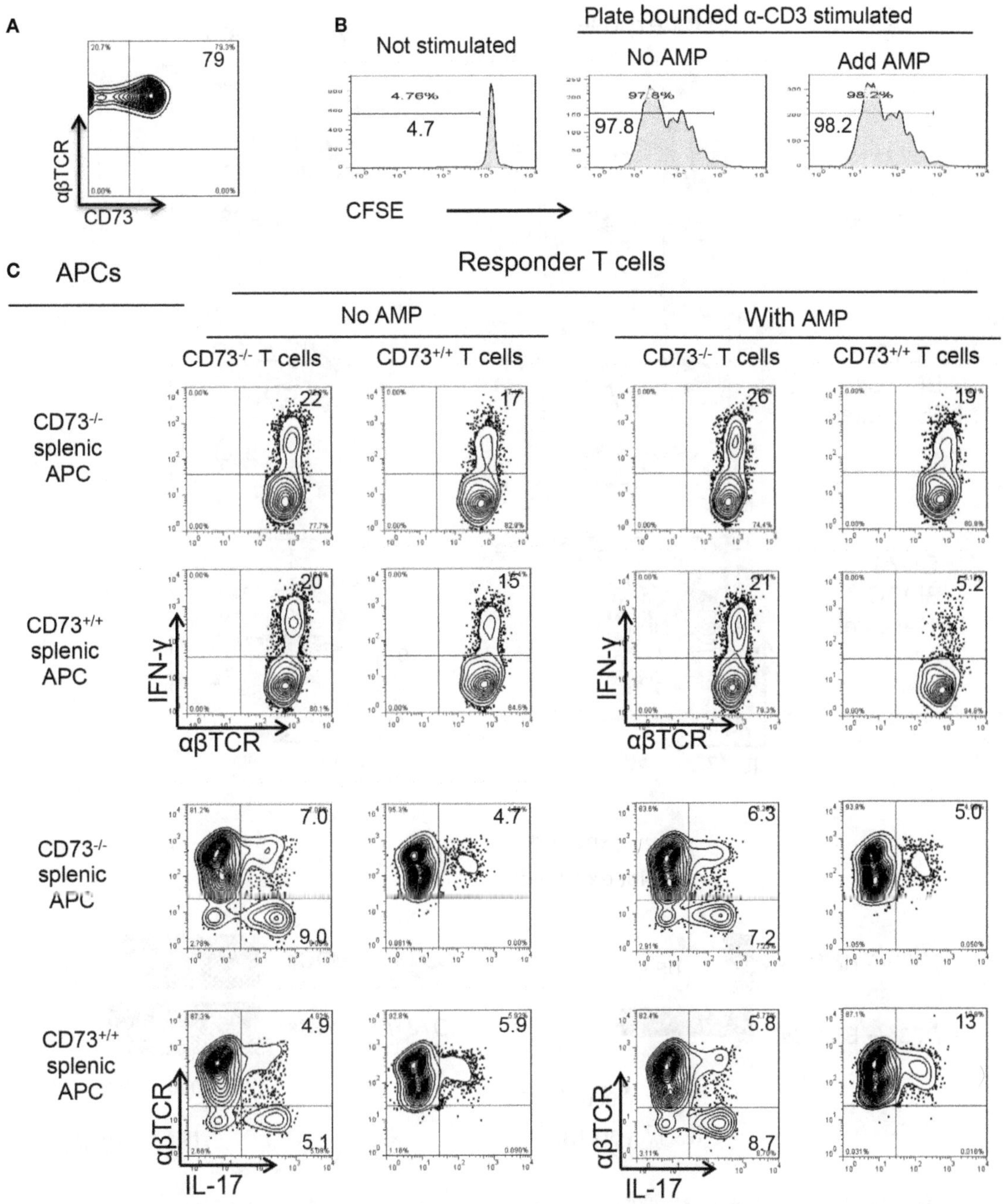

FIGURE 5 | Role of CD73 on splenic dendritic cells **(A)**. CD73 is constantly expressed in >60% of αβTCR+ T cells. MACS column enriched αβ T cells were stained with anti-αβ TCR and anti-mouse CD73, followed by FACS analysis **(B)**. CD73 expressed on αβ T cells is not responsible for adenosine monophosphate (AMP) enhancement of Th17 responses. MACS column enriched αβ T cells were CFSE (5 μM) stained. 1.5 × 10^6/well T cells were seeded into 24-well plate which were precoated with anti-CD3 antibodies. with or without AMP (1 μM). Some 48 h later the T cells were harvested and subjected to FACS analysis **(C)**. $CD73^{+/+}$ splenic dendritic cells (DCs), but not $CD73^{+/+}$ αβ T cells are responsible for AMP enhancement of Th17 responses. Crisscross test for determination of whether AMP has a direct effect on αβ responder T cells or splenic DCs. Responder αβ T cells and splenic DCs were isolated from $CD73^{+/+}$ (B6) and $CD73^{-/-}$ mice, respectively. The data are from one single experiment and are representative of those obtained in three independent experiments.

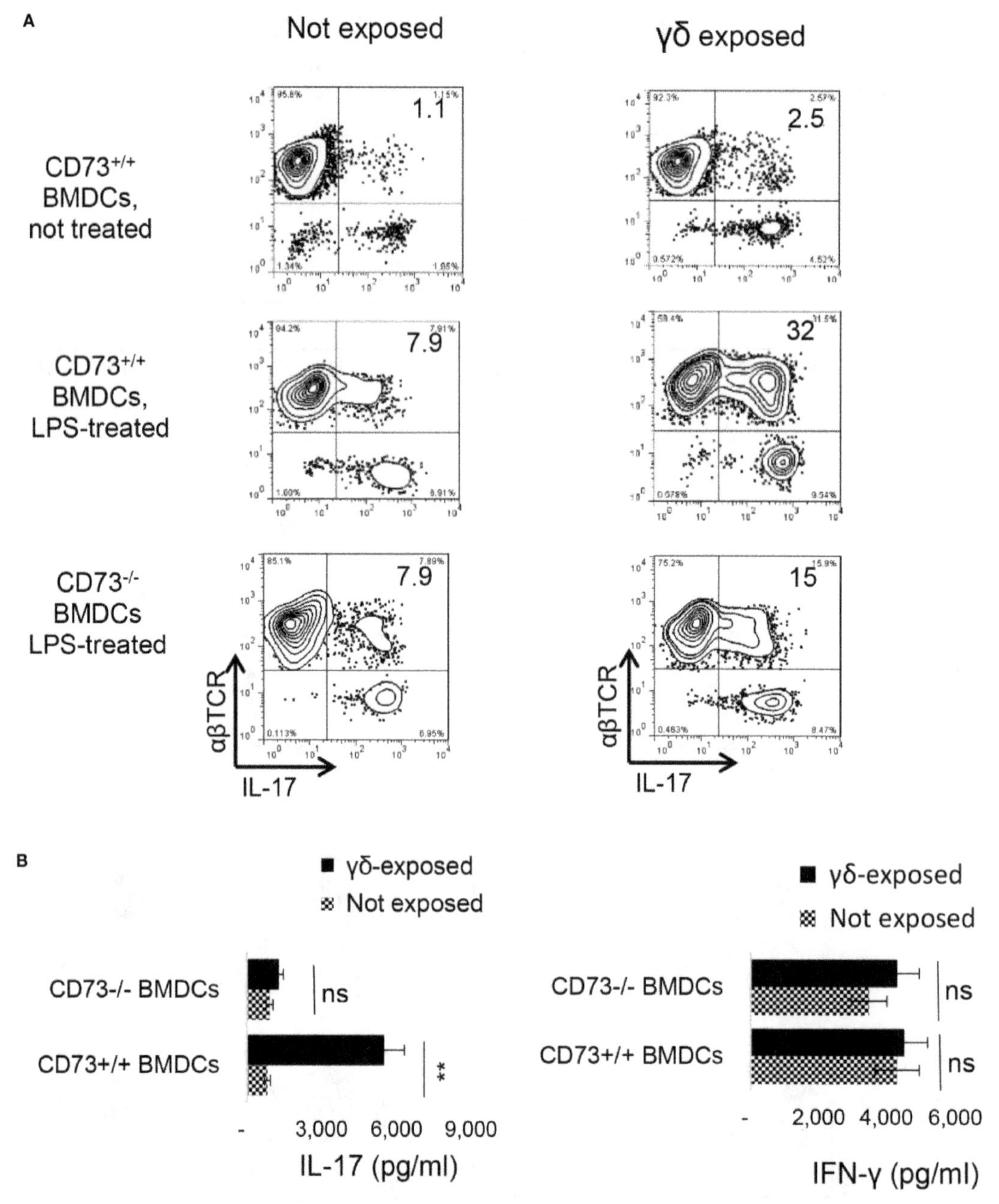

FIGURE 6 | Requirement of $CD73^{+/+}$ bone marrow dendritic cells in dendritic cell γδ T cell interaction **(A)**. Three differently prepared bone marrow dendritic cells (BMDCs) were compared for their interactive ability with γδ T cells—the BMDCs isolated from B6 mouse ($CD73^{+/+}$), with (mid panels) or without (top panels) a prior exposure to lipopolysaccharide (LPS, 100 ng/ml)), and the BMDCs isolated from $CD73^{-/-}$ mouse treated with LPS (lower panels). The γδ T cells were separated from immunized B6 mice using MACS column (38). After incubation with γδ T cells at a ratio of T: DC = 1:20 for 24 h. The γδ T cells were removed and the BMDCs were collected, irradiated, and seeded on to 24-well plates (5 × 10^5/well) for AP functional test. To determine antigen presenting function, responder T cells isolated from immunized B6 mice were co-cultured with BMDCs at a ratio of T: DC = 20:1, in the presence of immunizing antigen ($IRBP_{1-20}$) and under Th17 polarizing conditions. IFN-γ^+ and IL-17^+ T cells among responder T cells were examined after 5-day *in vitro* stimulation **(B)**. ELISA assays for IL-17 and IFN-γ production by responder T cells after 48 h stimulation by the immunizing antigen and $CD73^{+/+}$ or $CD73^{-/-}$ BMDCs. $CD73^{+/+}$ and $CD73^{-/-}$ BMDCs, with or without a prior exposure to γδ T cells. The data are from one single experiment and are representative of those obtained in three independent experiments. ns, not significant.

autoimmune diseases (61–63), and levels of extracellular adenosine increase greatly during inflammation (32, 33). The opposite effect of adenosine on Th1 and Th17 responses could certainly offset therapeutics targeting Th1 pathogenic reactions. As such, clarification of the conflicting effect of adenosine on Th1 and Th17 responses is of great importance.

Given the pivotal function of CD73 in adenosine-mediated immunoregulation (12, 15), and the previous finding that immune cells that express different levels of CD73 are functionally distinct (24, 25), we examined the role of CD73 on DCs and investigated whether $CD73^+$ DCs are functionally exceptional in Th1 and Th17 responses. Studies have reported that only ~2–10% of freshly isolated human monocytes express CD73 (64). In mouse BMDCs, CD73 was easier to find in immature BMDCs than in mature BMDCs (65). M1 macrophages have been reported to exhibit a modest decrease in the expression of both CD39 and CD73, while M2 macrophages express higher levels of both (11). Our results showed that GM-CSF-cultured BMDCs do not constantly express CD73; however, after exposure to TLR ligand or interaction with (γδ) T cells, a significantly increased number expressed CD73 which was closely associated with an increased ability to promote Th17 responses. We were also able to show that only a portion of the splenic DCs express CD73 (**Figure 4**). Functional comparisons between $CD73^+$ and $CD73^-$ APCs showed that while AMP has an enhancing effect on Th17 responses *via* splenic DCs, expression of CD73 on splenic DCs is required. Such observation agrees with previous findings that the mature mouse BMDCs and mature human monocyte derived DCs are less efficient than immature DCs in supporting Th17 differentiation (66, 67). Our observation complements the previous scenario by showing that adenosine diminishes the capacity of DCs to amplify Th1 immune responses (13, 14), we additionally show however adenosine augments Th17 responses in which $CD73^+$ DCs play an important role. Such an observation also supports our previous observation that adenosine tips the Th1/Th17 responses towards the latter (38, 39).

The previous conclusion that CD73 is important for the anti-inflammatory immune responses has mainly been proven in Th1 responses. To determine whether such a conclusion also applies to Th17 responses we have compared functions of $CD73^{+/+}$ and $CD73^{-/-}$ DCs in Th1 and Th17 responses. Our results showed that the $CD73^{+/+}$ DCs have significantly greater Th17 enhancing effects, particularly when AMP is provided. It is likely that the $CD73^+$ DCs have an increased ability to convert AMP to adenosine, leading to inhibited Th1 responses but enhanced Th17 responses. It is important to note, however, that CD73 molecules expressed on different immune cells are functionally different. We have previously reported that γδ T cells have a greater enhancing effect on Th17 responses when they express less CD73 (26, 27); in this study we show that BMDCs acquire a stronger Th17 stimulating activity when they express CD73. Given that Th17 cells uniquely express CD39/CD73 (42, 67, 68), it is likely that initiation of Th17 responses by $CD73^+$ DCs may trigger cascading responses in which activated Th17 cells become CD73-providing cells in the responses which further facilitate the conversion of AMP to adenosine. Given our previous observation that $CD73^+$ DCs have increased ability to activate γδ T cells and that CD73-expressing γδ T cells are much more potent in converting AMP to adenosine (26), we conclude that the induction of $CD73^+$ BMDCs cells will lead to cascading Th17 responses *via* several pathways.

In summary, stimulation of adenosine receptors skews DC differentiation (69–71). In this study, we show that conversion of AMP into adenosine by CD73 expressing DCs is an important pathway in triggering cascading T17 responses.

ETHICS STATEMENT

The animal study was reviewed and approved by Institutional Animal Care and Use Committee of University of California Los Angeles (Protocol number: ARC # 2014-029-21).

AUTHOR CONTRIBUTIONS

DS, HK, and HS designed research. DS and MK performed the experiments and analyzed data. DS and HK wrote the manuscript. All authors contributed to the article and approved the submitted version.

REFERENCES

1. Sitkovsky M, Lukashev D. Regulation of immune cells by local-tissue oxygen tension: HIF1α and adenosine receptors. *Nat Rev Immunol* (2005) 5:712–21. doi: 10.1038/nri1685
2. Linden J. Molecular appraoch to adenosine receotrs: Receptor-Mediated Mechanisms of Tissue Protection. *Ann Rev Pharmacol Toxicol* (2001) 41:775–87. doi: 10.1146/annurev.pharmtox.41.1.775
3. Dubyak GR, el-Moatassim C. Signal transduction via P2-purinergic receptors for extracellular ATP and other nucleotides. *Am J Physiol* (1993) 265:C577–606. doi: 10.1152/ajpcell.1993.265.3.C577
4. Pellegatti P, Raffaghello L, Bianchi G, Piccardi F, Pistoia V, Di Virgilio F. Increased Level of Extracellular ATP at Tumor Sites: In Vivo Imaging with Plasma Membrane Luciferase. *PloS One* (2008) 3:e2599. doi: 10.1371/journal.pone.0002599
5. Matzinger P. The Danger Model: A Renewed Sense of Self. *Science* (2002) 296:301–5. doi: 10.1126/science.1071059
6. Beigi RD, Kertesy SB, Aquilina G, Dubyak GR. Oxidized ATP (oATP) attenuates proinflammatory signaling via P2 receptor-independent mechanisms. *Br J Pharmacol* (2003) 140:507–19. doi: 10.1038/sj.bjp.0705470
7. Canaday DH, Beigi R, Silver RF, Harding CV, Boom WH, Dubyak GR. ATP and Control of Intracellular Growth of Mycobacteria by T Cells. *Infect Immun* (2002) 70:6456–9. doi: 10.1128/iai.70.11.6456-6459.2002
8. Wilkin F, Duhant X, Bruyns C, Suarez-Huerta N, Boeynaems J-M, Robaye B. The P2Y11 Receptor Mediates the ATP-Induced Maturation of Human Monocyte-Derived Dendritic Cells. *J Immunol* (2001) 166:7172–7. doi: 10.4049/jimmunol.166.12.7172
9. Hanley PJ, Musset B, Renigunta V, Limberg SH, Dalpke AH, Sus R, et al. Extracellular ATP induces oscillations of intracellular Ca2+ and membrane potential and promotes transcription of IL-6 in macrophages. *Proc Natl Acad Sci USA* (2004) 101:9479–84. doi: 10.1073/pnas.0400733101
10. Borsellino G, Kleinewietfeld M, Di Mitri D, Sternjak A, Diamantini A, Giometto R, et al. Expression of ectonucleotidase CD39 by Foxp3+ Treg cells: hydrolysis of extracellular ATP and immune suppression. *Blood* (2007) 110:1225–32. doi: 10.1182/blood-2006-12-064527
11. Zanin RF, Braganhol E, Bergamin LS, Campesato LFI, Filho AZ, Moreira JCF, et al. Differential Macrophage Activation Alters the Expression Profile of NTPDase and Ecto-5′-Nucleotidase. *PloS One* (2012) 7:e31205. doi: 10.1371/journal.pone.0031205
12. Beavis PA, Stagg J, Darcy PK, Smyth MJ. CD73: a potent suppressor of antitumor immune responses. *Trends Immunol* (2012) 33:231–7. doi: 10.1016/j.it.2012.02.009
13. Antonioli L, Pacher P, Vizi ES, Haskó G. CD39 and CD73 in immunity and inflammation. *Trends Mol Med* (2013) 19:355–67. doi: 10.1016/j.molmed.2013.03.005
14. Eltzschig HK, Carmeliet P. Hypoxia and Inflammation. *N Engl J Med* (2011) 364:656–65. doi: 10.1056/NEJMra0910283
15. Rabinovich GA, Gabrilovich D, Sotomayor EM. Immunosuppressive Strategies that are Mediated by Tumor Cells. *Annu Rev Immunol* (2007) 25:267–96. doi: 10.1146/annurev.immunol.25.022106.141609
16. Jin D, Fan J, Wang L, Thompson LF, Liu A, Daniel BJ, et al. CD73 on Tumor Cells Impairs Antitumor T-Cell Responses: A Novel Mechanism of Tumor-Induced Immune Suppression. *Cancer Res* (2010) 70:2245–55. doi: 10.1158/0008-5472.can-09-3109

17. Stagg J, Divisekera U, Duret H, Sparwasser T, Teng MWL, Darcy PK, et al. CD73-Deficient Mice Have Increased Antitumor Immunity and Are Resistant to Experimental Metastasis. *Cancer Res* (2011) 71:2892–900. doi: 10.1158/0008-5472.CAN-10-4246
18. Mills JH, Thompson LF, Mueller C, Waickman AT, Jalkanen S, Niemela J, et al. CD73 is required for efficient entry of lymphocytes into the central nervous system during experimental autoimmune encephalomyelitis. *Proc Natl Acad Sci U S A* (2008) 105:9325–30. doi: 10.1073/pnas.0711175105
19. Thompson LF, Eltzschig HK, Ibla JC, Van De Wiele CJ, Resta R, Morote-Garcia JC, et al. Crucial Role for Ecto-5′-Nucleotidase (CD73) in Vascular Leakage during Hypoxia. *J Exp Med* (2004) 200:1395–405. doi: 10.1084/jem.20040915
20. Kiss J, Yegutkin GG, Koskinen K, Savunen T, Jalkanen S, Salmi M. IFN-β protects from vascular leakage via up-regulation of CD73. *Eur J Immunol* (2007) 37:3334–8. doi: 10.1002/eji.200737793
21. Deaglio S, Dwyer KM, Gao W, Friedman D, Usheva A, Erat A, et al. Adenosine generation catalyzed by CD39 and CD73 expressed on regulatory T cells mediates immune suppression. *J Exp Med* (2007) 204:1257–65. doi: 10.1084/jem.20062512
22. Ryzhov S, Novitskiy SV, Goldstein AE, Biktasova A, Blackburn MR, Biaggioni I, et al. Adenosinergic Regulation of the Expansion and Immunosuppressive Activity of CD11b+Gr1+ Cells. *J Immunol* (2011) 187:6120–9. doi: 10.4049/jimmunol.1101225
23. Csóka B, Selmeczy Z, Koscsó B, Németh ZH, Pacher P, Murray PJ, et al. Adenosine promotes alternative macrophage activation via A2A and A2B receptors. *FASEB J* (2012) 26:376–86. doi: 10.1096/fj.11-190934
24. Naganuma M, Wiznerowicz EB, Lappas CM, Linden J, Worthington MT, Ernst PB. Cutting Edge: Critical Role for A2A Adenosine Receptors in the T Cell-Mediated Regulation of Colitis. *J Immunol* (2006) 177:2765–9. doi: 10.4049/jimmunol.177.5.2765
25. Zarek PE, Huang C-T, Lutz ER, Kowalski J, Horton MR, Linden J, et al. A2A receptor signaling promotes peripheral tolerance by inducing T-cell anergy and the generation of adaptive regulatory T cells. *Blood* (2008) 111:251–9. doi: 10.1182/blood-2007-03-081646
26. Liang D, Zuo A, Shao H, Chen M, Kaplan HJ, Sun D. Roles of the Adenosine Receptor and CD73 in the Regulatory Effect of γδ T Cells. *PloS One* (2014) 9: e108932. doi: 10.1371/journal.pone.0108932
27. Liang D, Zuo A, Zhao R, Shao H, Born WK, O'Brien RL, et al. CD73 Expressed on γδ T Cells Shapes Their Regulatory Effect in Experimental Autoimmune Uveitis. *PloS One* (2016) 11:e0150078. doi: 10.1371/journal.pone.0150078
28. Fedele G, Stefanelli P, Spensieri F, Fazio C, Mastrantonio P, Ausiello CM. Bordetella pertussis-Infected Human Monocyte-Derived Dendritic Cells Undergo Maturation and Induce Th1 Polarization and Interleukin-23 Expression. *Infect Immun* (2005) 73:1590–7. doi: 10.1128/IAI.73.3.1590-1597.2005
29. Lappas CM, Rieger JM, Linden J. A2A adenosine receptor induction inhibits IFN-gamma production in murine CD4+ T cells. *J Immunol* (2005) 174:1073–80. doi: 10.4049/jimmunol.174.2.1073
30. Ohta A, Gorelik E, Prasad SJ, Ronchese F, Lukashev D, Wong MKK, et al. A2A adenosine receptor protects tumors from antitumor T cells. *Proc Nat Acad Sci USA* (2006) 103:13132–7. doi: 10.1073/pnas.0605251103
31. Eltzschig HK, Sitkovsky MV, Robson SC. Purinergic Signaling during Inflammation. *N Engl J Med* (2012) 367:2322–33. doi: 10.1056/NEJMra1205750
32. Ohta A, Sitkovsky M. Role of G-protein-coupled adenosine receptors in downregulation of inflammation and protection from tissue damage. *Nature* (2001) 414:916–20. doi: 10.1038/414916a
33. Sitkovsky MV, Lukashev D, Apasov S, Kojima H, Koshiba M, Caldwell C, et al. Physiological Control of Immune Response and Inflammatory Tissue Damage by Hypoxia-Inducible Factors and Adenosine A2A Receptors. *Annu Rev Immunol* (2004) 22:657–82. doi: 10.1146/annurev.immunol.22.012703.104731
34. Mahamed DA, Toussaint LE, Bynoe MS. CD73-Generated Adenosine Is Critical for Immune Regulation during Toxoplasma gondii Infection. *Infect Immun* (2015) 83:721–9. doi: 10.1128/iai.02536-14
35. Inaba K, Inaba M, Romani N, Aya H, Deguchi M, Ikehara S, et al. Generation of large numbers of dendritic cells from mouse bone marrow cultures supplemented with granulocyte/macrophage colony-stimulating factor. *J Exp Med* (1992) 176:1693–702. doi: 10.1084/jem.176.6.1693
36. Lyons AB, Parish CR. Determination of lymphocyte division by flow cytometry. *J Immunol Methods* (1994) 171:131–7. doi: 10.1016/0022-1759(94)90236-4
37. Liang D, Zuo A, Shao H, Chen M, Kaplan HJ, Sun D. Anti-inflammatory or pro-inflammatory effect of an adenosine receptor agonist on the Th17 autoimmune response is inflammatory environmental-dependent. *J Immunol* (2014) 193:5498–505. doi: 10.4049/jimmunol.1401959
38. Liang D, Zuo A, Shao H, Born WK, O'Brien RL, Kaplan HJ, et al. IL-23 Receptor Expression on γδ T Cells Correlates with Their Enhancing or Suppressive Effects on Autoreactive T Cells in Experimental Autoimmune Uveitis. *J Immunol* (2013) 191:1118–25. doi: 10.4049/jimmunol.1300626
39. Nian H, Shao H, O'Brien RL, Born WK, Kaplan HJ, Sun D. Activated γδ cells promote the activation of uveitogenic T cells and exacerbate EAU development. *Invest Ophthalmol Vis Sci* (2011) 52:5920–7. doi: 10.1167/iovs.10-6758
40. Peng Y, Han G, Shao H, Wang Y, Kaplan HJ, Sun D. Characterization of IL-17 + Interphotoreceptor Retinoid-Binding Protein-Specific T Cells in Experimental Autoimmune Uveitis. *Invest Ophthalmol Vis Sci* (2007) 48:4153–61. doi: 10.1167/iovs.07-0251
41. Liang D, Zuo A, Shao H, Chen M, Kaplan HJ, Sun D. A2B adenosine receptor activation switches differentiation of bone marrow cells to a CD11c+Gr-1+ dendritic cell subset that promotes the Th17 response. *Immun Inflamm Dis* (2015) 3:360–73. doi: 10.1002/iid3.74
42. Ehrentraut H, Clambey ET, McNamee EN, Brodsky KS, Ehrentraut SF, Poth JM, et al. CD73+ regulatory T cells contribute to adenosine-mediated resolution of acute lung injury. *FASEB J* (2013) 27:2207–19. doi: 10.1096/fj.12-225201
43. Smyth LA, Ratnasothy K, Tsang JYS, Boardman D, Warley A, Lechler R, et al. CD73 expression on extracellular vesicles derived from CD4+CD25+Foxp3+ T cells contributes to their regulatory function. *Eur J Immunol* (2013) 43:2430–40. doi: 10.1002/eji.201242909
44. Conter LJ, Song E, Shlomchik MJ, Tomayko MM. CD73 Expression Is Dynamically Regulated in the Germinal Center and Bone Marrow Plasma Cells Are Diminished in Its Absence. *PloS One* (2014) 9:e92009. doi: 10.1371/journal.pone.0092009
45. Yegutkin GG, Auvinen K, Rantakari P, Hollmén M, Karikoski M, Grénman R, et al. Ecto-5′-nucleotidase/CD73 enhances endothelial barrier function and sprouting in blood but not lymphatic vasculature. *Eur J Immunol* (2015) 45:562–73. doi: 10.1002/eji.201444856
46. Synnestvedt K, Furuta GT, Comerford KM, Louis N, Karhausen J, Eltzschig HK, et al. Ecto-5′-nucleotidase (CD73) regulation by hypoxia-inducible factor-1 mediates permeability changes in intestinal epithelia. *J Clin Invest* (2002) 110:993–1002. doi: 10.1172/JCI15337
47. Mosser DM, Edwards JP. Exploring the full spectrum of macrophage activation. *Nat Rev Immunol* (2008) 8:958–69. doi: 10.1038/nri2448
48. Gordon S, Martinez FO. Alternative Activation of Macrophages: Mechanism and Functions. *Immunity* (2010) 32:593–604. doi: 10.1016/j.immuni.2010.05.007
49. Biswas SK, Mantovani A. Macrophage plasticity and interaction with lymphocyte subsets: cancer as a paradigm. *Nat Immunol* (2010) 11:889–96. doi: 10.1038/ni.1937
50. Yegutkin GG, Marttila-Ichihara F, Karikoski M, Niemelä J, Laurila JP, Elima K, et al. Altered purinergic signaling in CD73-deficient mice inhibits tumor progression. *Eur J Immunol* (2011) 41:1231–41. doi: 10.1002/eji.201041292
51. Fredholm BB, IJzerman AP, Jacobson KA, Linden J, Müller CE. International Union of Basic and Clinical Pharmacology. LXXXI. *Nomenclature and Classification of Adenosine Receptors—An Update. Pharmacol Rev* (2011) 63:1–34. doi: 10.1124/pr.110.003285
52. Jacobson KA, Gao Z-G. Adenosine receptors as therapeutic targets. *Nat Rev Drug Discov* (2006) 5:247–64. doi: 10.1038/nrd1983
53. Hasko G, Linden J, Cronstein B, Pacher P. Adenosine receptors: therapeutic aspects for inflammatory and immune diseases. *Nat Rev Drug Discov* (2008) 7:759–70. doi: 10.1038/nrd2638
54. Sauer AV, Brigida I, Carriglio N, Aiuti A. Autoimmune dysregulation and purine metabolism in adenosine deaminase (ADA)-deficiency. *Front Immunol* (2012) 3:265. doi: 10.3389/fimmu.2012.00265
55. Lappas CM, Sullivan GW, Linden J. Adenosine A2A agonists in development for the treatment of inflammation. *Expert Opin Invest Drugs* (2005) 14:797–806. doi: 10.1517/13543784.14.7.797
56. Panther EL, Idzko M, Herouy Y, Rheinen H, Gebrick-Haerter PJ, Mrowietz U, et al. Expression and function of adenosine receptors in human dendritic cells. *FASEB J* (2001) 15:1963–70. doi: 10.1096/fj.01-0169com

57. Hoskin DW, Mader JS, Furlong SJ, Conrad DM, Blay J. Inhibition of T cell and natural killer cell function by adenosine and its contribution to immune evasion by tumor cells (Review). *Int J Oncol* (2008) 32:527–35. doi: 10.3892/ijo.32.3.527
58. Fredholm BB, IJ AP, Jacobson KA, Klotz KN, Linden J. International Union of Pharmacology. XXV. Nomenclature and classification of adenosine receptors. *Pharmacol Rev* (2001) 53:527–52. doi: 10.1124/pr.110.003285
59. Varani K, Gessi S, Dalpiaz A, Borea PA. Pharmacological and biochemical characterization of purified A2a adenosine receptors in human platelet membranes by [3H]-CGS 21680 binding. *Br J Pharmacol* (1996) 117:1693–701. doi: 10.1111/j.1476-5381.1996.tb15341.x
60. Ehrentraut H, Westrich JA, Eltzschig HK, Clambey ET. Adora2b Adenosine Receptor Engagement Enhances Regulatory T Cell Abundance during Endotoxin-Induced Pulmonary Inflammation. *PloS One* (2012) 7:e32416. doi: 10.1371/journal.pone.0032416
61. Bettelli E, Carrier Y, Gao W, Korn T, Strom TB, Oukka M, et al. Reciprocal developmental pathways for the generation of pathogenic effector TH17 and regulatory T cells. *Nature* (2006) 441:235–8. doi: 10.1038/nature04753
62. Dong C. Diversification of T-helper-cell lineages: finding the family root of IL-17-producing cells. *Nat Rev Immunol* (2006) 6:329–34. doi: 10.1038/nri1807
63. Cua DJ, Sherlock J, Chen Y, Murphy CA, Joyce B, Seymour B, et al. Interleukin-23 rather than interleukin-12 is the critical cytokine for autoimmune inflammation of the brain. *Nature* (2003) 421:744–8. doi: 10.1038/nature01355
64. Sciaraffia E, Riccomi A, Lindstedt R, Gesa V, Cirelli E, Patrizio M, et al. Human monocytes respond to extracellular cAMP through A2A and A2B adenosine receptors. *J Leukoc Biol* (2014) 96:113–22. doi: 10.1189/jlb.3A0513-302RR
65. Silva-Vilches C, Ring S, Schrader J, Clausen BE, Probst H-C, Melchior F, et al. Production of Extracellular Adenosine by CD73+ Dendritic Cells Is Crucial for Induction of Tolerance in Contact Hypersensitivity Reactions. *J Invest Dermatol* (2019) 139:541–51. doi: 10.1016/j.jid.2018.10.016
66. Bouguermouh S, Fortin G, Baba N, Rubio M, Sarfati M. CD28 Co-Stimulation Down Regulates Th17 Development. *PloS One* (2009) 4:e5087. doi: 10.1371/journal.pone.0005087
67. Chalmin F, Mignot G, Bruchard M, Chevriaux A, Végran F, Hichami A, et al. Stat3 and Gfi-1 Transcription Factors Control Th17 Cell Immunosuppressive Activity via the Regulation of Ectonucleotidase Expression. *Immunity* (2012) 36:362–73. doi: 10.1016/j.immuni.2011.12.019
68. Doherty GA, Bai A, Hanidziar D, Longhi MS, Lawlor GO, Putheti P, et al. CD73 is a phenotypic marker of effector memory Th17 cells in inflammatory bowel disease. *Eur J Immunol* (2012) 42:3062–72. doi: 10.1002/eji.201242623
69. Novitskiy SV, Ryzhov S, Zaynagetdinov R, Goldstein AE, Huang Y, Tikhomirov OY, et al. Adenosine receptors in regulation of dendritic cell differentiation and function. *Blood* (2008) 112:1822–31. doi: 10.1182/blood-2008-02-136325
70. Desrosiers MD, Cembrola KM, Fakir MJ, Stephens LA, Jama FM, Shameli A, et al. Adenosine Deamination Sustains Dendritic Cell Activation in Inflammation. *J Immunol* (2007) 179:1884–92. doi: 10.4049/jimmunol.179.3.1884
71. Panther E, Corinti S, Idzko M, Herouy Y, Napp M, la Sala A, et al. Adenosine affects expression of membrane molecules, cytokine and chemokine release, and the T-cell stimulatory capacity of human dendritic cells. *Blood* (2003) 101:3985–90. doi: 10.1182/blood-2002-07-2113

7

Immune Phenotyping of Patients with Acute Vogt-Koyanagi-Harada Syndrome Before and After Glucocorticoids Therapy

Han Jiang[1†]*, Zhaohui Li*[2*†]*, Long Yu*[3]*, Ying Zhang*[4]*, Li Zhou*[5]*, Jianhua Wu*[2]*, Jing Yuan*[2]*, Mengyao Han*[2]*, Tao Xu*[2]*, Junwen He*[2]*, Shan Wang*[4]*, Chengfeng Yu*[2]*, Sha Pan*[2]*, Min Wu*[1]*, Hangyu Liu*[1]*, Haihong Zeng*[3]*, Zhu Song*[1]*, Qiangqiang Wang*[1]*, Shen Qu*[3]*, Junwei Zhang*[1]*, Yafei Huang*[3*] *and Junyan Han*[1*]

[1] *Department of Immunology, School of Basic Medicine, Tongji Medical College, Huazhong University of Science and Technology, Wuhan, China,* [2] *Retinal and Vitreous Diseases Department of Wuhan Aier Eye Hospital, Wuhan University, Wuhan, China,* [3] *Department of Pathogen Biology, School of Basic Medicine, Tongji Medical College, Huazhong University of Science and Technology, Wuhan, China,* [4] *Ophthalmic Imaging Department of Wuhan Aier Eye Hospital, Wuhan University, Wuhan, China,* [5] *Cataract Department of Wuhan Aier Eye Hospital, Wuhan University, Wuhan, China*

Correspondence:
Zhaohui Li
lizhaohui@whu.edu.cn
Junyan Han
hanj2014@hust.edu.cn
Yafei Huang
huangy2018@hust.edu.cn

[†]*These authors have contributed equally to this work*

Previous studies have established that disturbed lymphocytes are involved in the pathogenesis of Vogt-Koyanagi-Harada (VKH) syndrome. Accordingly, glucocorticoids (GCs), with their well-recognized immune-suppressive function, have been widely used for treatment of VKH patients with acute relapses. However, the systemic response of diverse immune cells to GC therapy in VKH is poorly characterized. To address this issue, we analyzed immune cell subpopulations and their phenotype, as well as cytokine profiles in peripheral blood from VKH patients (n=25) and health controls (HCs, n=21) by flow cytometry and luminex technique, respectively. For 16 patients underwent GC therapy (methylprednisolone, MP), the aforementioned measurements as well as the transcriptome data from patients before and after one-week's GC therapy were also compared to interrogate the systemic immune response to GC therapy. Lymphocyte composition in the blood was different in VKH patients and HCs. VKH patients had significantly higher numbers of T cells with more activated, polarized and differentiated phenotype, more unswitched memory B cells and monocytes, as compared to HCs. MP treatment resulted in decreased frequencies of T cells and NK cells, inhibited NK cell activation and T cell differentiation, and more profoundly, a marked shift in the distribution of monocyte subsets. Collectively, our findings suggest that advanced activation and differentiation, as well as dysregulated numbers of peripheral lymphocytes are the major immunological features of VKH, and GC therapy with MP not only inhibits T cell activation directly, but also affects monocyte subsets, which might combinatorically result in the inhibition of the pathogenic immune response.

Keywords: immunopathogenesis, lymphocyte subsets, monocytes, VKH, autoimmunity, cytokine

INTRODUCTION

Vogt-Koyanagi-Harada syndrome (VKH syndrome) is an acute diffuse uveitis characterized by bilateral, diffuse granulomatous resulted from stromal choroiditis, accompanied by neurologic manifestations consisting of headache and nausea (1). Ocular manifestations of this disease include retinal detachment or subretinal fluid, papilledema and hyperemia of the optic disk at initial onset. The prevalence of VKH varies among different countries and ethnic groups. In Asian, VKH represents one of the most common uveitis entities (2).

The pathogenesis of VKH has been extensively studied during the past decades. It is well established that an autoimmune response against melanocytes is considered to be involved in the pathogenesis of this disease (3). Early studies found that peripheral lymphocytes from patients with VKH could be activated by bovine uveal pigment (4). Subsequently, activated T cells were demonstrated as the predominant cell types in choroidal inflammation, accompanied by the presence of choroidal melanocytes that express HLA-DR, a major histocompatibility complex class II (MHC II) molecule, suggesting activated T cells as the pathogenic cells and the potential role of choroidal melanocytes in antigen presentation and T cell activation (5, 6). Later, different T cell subsets, including cytotoxic T cells (7), T helper (Th) 1 cells (8), and Th17 cells (9), were identified to be pathogenic in the settings of experimental autoimmune uveitis (EAU), a classical animal model for human uveitis, and/or clinical uveitis. In addition to T cells, other immune cells also contribute, including NK cells, B cells and myeloid cells (6). However, the role of these cells in the pathogenesis of VKH is not systemically addressed.

Tissue resident dendritic cells and macrophages are the major professional APCs, while monocytes are regarded as their counterparts in peripheral blood. In addition to antigen presentation (10), monocytes can also release inflammatory cytokines such as interleukin (IL)-6, IL-1β, and TNF-α, thereby directly mediating inflammation. Human monocyte is a heterogeneous cell population that can be classified into three subpopulations based on the differential expression levels of CD14 and CD16 (11). Classical monocytes, which is the major population of human monocytes (~90%), express high levels of CD14 but lack CD16 expression ($CD14^{++}CD16^{-}$). The remaining ~10% of human monocytes are further subdivided into the intermediate subset, with low CD16 and high CD14 expression ($CD14^{++}CD16^{+}$), and the non-classical subset, with high CD16 but relatively lower CD14 expression ($CD14^{+}CD16^{++}$). Classical monocytes express high levels of chemokine receptor CCR2 and low levels of CX3CR1, and perform better in phagocytosis compared to other monocyte subsets, thus contribute to anti-microbial responses (12–14). In contrast to this major subset, human intermediate monocytes express high levels of CCR5, CX3CR1 and HLA-DR, and low levels of CCR2 (13, 15), thus are specialized in antigen processing and presentation. Non-classical monocytes are less characterized, nevertheless, they are demonstrated to have the capacity to patrol blood vessels, resist viruses and stimulate T cell proliferation (16, 17). Although the involvement of these monocyte subsets has been reported in various inflammatory conditions, such as tuberculosis (18), asthma (19), rheumatoid arthritis (RA) (20) and Crohn's disease (21), their contributions to the pathogenesis of VKH are not fully understood. In addition, a new monocyte subset, $CD56^{+}$ monocyte, was identified and found to be expanded in certain autoimmune diseases such as rheumatoid arthritis and Crohn's disease (21–23), but their role in VKH remains unclear.

Although numerous new drugs have been developed within the last few decades, the most widely used treatment for acute VKH remains high-dose MP pulse therapy, to which most patients respond well and achieve an amelioration of symptoms within a few days (24, 25). It has been reported that GCs downregulate the expression levels of pro-inflammatory cytokines and adhesion molecules, which are required for cells to pass the blood-brain barrier (BBB). The GC response was reported to be highly cell type-specific in magnitude, and even in terms of the direction of transcriptional regulation (26). It is believed that patients profit most from the direct or indirect dampening effects on T cells by GC treatment, which can inhibit T cell activation, promote apoptosis in immune cells, and additionally exert inhibitory effects on inflammatory mediators such as nitric oxide (NO) (27). However, the effect of GCs on other immune cells including monocytes in VKH is not well characterized. Although it has been demonstrated that *in vitro* treatment of monocytes from healthy donors with GC induced an upregulation of transcripts associated with an anti-inflammatory phenotype, as well as enhanced cell survival, phagocytosis, and chemotaxis (28), the subset-specific response of monocytes to GC treatment and the underlying mechanism in VKH remain to be defined.

This study was designed to systemically characterize and compare the immunological profiles of peripheral blood from patients with VKH and healthy controls. The influence of MP, which has been the most widely prescribed GC in VKH therapy, on immune phenotypes in peripheral blood from VKH patients was also evaluated. Our investigation will offer a better understanding of the function, activation and differentiation status of the leukocyte subpopulations during autoimmune VKH and after GC therapy, and may facilitate a more specific therapeutic regimen for this particular disease, which is a major cause of visual impairment.

MATERIALS AND METHODS

Patients

All patients with uveitis were recruited at the retinal and vitreous diseases department of Wuhan Aier Eye Hospital from April 8, 2017 to December 17, 2020. Healthy controls (HCs) matched for gender and age were recruited among the employees of the hospital. The study protocol was approved by the Ethics Committee of Wuhan Aier Eye Hospital (Clinical Ethical Approval No. 2019IRBKY04). The diagnosis of VKH was based on the newly revised diagnostic criteria of the International Uveitis Conference. Written informed consent was obtained from all patients and HCs before study entry. A venous blood sample was taken from acute VKH patients prior to MP therapy (n=25), after MP therapy for seven consecutive days (n=16), as well as HCs (n=21) (**Tables 1** and **2**). The numbers of subjects used for each assay were indicated in the relevant tables or figures.

PBMC Isolation

Peripheral blood samples were collected in heparinized vacutainer tubes (BD bioscience, San Jose, CA, USA). After diluted two times by PBS, the blood was added carefully onto the Ficoll-Hypaque layer (3 ml Ficoll-Hypaque per 10 ml blood/PBS mixture), and centrifuged at 800 × g for 30 minutes with brake off, room temperature. Mononuclear layer was obtained and washed twice by PBS. The PBMC aliquots were used immediately for flow cytometry staining, or stocked frozen in fetal calf serum containing 10% DMSO and 5% dextran at -80°C for further test.

Cell Staining and Flow-Cytometric Analysis

Flow-cytometric analysis was performed according to our standard institutional protocols. All reagents were obtained from BD bioscience unless otherwise indicated. For surface staining, 50 µl freshly collected blood was aliquoted and stained by fluorochrome-conjugated monoclonal antibodies (FCmAbs) against CD45 (HI30), CD14 (M5E2), CD56 (NCAM16.2), CD3 (HIT3a), CD19 (HIB19), CD4 (RPA-T4), CD8 (RPA-T8), HLA-DR (G46-6), CD314 (NKG2D, 1D11), CD25 (M-A251), CD127 (HIL-7R-M21), CCR7 (3D12), CD45RA (HI100), IgD (IA6-2), CD27 (M-T271), CD335 (NKp46, 9E2/NKp46) and CD16 (3G8), to characterize general leukocyte populations and the phenotype of and T, B, NK and monocyte subsets using different staining panels (**Table S1**). After incubated with indicated mAbs for 30 minutes at 4°C in dark, blood samples were lysed by 2 ml red blood cell lysis buffer for 8 minutes, washed twice with 2 ml ice-cold staining buffer (2% FCS and 0.1% sodium azide in 1 × PBS), and then fixed in 300 µl of 1% paraformaldehyde (PFA) for flow cytometric analysis. For intracellular cytokine staining, 5×10^5 PBMCs were stimulated by a cocktail containing phorbol myristate acetate (PMA), ionomycin and brefeldin A for 5 hours in 24-well flat-bottom plates, thereafter the cells were harvested and washed once with PBS. The cells were then stained by fixable viability staining dye (FVS), FCmAbs against CD3 and CD8 for 30 minutes at 4°C in dark, followed by intracellular staining with FCmAbs against IFN-γ (B27), IL-17A (N49-653), and IL-4 (8D4-8) after fixation and permeabilization. Finally, cells were washed twice and re-suspended in 300 µl of 1% PFA. Flow cytometric analysis was performed on a BD Verse instrument and data were analyzed by FlowJo V10 (BD bioscience, San Jose, CA, USA).

TABLE 1 | Clinical features of VKH patients and healthy controls.

Clinical features	Acute VKH	Healthy control
Participants (n)	25	21
Age (mean ± SD)	42.1 ± 12.2	41.4 ± 12.9
Gender	9 (36.0%)	9 (42.9%)
Female		
Male	16 (64.0%)	12 (57.1%)
Subretinal fluid	18 (72%)	n.a.
Bullous serous retinal detachment	2 (8%)	n.a.
Papilledema	15 (60.0%)	n.a.
Hearing loss	5 (20.0%)	n.a.
Tinnitus	4 (16.0%)	n.a.
Headache	13 (52.0%)	n.a.

TABLE 2 | Clinical features of VKH patients before and after GC treatment.

Clinical features	Before GC	After GC
Patients (n)	16	
Age (mean ± SD)	44.9 ± 11.8	
Gender	6 (37.5%)	
Female		
Male	10 (62.5%)	
Subretinal fluid	10 (62.5%)	6 (37.5%)
Bullous serous retinal detachment	2 (12.5%)	0
Papilledema	8 (50.0%)	5 (31.3%)
Hearing loss	4 (25.0%)	0 (0.0%)
Tinnitus	3 (18.8%)	0 (0.0%)
Headache	10 (62.5%)	0 (0.0%)

Cytokine Measurements

Blood samples were collected from HCs and VKH patients. After centrifugation, plasma was extracted and stored at −80°C. A human Premixed Multi-Analyte kit (LXSAHM-21 R&D Systems) was used to measure the concentrations of a panel of soluble factors (TNF-α, IL-6, IL-8, CXCL10, IL-10, CCL2, IL-1-β, IFN-γ, CCL20, CCL3, CCL22, IL-4, IL-17, IL-2, IL-13, CXCL9, IL-12, CCL17, IL-21, IL-23, IL-18) in one sample at the same time. Since the concentration of some cytokines from most plasma samples is lower than the detection limit of this assay, as determined by our preliminary experiment, 250 µl plasma is lyophilized and re-suspended in 50 µl PBS (5:1 concentrated). Luminex assays were performed according to the manufacturer's protocol with standard curves and quality and background controls included. Samples and standards were run in duplicate and mean values were used for data analysis. The concentrations of TGF-β1 in the plasma were assayed using human ELISA kits (Cat# 88-8350, Invitrogen) according to the manufacturer's instructions.

RNA Sequencing

Total RNAs of whole blood cells were extracted in accordance with the manual of PAXgene tube (BD bioscience, San Jose, CA, USA). Preparation of library and transcriptomic sequencing were carried out using Illumina Novaseq 6000 (Novogene Bioinformatics Technology Co., Ltd., Beijing, China). Differential expression analysis of two conditions/groups (two biological replicates per condition) was performed using the DESeq2 R package (1.16.1). DESeq2 provide statistical routines for determining differential expression in digital gene expression data using a model based on the negative binomial distribution. The resulting *P* values were adjusted using the Benjamini and Hochberg's approach for controlling the false discovery rate. Genes with an adjusted P value < 0.05 found by DESeq2 were assigned as differentially expressed.

Gene Ontology (GO) enrichment analysis of differentially expressed genes was implemented by the cluster Profiler R package, in which gene length bias was corrected. GO terms with corrected P value less than 0.05 were considered significantly enriched by differential expressed genes.

Kyoto Encyclopedia of Genes and Genomes (KEGG) is a database resource for understanding high-level functions and utilities of the biological system, such as the cell, the organism and the ecosystem, from molecular-level information, especially large-scale molecular datasets generated by genome sequencing and other high-throughput experimental technologies (http://www.genome.jp/kegg/). We used cluster Profiler R package to test the statistical enrichment of differential expression genes in KEGG pathways.

Statistical Analysis

General statistical analysis was performed using GraphPad Prism software. Throughout the study, n refers to the number of subjects where every subject is one data point. Unpaired two-group comparisons were done with Mann–Whitney U-test. Paired group comparisons were done with Wilcoxon test. $P < 0.05$ was considered statistically significant.

RESULTS

Dysregulated Peripheral Leukocyte Compartment in Acute VKH Patients

To explore immune cell-mediated mechanisms in the development and progression of VKH disease, we examined leukocyte populations in patients with active VKH by flow cytometry (**Figure 1A**). Compared with healthy controls, the number of total leukocytes in peripheral blood of acute VKH patients was increased significantly (**Figure 1B**). There were no significant changes in granulocytes, total lymphocytes and $CD3^+CD56^+$ T cells in terms of both absolute number and relative frequency (**Figures S1A, B**), however, the numbers of T cells and B cells displayed an increased tendency, although this difference failed to reach statistical significance (**Figures 1C, D**). Interestingly, markedly decreased proportion but not absolute

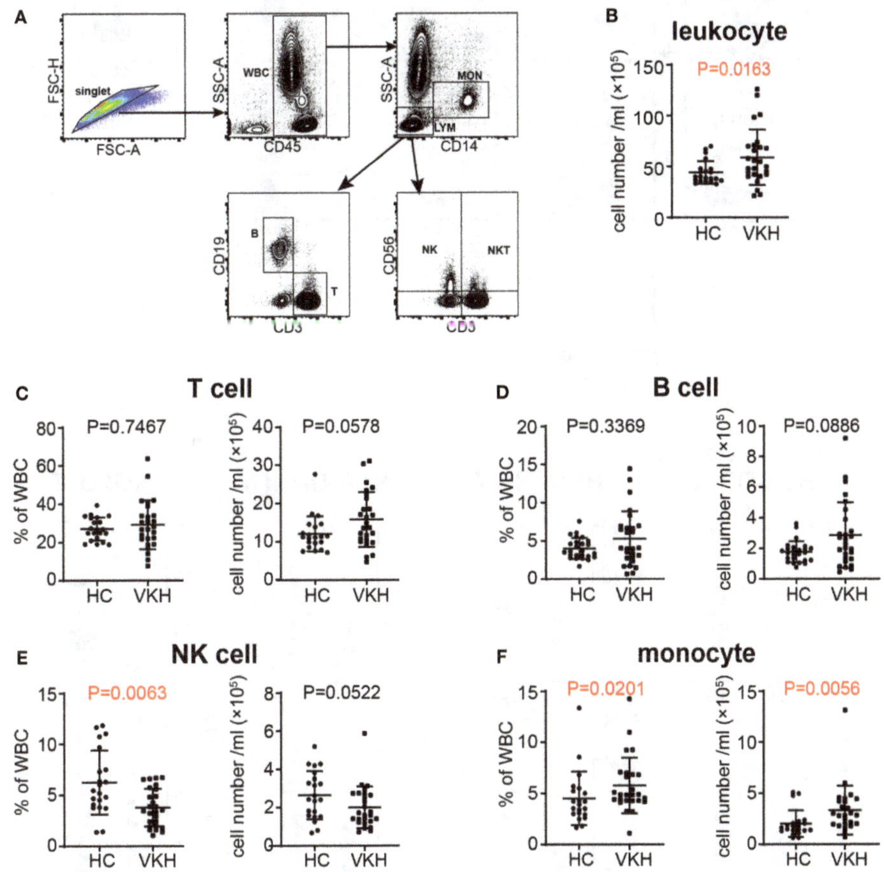

FIGURE 1 | Changes of white blood cells in peripheral blood of VKH patients compared with healthy controls. **(A)** Gating strategy used for the characterization of leukocyte subpopulations. **(B)** The absolute number of leukocytes. **(C)** The absolute number and proportion of T cells. **(D)** the absolute number and proportion of B cells. **(E)** The absolute number and proportion of NK cells. **(F)** the absolute number and proportion of monocytes. Statistical analysis was performed using Mann–Whitney test. WBC, white blood cells; LYM, lymphocytes; MON, monocytes; T, T lymphocytes; B, B lymphocytes; NK, natural killer cells; NKT, natural killer T cells.

number of NK cells was found in VKH patients (P = 0.0063) (**Figure 1E**). Finally, both the absolute number and relative frequency of monocytes were significantly increased in VKH patients, as compared to that in HCs (P = 0.0201 and P = 0.0056, respectively) (**Figure 1F**). Thus, our results in VKH elaborate the proposed notion that T cells and B cells might be pathogenic and NK cells could be protective in most autoimmune diseases, and also raise a question regarding the functional role of increased monocytes.

Over-Activation of Peripheral T Cells in VKH Patients

Activation is a necessary step through which lymphocytes differentiate and exert their function. In this regard, we next determined the activation status of lymphocyte populations by analysis of the expression levels of established T cell and NK cell activation markers HLA-DR, NKG2D and NKp46 (**Figure 2A**). HLA-DR$^+$ cytotoxic T lymphocytes (CTLs) have been shown to be increased in patients with HIV infection (29) and in systemic lupus erythematosus (30). In our study, the percentage and absolute number of HLA-DR$^+$ T cells in peripheral blood of VKH patients were increased (**Figure 2B**), and these changes were observed in both CD8$^+$ and CD4$^+$ T cell compartments (**Figures 2C, D**), whereas NKG2D$^+$ and NKp46$^+$ NK cells did not show much difference (**Figures S2A, B**). NKG2D and NKp46 expression can also be used to reflect the activation status of T cells. In humans, naïve CD8$^+$ T cells express NKG2D, whereas CD4$^+$ T cells generally do not express NKG2D even after activation, but its expression can be induced under certain pathological conditions, such as Crohn's disease, juvenile-onset lupus and cytomegalovirus infection (31, 32). In this study, we found that the absolute number of NKG2D$^+$ T cells was upregulated (**Figure 2E**), whereas no difference was observed for NKp46$^+$ T cells in VKH patients. Together, the elevated

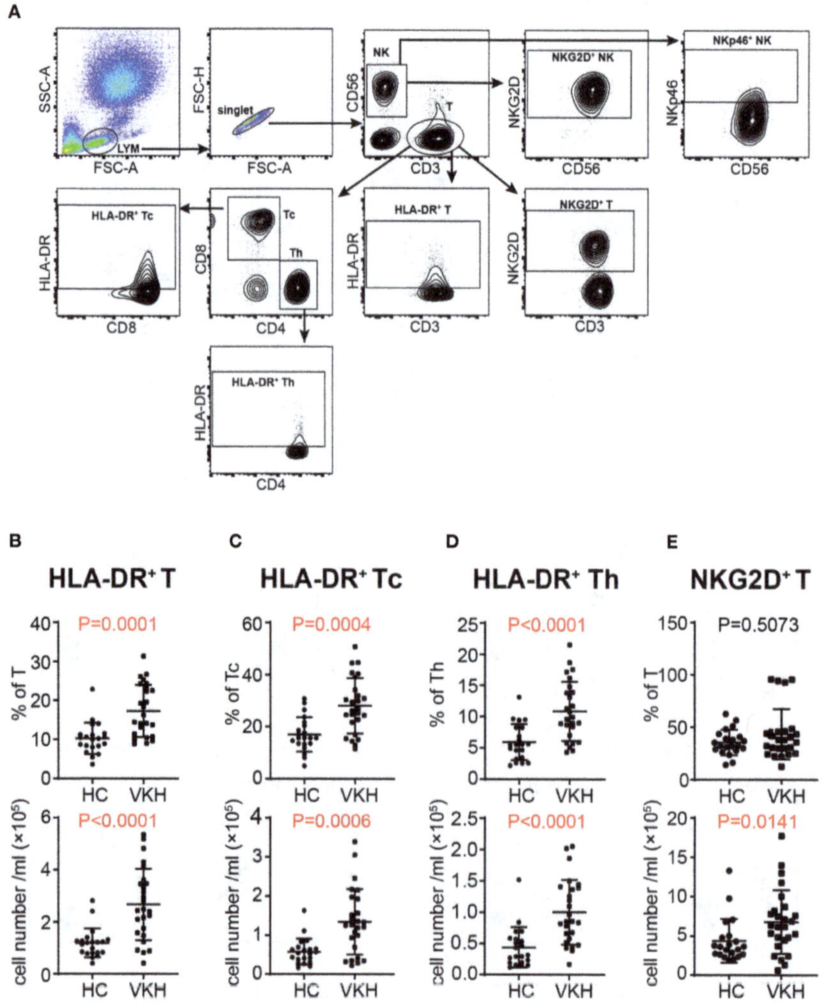

FIGURE 2 | Comparison of activated immune cells between VKH patients and healthy controls. **(A)** Gating strategy used for analysis of activated immune cells. **(B)** The absolute number and proportion of HLA-DR$^+$ CD3$^+$ T cells. **(C)** The absolute number and proportion of HLA-DR$^+$ CD8$^+$ T cells. **(D)** The absolute number and proportion of HLA-DR$^+$ CD4$^+$ T cell. **(E)** The absolute number and proportion of NKG2D$^+$ T cells. Statistical analysis was performed using Mann–Whitney test. Th, helper T cells; Tc, cytotoxic T cells.

expression of HLA-DR and NKG2D in T cells suggested that T cells are over-activated in the context of VKH.

Advanced Differentiation of T Cells in VKH Patients

Th1 and Th17 cells have been shown to be critical in the pathogenesis of VKH (33, 34). Thus, we next sought to determine the polarization status of peripheral T cells in VKH patients (**Figure 3A**). Compared with healthy controls, VKH patients had significantly increased number of IFN-γ^+ cytotoxic T cells (Tc), and regulatory T cells (Tregs) (**Figures 3B, C**), whereas Th1, Th2, Th17, IL-4$^+$ Tc and IL-17$^+$ Tc did not show much difference, in terms of both relative frequency and absolute number (**Figures S3A–E**). Furthermore, after examining the concentration of various cytokines in the plasma of VKH patients and HCs (**Table 3**), we found that CCL17, a chemokine with the potential to recruit Tregs, and TGF-β, a regulatory cytokine mainly secreted by Treg, were also increased in VKH patients (**Figure 3D**).

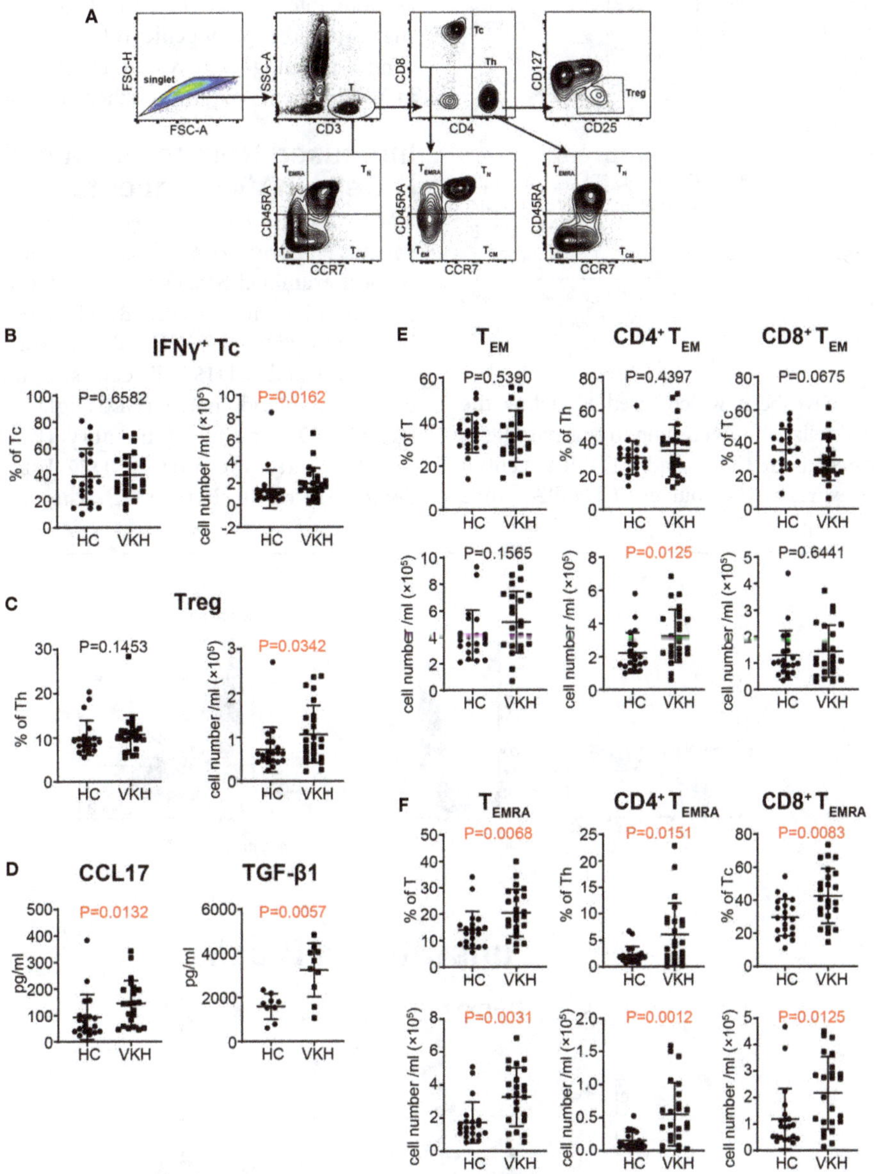

FIGURE 3 | Comparison of T cell subsets defined by cytokine profile and differential status between VKH patients and healthy controls. **(A)** Gating strategy used for T cell classification. **(B)** The absolute number and proportion of IFN-γ^+ CD8$^+$ T cell. **(C)** The absolute number and proportion of Treg. **(D)** plasma levels of CCL17 and TGF-β1 (pg/ml) of HCs and VKH patients. **(E)** The absolute number and proportion of T_{EM} in total T cells, CD4$^+$ T and CD8$^+$ T cells in HCs and VKH patients. **(F)** The absolute number and proportion of T_{EMRA} in total T cells, CD4$^+$ T and CD8$^+$ T in HCs and VKH patients. Statistical analysis was performed using Mann–Whitney test. Treg, regulatory T cells; T_N, naïve T cells; T_{CM}, central memory T cells; T_{EM}, effector memory T cells; T_{EMRA}, CD45RA$^+$ effector memory T cells.

TABLE 3 | Comparison of plasma cytokines between VKH patients and healthy controls.

	VKH (n=22)	HC (n=20)	*P* value
TNF-α	0.73 (0.34-1.64)	0.57 (0.32-1.15)	0.1112
IL-6	0.40 (0.16-1.67)	0.34 (0.16-0.75)	0.6305
IL-8	13.35 (0.12-199.20)	1.97 (0.19-13.14)	0.0002***
CXCL10	21.98 (7.78-124.40)	30.02 (14.94-86.93)	0.1116
IL-10	0.10 (0-3.85)	0.09 (0.01-0.57)	0.9255
CCL2	91.16 (19.43-202.33)	89.61 (49.95-161.87)	0.9752
IL-1β	0.63 (0.38-2.94)	0.61 (0.29-5.47)	0.6218
IFN-γ	3.53 (1.97-22.88)	3.88 (1.63-22.49)	0.9751
CCL20	15.95 (1.85-85.75)	14.64 (5.60-204.19)	0.8273
CCL3	14.73 (5.90-44.47)	8.00 (4.60-49.30)	0.0621
CCL22	94.13 (9.30-284.07)	95.29 (56.21-259.00)	0.9305
IL-4	4.33 (0.11-21.70)	4.79 (3.83-7.75)	0.0936
IL-17A	0.54 (0.35-5.24)	0.47 (0.24-1.32)	0.5343
IL-2	1.15 (0.84-4.34)	1.06 (0.69-1.66)	0.0604
IL-13	16.80 (9.70-48.79)	16.43 (5.14-27.31)	0.5860
CXCL9	49.52 (39.09-129.64)	47.58 (36.46-111.30)	0.5279
IL-12	3.58 (2.33-4.71)	4.14 (2.94-7.32)	0.0599
CCL17	144.12 (44.85-342.22)	67.19 (23.16-383.50)	0.0132*
IL-21	1.72 (1.05-8.52)	1.85 (1.00-8.52)	0.7884
IL-23	25.37 (5.90-136.11)	34.25 (7.41-88.04)	0.2518
IL-18	83.20 (36.80-152.98)	64.29 (5.57-166.69)	0.2171

*Cytokine concentrations are expressed in pg/ml as median (min-max). Data were analyzed by Mann–Whitney test; *P < 0.05; **P < 0.01; ***P < 0.001; ****P < 0.0001.*

CCR7 and CD45RA have been widely used to define the differentiation status of T cells (35). According to this paradigm, naïve T cells (T_N) express both CCR7 and CD45RA, central memory T cells (T_{CM}) express CCR7 but not CD45RA, while effector memory T cells (T_{EM}) lack the expression of both CCR7 or CD45RA. In humans, there is a third memory T cell subset, T_{EMRA} cell, which expresses CD45RA but lack CCR7 expression. Further analysis of T cell subpopulations demonstrated that certain differentiated subsets were variably affected in VKH patients. Although there were no significant changes in naïve T cells and T_{CM} cells in terms of both absolute number and relative frequency (**Figures S3F, G**), the number of $CD4^+$ T_{EM} cells was increased (**Figure 3E**), and the frequencies of T_{EMRA} cells were also increased in both $CD8^+$ and $CD4^+$ T cell compartments in VKH patients (**Figure 3F**). In sum, these results demonstrated that VKH patients harbor more polarized IFN-γ^+ Tc cells, as well as more differentiated T_{EM} and T_{EMRA} cells in peripheral blood, suggesting the pathogenic role of these cells. However, the clinical meaning of increased Tregs and Treg-related cytokines in VKH patients requires further investigation.

Increased Number of Unswitched Memory B Cells in VKH Patients

Since we observed an increased tendency of B cells in VKH patients (**Figure 1D**), and because of the heterogeneity of B cells, we next examined B cell subsets by flow cytometry (**Figure 4A**), to determine the specific B cell subsets that may play an important role in VKH. There are four relatively well-characterized $CD19^+$ B cell subpopulations in human peripheral blood, naïve ($CD27^-IgD^+$), unswitched memory ($CD27^+IgD^+$), switched memory ($CD27^+IgD^-$) and double negative late memory ($CD27^-IgD^-$) B cells (36). As demonstrated in **Figure 4B**, the number of unswitched

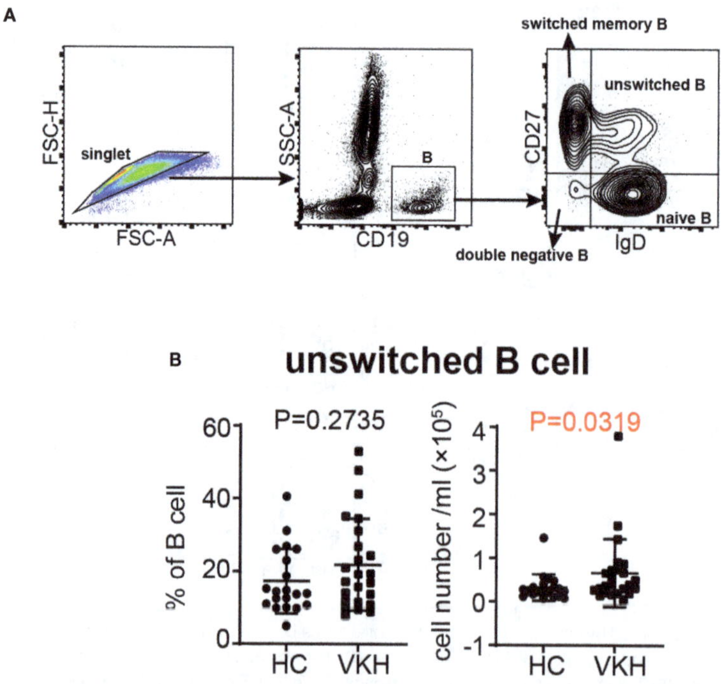

FIGURE 4 | Comparison of B cell subsets between VKH patients and healthy controls. **(A)** Gating strategy used for the characterization of B cell subsets. **(B)** The absolute number and proportion of unswitched B cells. Statistical analysis was performed using Mann–Whitney test.

memory B cells was markedly increased in VKH patients. The numbers of naïve B cells, switched memory B cells and late memory B cells tended to be increased as well, but these differences failed to reach statistical significance (**Figures S4A–C**). Our findings thus suggest the pathogenic role of B cells, especially unswitched memory B cells, in VKH.

Alteration of Monocyte Subsets in VKH Patients

Monocytes have been considered as the precursors of tissue macrophages and monocyte derived DC in periphery. Increased number of monocytes was noted in VKH patients (**Figure 1C**). Therefore, we went on to examine the changes of monocyte subsets in the peripheral blood (**Figure 5A**) and concentration of cytokines related to monocyte in the plasma of VKH patients. We found that IL-8, which could be secreted by monocytes and other cells in the peripheral blood, was increased in VKH patients (**Figure 5B**). This result is consistent with the increased number of monocytes in VKH patients. Moreover, the numbers of classical, non-classical and CD56$^+$ monocytes were all significantly increased in VKH patients as compared to HCs (**Figures 5C–E**). However, both the proportion and number of intermediate monocytes were not statistically different between these two groups (**Figure S4D**).

GC Treatment Influences White Blood Cells in VKH Patients

Previous studies have found that treating healthy subjects with high dose of GC (400 mg) resulted in transient neutrophil demargination and a decrease in circulating lymphocytes peaking at 4 hours post treatment (37). In our study, we examined the changes of leukocyte subpopulations in VKH patients after GC therapy for seven consecutive days. The total number of white blood cells in peripheral blood of patients was increased after GC therapy (**Figure 6A**), which was mainly ascribed to the increase of granulocytes, the most abundant leukocytes in human peripheral blood (**Figure 6B**). The average number of total monocytes was increased from 3×10^5 to 5×10^5 after GC treatment (**Figure 6C**). In contrast, the number of total lymphocytes did not change significantly, whereas the percentage

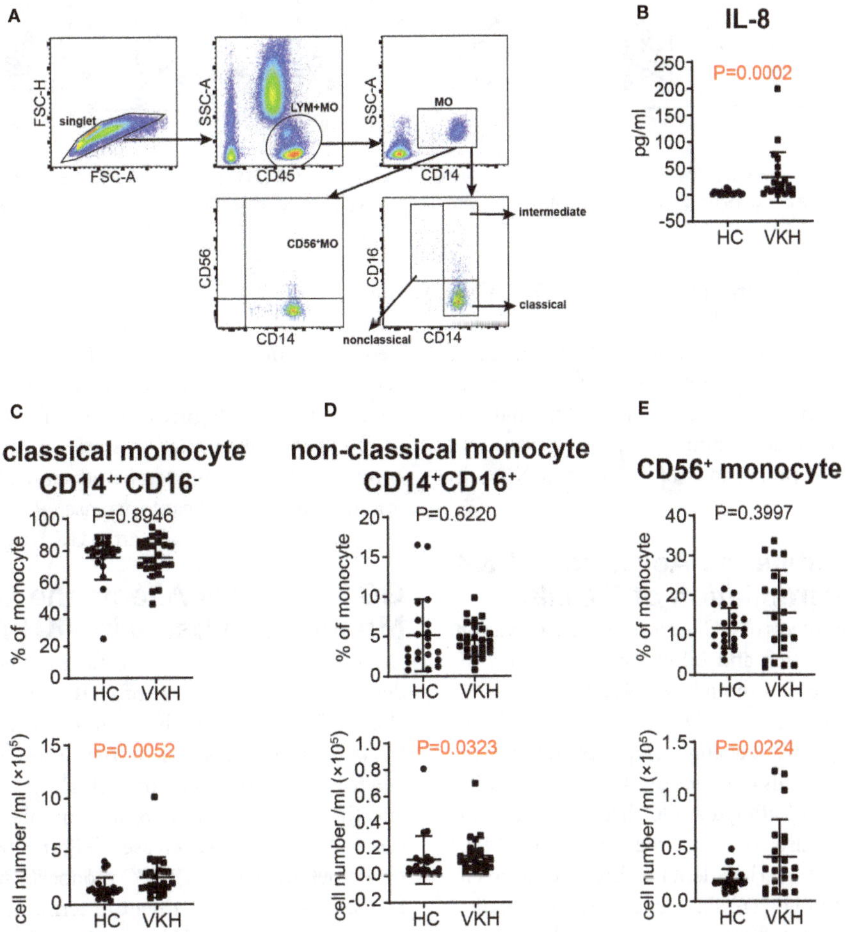

FIGURE 5 | Changes of monocyte subsets in VKH patients compared with healthy controls. **(A)** Gating strategy used for the characterization of monocyte subsets. **(B)** Plasma level of IL-8 (pg/ml) of HCs and VKH patients. The absolute number and proportion of **(C)** classical monocytes, **(D)** non-classical monocytes and **(E)** CD56$^+$ monocytes. Statistical analysis was performed using Mann–Whitney test.

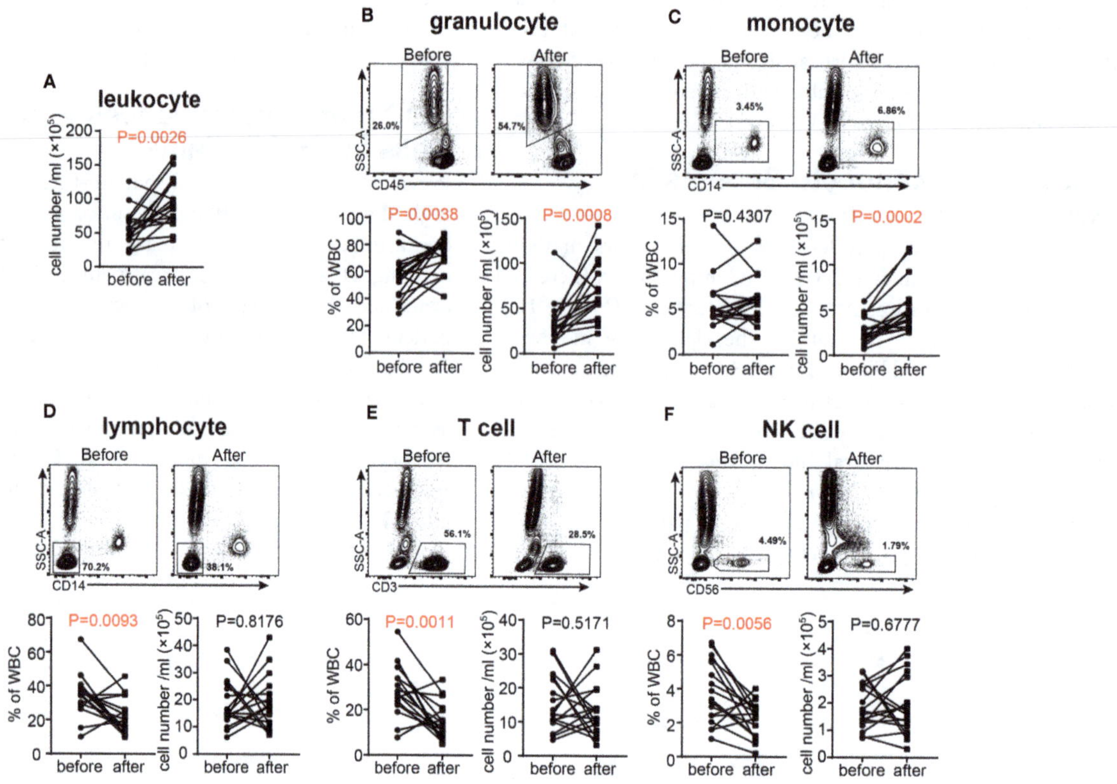

FIGURE 6 | Changes of white blood cells in acute VKH patients before and after GC treatment (n = 16). **(A)** Changes in the total number of white blood cells. The absolute number and proportion of granulocytes **(B)**, monocytes **(C)**, lymphocytes **(D)**, T cells **(E)** and NK cells **(F)**. Statistical analysis was performed using Wilcoxon test.

of lymphocytes decreased after treatment (**Figure 6D**). When lymphocyte subsets were compared, the proportion of T cells and NK cells were decreased (**Figures 6E, F**), whereas B cells and NKT cells did not change significantly in response to GC treatment (**Figures S5A, B**). In together, our results indicated that GC treatment resulted in increased numbers of monocytes and granulocytes, but decreased proportions of T cells and NK cells in VKH patients.

GC Treatment Inhibits the Activation of NK Cells and the Differentiation of T Cells

In order to determine the effects of GC therapy on cell activation, we next analyzed the activation and inhibition markers on the surface of T cells and NK cells. Although NKp46$^+$ NK, HLA-DR$^+$ T, HLA-DR$^+$ Th, HLA-DR$^+$ Tc, NKG2D$^+$ T, NKp46$^+$ T and Treg cells did not show any significant changes (**Figures S6A–G**), the percentage of NKG2D$^+$ NK cells was decreased significantly after GC therapy (**Figure 7A**), indicating that GC therapy inhibits the activation of NK cells. We also compared the content of various cytokines in the plasma of VKH patients before and after GC therapy (**Table 4**), and found that CCL22, one of the chemokines with the potential to recruit Tregs, was decreased after GC treatment (**Figure 7B**). Next, we focused on cytokine profile-defined T cell subsets, GC treatment did not change both the absolute numbers and relative frequencies of Th1, Th2, Th17, IFN-γ^+ Tc, IL-4$^+$ Tc and IL-17$^+$ Tc subsets (**Figures S7A–F**). When T cell differentiation status was examined, the relative frequencies of CD4$^+$ T_N, T_{CM} (within both CD4$^+$ and CD8$^+$ T cell compartments) and CD8$^+$ T_{EM} cells changed significantly after GC therapy (**Figures S8A–C**). T_{CM}/T_{EM} ratio has been used to reflect the differentiation status of T cells (38), We therefore compared this parameter before and after GC treatment and found a highly significant increase ($P = 0.0004$) of the T_{CM}/T_{EM} ratio among CD8$^+$ T cells after GC treatment (**Figure 7C**).

GC Treatment Affects the Distribution of Monocyte Subsets in VKH Patients

After GC treatment, the proportions of the three monocyte subsets defined by the expression of CD14 and CD16 were significantly altered (**Figure 8A**). Both the proportion and absolute number of CD14^{++}CD16$^-$ classical subset were increased (**Figure 8B**), whereas the proportion of CD14^{++}CD16$^+$ intermediate subset, and the proportion and absolute number of CD14$^+$CD16$^+$ non-classical subset were decreased (**Figures 8C, D**). Interestingly, the newly defined CD14$^+$CD56$^+$ monocyte subset were significantly increased after GC treatment in terms of both relative frequency and absolute number (**Figure 8E**), indicating that this monocyte subset might play a role in the remission of VKH. Additionally, we examined the concentration of cytokines related to monocyte in the plasma of VKH patients before and after GC treatment, and

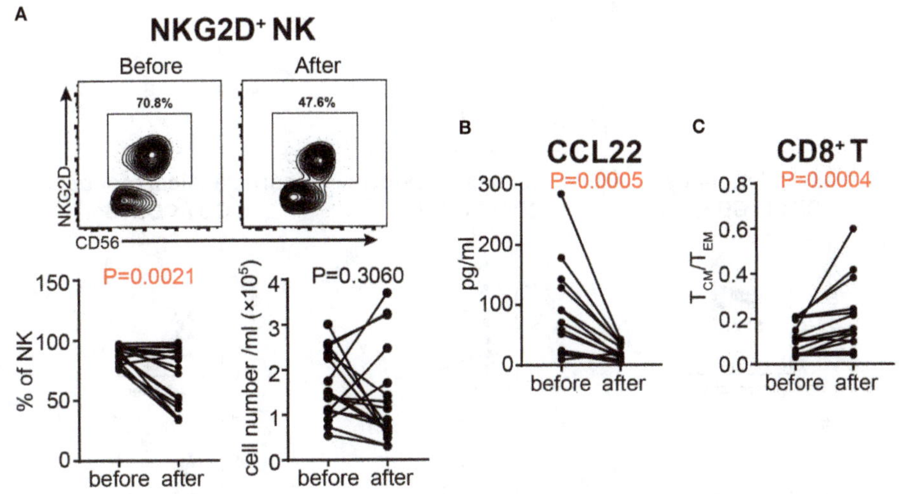

FIGURE 7 | Assessment of the activation status of NK cells and the differentiation status of T cells in VKH patients before and after GC treatment. **(A)** The absolute number and proportion of NKG2D⁺ NK cells. **(B)** plasma level of CCL22 (pg/ml) in HCs and VKH patients. **(C)** The T_{CM}/T_{EM} ratio of CD8⁺ T cells. Statistical analysis was performed using Wilcoxon test.

TABLE 4 | Comparison of plasma cytokines in VKH patients before and after GC treatment.

	Before GC (n=13)	After GC (n=13)	*P* value
TNF-α	0.61 (0.32-6.85)	0.57 (0.32-1.34)	0.1099
IL-6	0.35 (0.16-2.48)	0.30 (0.16-1.29)	0.1465
IL-8	11.65 (0.12-243.18)	11.65 (0.41-243.18)	0.9460
CXCL10	27.95 (4.98-151.14)	16.00 (4.98-151.14)	0.0681
IL-10	0.13 (0-74.61)	0.06 (0-2.81)	0.0425*
CCL2	85.77 (19.43-161.87)	57.79 (39.28-129.49)	0.0398*
IL-1β	0.61 (0.29-5.86)	0.52 (0.37-5.86)	0.5879
IFN-γ	3.00 (1.00-51.20)	3.16 (1.86-6.67)	0.2925
CCL20	14.64 (1.85-204.19)	7.37 (1.85-31.15)	0.4973
CCL3	11.26 (4.60-59.54)	11.26 (4.60-59.54)	0.6221
CCL22	41.98 (2.83-259.00)	18.74 (2.83-41.98)	0.0005***
IL-4	5.13 (0.11-10.55)	5.13 (2.10-10.55)	0.3850
IL-17A	0.54 (0.22-5.81)	0.54 (0.22-5.81)	0.3481
IL-2	1.21 (0.69-6.40)	1.21 (0.81-6.40)	0.8145
IL-13	17.56 (5.14-69.60)	17.56 (9.70-39.72)	0.7646
CXCL9	48.88 (36.46-264.50)	44.33 (39.09-71.09)	0.3613
IL-12	4.14 (2.33-42.03)	3.36 (2.53-28.36)	0.8066
CCL17	64.32 (23.16-383.50)	64.32 (30.22-221.36)	0.3757
IL-21	1.85 (1.00-20.10)	1.39 (1.00-3.45)	0.1851
IL-23	34.25 (3.94-88.04)	10.83 (3.94-83.63)	0.0681
IL-18	76.99 (5.57-215.64)	76.99 (27.02-215.64)	0.3804

*Cytokine concentrations are expressed in pg/ml as median (min-max). Data were analyzed by Wilcoxon test; *P < 0.05; ***P < 0.001.*

found that CCL2, a chemokine with the potential to recruit monocyte and T cell to the sites of inflammation induced by either tissue injury or infection (39), were also decreased after GC treatment. In addition, IL-10, a regulatory cytokine secreted by monocyte and Treg, was decreased after GC treatment as well, however, plasma IL-10 levels were extremely low in both groups and the biological meaning of this difference is questionable (**Figures 8F, G**). Therefore, whether IL-10 and CCL2 are involved in the function of CD14⁺CD56⁺ monocytes in GC treatment of VKH patients warrants further investigations.

GC Treatment Affects the Proliferation, Activation, Differentiation and Migration of Immune Cells at the Transcriptomic Level

To further interrogate the effects of GC treatment on peripheral immune cells in the context of VKH, we analyzed transcriptomic changes in peripheral blood from healthy controls and VKH patients before and after GC treatment. For this purpose, peripheral blood samples were collected from HCs, as well as patients before and after GC treatment for one week (seven samples per group). Transcriptomic profiles of these samples were examined by RNA sequencing. Our RNA-seq analysis revealed 1268 differentially expressed genes (DEGs), of which 676 genes were upregulated and 592 genes were downregulated in VKH patients compared to healthy controls ($P < 0.05$) (**Figure 9A**). NK cell-related genes in VKH patients were significantly downregulated, which is in agreement with our finding by flow cytometry that the percentage of CD56⁺ NK cells was significantly reduced in the VKH patients (**Figure 1E**). However, genes that are associated with NK cell activation (e.g., *SH2D1B* and *KLRF1*) and inhibition (e.g., *KIR2DL3* and *KIR3DL2*) were both reduced, suggesting the complex role of NK cells in the pathogenesis of VKH diseases. In addition, *BOK*, the gene related to apoptosis, was down-regulated, and genes related to inflammation (e.g., *SLPI* and *VNN1*) were upregulated in VKH patients (**Figure 9B**).

Differential gene expression analysis of VKH patients before and after GC treatment revealed that 1925 genes were upregulated and 2015 genes were downregulated with P value less than 0.05 after GC treatment (**Figure 9C**). GO enrichment analysis showed that genes associated with lymphocyte (especially T cell) activation and differentiation were downregulated (**Figure 9D**). KEGG enrichment analysis of the differential genes revealed that gene modules associated with Th1, Th2 and Th17 cell differentiation, as well as 'chemokines and chemokine receptor interaction' were all

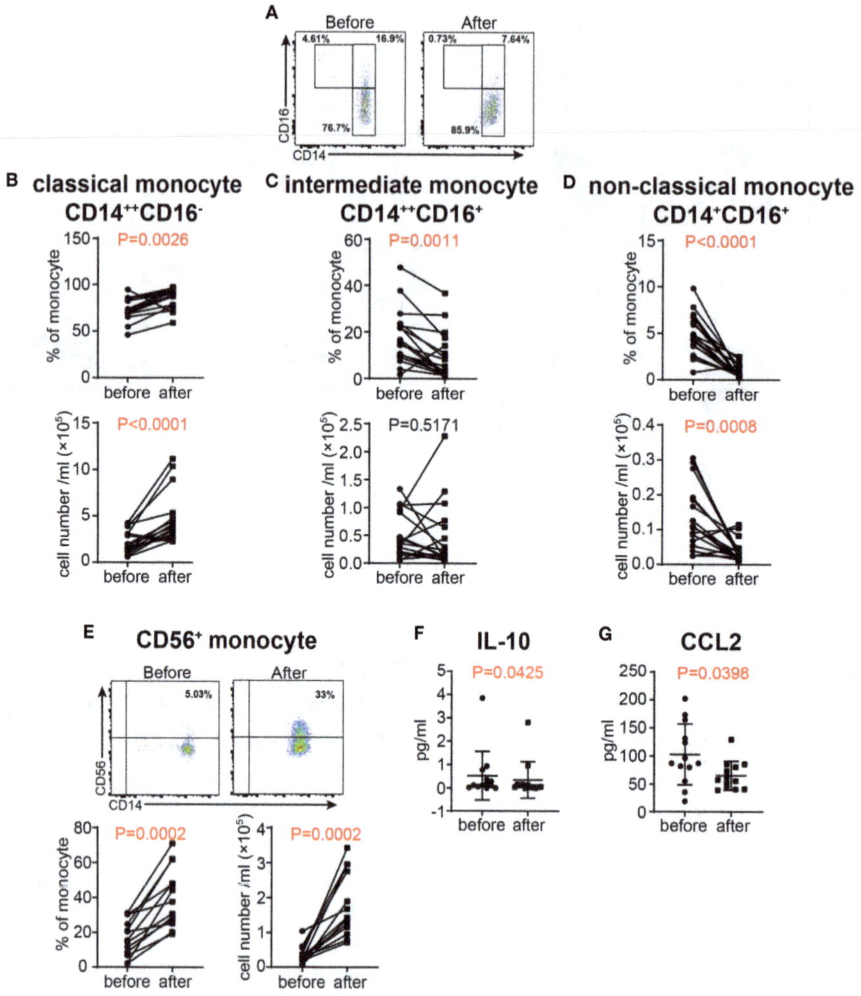

FIGURE 8 | Changes of monocyte subsets in VKH patients before and after GC treatment. **(A)** Monocyte subsets in a VKH patient before and after GC treatment. The absolute number and proportion of classical monocytes **(B)**, intermediate monocytes **(C)**, non-classical monocytes **(D)** and **(E)** $CD56^+$ monocytes. Statistical analysis was performed using Wilcoxon test. Plasma levels of IL-10 **(F)** andCCL2 (pg/ml) **(G)** in VKH patients before and after GC treatment.

downregulated (**Figure 9E**). Therefore, these results indicated that GC treatment might counteract VKH disease through inhibiting T cell activation, differentiation and cytokine/chemokine interaction, which is consistent with our results that the total number of T cells, the number and proportion of activated T cells were increased in the peripheral blood of VKH patients (**Figure 1C** and **Figures 2A–E**). GO pathway analysis also revealed that genes associated with granulocyte activation and degranulation were mostly upregulated after GC therapy, which is consistent with the increased number of granulocytes after GC therapy found by flow cytometry (**Figure S9A**). In addition, KEGG analysis indicated that pathways associated with apoptosis were upregulated after GC therapy (**Figure S9B**). Together, these results demonstrated that GC treatment of VKH may function through inhibiting the activation, proliferation and differentiation, and promoting the apoptosis of immune cells.

In order to identify the key genes that contribute to both the occurrence of VKH and the effects of GC treatment, we performed integrated analysis of DEGs in all three groups. We found that 66 genes were upregulated in VKH patients but downregulated after GC therapy (**Figure 9F**), and 40 genes were downregulated in VKH patients but upregulated after GC therapy (**Figure 9G**). Among these 106 genes, a key gene *NOS3* (Nitric oxide synthase), which plays crucial roles in regulating vascular tone, cellular proliferation, leukocyte adhesion and platelet aggregation through production of NO in the vascular endothelium (40), was elevated in VKH patients and can be reduced after GC therapy (**Figure 9H**), suggesting the dysregulated inflammatory response in VKH patients, and the anti-inflammatory effect of GC treatment in VKH.

DISCUSSION

VKH is a complex disease involving multiple interactions between different immune cell populations. Although much

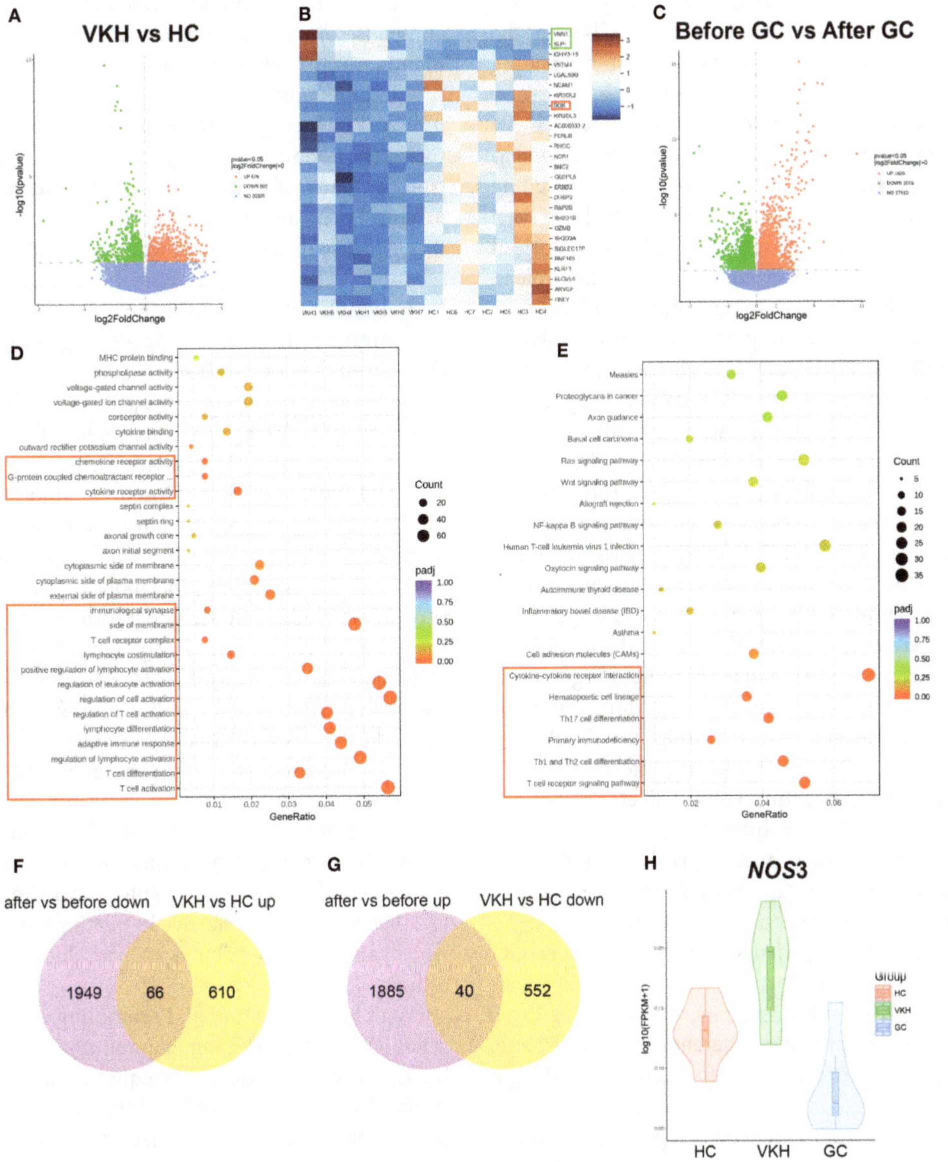

FIGURE 9 | Gene expression in the peripheral blood from VKH patients before (before, n=7) and after (after, n=7) GC treatment for one week, as well as healthy controls (HC, n=7). **(A)** Volcano plots illustrating the differential RNA expression levels between VKH patients and healthy controls. **(B)** Heatmap shows differentially expressed genes in VKH patients and HCs. **(C)** Volcano plots illustrating the differential RNA expression levels between patients before and after GC treatment. Functional enrichment analysis revealing differentially expressed genes in VKH patients before and after GC by KEGG **(D)** and GO enrichment **(E)**. **(F)** Genes up-regulated in VKH and down-regulated after GC therapy. **(G)** Genes down-regulated in VKH and up-regulated after GC therapy. **(H)** Violin plot of *NOS3* expression in HCs, VKH patients before and after GC treatment.

effort has been made in elucidating the pathogenesis of VKH (3), the role of different leukocytes in this disease remains incompletely understood. In addition, despite the widely use of GCs in clinical management of VKH, the specific anti-inflammatory effects of GCs (i.e. MP) on different cellular compartments in VKH disease are yet to be defined. In this observational study, we performed a comprehensive analysis of the peripheral immune system in VKH patients before and after GC treatment. Our analysis included the subsets of T lymphocytes, NK cells, B cells, monocytes and granulocytes, as well as the functional potential of these cell subsets. The major findings of this study are presented as follows: Firstly, VKH patients harbor a dysregulated lymphocyte compartment in peripheral blood, including higher numbers of T cells, unswitched memory B cells and monocytes, as compared to healthy controls. Secondly, peripheral T cells from VKH patients are more activated, polarized and differentiated than those from HCs. Thirdly, leukocytes from VKH patients are generally more inflammatory and less prone to apoptosis than those from HCs, as indicated by transcriptomic analysis. Finally, GC treatment is not only able to inhibit the activation of NK cells and the differentiation of T cells, but also capable of polarizing monocytes toward an inhibitory phenotype, thereby counteracting the pathogenic immune response in VKH.

Dysregulated T cell compartment has been well-recognized as a prominent feature of multiple autoimmune diseases including VKH. Increased numbers of activated T lymphocytes have been reported in patients with active uveitis (41, 42), and polarized Th1 and/or Th17 lymphocytes are thought to play a major role in the pathogenesis of VKH (9, 33, 34). In our study, total T cells are elevated in VKH patients, and the percentages of $CD4^+HLA\text{-}DR^+$, $CD8^+HLA\text{-}DR^+$ and $NKG2D^+$ T cells are significantly higher in VKH patients than that in HCs, elaborating previous findings that activated T cells play a pathogenic role in VKH. With regard to T cell polarization, the number of Th1 cells in VKH patients is only slightly higher than in controls, and the difference was not significant. However, we do notice an increase in the number of IFN-γ-secreting $CD8^+$ T cells, suggesting that T cells from patients with VKH disease are apt to produce IFN-γ, thereby promoting inflammation. Upon antigen challenge, naïve T cells further differentiate into central memory T cells (T_{CM}), which home to T cell areas of secondary lymphoid organs and have little effector function, but are able to readily proliferate and differentiate to effector cells in response to antigenic stimulation, and effector memory T cells (T_{EM}) that migrate to inflamed peripheral tissues and display immediate effector function. Another memory T cell subset in human, T_{EMRA} cells, which express CD45RA but lack CCR7 expression, is also thought to be able to exert rapid effector function (43). Our results demonstrated a significant increase in the percentage of T_{EMRA} and $CD4^+$ T_{EM} cells in VKH patients. Furthermore, after GC treatment, we found that $CD8^+$ T_{CM} was increased while $CD8^+$ T_{EM} was decreased, which resulted in an increased ratio of T_{CM}/T_{EM}, suggesting that T cells are more differentiated in VKH, and switch to a relatively static memory state from an activated state upon GC treatment.

Regarding the changes of peripheral Tregs (e.g., number, frequency and functionality) in autoimmunity, conflicting results have been reported in a variety of autoimmune diseases, including type 1 diabetes, multiple sclerosis, systemic lupus erythematosus (SLE), myasthenia gravis, rheumatoid arthritis (RA) (44–47). In this study, we observed that the number of $CD4^+CD127^-CD25^{++}$ Tregs was increased, accompanied by elevated plasma levels of chemokines and cytokines that recruit and induce differentiation of Tregs, such as CCL17 and TGF-β. Moreover, CCL22, another chemokine with the potential to recruit Tregs, was decreased after GC treatment. The increase of Tregs in VKH is somewhat counterintuitive given the well-established protective role of these cells in autoimmunity. Several interpretations could be applied to these results: Firstly, the number of peripheral Tregs is simply not reflective of that of tissue Tregs, which are more related to autoimmunity. Secondly, in addition to CD4, CD127 and CD25, other markers are needed to identify functional subsets of Tregs, especially those autoimmune-protective Treg subsets. Finally, the increased number of these cells in VKH patients may simply reflect a compensatory response of our immune system in an effort to maintain immune homeostasis but unfortunately fail to control the inflammatory response (48), either due to the still limited numbers or their potential functional impairment. In support of the latter notion, recent reports have demonstrated that APCs from patients with autoimmune diseases (such as RA) could inhibit the function of Tregs in their peripheral blood, suggesting that APCs (e.g., monocytes, will discuss later) may be critical for secondary Treg cell dysfunction in autoimmune patients (49).

B lymphocytes could contribute to the pathogenesis of autoimmune diseases by producing autoantibodies and/or through acting as APCs (50). B cell infiltration was found in uveal tissues obtained from two patients with VKH, indicating its involvement in VKH (51). Here we found that peripheral B cells were increased in VKH patients, further support the pathogenic role of B cells in VKH. Moreover, among all B cell subsets, IgD^+CD27^+ B cell was the most increased subset. As a typical memory B cell subset, IgD^+CD27^+ B cell has key features of enhanced responsiveness, metabolism, proliferation, as well as a propensity to differentiate into plasmablast, together arguing for these cells being antigen-experienced. In various functional activation assays, the IgD^+CD27^+ B cells showed a higher and faster reactivity than naïve B cells (52). Thus, the increase of IgD^+CD27^+ memory B cells may suggest a prominent role of memory B cells in the pathogenesis of VKH. However, we did not find significant changes of B cell subsets after GC treatment (**Figures S10A–E**). It's likely that GC treatment may not be able to counteract the dysregulation of B cell subsets, although B cells express the glucocorticoid receptor throughout development and GC therapy has been effective in treating autoimmune diseases in which antibody contributes to pathology, such as rheumatoid arthritis (53).

With both regulatory and promoting effects, NK cells seem to act as a two-edged weapon in autoimmune disorders. On the one hand, decreased NK cell frequency and impaired NK cell cytotoxicity were observed in a variety of autoimmune diseases (e.g., systemic juvenile rheumatoid arthritis, SLE, psoriasis and Graves' disease), implying a protective role of NK cells in controlling autoimmunity (54, 55). NK cells may limit autoimmune responses by inhibiting the proliferation and activation of auto-reactive T lymphocytes, and hampering the activation of monocytes. Accordingly, deficiency or decreased NK cell activity might result in sustained activation of auto-reactive T cell and increased monocytes, thus aggravate inflammatory responses and tissue injury. On the other hand, NK cells also have deleterious roles in the pathogenesis of autoimmune diseases. Increasing evidence has demonstrated that NK cells may participate in nearly all steps in the pathogenesis of autoimmunity, including direct killing, leading to the release of self-antigens, priming T cell activation at the initial and late stages, and finally resulting in tissue destruction (56). In this study, the proportion of NK cells was decreased, accompanied by the downregulation of NK cell-related genes in VKH patients, supporting the overall regulatory role of NK cells in VKH, and the decrease of these cells may result in sustained activation of autoimmune T cells. However, NKG2D$^+$ NK cells were decreased after GC treatment, suggesting the complex role of NK cells in VKH. NKG2D$^+$ NK cells may represent a pro-inflammatory NK cell subset, which could be eliminated by GC treatment.

It has been well-established that GCs increase bone marrow-derived granulocytes in the blood stream. This effect is utilized clinically to combat granulocytopenia, usually in combination with G-CSF (57). In this study, GC treatment resulted in elevated neutrophils in VKH patients, which is in agreement with previous reports. The increased number of peripheral neutrophils in response to GC treatment could result from the release of these cells from marginal pool to circulation. In fact, it has been reported that GCs could suppress cell adhesion *via* reducing L-selectin expression in PMNs and E-and P-selectin in endothelial cells (58, 59). This notion is further supported by our transcriptomic analysis in which the upregulated expression of genes related to granulocytes, and the decreased expression of cell adhesion molecules were simultaneously observed following GC treatment. Similar mechanisms could also be used to explain the changes of blood monocytes in VKH patients after GC treatment.

Monocytes are rapidly mobilized in large numbers to inflamed sites, where they exert both T cell-dependent function through antigen presentation, and T cell-independent effects such as phagocytic activity as well as secretion of pro-inflammatory cytokines and chemokines. The three major monocyte subsets had differential functional properties (12). Classical monocytes are particularly potent in phagocytosis and resisting bacterial infection, intermediate monocytes are more capable of antigen presentation and stimulating T cell differentiation, whereas non-classical monocytes are specialized in patrolling blood vessels, resisting viruses and stimulating T cell proliferation (12, 60). In contrast to these three major monocyte subsets, the function of the newly identified human CD14$^+$CD56$^+$ monocytes remains undefined, despite increased number of these cells found in certain pathological conditions, such as Crohn's disease and rheumatoid arthritis (21, 23). In this study, peripheral monocytes, especially classical monocytes and CD56$^+$ monocytes were expanded in VKH patients. Intermediate and non-classical monocytes are also showing a tendency to increase in VKH patients. These findings suggest that the overall effect of peripheral monocytes in VKH patients may be pro-inflammatory. Furthermore, IL-8, a chemokine produced by multiple cell types including peripheral monocytes, was upregulated in VKH patients. IL-8 is the primary cytokine involved in the recruitment of neutrophils to the site of damage or infection and plays important roles in the ocular inflammation and inducing ocular angiogenesis in any parts of the eyes (61). This result suggests that IL-8 may be responsible for the overall pro-inflammatory effect of monocytes in VKH.

Widely used in clinic practice to contain inflammation-related diseases, GCs are well-recognized as an anti-inflammatory agent. With regard to monocytes, GC treatment not just suppresses the pro-inflammatory properties of monocytes but rather induces a distinct functional phenotype. Transcriptomic analysis found that GC-treated monocytes are able to limit tissue damage by improving the anti-oxidative properties and increasing the capacity for phagocytosis in response to pro-inflammatory stimuli (e.g., microbial agents, particles, and cellular debris) (62). Our data elaborate this finding at the cellular level, indicating that GC treatment results in significantly increased number of classical monocytes that have strong phagocytic capacity, accompanied by the decreased proportion of intermediate and non-classical monocytes which possess stronger antigen presentation capacity. These results are in agreement with previous *in vivo* studies in healthy individuals and patients with certain autoimmune disorders (63), but are contradictory to the findings by the Nussenblatt group, which showed that the proportion of intermediate monocytes are increased in uveitis patients received GC therapy, and after *in vitro* treatment of purified monocytes with dexamethasone (64). However, the *in vivo* short-term effect of GCs on monocyte subsets observed by us and others may be different from the long-term effect of GCs described by the Nussenblatt group. In addition, *in vitro* treatment of purified monocyte or monocyte subsets with GCs may not faithfully recapitulate what happened *in vivo*, in which multiple cell types and cell-cell interactions are all subject to the regulation of GCs, and the combined effects could be fundamentally different. Our finding that GC treatment resulted in a further increase of the already expanded CD56$^+$ monocytes in VKH patients is not reported in the literature, to the best of our knowledge. It is possible that these cells are regulatory and are increased in VKH patients in an effort to inhibit exaggerated inflammatory response, while in response to GC treatment, these cells quickly improve their quantity and quality, thereby contributing to the successful control of VKH. However, the exact functional properties of CD56$^+$ monocytes and underlying mechanisms of their response to GC treatment in VKH require further investigations.

NOS3 is one of the several forms of nitric oxide synthase, which catalyzes the formation of nitric oxide (NO). It has been already known that NO is synthesized by many cell types that are involved in immune responses and inflammatory reactions (40), but the role of NO in immune diseases and inflammation is still unclear. It has been reported that the increased serum nitrite (NO surrogate) in patients suffering from active RA is associated with disease activity, inflammatory cytokines, and endothelial function (65). As demonstrated by our RNA-Seq results, *NOS3* was increased in VKH patients, but decreased after GC treatment, indicating that the concentration of nitrite in peripheral blood may be related to VKH activity, and the measurement of nitrite could be a diagnostic and prognostic candidate for the management of VKH patients.

In conclusion, the comprehensive analysis of blood leukocytes from VKH patients and HCs described in this study reveals a perturbation of the lymphocyte compartment in VKH, exemplified by the increased activation and proliferation of T cells in VKH patients. GC therapy not only affects the proliferation and apoptosis of lymphocytes, especially T cells, but also affects the distribution of monocyte subsets. Our results also indicate that $CD56^{+}$ monocytes may be involved in the remission of inflammatory autoimmune diseases such as VKH, suggesting that this monocyte subset could represent a potentially useful cellular therapeutic target in certain inflammatory diseases, especially when patients have strong side effects in response to GC therapy.

ETHICS STATEMENT

The studies involving human participants were reviewed and approved by Ethics Committee of Wuhan Aier Eye Hospital (Clinical Ethical Approval No. 2019IRBKY04). The patients/ participants provided their written informed consent to participate in this study.

AUTHOR CONTRIBUTIONS

YH, ZL, HJ, and JHa designed the study and wrote the manuscript. YZ, LZ, JW, JY, MH, TX, JHe, SW, CY, and SP collected the peripheral blood samples and provided clinical data. LY and HJ performed the experiments and analyzed the data. All authors critically reviewed the manuscript and made key contributions to the analysis and interpretations of the results. All authors contributed to the article and approved the submitted version.

ACKNOWLEDGMENTS

The authors thank members from the Lei Yin laboratory, College of Life Sciences, Wuhan University for conducting the RNA-seq analysis. We thank all volunteers and VKH patients for supporting the project.

REFERENCES

1. Burkholder BM. Vogt-Koyanagi-Harada Disease. *Curr Opin Ophthalmol* (2015) 26(6):506–11. doi: 10.1097/icu.0000000000000206
2. Chang JH, Wakefield D. Uveitis: A Global Perspective. *Ocul Immunol Inflamm* (2002) 10(4):263–79. doi: 10.1076/ocii.10.4.263.15592
3. Du L, Kijlstra A, Yang P. Vogt-Koyanagi-Harada Disease: Novel Insights Into Pathophysiology, Diagnosis and Treatment. *Prog Retin Eye Res* (2016) 52:84–111. doi: 10.1016/j.preteyeres.2016.02.002
4. Hammer H. Cellular Hypersensitivity to Uveal Pigment Confirmed by Leucocyte Migration Tests in Sympathetic Ophthalmitis and the Vogt-Koyanagi-Harada Syndrome. *Br J Ophthalmol* (1974) 58(9):773–6. doi: 10.1136/bjo.58.9.773
5. Okada T, Sakamoto T, Ishibashi T, Inomata H. Vitiligo in Vogt-Koyanagi-Harada Disease: Immunohistological Analysis of Inflammatory Site. *Graefe's Arch Clin Exp Ophthalmol = Albrecht von Graefes Archiv fur Klinische und Exp Ophthalmol* (1996) 234(6):359–63. doi: 10.1007/bf00190711
6. Sakamoto T, Murata T, Inomata H. Class II Major Histocompatibility Complex on Melanocytes of Vogt-Koyanagi-Harada Disease. *Arch Ophthalmol (Chicago Ill 1960)* (1991) 109(9):1270–4. doi: 10.1001/archopht.1991.01080090096030
7. Maezawa N, Yano A, Taniguchi M, Kojima S. The Role of Cytotoxic T Lymphocytes in the Pathogenesis of Vogt-Koyanagi-Harada Disease. *Ophthalmol J Int d'ophtalmologie Int J Ophthalmol Z fur Augenheilkunde* (1982) 185(3):179–86. doi: 10.1159/000309240
8. Egwuagu CE, Sztein J, Mahdi RM, Li W, Chao-Chan C, Smith JA, et al. IFN-Gamma Increases the Severity and Accelerates the Onset of Experimental Autoimmune Uveitis in Transgenic Rats. *J Immunol (Baltimore Md 1950)* (1999) 162(1):510–7.
9. Chi W, Yang P, Li B, Wu C, Jin H, Zhu X, et al. Il-23 Promotes CD4+ T Cells to Produce IL-17 in Vogt-Koyanagi-Harada Disease. *J Allergy Clin Immunol* (2007) 119(5):1218–24. doi: 10.1016/j.jaci.2007.01.010
10. Jakubzick CV, Randolph GJ, Henson PM. Monocyte Differentiation and Antigen-Presenting Functions. *Nat Rev Immunol* (2017) 17(6):349–62. doi: 10.1038/nri.2017.28
11. Ziegler-Heitbrock L, Ancuta P, Crowe S, Dalod M, Grau V, Hart DN, et al. Nomenclature of Monocytes and Dendritic Cells in Blood. *Blood* (2010) 116 (16):e74–80. doi: 10.1182/blood-2010-02-258558
12. Cros J, Cagnard N, Woollard K, Patey N, Zhang SY, Senechal B, et al. Human CD14dim Monocytes Patrol and Sense Nucleic Acids and Viruses Via TLR7 and TLR8 Receptors. *Immunity* (2010) 33(3):375–86. doi: 10.1016/j.immuni.2010.08.012
13. Geissmann F, Jung S, Littman DR. Blood Monocytes Consist of Two Principal Subsets With Distinct Migratory Properties. *Immunity* (2003) 19(1):71–82. doi: 10.1016/s1074-7613(03)00174-2
14. Weber C, Belge KU, von Hundelshausen P, Draude G, Steppich B, Mack M, et al. Differential Chemokine Receptor Expression and Function in Human Monocyte Subpopulations. *J Leukoc Biol* (2000) 67(5):699–704. doi: 10.1002/jlb.67.5.699
15. Ancuta P, Rao R, Moses A, Mehle A, Shaw SK, Luscinskas FW, et al. Fractalkine Preferentially Mediates Arrest and Migration of CD16+ Monocytes. *J Exp Med* (2003) 197(12):1701–7. doi: 10.1084/jem.20022156
16. Wong KL, Tai JJ, Wong WC, Han H, Sem X, Yeap WH, et al. Gene Expression Profiling Reveals the Defining Features of the Classical, Intermediate, and Nonclassical Human Monocyte Subsets. *Blood* (2011) 118(5):e16–31. doi: 10.1182/blood-2010-12-326355
17. Kapellos TS, Bonaguro L, Gemünd I, Reusch N, Saglam A, Hinkley ER, et al. Human Monocyte Subsets and Phenotypes in Major Chronic Inflammatory Diseases. *Front Immunol* (2019) 10:2035. doi: 10.3389/fimmu.2019.02035
18. Vanham G, Edmonds K, Qing L, Hom D, Toossi Z, Jones B, et al. Generalized Immune Activation in Pulmonary Tuberculosis: Co-Activation With HIV Infection. *Clin Exp Immunol* (1996) 103(1):30–4. doi: 10.1046/j.1365-2249.1996.907600.x
19. Rivier A, Pène J, Rabesandratana H, Chanez P, Bousquet J, Campbell AM. Blood Monocytes of Untreated Asthmatics Exhibit Some Features of Tissue Macrophages. *Clin Exp Immunol* (1995) 100(2):314–8. doi: 10.1111/j.1365-2249.1995.tb03670.x
20. Rossol M, Kraus S, Pierer M, Baerwald C, Wagner U. The CD14(bright) CD16 + Monocyte Subset is Expanded in Rheumatoid Arthritis and Promotes Expansion of the Th17 Cell Population. *Arthritis Rheum* (2012) 64(3):671–7. doi: 10.1002/art.33418
21. Grip O, Bredberg A, Lindgren S, Henriksson G. Increased Subpopulations of CD16(+) and CD56(+) Blood Monocytes in Patients With Active Crohn's Disease. *Inflamm Bowel Dis* (2007) 13(5):566–72. doi: 10.1002/ibd.20025
22. Sconocchia G, Keyvanfar K, El Ouriaghli F, Grube M, Rezvani K, Fujiwara H, et al. Phenotype and Function of a CD56+ Peripheral Blood Monocyte. *Leukemia* (2005) 19(1):69–76. doi: 10.1038/sj.leu.2403550
23. Krasselt M, Baerwald C, Wagner U, Rossol M. CD56+ Monocytes Have a Dysregulated Cytokine Response to Lipopolysaccharide and Accumulate in Rheumatoid Arthritis and Immunosenescence. *Arthritis Res Ther* (2013) 15 (5):R139. doi: 10.1186/ar4321
24. Sasamoto Y, Ohno S, Matsuda H. Studies on Corticosteroid Therapy in Vogt-Koyanagi-Harada Disease. *Ophthalmol J Int d'ophtalmologie Int J Ophthalmol Z fur Augenheilkunde* (1990) 201(3):162–7. doi: 10.1159/000310145
25. Read RW, Rechodouni A, Butani N, Johnston R, LaBree LD, Smith RE, et al. Complications and Prognostic Factors in Vogt-Koyanagi-Harada Disease. *Am J Ophthalmol* (2001) 131(5):599–606. doi: 10.1016/s0002-9394(01)00937-0
26. Meijsing SH. Mechanisms of Glucocorticoid-Regulated Gene Transcription. *Adv Exp Med Biol* (2015) 872:59–81. doi: 10.1007/978-1-4939-2895-8_3
27. Sloka JS, Stefanelli M. The Mechanism of Action of Methylprednisolone in the Treatment of Multiple Sclerosis. *Mult Scler (Houndmills Basingstoke England)* (2005) 11(4):425–32. doi: 10.1191/1352458505ms1190oa

28. Ehrchen J, Steinmüller L, Barczyk K, Tenbrock K, Nacken W, Eisenacher M, et al. Glucocorticoids Induce Differentiation of a Specifically Activated, Anti-Inflammatory Subtype of Human Monocytes. *Blood* (2007) 109(3):1265–74. doi: 10.1182/blood-2006-02-001115
29. Sáez-Cirión A, Lacabaratz C, Lambotte O, Versmisse P, Urrutia A, Boufassa F, et al. HIV Controllers Exhibit Potent CD8 T Cell Capacity to Suppress HIV Infection Ex Vivo and Peculiar Cytotoxic T Lymphocyte Activation Phenotype. *Proc Natl Acad Sci U S A* (2007) 104(16):6776–81. doi: 10.1073/pnas.0611244104
30. Viallard JF, Bloch-Michel C, Neau-Cransac M, Taupin JL, Garrigue S, Miossec V, et al. Hla-DR Expression on Lymphocyte Subsets as a Marker of Disease Activity in Patients With Systemic Lupus Erythematosus. *Clin Exp Immunol* (2001) 125(3):485–91. doi: 10.1046/j.1365-2249.2001.01623.x
31. Sáez-Borderías A, Gumá M, Angulo A, Bellosillo B, Pende D, López-Botet M. Expression and Function of NKG2D in CD4+ T Cells Specific for Human Cytomegalovirus. *Eur J Immunol* (2006) 36(12):3198–206. doi: 10.1002/eji.200636682
32. Allez M, Tieng V, Nakazawa A, Treton X, Pacault V, Dulphy N, et al. Cd4 +Nkg2d+ T Cells in Crohn's Disease Mediate Inflammatory and Cytotoxic Responses Through MICA Interactions. *Gastroenterology* (2007) 132 (7):2346–58. doi: 10.1053/j.gastro.2007.03.025
33. Liang L, Peng XY, Wang H. Th Lymphocyte Subsets in Patients With Vogt-Koyanagi-Harada Disease. *Int J Ophthalmol* (2019) 12(2):207–11. doi: 10.18240/ijo.2019.02.04
34. Wang C, Tian Y, Lei B, Xiao X, Ye Z, Li F, et al. Decreased IL-27 Expression in Association With an Increased Th17 Response in Vogt-Koyanagi-Harada Disease. *Invest Ophthalmol Visual Sci* (2012) 53(8):4668–75. doi: 10.1167/iovs.12-9863
35. Rocha B, Tanchot C. Cd8 T Cell Memory. *Semin Immunol* (2004) 16(5):305–14. doi: 10.1016/j.smim.2004.08.011
36. Blomberg BB, Frasca D. Age Effects on Mouse and Human B Cells. *Immunol Res* (2013) 57(1-3):354–60. doi: 10.1007/s12026-013-8440-9
37. Dale DC, Fauci AS, Guerry DI, Wolff SM. Comparison of Agents Producing a Neutrophilic Leukocytosis in ManHydrocortisone, Prednisone, Endotoxin, and Etiocholanolone. *J Clin Invest* (1975) 56(4):808–13. doi: 10.1172/jci108159
38. Busch A, Zeh D, Janzen V, Mügge LO, Wolf D, Fingerhut L, et al. Treatment With Lenalidomide Induces Immunoactivating and Counter-Regulatory Immunosuppressive Changes in Myeloma Patients. *Clin Exp Immunol* (2014) 177(2):439–53. doi: 10.1111/cei.12343
39. Xu LL, Warren MK, Rose WL, Gong W, Wang JM. Human Recombinant Monocyte Chemotactic Protein and Other C-C Chemokines Bind and Induce Directional Migration of Dendritic Cells In Vitro. *J Leukoc Biol* (1996) 60 (3):365–71. doi: 10.1002/jlb.60.3.365
40. Król M, Kepinska M. Human Nitric Oxide Synthase-Its Functions, Polymorphisms, and Inhibitors in the Context of Inflammation, Diabetes and Cardiovascular Diseases. *Int J Mol Sci* (2020) 22(1). doi: 10.3390/ijms22010056
41. Deschênes J, Char DH, Kaleta S. Activated T Lymphocytes in Uveitis. *Br J Ophthalmol* (1988) 72(2):83–7. doi: 10.1136/bjo.72.2.83
42. Wang XC, Norose K, Yano A, Ohta K, Segawa K. Two-Color Flow Cytometric Analysis of Activated T Lymphocytes in Aqueous Humor of Patients With Endogenous vs. Exogenous Uveitis. *Curr Eye Res* (1995) 14(6):425–33. doi: 10.3109/02713689509003752
43. Sallusto F, Geginat J, Lanzavecchia A. Central Memory and Effector Memory T Cell Subsets: Function, Generation, and Maintenance. *Annu Rev Immunol* (2004) 22:745–63. doi: 10.1146/annurev.immunol.22.012703.104702
44. Göschl L, Scheinecker C, Bonelli M. Treg Cells in Autoimmunity: From Identification to Treg-based Therapies. *Semin Immunopathol* (2019) 41 (3):301–14. doi: 10.1007/s00281-019-00741-8
45. Mesquita D, de Melo Cruvinel W, Araujo J, Pucci F, Salmazi K, Kallas E, et al. Systemic Lupus Erythematosus Exhibits a Dynamic and Continuum Spectrum of Effector/Regulatory T Cells. *Scand J Rheumatol* (2011) 40(1):41–50. doi: 10.3109/03009742.2010.489229
46. Yan B, Ye S, Chen G, Kuang M, Shen N, Chen S. Dysfunctional CD4+,CD25+ Regulatory T Cells in Untreated Active Systemic Lupus Erythematosus Secondary to Interferon-Alpha-Producing Antigen-Presenting Cells. *Arthritis Rheum* (2008) 58(3):801–12. doi: 10.1002/art.23268
47. Vitales-Noyola M, Layseca-Espinosa E, Baranda L, Abud-Mendoza C, Niño-Moreno P, Monsiváis-Urenda A, et al. Analysis of Sodium Chloride Intake and Treg/Th17 Lymphocytes in Healthy Individuals and Patients With Rheumatoid Arthritis or Systemic Lupus Erythematosus. *J Immunol Res* (2018) 2018:9627806. doi: 10.1155/2018/9627806
48. Scheinecker C, Göschl L, Bonelli M. Treg Cells in Health and Autoimmune Diseases: New Insights From Single Cell Analysis. *J Autoimmun* (2020) 110:102376. doi: 10.1016/j.jaut.2019.102376
49. van Amelsfort JM, van Roon JA, Noordegraaf M, Jacobs KM, Bijlsma JW, Lafeber FP, et al. Proinflammatory Mediator-Induced Reversal of CD4+, CD25+ Regulatory T Cell-Mediated Suppression in Rheumatoid Arthritis. *Arthritis Rheum* (2007) 56(3):732–42. doi: 10.1002/art.22414
50. Yanaba K, Bouaziz JD, Matsushita T, Magro CM, St Clair EW, Tedder TF. B-Lymphocyte Contributions to Human Autoimmune Disease. *Immunol Rev* (2008) 223:284–99. doi: 10.1111/j.1600-065X.2008.00646.x
51. Inomata H, Sakamoto T. Immunohistochemical Studies of Vogt-Koyanagi-Harada Disease With Sunset Sky Fundus. *Curr Eye Res* (1990) 9(Suppl):35–40. doi: 10.3109/02713689008999417
52. Seifert M, Przekopowitz M, Taudien S, Lollies A, Ronge V, Drees B, et al. Functional Capacities of Human IgM Memory B Cells in Early Inflammatory Responses and Secondary Germinal Center Reactions. *Proc Natl Acad Sci United States America* (2015) 112(6):E546–55. doi: 10.1073/pnas.1416276112
53. Cain DW, Cidlowski JA. Immune Regulation by Glucocorticoids. *Nat Rev Immunol* (2017) 17(4):233–47. doi: 10.1038/nri.2017.1
54. Perricone R, Perricone C, De Carolis C, Shoenfeld Y. NK Cells in Autoimmunity: A Two-Edg'd Weapon of the Immune System. *Autoimmun Rev* (2008) 7(5):384–90. doi: 10.1016/j.autrev.2008.03.002
55. Flodström-Tullberg M, Bryceson YT, Shi FD, Höglund P, Ljunggren HG. Natural Killer Cells in Human Autoimmunity. *Curr Opin Immunol* (2009) 21 (6):634–40. doi: 10.1016/j.coi.2009.09.012
56. Lünemann A, Lünemann JD, Münz C. Regulatory NK-cell Functions in Inflammation and Autoimmunity. *Mol Med (Cambridge Mass)* (2009) 15(9-10):352–8. doi: 10.2119/molmed.2009.00035
57. Stroncek DF, Yau YY, Oblitas J, Leitman SF. Administration of G–CSF Plus Dexamethasone Produces Greater Granulocyte Concentrate Yields While Causing No More Donor Toxicity Than G–CSF Alone. *Transfusion* (2001) 41(8):1037–44. doi: 10.1046/j.1537-2995.2001.41081037.x
58. Pitzalis C, Pipitone N, Bajocchi G, Hall M, Goulding N, Lee A, et al. Corticosteroids Inhibit Lymphocyte Binding to Endothelium and Intercellular Adhesion: An Additional Mechanism for Their Anti-Inflammatory and Immunosuppressive Effect. *J Immunol (Baltimore Md 1950)* (1997) 158(10):5007–16.
59. Pitzalis C, Pipitone N, Perretti M. Regulation of Leukocyte-Endothelial Interactions by Glucocorticoids. *Ann New York Acad Sci* (2002) 966:108–18. doi: 10.1111/j.1749-6632.2002.tb04208.x
60. Sampath P, Moideen K, Ranganathan UD, Bethunaickan R. Monocyte Subsets: Phenotypes and Function in Tuberculosis Infection. *Front Immunol* (2018) 9:1726. doi: 10.3389/fimmu.2018.01726
61. Ghasemi H, Ghazanfari T, Yaraee R, Faghihzadeh S, Hassan ZM. Roles of IL-8 in Ocular Inflammations: A Review. *Ocul Immunol Inflamm* (2011) 19 (6):401–12. doi: 10.3109/09273948.2011.618902
62. Ehrchen JM, Roth J, Barczyk-Kahlert K. More Than Suppression: Glucocorticoid Action on Monocytes and Macrophages. *Front Immunol* (2019) 10:2028. doi: 10.3389/fimmu.2019.02028
63. Zeng Q, Dong X, Ruan C, Hu B, Luo Y, Luo Z, et al. CD14(+)CD16(++) Monocytes are Increased in Patients With NMO and are Selectively Suppressed by Glucocorticoids Therapy. *J Neuroimmunol* (2016) 300:1–8. doi: 10.1016/j.jneuroim.2016.09.011
64. Liu B, Dhanda A, Hirani S, Williams EL, Sen HN, Martinez Estrada F, et al. Cd14++Cd16+ Monocytes are Enriched by Glucocorticoid Treatment and Are Functionally Attenuated in Driving Effector T Cell Responses. *J Immunol (Baltimore Md 1950)* (2015) 194(11):5150–60. doi: 10.4049/jimmunol.1402409
65. Garg N, Syngle A, Krishan P. Nitric Oxide: Link Between Inflammation and Endothelial Dysfunction in Rheumatoid Arthritis. *Int J angiology* (2017) 26 (3):165–9. doi: 10.1055/s-0036-1597577

8

Systemic Regulatory T Cells and IL-6 as Prognostic Factors for Anatomical Improvement of Uveitic Macular Edema

Jessica Matas[1], Victor Llorenç[1], Alex Fonollosa[2], David Díaz-Valle[3], Cristina Esquinas[4], Maria Teresa Sainz de la Maza[1], Marc Figueras-Roca[1], Joseba Artaraz[2], Barbara Berasategui[2], Marina Mesquida[1], Alfredo Adán[1] and Blanca Molins[1]*

[1] Group of Ocular Inflammation, Institut d'Investigacions Biomèdiques Agustí Pi i Sunyer (IDIBAPS), Hospital Clínic de Barcelona, Barcelona, Spain, [2] Department of Ophthalmology, BioCruces Health Research Institute, Hospital Cruces, University of the Basque Country, Baracaldo, Spain, [3] Ophthalmology Department and Health Research Institute (IdISSC), Hospital Clinic of San Carlos, Madrid, Spain, [4] Valle Hebron Research Institute, Autonomous University of Barcelona, Barcelona, Spain

Correspondence:
Blanca Molins
bmolins@clinic.cat

Purpose: To investigate whether systemic immune mediators and circulating regulatory T cells (Tregs) could be prognostic factors for anatomic outcomes in macular edema secondary to non-infectious uveitis (UME).

Methods: Multicenter, prospective, observational, 12-month follow-up study of 60 patients with UME. Macular edema was defined as central subfield thickness (CST) > 300 μm measured with spectral domain optical coherence tomography (SD-OCT). Serum samples and peripheral blood mononuclear cells (PBMC) were obtained from venous blood extraction at baseline. Serum levels of IL-1β, IL-6, IL-8, IL-17, MCP-1, TNF-α, IL-10, and VEGF were determined by Luminex. Tregs population, defined as $CD3^{+}CD4^{+}FoxP3^{+}$ in PBMC, was determined by flow cytometry. Main outcome measure was the predictive association between searched mediators and CST sustained improvement, defined as CST < 300 microns or a 20% CST decrease, at 6 months maintained until 12-months compared to baseline levels.

Results: Multivariate logistic regression analysis showed an association between CST sustained improvement at 12 months follow-up and IL-6 and Tregs baseline levels. Higher IL-6 levels were associated with less events of UME improvement (OR: 0.67, 95% CI (0.45–1.00), P = 0.042), whereas higher levels of Tregs favored such improvement (OR: 1.25, 95% CI: 1.12–2.56, P = 0.049).

Conclusions: Increased levels of Tregs and reduced levels of IL-6 in serum may be prognostic factors of sustained anatomical improvement in UME. These findings could enforce the opportunity to develop more efficient and personalized therapeutic approaches to improve long-term visual prognosis in patients with UME.

Keywords: macular edema, uveitis, cytokines, regulatory T cells, biomarkers

INTRODUCTION

Non-infectious uveitis accounts for 10% of cases of total blindness in developed world and may result in persistent visual impairment in untreated patients (1). Uveitis may affect people of all ages but most frequently occurs in the working age population, thus implying a high socioeconomical burden (2). Macular edema remains the most commonly found structural complication of uveitis that results in central visual impairment although only one third of uveitis patients develop it (3). The pathogenesis of uvetitic macular edema (UME) involves breakdown of the blood-retinal barrier, followed by both intracellular and extracellular fluid accumulation within the macular retina (4). However, the underlying pathophysiology as well as the molecular mediators involved are not fully understood, therefore making UME a controversial topic.

Chronic retinal inflammation has been observed in early phases and also in the sight-threatening advanced forms of UME. The uveitic retina is characterized by a complex milieu of dysregulated proinflammatory factors. Increased levels of certain proinflammatory cytokines, such as interleukin-6 (IL-6), IL-8, and tumor necrosis factor-α (TNF-α), both in serum and aqueous humor, have been found in patients with UME (5). Vascular endothelial growth factor (VEGF) may also play a major role as it can be increased in aqueous humor of patients with UME and in other forms of macular edema (5, 6). On the other hand, in the last years, the interest in regulatory T cells (Tregs) as markers of activity and modulators of autoreactive T lymphocytes in uveitis and other inflammatory diseases has gained attention (7). Patients with active uveitis have reduced circulating levels of Tregs compared to healthy subjects, with Tregs levels being significantly upregulated during quiescent disease (8, 9). Moreover, adoptive transfer of Tregs has resulted in greater protection against intraocular inflammation in experimental models of uveitis (10, 11). However, it is unknown whether Tregs are also involved in the pathophysiology of UME.

UME may persist despite adequate control of activity, thus leading to permanent photoreceptor damage and loss of central visual acuity (12). After the acute phase, UME may either subside spontaneously or respond to treatment intended to reduce local inflammatory mediators. Moreover, in relapsing and chronic forms of UME, especially in bilateral forms, systemic treatment should be started, usually consisting of corticosteroids and/or immunomodulators (13). However, despite these options, a number of patients still remain refractory to treatment and UME may lead to severe visual impairment.

In summary, there is scarce data regarding the factors influencing sustained anatomic and visual recovery in eyes with UME. A better understanding of the prognostic biomarkers in patients with UME would allow the use of more efficient and selective pharmacological approaches to improve long-term visual prognosis and minimizing unnecessary drug-induced toxicity. In this prospective study, we aimed to investigate the association of several systemic immune mediators and Tregs with the anatomic outcome of UME after 12 months of follow-up.

MATERIALS AND METHODS

Study Design and Selection Criteria

We conducted a multicenter, prospective, observational, 12-month follow-up study to analyze the association of peripheral blood immune mediators and Tregs with the clinical evolution of UME. Adult (>18 years-old) patients with non-infectious UME in at least one eye were proposed for inclusion. UME was defined as central subfield thickness (CST) of >300 μm as measured by SD-OCT (HD-Cirrus, Carl Zeiss Meditec, Dublin, CA) and presence of fluid (intraretinal and/or subretinal) in the macula. Whenever bilateral UME was present, the eye with the higher CST value in the fovea according to OCT measurements in μm was selected as the study eye. Exclusion criteria were limited to infectious uveitis, highly hazy ocular media, concurrent ocular diseases, exclusive tractional UME, pregnancy, immunocompromising systemic diseases (including, but not limited to HIV, leukemia, lymphoma, and chemotherapy), and eyes with any intervention (intraocular surgery, laser, and intravitreal therapy) in the previous 4 months.

Three referral centers for ocular inflammatory diseases in Spain (Clínic Hospital of Barcelona, Cruces Hospital of Bilbao and Clínico San Carlos Hospital of Madrid) participated in the recruitment of patients from January 2015 to January 2017. Local ethics committees approved the study (Comité Ético de Investigación Clínica del Hospital Clínic de Barcelona 2013/8574; Comité de Ética de la Investigación con Medicamentos de Euskadi, Hospital Universitario Cruces PI201406; Comité Ético de Investigación Clínica del Hospital Clínico San Carlos de Madrid 13/244-E). All patients provided written informed consent, and the research followed the regulations of the Declaration of Helsinki.

Data Collection and Ophthalmic Assessment

Patients were evaluated at each clinical site, and protocol-based assessments were performed at different time-points: baseline, month 1, month 6, and month 12 of follow-up. Other visits at different time-points were allowed at the discretion of the treating physician. Data were recorded in an electronic case report form designed *ad hoc*.

Medical record data from each patient included demographics (age, race, and sex), diagnosis classified by anatomic location according to the Standardization of Uveitis Nomenclature (SUN) criteria (14), laterality of disease, systemic or isolated ocular inflammatory disease classification, and a complete ophthalmic examination.

Data gathered from evaluation of each patient included best-corrected visual acuity (BCVA, with Snellen charts in decimal scale at a test distance of 6 m), the presence or absence of disease activity, categorical and quantitative OCT findings, and UME treatment. The SUN recommendations were used for anterior chamber and vitreous inflammatory activity gradations. SD-OCT exploration was used as determination of UME using Macular cube 512 × 128 A-scan, within a 6 × 6 mm area centered on the fovea. Imaging assessment was performed by two investigators who were masked to clinical data of the corresponding patients. In the event of discrepancies, the two graders made the assessment together and reached a consensus. Masked investigators were asked to determine the CST and the pattern of UME (sub-retinal fluid, cystoid, diffuse, or tractional components). Macular volume, subfoveal choroidal thickness (enhanced deep imaging mode), maximum diameter of the greatest cyst if present, subretinal fluid pocket's length in a transfoveal B-scan were also recorded. Ancillary tests to rule out infectious origin (including but not limited to luetic serology, quantiFERON-TB Gold and toxoplasma serology) and to appropriately classify the uveitis were ordered at the investigator discretion.

Sample Collection

Two peripheral blood samples were obtained at the time of patient inclusion in the presence of UME according to the aforementioned definition. Serum was obtained from sample 1 as follows: blood was centrifugated at 1600 g within 20 min and stored at -80°C until inflammatory mediators were determined. The levels of Tregs in peripheral blood were determined from sample 2: peripheral blood mononuclear cells (PBMCs) were obtained by Ficoll (Ficoll-Plaque Plus, GE Healthcare) gradient centrifugation, washed twice with RPMI 1640 containing 2% heat-inactivated fetal calf serum and cryopreserved for further staining and analysis by flow cytometry. Cryopreserved serum and PBMC samples were then shipped to the Ocular Inflammation Laboratory (Hospital Clinic of Barcelona) where they were analyzed.

Cytokine Determination

Eight immune mediators were determined: IL-1β, IL-6, IL-8, IL-17, MCP-1, TNF-α, IL-10, and VEGF. These molecules were chosen based on published results of previous studies regarding both local and systemic biomarkers in uveitis and UME. Selected immune mediators were determined by a Luminex platform (Millipore's MilliPlex Human Cytokine/Chemokine kit) used to measure cytokine and chemokine levels in serum samples using an assay plate layout consisting of seven standards in duplicate (3.2–2,000 pg/mL), one blank well (for background fluorescence subtraction), two internal quality control samples in duplicate, and 25-μL duplicates of each serum sample. The MilliPlex method was performed as recommended by the manufacturer. Zero values were statistically handled as a third of the provided detection limit.

Treg Determination by Flow Cytometry

FoxP3 levels in $CD3^+CD4^+$ cells from cryopreserved PBMCs were determined by flow cytometry. A live/dead Fixable Dead Cell Stain (Invitrogen) was used to exclude dead cells from the analysis, followed by incubation for 30 min on ice with AF700-CD3 (clone OKT3) and FITC-CD4 (OKT4) (eBiosciences). Cells were then washed, fixed and permeabilized before adding PE-FOXP3 (clone 236A/E7) (eBiosciences) for 30 min. Appropriate isotype controls were included in each experiment. Flow cytometric analyses were performed on a Fortessa flow cytometer (BD Biosciences) with a total of 50,000 events recorded for each sample through a live $CD3^+CD4^+$ lymphocyte gate. Analysis of flow cytometry data was performed using FlowJo software. Tregs were defined as $CD3^+CD4^+FoxP3^+$ cells.

Outcome Measures

To determine whether Tregs and serum immune mediators can be predictive factors for anatomic outcomes in UME, we analyzed the association between baseline levels of the above-mentioned immune mediators and Tregs with sustained anatomical improvement of UME. Improvement of UME was defined as a 20% CST decrease or CST < 300 μm at 6 months and maintained at 12 months of follow-up compared to baseline.

Statistical Analysis

To describe the qualitative variables, absolute frequencies and percentages were used. The description of quantitative variables was performed using the mean and standard deviation (SD). The Kolmogorov-Smirnov test was used to assess the normality of distributions. In the case of quantitative variables, the comparison of the characteristics of the eyes depending on the presence of sustained anatomical improvement was carried out using the Student t-test (or Mann-Whitney U-test if normality was not assumed). The Chi-squared test (Fisher test for frequencies < 5) was used for the comparison of categorical variables. Wilcoxon test was performed in order to analyze changes in CST during follow up.

A back stepwise logistic regression analysis was developed including the defined and CST-based favorable anatomical outcome item as the dependent variable, and as independent variables, those cytokines and clinical variables with a P-value < 0.2 in the univariate analysis and clinical pertinence (evolution time of the EMU to baseline, age at baseline, and sex). The results have been described with odds ratios (OR), 95% confidence intervals (CI), and P-values. Linear relationships between defined biomarkers were assessed using Spearman tests. For all tests, values of P <0.05 were considered statistically significant. The R Studio statistical package (version 2.5) was used for statistical analysis.

RESULTS

Sixty eyes of sixty patients were included. The mean age of the group was 51.1 years (SD, 15.1; range, 21–89). The mean previous duration of UME at the inclusion time was 17.37 months (SD, 31.5; range, 0–144 months). **Table 1** shows patients' demographics and clinical data. The description of etiological diagnosis showed that systemic disorders were the predominant ones (n = 24), followed by isolated ocular syndromes (n = 21), and unclassified uveitis (n = 15).

The overall mean CST was 437.8 ± 122.2 (SD) μm at baseline and decreased significantly after 1 month to 357.4 ± 118.9 μm (P < 0.001), reaching 337.73 ± 135.5 μm at 6 months and 329.6 ± 108.1 μm at 12 months (P < 0.001). Reduction in CST followed a similar pattern in systemically treated patients and non-

TABLE 1 | Baseline ophthalmic characteristics in eyes with uveitic macular edema.

Baseline characteristics	
Eyes/Patients (n/n)	60/60
Evolution time to baseline (months, mean ± SD)	17 ± 31
Follow-up (months)	12
Age (years, mean ± SD)	51 ± 15
Female, n (%)	35 (58.3)
Bilateral, n (%)	23 (38.3)
Patterns of UME[1]	
Cystoid, n (%)	47 (78.3)
Diffuse, n (%)	14 (23.3)
Subretinal fluid, n (%)	21 (35)
Tractional component[2], n (%)	18 (30)
Anatomical classification (SUN)	
Anterior, n (%)	16 (26.6)
Intermediate, n (%)	9 (15)
Posterior, n (%)	22 (36.7)
Panuveitis, n (%)	13 (21.7)
Etiologic classification	
Unclassifiable (undifferentiated), n (%)	15 (25)
Seronegative spondyloarthropathies, n (%)	12 (20)
Ankylosing spondylitis, n	6
HLA-B27 + (without SA), n	3
Inflammatory bowel disease, n	1
Psoriatic arthritis, n	1
Reactive arthritis, n	1
White dot syndromes,n (%)	14 (23.3)
Birdshot, n	13
Serpiginous, n	1
Other etiologies, n (%)	19 (31.6)
Sarcoidosis, n	6
Vogt-Koyanagi-Harada, n	5
Juvenile idiopathic arthritis	2
Multiple sclerosis, n	2
Pars planitis, n	2
Sympathetic ophthalmia, n	1
IRVAN, n	1
Treatment/s for UME[1]	
Topical, n (%)	2 (3.3)
Local (only), n (%)	14(23.3)
TCA (peri/intraocular), n	5
Dexamethasone implant, n	11
Systemic ± local, n (%)	40 (66.7)
Oral Corticosteroids, n	37
Classic Immunomodulators, n	19
Biologics, n	13
Previous vitrectomy, n (%)	2 (3.3)

[1]One eye may belong to more than one category (four eyes did not receive any treatment). [2]It refers to qualitatively thickened vitreo-macular interface.
UME, uveitis macular edema; SUN, standardization of uveitis nomenclature classification; SA, spondyloarthropaties; IRVAN, idiopathic retinal vasculitis, aneurisms and neuroretinitis syndrome; TCA, triamcinolone acetonide injections.

systemically treated eyes, reaching a significant reduction already at month 1 and maintaining a sustained reduction throughout the 12-month follow-up (**Figure 1**).

Cytokines and Tregs levels were compared between patients with and without systemic treatment. In our cohort, 66.7% of patients had received systemic treatment for their underlying disease (non-infectious uveitis), and 33.3% had not received systemic treatment for at least 6 months before inclusion. There were no significant differences in the levels of cytokines and Tregs between both groups (**Table 2**). However, differences among specific treatments could not properly be evaluated due to the reduced sample size in each specific treatment subgroup.

In the univariate analysis, qualitatively assessed significant tractional component of the UME was associated to non-sustained anatomical improvement, whereas presence of subretinal fluid was associated to sustained improvement in UME (**Table 3**). To evaluate prognostic factors for UME outcome, variables were analyzed according to the pre-defined CST improvement event with a Step Backwise Logistic Regression Model. Higher macular volume at baseline was the only clinical variable that precluded favorable UME outcome (OR: 1.41, 95% CI: 0.97–2.03, $P = 0.032$). Interestingly, higher baseline levels of IL-6 were associated with no sustained anatomical improvement of UME at 12 months of follow-up

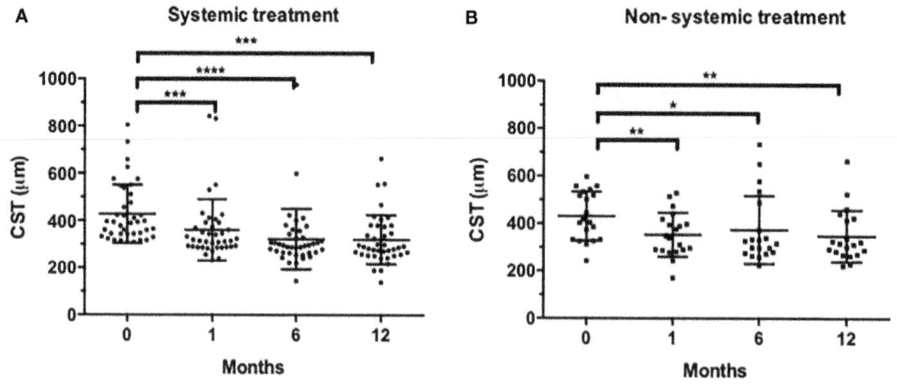

FIGURE 1 | Evolution of central subfield thickness (CST) in systemically treated eyes **(A)** and non-systemically treated eyes **(B)**. Statistical analysis was conducted using the Wilcoxon test (*P < 0.05, **P < 0.001, ***P < 0.001 ****P < 0.0001, vs. baseline).

TABLE 2 | Inflammatory mediators in patients with or without systemic treatment at baseline.

Mediator, mean ± SD	No systemic treatment	Systemic treatment	P-value
n (eyes/patients)	20/20	40/40	
TNF-α (pg/mL)	8.83 ± 6.17	9.39 ± 10.44	0.551
IL-1β (pg/mL)	0.91 ± 1.69	0.46 ± 0.52	0.432
IL-6 (pg/mL)	3.10 ± 5.86	6.44 ± 16.43	0.545
IL-8 (pg/mL)	13.66 ± 21.02	12.70 ± 11.57	0.960
IL-10 (pg/mL)	2.01 ± 6.52	0.52 ± 0.97	0.276
IL-17 (pg/mL)	10.7 ± 19.91	15.48 ± 30.68	0.778
MCP-1 (pg/mL)	617.41 ± 404.47	676.45 ± 409.43	0.846
VEGF (pg/mL)	275.58 ± 216.92	226.82 ± 155.29	0.389
Tregs (% $CD3^+$ $CD4^+$ $PoxP3^+$)	3.78 ± 2.46	4.53 ± 2.76	0.392

TNF, tumor necrosis factor; IL, interleukin; MCP, monocyte chemoattractant protein; VEGF, vascular endothelial growth factor; Tregs, regulatory T lymphocytes.

(OR: 0.67, 95% CI: 0.45–1.00); P = 0.042). In contrast, higher baseline levels of Tregs were associated with UME sustained anatomical improvement (OR: 1.25, 95% CI: 1.12–2.56, P = 0.049). The final model showed good goodness-of-fit (Lemeshow P = 0.13) (**Figure 2**). Given the observed associations, the inverse relationship between Tregs and IL-6 was evaluated. Spearman correlation showed no linear association between baseline levels of Tregs and IL-6 (r = 0.254, P = 0.109).

DISCUSSION

In this prospective study, we evaluated the association of several inflammatory cytokines and Tregs with anatomical improvement of UME. We analyzed the systemic levels of Tregs and eight serum immune mediators in a large group of patients who presented with macular edema secondary to non-infectious uveitis. Our findings show that high baseline serum levels of IL-6 were associated with poorer anatomical response in UME, whereas high levels of circulating Tregs were associated with UME sustained resolution throughout 12-month follow up.

The involvement of Tregs in controlling inflammation has gained considerable attention in uveitis as well as in other systemic autoimmune conditions (15, 16). To our knowledge, this is the first study that describes the association of Tregs with anatomical outcome in UME. Previous studies have compared Tregs levels between active uveitis, inactive uveitis and healthy control subjects. Some studies reported decreased levels of Tregs in active uveitis compared to inactive or quiescent status (9, 17) or healthy subjects (18), while others observed no differences (19) or even increased levels. Indeed, a previous study by our group showed no differences in Tregs levels between patients with active non-infectious uveitis and healthy subjects (20). Regarding the potential association of UME and Tregs levels, Yeh et al. did not observe differences between uveitis patients with and without UME (9). These discrepancies between studies could partly be attributed to the heterogeneity of uveitis subsets, clinical immunophenotyping and to the different strategies used to characterize Tregs. FoxP3 is the canonical transcription factor for naturally-occurring Tregs and is enriched in human $CD4^+CD25^{hi}$ T cells. Nevertheless, the $CD4^+CD25^{hi}$ population does not necessarily capture all $FoxP3^+$ cells, therefore we defined $CD3^+CD4^+FoxP3^+$ as Tregs. The existence of several subtypes of Tregs involved in the modulation of the inflammatory response, could also explain such discrepancies. Thymus originated tTregs inhibit T effector cell trafficking, whereas inducible iTregs primarily prevent T cell priming by acting on antigen-presenting dendritic cells (21). The expression

TABLE 3 | Clinical variables in UME with and without anatomical improvement.

Clinical variables at baseline		Total	No improvement	Improvement[1]	P-value[2]
Total (eyes/patients)		60/60	38/38	22/22	
Clinical imputs					
Age (years, mean ± SD)		51.1 ± 15.1	54 ± 14.7	46.1 ± 14.8	0.063
Female, n (%)		35 (58.3)	24 (63.2)	11 (50)	0.319
Evolution time (months, mean ± SD)		17.3 ± 31.5	12.5 ± 22.49	25.7 ± 42.2	0.357
Bilateral, n (%)		23 (38.3)	14 (36.8)	9 (40.9)	0.755
ACC (SUN) > 0.5+, n (%)		29 (48.3)	17 (44.7)	12 (54.5)	0.464
Keratic precipitates, n (%)	Fines	10 (16.9)	7 (18.9)	3 (13.6)	0.725
	Granulomatous	6 (10.2)	3 (8.1)	3 (13.6)	
Vitreous haze (NEI) > 0.5+, n (%)		29 (48.3)	20 (52.6)	9 (40.9)	0.381
Chorioretinal lesions (any), (%)		15 (25)	12 (31.6)	3 (13.6)	0.122
Anterior uveitis (SUN), n (%)		16 (26.7)	9 (23.7)	7 (31.8)	0.492
Unclassifiable uveitis, n (%)		7 (20.6)	5 (23.8)	2 (15.4)	0.654
Ocular comorbidities, n (%)	Cataract	16 (26.7)	8 (21.1)	8 (36.4)	0.196
	Glaucoma	11 (18.3)	7 (18.4)	4 (18.2)	0.982
Treatments for UME, n (%)	None	4 (6.9)	4 (10.8)	0 (0)	
	Local only	14 (23.3)	10 (27)	4 (19)	0.191
	Systemic	40 (66.7)	23 (62.2)	17 (81)	
SD-OCT imputs					
Macular volume (mm3, mean ± SD)		11.9 ± 1.9	11.5 ± 1.3	12.6 ± 2.6	0.063
Thickened vitreo-macular interface, n (%)		18(30)	14 (36.8)	4 (18.2)	0.129
Unaltered ellipsoid layer, n (%)		35 (58.3)	25 (65.8)	10 (45.5)	0.124
Significant Tractional component, n (%)		7 (11.7)	7 (18.4)	0 (0)	0.032
UME cystoid component, n (%)		47 (78.3)	29 (76.3)	18 (81.8)	0.618
Diameter of major cyst (µm, mean ± SD)		330.1 ± 475.5	266.8 ± 208.8	433.5 ± 723.2	0.706
UME diffuse component, n (%)		14 (23.3)	11 (28.9)	3 (13.6)	0.177
SRF transverse extent (µm, mean ± SD)		363.1 ± 520.2	169 ± 271.6	621.9 ± 665.8	0.021
Choroidal thickness (µm, mean ± SD)		272.8 ± 97.7	258.5 ± 80.6	297.4 ± 119.9	0.137
Immune imputs					
Tregs (% $CD3^+$ $CD4^+$ $PoxP3^+$)		4.2 ± 2.6	4.0 ± 2.3	4.9 ± 2.9	0.153
TNFα (pg/mL)		8.9 ± 8.2	10.1 ± 9.3	7.1 ± 5.9	0.136
IL-1β (pg/mL)		0.7 ± 1.4	1.0 ± 1.7	0.3 ± 0.3	0.075
IL-6 (pg/mL)		4.7 ± 11.9	6.2 ± 14.2	2.3 ± 6.7	0.064
IL-8 (pg/mL)		12.9 ± 18.5	14.7 ± 21.8	10.0 ± 11.1	0.281
IL-10 (pg/mL)		1.5 ± 5.4	1.1 ± 2.4	2.1 ± 8.3	0.281
IL-17 (pg/mL)		12.7 ± 25.4	9.5 ± 14.3	17.9 ± 36.9	0.589
MCP-1 (pg/mL)		640.0 ± 390.0	650.0 ± 410.0	628.4 ± 381.0	0.822
VEGF (pg/mL)		263.8 ± 195.8	282.5 ± 178.8	233.6 ± 221.7	0.127

[1]*Improvement, defined as per decrease ≥20% or reach <300 µm in central subfield thickness at 6 months and maintained through month 12.*

[2]*Chi-square or Fisher (categorical), Mann-Whitney (continuous).*

ACC, anterior chamber cells; SUN standardization of uveitis nomenclature; NEI, National Eye Institute scale; UME, uveitic macular edema; SD-OCT, spectral-domain optical coherence tomography; SRF, subretinal fluid; TNF, tumor necrosis factor; IL, interleukin; MCP, monocyte chemoattractant protein; VEGF, vascular endothelial growth factor; Tregs, regulatory T cells.

of the transcription factor Helios is a useful marker for the identification of stable tTregs. However, we did not include Helios in our flow cytometry panel to characterize Tregs subtype. Previous studies determined Tregs levels in patients with and without UME in a cross-sectional manner, whereas the present study is prospective in nature, with the aim to investigate the predictive value of Tregs levels in the anatomical response after 12 months.

The differences observed in Tregs levels according to the anatomical event of UME improvement suggest that Tregs could be associated with the protective processes underlying UME resolution. In line with our findings, preclinical evidence shows that in experimental autoimmune uveoretinitis (EAU), the adoptive transfer of Tregs appears to confer protection from uveitis induced by the uveitogenic retinal antigen interphotoreceptor binding protein (IRBP) (22), and another study showed that retinal antigen-specific Foxp3+ Tregs contribute to the natural resolution of EAU and the maintenance of remission (23). Interestingly, Gilbert et al. recently showed that clinical remission of non-infectious uveitis is characterized by an upregulation of peripheral Tregs polarized toward TIGIT and T-bet (24). TIGIT is a co-inhibitory molecule expressed by Tregs. $TIGIT^+$ Tregs seem to selectively inhibit Th17 and Th1, but not Th2 responses (25). Since it is known that the Th17 and Th1 subsets are pivotal in the pathogenesis of autoimmune disorders, TIGIT could be a biomarker of stable, functionally suppressive Tregs in such disorders. Even though we did not specifically analyze the suppressive function of Tregs, we observed an independent association between increased Tregs and anatomical improvement or resolution of UME, which was a 25% more frequently found for each unitary increase in Tregs log levels. Almost 67% of recruited patients received systemic treatment showing a good clinical ocular response, supporting the fact that systemic peripheral blood Tregs and their associated microenvironment influence ocular immunity and that, therefore, peripheral blood biomarkers can be useful in predicting ocular outcomes.

Outcome = "Sustained anatomical improvement in uveitic macular edema at 12 months".

	Univariate		Multivariate		
	p-value	OR	95% CI		p-value
Age (+1 year)	0.063	0.96	0.93	1.00	ns
Female	0.321	0.58	0.20	1.69	ns
EMU evolution time (+1 month)	0.133	1.01	1.00	1.03	ns
Chorioretinal lesions	0.122	0.34	0.09	1.38	ns
Cataract	0.196	2.14	0.67	6.89	ns
Systemic treatment	0.191	1.00	-	-	out
Macular volume (+1 μm)	0.063	**1.41**	**1.01**	**2.03**	**0.032**
Normal vitreo-macular interface	0.129	2.63	0.74	9.33	ns
UME diffuse component	0.177	0.39	0.10	1.58	ns
SRF transverse extent (+25 μm)	0.021	1.06	0.99	1.14	ns
Unaltered ellipsoid layer	0.124	0.43	0.15	1.27	ns
Choroidal thickness (+25 μm)	0.137	1.11	0.97	1.27	ns
Log Tregs (+1 unit)	0.032	**1.25**	**1.12**	**2.56**	**0.049**
Log TNFα (+1 unit)	0.136	0.78	0.45	1.36	ns
Log IL-1ß (+1 unit)	0.075	0.65	0.36	1.17	ns
Log IL-6 (+1 unit)	0.064	**0.67**	**0.45**	**1.00**	**0.042**
Log VEGF (+1 unit)	0.127	0.78	0.48	1.29	ns

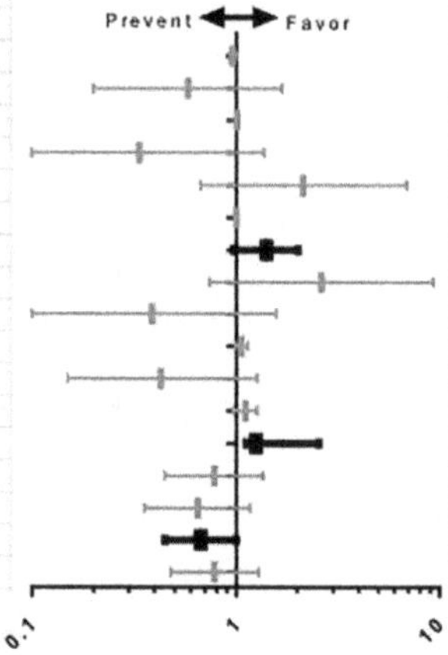

FIGURE 2 | Uni and multivariate regression model of variables as predictors of anatomic outcome in uveitic macular edema. Outcome: "sustained anatomical improvement", defined as per decrease ≥20% or reaches <300 μm in central subfoveal thickness at 6 months and maintained through month 12. All covariates ($P < 0.20$) included in the multivariable model are shown. Quantitative variables were transformed to log scale. Statistically significant associations (P-value < 0.05) are noted in bold. Hosmer-Lemeshow goodness-of-fit test, $P = 0.13$. Abbreviations: CI, confidence interval; OR, odds ratio; UME, uveitic macular edema; SRF, subretinal fluid; TNF, tumor necrosis factor; IL, interleukin; VEGF, vascular endothelial growth factor; Tregs, regulatory T lymphocytes.

On the other hand, the cytokine milieu in non-infectious uveitis has been extensively investigated (26–30). In the present study our focus was investigating the relationship between serum cytokines and anatomical improvement of UME. We therefore selected defined outcomes that may influence UME prognosis and can be easily and objectively assessed. BCVA, although a major clinical end result of UME, is not one of these features, since it can be easily biased by other parameters such as UME duration, presence of cataract, retinal scarring, or macular non-perfusion. We investigated whether anatomical improvement of UME could be predicted by immunological variables besides Tregs after adjusting for covariates in the model. The multivariate model showed that higher baseline levels of IL-6 were associated with lower CST improvement, which was a 33% less frequent for each unitary increase in IL-6 log-levels. IL-6 is a cytokine produced by several immune cells, in response to molecular patterns and affects multiple inflammatory cells and pathways. IL-6 is responsible for the induction of acute-phase proteins, differentiation of adaptive T cell responses, trafficking of acute and chronic inflammatory cells, regulation of homeostasis, and tissue regeneration (31). In the eye, significant elevation of IL-6 has been observed in ocular fluids (vitreous and aqueous) derived from retinal vein occlusion, diabetic macular edema, and refractory/chronic uveitis patients (32–34). Our group and others have previously reported that in patients with UME refractory to conventional therapies, systemic inhibition of IL-6 signaling with the IL-6 receptor (IL-6R) monoclonal antibody tocilizumab (TCZ–Actemra; Hoffmann-La Roche Ltd, Basel, Switzerland) was beneficial at 6, 12, and 24 months (35, 36), in particular with regards to achieving a reduction in CST. Indeed, IL-6 signaling blockade suppresses EAU (37), and it has been recently described that IL-6 reversibly disrupts the integrity of the blood-retinal barrier *in vitro* (38), a key feature of the pathophysiology of macular edema. Our current study actually reinforces the concept of targeting systemic IL-6 in UME, as patients with higher baseline serum levels of IL-6 showed a less favorable anatomical response.

Despite the association of increased Tregs and reduced IL-6 levels with UME anatomical improvement, no linear association between IL-6 and Tregs was observed. The exact relationship between IL-6 and Tregs in modulating uveitis is not clearly understood. IL-6 is involved in the differentiation of $CD4^+$ T cells into Th17 cells known to play a pivotal role in uveitis. Moreover, blockade of IL-6 signaling not only suppresses Th17 but also promotes Tregs in EAU (39). In other autoimmune disorders such as psoriasis, IL6 signaling prevents immune suppression by Tregs (40). Other authors have shown that IL6 overproduction *in vivo* inhibits inducible Treg generation from naïve T cells, but does not affect the development and function of natural Tregs (41). The inverse association of IL-6 and Tregs might occur only at the local site within the eye, but not in the systemic circulation, which could explain why we did not observe any association. Alternatively, the limited number of samples could also explain the lack of association. Thus, how IL6 modulates Treg function in the eye warrants further investigation.

Regarding the therapeutic approach, one may expect a relationship between systemic treatment and serum cytokine levels, as immunomodulatory agents are used to treat non-infectious uveitis. However, we did not observe significant differences in cytokine levels between none of the initial treatment modalities, either local, systemic, or a combination of both.

The main limitations of the present study include the sample size of eyes included in the analysis, the heterogeneity of uveitic conditions and immunomodulatory treatments, and the interindividual variability of cytokine levels. Despite these concerns, the strengths of the study include a prospective design, the use of standardized masked data collection protocols, a centralized center for the cytokine and Tregs determination, and the recruitment from multiple uveitis referral centers.

In conclusion, the results presented herein suggest that higher levels of Tregs may contribute to sustained anatomical improvement of UME, whereas increased systemic levels of IL-6 may be a prognostic factor of poor anatomical outcome of UME. These findings could open the opportunity to more efficient and personalized therapeutic approaches to improve long-term visual prognosis in patients with macular edema secondary to non-infectious uveitis.

ETHICS STATEMENT

The studies involving human participants were reviewed and approved by Comité Ético de Investigación Clínica del Hospital Clínic de Barcelona 2013/8574; Comité de Ética de la Investigación con Medicamentos de Euskadi, Hospital Universitario Cruces PI201406; and Comité Ético de Investigación Clínica del Hospital Clínico San Carlos de Madrid 13/244-E. The patients/participants provided their written informed consent to participate in this study.

AUTHOR CONTRIBUTIONS

VL, MM, AF, DD-V, AA, and BM contributed to the design of the study and experiments. JM, VL, AF, DD-V, CE, JA, BB, MS, AA, and BM performed the experiments, data capture, and analysis. JM, VL, MF-R, and BM performed the data interpretation. All authors contributed to the article and approved the submitted version.

REFERENCES

1. Nussenblatt RB. The natural history of uveitis. *Int Ophthalmol* (1990) 14(5-6):303–8. doi: 10.1007/BF00163549
2. Suttorp-Schulten MSA, Rothova A. The possible impact of uveitis in blindness: A literature survey. *Br J Ophthalmol* (1996) 80(9):844–8. doi: 10.1136/bjo.80.9.844
3. Dick AD. Doyne lecture 2016: Intraocular health and the many faces of inflammation. *Eye* (2017) 31(1):87–96. doi: 10.1038/eye.2016.177
4. Munk MR, Kiss CG, Steiner I, Sulzbacher F, Roberts P, Kroh M, et al. Systematic correlation of morphologic alterations and retinal function in eyes with uveitis-associated cystoid macular oedema during development, resolution and relapse. *Br J Ophthalmol* (2013) 97:1289–96. doi: 10.1136/bjophthalmol-2012-303052
5. Rothova A. Medical treatment of cystoid macular edema. *Ocul Immunol Inflammation* (2002) 10(4):239–46. doi: 10.1076/ocii.10.4.239.15589
6. Jeon S, Lee WK, Jung Y. Changes in the intraocular cytokine levels after intravitreal bevacizumab in uveitic macular edema. *Ocul Immunol Inflammation* (2012) 20(5):360–4. doi: 10.3109/09273948.2012.709576
7. Valencia X, Lipsky PE. CD4+CD25+FoxP3+regulatory T cells in autoimmune diseases. *Nat Clin Pract Rheumatol* (2007) 3(11):619–26. doi: 10.1038/ncprheum0624
8. Ruggieri S, Frassanito MA, Dammacco R, Guerriero S. T reg lymphocytes in autoimmune uveitis. *Ocul Immunol Inflammation* (2012) 20(4):255–61. doi: 10.3109/09273948.2012.681830
9. Yeh S, Li Z, Forooghian F, Hwang FS, Cunningham MA, Pantanelli S, et al. CD4 +foxp3 + T-regulatory cells in noninfectious uveitis. *Arch Ophthalmol* (2009) 127(4):407–13. doi: 10.1001/archophthalmol.2009.32
10. Keino H, Takeuchi M, Usui Y, Hattori T, Yamakawa N, Kezuka T, et al. Supplementation of CD4+CD25+ regulatory T cells suppresses experimental autoimmune uveoretinitis. *Br J Ophthalmol* (2007) 91(1):105–10. doi: 10.1136/bjo.2006.099192
11. Siepmann K, Biester S, Plšková J, Muckersie E, Duncan L, Forrester JV. CD4+CD25+ T regulatory cells induced by LPS-activated bone marrow dendritic cells suppress experimental autoimmune uveoretinitis in vivo. *Graefe's Arch Clin Exp Ophthalmol* (2007) 245(2):221–9. doi: 10.1007/s00417-006-0356-9
12. Levin MH, Pistilli M, Daniel E, Gangaputra SS, Nussenblatt RB, Rosenbaum JT, et al. Incidence of visual improvement in uveitis cases with visual impairment caused by macular edema. *Ophthalmology* (2014) 121:588–95.e1. doi: 10.1016/j.ophtha.2013.09.023
13. Ossewaarde-Van Norel A, Rothova A. Clinical review: Update on treatment of inflammatory macular edema. *Ocul Immunol Inflammation* (2011) 19(1):75–83. doi: 10.3109/09273948.2010.509530
14. Jabs DA, Nussenblatt RB, Rosenbaum JT, Atmaca LS, Becker MD, Brezin AP, et al. Standardization of uveitis nomenclature for reporting clinical data. Results of the first international workshop. *Am J Ophthalmol* (2005) 140 (3):509–16. doi: 10.1016/j.ajo.2005.03.057
15. Rizzo LV, Xu H, Chan CC, Wiggert B, Caspi RR. IL-10 has a protective role in experimental autoimmune uveoretinitis. *Int Immunol* (1998) 10(6):807–14. doi: 10.1093/intimm/10.6.807
16. Roncarolo MG, Bacchetta R, Bordignon C, Narula S, Levings MK. Type 1 T regulatory cells. *Immunol Rev* (2001) 182:68–79. doi: 10.1034/j.1600-065X.2001.1820105.x
17. Chen L, Yang P, Zhou H, He H, Ren X, Chi W, et al. Diminished frequency and function of CD4+CD25high regulatory T cells associated with active uveitis in Vogt-Koyanagi-Harada syndrome. *Invest Ophthalmol Vis Sci* (2008) 49(8):3475–82. doi: 10.1167/iovs.08-1793
18. Sugita S, Yamada Y, Kaneko S, Horie S, Mochizuki M. Induction of regulatory T cells by infliximab in behçet's disease. *Invest Ophthalmol Vis Sci* (2011) 52 (1):476–84. doi: 10.1167/iovs.10-5916
19. Commodaro AG, Peron JPS, Genre J, Arslanian C, Sanches L, Muccioli C, et al. IL-10 and TGF-β immunoregulatory cytokines rather than natural regulatory T cells are associated with the resolution phase of Vogt-Koyanagi-Harada (VKH) syndrome. *Scand J Immunol* (2010) 72(1):31–7. doi: 10.1111/j.1365-3083.2010.02401.x
20. Molins B, Mesquida M, Lee RWJ, Llorenç V, Pelegrín L, Adán A. Regulatory T cell levels and cytokine production in active non-infectious uveitis: In-vitro effects of pharmacological treatment. *Clin Exp Immunol* (2015) 179(3):529–38. doi: 10.1111/cei.12479
21. Shevach EM, Thornton AM. tTregs, pTregs, and iTregs: Similarities and differences. *Immunol Rev* (2014) 259(1):88–102. doi: 10.1111/imr.12160
22. Silver PB, Agarwal RK, Su S-B, Suffia I, Grajewski RS, Luger D, et al. Hydrodynamic Vaccination with DNA Encoding an Immunologically Privileged Retinal Antigen Protects from Autoimmunity through Induction of Regulatory T Cells. *J Immunol* (2007) 179(8):5146–58. doi: 10.4049/jimmunol.179.8.5146
23. Silver PB, Horai R, Chen J, Jittayasothorn Y, Chan C-C, Villasmil R, et al. Retina-Specific T Regulatory Cells Bring About Resolution and Maintain Remission of Autoimmune Uveitis. *J Immunol* (2015) 194(7):3011–9. doi: 10.4049/jimmunol.1501038
24. Gilbert RM, Zhang X, Sampson RD, Ehrenstein MR, Nguyen DX, Chaudhry M, et al. Clinical remission of sight-threatening non-infectious uveitis is characterized by an upregulation of peripheral T-regulatory cell polarized towards T-bet and TIGIT. *Front Immunol* (2018) 9:907. doi: 10.3389/fimmu.2018.00907
25. Joller N, Lozano E, Burkett PR, Patel B, Xiao S, Zhu C, et al. Treg cells expressing the coinhibitory molecule TIGIT selectively inhibit proinflammatory Th1 and Th17 cell responses. *Immunity* (2014) 40(4):569–81. doi: 10.1016/j.immuni.2014.02.012
26. Torun N, Callizo J, Orlic N, Scherer M, Hartmann C, Pleyer U. Serum cytokine receptor levels in noninfectious uveitis. *Ophthalmic Res* (2005) 37 (2):112–6. doi: 10.1159/000084271

(VKH) syndrome. *Scand J Immunol* (2010) 72(1):31–7. doi: 10.1111/j.1365-3083.2010.02401.x

20. Molins B, Mesquida M, Lee RWJ, Llorenç V, Pelegrín L, Adán A. Regulatory T cell levels and cytokine production in active non-infectious uveitis: In-vitro effects of pharmacological treatment. *Clin Exp Immunol* (2015) 179(3):529–38. doi: 10.1111/cei.12479
21. Shevach EM, Thornton AM. tTregs, pTregs, and iTregs: Similarities and differences. *Immunol Rev* (2014) 259(1):88–102. doi: 10.1111/imr.12160
22. Silver PB, Agarwal RK, Su S-B, Suffia I, Grajewski RS, Luger D, et al. Hydrodynamic Vaccination with DNA Encoding an Immunologically Privileged Retinal Antigen Protects from Autoimmunity through Induction of Regulatory T Cells. *J Immunol* (2007) 179(8):5146–58. doi: 10.4049/jimmunol.179.8.5146
23. Silver PB, Horai R, Chen J, Jittayasothorn Y, Chan C-C, Villasmil R, et al. Retina-Specific T Regulatory Cells Bring About Resolution and Maintain Remission of Autoimmune Uveitis. *J Immunol* (2015) 194(7):3011–9. doi: 10.4049/jimmunol.1501038
24. Gilbert RM, Zhang X, Sampson RD, Ehrenstein MR, Nguyen DX, Chaudhry M, et al. Clinical remission of sight-threatening non-infectious uveitis is characterized by an upregulation of peripheral T-regulatory cell polarized towards T-bet and TIGIT. *Front Immunol* (2018) 9:907. doi: 10.3389/fimmu.2018.00907
25. Joller N, Lozano E, Burkett PR, Patel B, Xiao S, Zhu C, et al. Treg cells expressing the coinhibitory molecule TIGIT selectively inhibit proinflammatory Th1 and Th17 cell responses. *Immunity* (2014) 40(4):569–81. doi: 10.1016/j.immuni.2014.02.012
26. Torun N, Callizo J, Orlic N, Scherer M, Hartmann C, Pleyer U. Serum cytokine receptor levels in noninfectious uveitis. *Ophthalmic Res* (2005) 37 (2):112–6. doi: 10.1159/000084271

edema. *Curr Diabetes Rep* (2013) 13:476–80. doi: 10.1007/s11892-013-0382-z

33. Noma H, Funatsu H, Mimura T, Harino S, Hori S. Vitreous Levels of Interleukin-6 and Vascular Endothelial Growth Factor in Macular Edema with Central Retinal Vein Occlusion. *Ophthalmology* (2009) 116:87–93. doi: 10.1016/j.ophtha.2008.09.034
34. van Kooij B, Rothova A, Rijkers GT, de Groot-Mijnes JDF. Distinct cytokine and chemokine profiles in the aqueous of patients with uveitis and cystoid macular edema. *Am J Ophthalmol* (2006) 142:192–4. doi: 10.1016/j.ajo.2006.02.052
35. Mesquida M, Molins B, Llorenç V, Hernández MV, Espinosa G, Sainz de la Maza M, et al. Twenty-Four Month Follow-Up Of Tocilizumab Therapy For Refractory Uveitis-Related Macular Edema. *Retina* (2018) 38(7):1361–70. doi: 10.1097/IAE.0000000000001690
36. Mesquida M, Molins B, Llorenç V, Sainz de la Maza M, Adán A. Long-term effects of tocilizumab therapy for refractory uveitis-related macular edema. *Ophthalmology* (2014) 121:2380–6. doi: 10.1016/j.ophtha.2014.06.050
37. Rochfort KD, Collins LE, Murphy RP, Cummins PM. Downregulation of blood-brain barrier phenotype by proinflammatory cytokines involves NADPH oxidase-dependent ROS generation: Consequences for interendothelial adherens and tight junctions. *PLoS One* (2014) 9(7): e101815. doi: 10.1371/journal.pone.0101815
38. Mesquida M, Drawnel F, Lait PJ, Copland DA, Stimpson ML, Llorenç V, et al. Modelling macular edema: The effect of IL-6 and IL-6r blockade on human blood-retinal barrier integrity in vitro. *Transl Vis Sci Technol* (2019) 8(5):32. doi: 10.1167/tvst.8.5.32
39. Hohki S, Ohguro N, Haruta H, Nakai K, Terabe F, Serada S, et al. Blockade of interleukin-6 signaling suppresses experimental autoimmune uveoretinitis by the inhibition of inflammatory Th17 responses. *Exp Eye Res* (2010) 91:162–70. doi: 10.1016/j.exer.2010.04.009
40. Goodman WA, Levine AD, Massari JV, Sugiyama H, McCormick TS, Cooper KD. IL-6 Signaling in Psoriasis Prevents Immune Suppression by Regulatory T Cells. *J Immunol* (2009) 183(5):3170–6. doi: 10.4049/jimmunol.0803721
41. Fujimoto M, Nakano M, Terabe F, Kawahata H, Ohkawara T, Han Y, et al. The Influence of Excessive IL-6 Production In Vivo on the Development and Function of Foxp3 + Regulatory T Cells. *J Immunol* (2011) 186(1):32–40. doi: 10.4049/jimmunol.0903314

9

Genetic Association of Interleukin 33/ST2 Polymorphisms with Behcet's Uveitis

Minghang Pei[1], Xinshu Liu[2], Peizeng Yang[3], Chan Zhao[4], Fei Gao[4], Yi Qu[4], Anyi Liang[4], Junyan Xiao[4] and Meifen Zhang[4]*

[1] *Department of Ophthalmology, The First Affiliated Hospital of Zhengzhou University, Zhengzhou, China,* [2] *Department of Ophthalmology, The Fourth People's Hospital of Shenyang, Shenyang, China,* [3] *The First Affiliated Hospital of Chongqing Medical University, Chongqing Key Lab of Ophthalmology, Chongqing Eye Institute, Chongqing Branch of National Clinical Research Center for Ocular Diseases, Chongqing, China,* [4] *Department of Ophthalmology, Peking Union Medical College Hospital, Chinese Academy of Medical Sciences and Peking Union Medical College, Beijing, China*

***Correspondence:**
Meifen Zhang
meifen_zhang@hotmail.com

Interleukin (IL)33, a member of the IL1 superfamily, functions as a nuclear factor and mediates biological effects by interacting with the ST2 receptor. Recent studies have described IL33 as an emerging pro-inflammatory cytokine in the immune system, and *IL33/ST2* gene polymorphisms have been implicated in the pathogenesis of various immune diseases. However, the underlying mechanisms of *IL33/ST2* in Behcet's disease (BD) remain to be defined. Here, we investigated the association between *IL33/ST2* gene polymorphisms and BD in 585 BD uveitis (BDU) patients and 834 healthy controls using Agena MassARRAY iPLEX platform. We found that rs3821204 was associated with the development of BDU. Moreover, the frequency of rs2210463 G allele was lower in patients with genital involvement. Association analysis revealed a much greater genetic difference between complete-type and incomplete-type BD groups, including three SNPs (rs7044343, rs1048274, and rs2210463). Our findings suggest that *IL33/ST2* gene polymorphisms are involved in the pathogenesis of BDU. Different genetic backgrounds may exist in complete-type and incomplete-type BD patients.

Keywords: Behcet's disease, Behcet's uveitis, uveitis, gene polymorphism, single nucleotide polymorphism, interleukin 33, ST2

INTRODUCTION

Behçet's disease (BD) is a chronic, relapsing, systemic vasculitis involving complex pathologic processes characterized by recurrent episodes of uveitis, oral and genital ulcers, and skin lesions (1). It may also affect the digestive, cardiovascular, and nervous systems and involve joints and large vessels (1). Eye involvement is one of the most serious manifestations of BD with high incidence of disability. It affects about 70% of patients and is characterized by uveitis (BDU) (2). The onset of BD usually occurs in the third or fourth decade of life and is rare in children or individuals over the age of 40 years. The etiology of BD is still unclear, although, an inflammatory response triggered by immune and unknown environmental factors in a genetically susceptible individual has been proposed as its cause. Among all genetic factors, HLA-B51 has been confirmed as the strongest risk factor for BD. However, the presence of HLA-B51 alone is not sufficient to explain all the symptoms of BD patients (3).

Interleukin (IL)33, a member of the IL-1 family, is evolutionarily conserved in mammals and a ligand for the orphan receptor ST2. It is constitutively expressed by tissue barrier cells, such as epithelial and endothelial cells, and various innate immune cells, such as macrophages and dendritic cells. Both enhanced innate immunity and neutrophil hyperactivity with endothelial damage, which are part of BD pathogenesis (4), are related to disrupted IL33 levels. Therefore, we hypothesized that BD may be associated with *IL33/ST2* genetic abnormalities.

In the present study, we aimed to establish the role of *IL33* and *ST2* genes in the risk of developing BDU in a well-characterized Chinese cohort by genotyping and association analysis. We analyzed single nucleotide polymorphisms (SNPs) of *IL33* (rs1891385, rs2210463, rs11792633, rs7044343, rs1048274) and *ST2* (rs3821204, rs12712142, rs2058660) with respect to BDU pathogenesis and characteristic BDU phenotypes in these patients.

MATERIALS AND METHODS

Patients

This study was approved by the Ethics Committee of Peking Union Medical College Hospital. A total of 585 patients with BDU were recruited from the Peking Union Medical College Hospital (PUMCH, 190 patients) and the First Affiliated Hospital of Chongqing Medical University (395 patients) between January 2018 and June 2019. All patients with BD were diagnosed according to the International BD Study Group criteria. Eight hundred and thirty-four healthy controls with no previous history of immune-related diseases were enrolled from the health examination center of PUMCH. All participants were self-reported as Han Chinese and were unrelated.

Of the 585 BD patients included, detailed clinical data for 553 patients was recorded. Based on their clinical characteristics, patients were divided into the following subgroups: complete-type and incomplete-type BD groups (1); severe and non-severe BD groups; early-onset and late-onset BD groups.

In case of complete-type BD, all four main symptoms (ocular lesion, recurrent aphthous ulcers on the oral mucosa, genital ulcers, and skin lesion) appeared during the clinical course. In case of incomplete-type BD, either of the following conditions was met: 1. Three of the four main symptoms, or two main symptoms and two additional symptoms (arthritis without deformity or sclerosis, epididymitis, gastrointestinal lesion represented by ileocecal ulceration, vascular lesions, and central nervous system lesions including and above middle class of severity) appeared during the clinical course; 2. Typical ocular lesions and other main symptoms, or two additional symptoms appeared during the clinical course.

Severe and non-severe BD were classified based on clinical severity score ≥7 or <7 points, respectively. Clinical severity score was determined as previously described (5, 6): 1 point for each of the mild symptoms (oral ulcers, genital ulcers, arthralgia, typical skin lesions such as erythema, nodosum-like lesions, papulopustular lesions, and folliculitis), 2 points for each of the moderate symptoms (arthritis, deep vein thrombosis of the legs, anterior uveitis, gastrointestinal involvement), and 3 points for each of the severe symptoms (posterior/panuveitis, retinal vasculitis, arterial thrombosis, neuro Behcet's disease, bowel perforation).

In case of early-onset BD, the age of first BD attack was <40 years, while in late-onset BD group, the age of first BD attack was ≥40 years.

Selection of SNPs

Considering the vital effects of IL33 and ST2 in immune-mediated diseases, eight SNPs (rs1891385, rs2210463, rs11792633, rs7044343, rs1048274, rs2058660, rs3821204, rs12712142), which were reported to show a positive association with systemic lupus erythematosus, ankylosing spondylitis (AS), or other immune-related diseases, based on GWAS and candidate gene association studies, were selected for further analysis.

Sample Collection and SNP Analysis

A total of 2 ml blood sample was collected in an ethylenediaminetetraacetic acid (EDTA) anticoagulant tube from each subject. Genomic DNA was extracted from peripheral blood cells using a kit from Thermo Fisher Scientific Inc. according to the manufacturer's instructions. DNA concentration was determined by using a Nanodrop spectrophotometer (Thermo, Wilmington, DE, USA) using the 260/280 nm ratio and diluted to a working concentration of 15–20 ng/μl. The SNPs of *IL33* and *ST2* were genotyped using Agena MassArray system (Agena iPLEX assay, San Diego, CA, USA) following the manufacturer's instructions. Both polymerase chain reaction (PCR) and single-base extension primers for *IL33* (rs1891385, rs2210463, rs11792633, rs7044343, rs1048274) and *ST2* (rs3821204, rs12712142, rs2058660) were designed by the Assay Design Suite (ADS, Agena). After multiplex PCR amplifications, the products were used for locus specific single base extension reactions and the final products were desalted and transferred on to a 384-element SpectroCHIP array. Allele detection was conducted by matrix-assisted laser desorption ionization time of flight mass spectrometry (MALDI-TOF MS). The mass spectrogram data were analyzed using MassArray Typer 4.0 software (Agena).

The current SNP assay method is based on primer extension and offers two levels of specificity. First, a locus-specific PCR reaction takes place, followed by a locus-specific primer extension reaction (iPLEX assay) in which an oligonucleotide primer anneals immediately upstream of the polymorphic site being genotyped. In the iPLEX assay, the primer and amplified target DNA are incubated with mass-modified dideoxynucleotide terminators. The primer extension is made according to the sequence of the variant site, and is a single complementary mass-modified base. Through the use of MALDI-TOF mass spectrometry, the mass of the extended primer is determined. The primer's mass indicates the sequence and, therefore, the alleles present at the polymorphic site of interest (7).

Duplicate samples, negative controls, and blank controls were included on the plates to ensure the accuracy of genotyping.

Statistical Analysis

Statistical analyses were performed using PLINK 1.07 software (Shaun Purcell, Boston, MA, USA). The Hardy-Weinberg equilibrium (HWE) of each SNP was examined by using the Chi-square (χ^2) test in healthy controls. Any SNPs that deviated from the HWE ($P < 0.05$ in the control groups) would be excluded from subsequent analysis. Differences in genotype and allele frequencies between cases and controls, and between different BD subgroups and phenotypes were analyzed using χ^2 test. The odds ratio (OR) and 95% confidence interval (95% CI) of associations were calculated. For multiple comparisons, Pc values (corrected for multiple comparisons by the Bonferroni adjustment test) <0.05 were deemed to be statistically significant. For genetic model testing (additive, dominant, and recessive model), logistic regression analyses were used.

RESULTS

Patient Characteristics and Sequencing Analysis

The characteristics of the controls and patients with BD are shown in **Table 1.** The gender distributions in both controls and cases were similar (p = 0.127). The median age was 36.0 (31.0–42.0) years and 32.0 (26.0–39.0) years for controls and cases respectively. The success rate for sequencing of each SNP was more than 99%. The eight SNPs of *IL33* and *ST2* selected in the present study did not show any deviation from HWE (all P > 0.05) in controls, and thus, the data were suitable for further comparisons.

ST2 rs3821204 SNP Was Associated With BD Development

ST2 SNPs rs3821204, rs12712142, and rs2058660 were analyzed in both cases and controls and rs3821204 G allele was found to be associated with BDU development (X2 = 7.94, Pc = 0.039; **Table 2**). Although the frequency of GG genotype of *ST2* rs3821204 was higher in the control group than that in the BDU group (10.71 *vs* 6.16%), genotype frequency analysis failed to reach the statistical significance threshold as the trend was not statistically significant after Bonferroni correction (Pc = 0.051; **Table 2**). Logistic analysis with three models (i.e., additive, dominant, and recessive) revealed significant differences in the genotypic distributions of rs3821204 in both additive (Pc = 0.036) and recessive (Pc = 0.027) models (**Table 3**).

TABLE 1 | Clinical and demographic characteristics of the study population.

Characteristic	Patients with BDU	Controls
Male, n (%)	484 (82.7%)	663 (79.5%)
Age (years)	32.0 (26.0–39.0)	36.0 (31.0–42.0)
BD subgroups		
Complete BD, n	334	/
Incomplete BD, n	219	/
Severe BD, n	132	/
Un-severe BD, n	421	/
Early-onset BD, n	423	/
Late-onset BD, n	130	/
Phenotypes		
Uveitis	553	/
Genital ulcer	285	/
Erythema nodosum	233	/
Arthritis	250	/
Aphthous ulcer	545	/

BD, Behcet's disease; BDU, Behcet's uveitis.
Five hundred and fifty-three BD patients with detailed clinical data were included in the subgroup and phenotype association analysis.

IL33 SNPs Were Not Associated With BD Development

We then detected *IL33* SNPs (rs11792633, rs1048274, rs7044343, rs2210463, and rs1891385) in the study population. Our study showed that neither genotype nor allele frequencies of these five SNPs were statistically significant between patients and healthy controls (Pc > 0.05; **Table 2**). Moreover, logistic regression analysis with three genetic models (i.e., additive, dominant, and recessive) also did not reveal any statistical difference between patient and control groups (Pc > 0.05; **Table 3**).

Correlation of *ST2* and *IL33* SNPs With the Phenotype Subgroups of BD

Association analyses of *ST2* and *IL33* SNPs with different BD subgroups and phenotypes were also performed (**Tables 4A** and **4B**). The allele frequencies of *IL33* SNPs rs2210463 (P = 0.0028, Pc = 0.022), rs7044343 (P = 0.0034, Pc = 0.027), and rs1048274 (P = 0.0050, Pc = 0.040) were all significantly different between the complete-type and incomplete-type BDU groups. The allele frequency of *IL33* SNP rs2210463 (P = 0.006, Pc = 0.048) was significantly different between patients with and without genital ulcers. No allele frequency differences were found between the early- and late-onset or severe and non-severe BDU groups in any *ST2* or *IL33* SNP. Moreover, no association was found between erythema nodosum, or arthritis and *IL33* or *ST2* SNPs.

DISCUSSION

Although the etiopathogenesis of BD remains uncertain, microbial agent triggers, environmental factors, genetic predisposition, and immunological abnormalities have been implicated (8–10). Complex disorders implicating innate and adaptive immunity in humoral and cellular immunity settings are observed in BD. IL33, a member of the IL1 family that potently drives the production of T helper (Th)-2-associated cytokines and promotes responses by cytotoxic NK cells, Th1 cells, and CD8+ T cells (11), has been associated with various immune-related diseases (12, 13). ST2, the receptor of IL33, is highly expressed in many immunocytes (14).

In the present study, we demonstrated significant association between the *IL33/ST2* pathway SNP rs3821204 and the development of BDU. The rs3821204 polymorphism occurs in the 3′ untranslated region of *ST2*, which was found to be functional with the rs3821204 gene mutation by disrupting the binding site of miR-202-3p, resulting in plasma level changes of sST2 (15, 16). sST2 is the soluble form of ST2, which together with the membrane-bound form (ST2L), comprise the two main ST2 existing forms (17). ST2L functions as a transmembrane signaling receptor of IL33, mediating the effect of IL33 on

TABLE 2 | Allele and genotype distribution of the IL-33 and ST2 gene markers in BDU patients and controls.

SNPs	Groups	Allele (%)		OR (95% CI)	χ^2	P	Pc	Genotype (%)			χ^2	P	Pc
		C	A					CC	CA	AA			
rs1891385	BDU	318 (27.3)	846 (72.7)	0.991 (0.838,1.172)	0.012	0.914	1	41 (7.0)	236 (40.5)	305 (52.4)	0.052	0.974	1
	Controls	456 (27.5)	1202 (72.5)					61 (7.4)	334 (40.3)	434 (52.4)			
		G	A					GG	GA	AA			
rs2210463	BDU	474 (40.7)	690 (59.3)	1.032 (0.886,1.202)	0.164	0.686	1	98 (16.8)	278 (47.8)	206 (35.4)	1.022	0.600	1
	Controls	665 (40.0)	999 (60.0)					145 (17.4)	375 (45.1)	312 (37.5)			
		C	T					CC	CT	TT			
rs11792633	BDU	537 (45.9)	633 (54.1)	1.118 (0.962,1.299)	2.103	0.147	1	125 (21.4)	287 (49.1)	173 (29.6)	2.397	0.302	1
	Controls	718 (43.1)	946 (56.9)					164 (19.7)	390 (46.9)	278 (33.4)			
		T	C					TT	TC	CC			
rs7044343	BDU	574 (49.1)	596 (50.9)	1.121 (0.965,1.302)	2.226	0.136	1	140 (23.9)	294 (50.3)	151 (25.8)	3.980	0.137	1
	Controls	770 (46.2)	896 (53.8)					192 (23.0)	386 (46.3)	255 (30.6)			
		G	A					GG	GA	AA			
rs1048274	BDU	588 (50.3)	580 (49.7)	1.136 (0.978,1.320)	2.779	0.096	0.764	148 (25.3)	292 (50.0)	144 (24.7)	4.247	0.120	0.957
	Controls	780 (47.2)	874 (52.8)					198 (23.9)	384 (46.4)	245 (29.6)			
		A	G					AA	AG	GG			
rs2058660	BDU	511 (43.7)	659 (56.3)	0.844 (0.726,0.980)	4.93	0.026	0.211	120 (20.5)	271 (46.3)	194 (33.2)	4.72	0.095	0.756
	Controls	797 (47.9)	867 (52.1)					201 (24.2)	395 (47.5)	236 (28.4)			
		G	C					GG	GC	CC			
rs3821204	BDU	321 (37.9)	526 (62.1)	0.790 (0.670,0.931)	7.94	0.005	0.039	36 (6.2)	249 (42.6)	299 (51.2)	10.12	0.006	0.051
	Controls	539 (48.0)	584 (52.0)					89 (10.7)	361 (43.4)	381 (45.8)			
		A	C					AA	AC	CC			
rs12712142	BDU	358 (44.2)	452 (55.8)	0.826 (0.704,0.970)	5.48	0.019	0.154	54 (9.2)	250 (42.8)	280 (47.9)	6.53	0.038	0.306
	Controls	580 (53.5)	504 (46.5)					112 (13.4)	356 (42.8)	364 (43.8)			

BDU, Behcet's uveitis; OR, odds ratio; CI, confidence interval; $\chi2$, Chi-square test; Pc, P values adjusted by Bonferroni correction, Pc = P × 8.

TABLE 3 | Analysis of the eight SNPs based on three genetic models.

Gene	SNPs	Additive model			Dominant model			Recessive mode		
		P	Pc	OR (95% CI)	P	Pc	OR (95% CI)	P	Pc	OR (95% CI)
ST2	rs3821204	0.005	0.036	0.786 (0.665–0.928)	0.047	0.380	0.807 (0.653–0.998)	0.003	0.027	0.548 (0.366–0.819)
ST2	rs12712142	0.022	0.172	0.831 (0.710–0.973)	0.119	0.950	0.844 (0.683–1.044)	0.016	0.126	0.655 (0.465–0.924)
ST2	rs2058660	0.031	0.247	0.851 (0.735–0.985)	0.053	0.427	0.798 (0.634–1.003)	0.107	0.854	0.810 (0.627–1.046)
IL33	rs1891385	0.914	1	0.991 (0.836–1.173)	0.984	1	0.998 (0.807–1.234)	0.823	1	0.954 (0.633–1.439)
IL33	rs2210463	0.692	1	1.031 (0.888–1.197)	0.419	1	1.095 (0.879–1.365)	0.773	1	0.959 (0.724–1.271)
IL33	rs11792633	0.154	0.534	1.114 (0.961–1.292)	0.127	1	1.195 (0.951–1.502)	0.446	1	1.107 (0.852–1.437)
IL33	rs7044343	0.143	0.524	1.116 (0.963–1.293)	0.049	0.394	1.268 (1.001–1.607)	0.699	1	1.050 (0.819–1.347)
IL33	rs1048274	0.103	0.477	1.130 (0.976–1.310)	0.399	0.320	1.286 (1.012–1.635)	0.547	1	1.078 (0.844–1.378)

OR, odds ratio; CI, confidence interval; Pc, P values adjusted by Bonferroni correction, Pc = P × 8.

TABLE 4A | Analysis of eight SNPs based on different BD subgroups.

Gene	SNPs	Severe BD			Complete BD			Early-onset BD		
		OR	95% CI	Pc	OR	95% CI	Pc	OR	95% CI	Pc
ST2	rs3821204	0.897	0.657–1.225	1	0.799	0.609–1.049	0.845	0.735	0.545–0.993	0.354
ST2	rs12712142	1.070	0.796–1.439	1	0.951	0.734–1.233	1	0.708	0.529–0.948	0.161
ST2	rs2058660	1.141	0.865–1.506	1	1.066	0.836–1.358	1	0.844	0.639–1.116	1
IL33	rs1891385	0.995	0.728–1.359	1	1.132	0.864–1.483	1	1.098	0.799–1.509	1
IL33	rs2210463	0.693	0.518–0.926	0.102	0.684	0.533–0.878	0.022	0.823	0.621–1.091	1
IL33	rs11792633	0.839	0.635–1.109	1	0.760	0.596–0.969	0.213	0.849	0.643–1.121	1
IL33	rs7044343	0.801	0.607–1.058	0.941	0.697	0.547–0.887	0.027	0.925	0.700–1.221	1
IL33	rs1048274	0.138	0.614–1.070	1	0.707	0.555–0.901	0.040	0.895	0.677–1.182	1

BD, Behcet's disease; OR, odds ratio; CI, confidence interval; Pc, P values adjusted by Bonferroni correction, Pc = P × 8.

TABLE 4B | Analysis of eight SNPs based on different phenotypes of BD patients.

	SNPs	Genital ulcer			Arthritis			Erythema nodosum		
		OR	95% CI	Pc	OR	95% CI	Pc	OR	95% CI	Pc
ST2	rs3821204	0.898	0.691–1.167	1	1.097	0.844–1.427	1	0.934	0.716–1.219	1
ST2	rs12712142	1.022	0.793–1.317	1	1.247	0.967–1.609	0.705	0.965	0.746–1.247	1
ST2	rs2058660	1.115	0.880–1.414	1	1.240	0.977–1.574	0.611	1.073	0.844–1.364	1
IL33	rs1891385	0.993	0.761–1.295	1	0.959	0.734–1.252	1	0.971	0.741–1.271	1
IL33	rs2210463	0.713	0.560–0.908	0.048	0.757	0.594–0.966	0.199	0.867	0.679–1.107	1
IL33	rs11792633	0.805	0.636–1.021	0.586	0.784	0.618–0.994	0.358	0.958	0.754–1.217	1
IL33	rs7044343	0.761	0.600–0.963	0.185	0.731	0.577–0.927	0.078	0.948	0.746–1.203	1
IL33	rs1048274	0.759	0.599–0.961	0.175	0.781	0.616–0.990	0.327	0.973	0.766–1.236	1

BD, Behcet's disease; OR, odds ratio; CI, confidence interval; Pc, P values adjusted by Bonferroni correction, Pc = P × 8.

inflammatory processes, while sST2 acts as a decoy receptor that prevents the interaction of ST2L with IL33 (18, 19).

Several studies have reported associations between *IL33* rs7044343 polymorphism and autoimmune diseases, including rheumatoid arthritis, systemic sclerosis, and BD in Turkey (20–22). Previous case-control study revealed a significant association between the rs7044343 TT genotype and Turkish BD patients in the discovery population (22). However, in the present study, rs7044343 SNP was not found to be associated with the development of BD in patients belonging to Chinese Han ethnicity. Ethnic differences may be a reason for this discrepancy, as genetic heterogeneity between races has been reported to be 58% in a previous research (23).

The association of *IL33/ST2* SNPs with different BD phenotype subgroups were also investigated. No associations were found except for genital ulcer and the BD of the complete-type. As compared with the other phenotype-based subgroups, greater genetic differences were found between the complete-type and incomplete-type BD groups, which indicated that different genetic backgrounds may exist in these groups of BD patients. Although previous studies reported that similar gene mechanisms underlie the pathogenesis of different immune diseases (24, 25), in the present study, rs2058660 [inflammatory bowel disease-associated (26)], rs1891385 [AS-associated (27)], and rs11792633 [systemic sclerosis-associated (28)] SNPs were not associated with either onset or phenotypes of BD. Compared with the classical immune diseases, BD presents more extensive pathological changes in tissues and organs with featured spontaneous exacerbation and remission clinical courses (29), which, together with the genetic findings, indicate that different molecular mechanisms may exist in BD pathology as compared to classical immune diseases.

Our study had several limitations. First, genetic variants may have different effects in diverse ethnicities. In this study, only Chinese Han individuals were recruited, thus, our results may not be generalizable to other ethnicities. Second, all the study subjects were enrolled from two tertiary ophthalmologic centers, therefore, selection bias may exist. Third, the mRNA expressions of BD patients with different SNP genotypes were not analyzed in this study, further studies are needed to validate our findings.

In conclusion, we reported the association of rs3821204, rs2210463, rs7044343, rs1048274 with the development or phenotypes of BDU, and for the first time revealed significant genetic differences between patients with complete-type and incomplete-type BD. Our findings indicate that *IL33/ST2* polymorphisms have a close and probable causal association with BDU, and different genetic backgrounds may exist in complete-type and incomplete-type BD patients.

ETHICS STATEMENT

The studies involving human participants were reviewed and approved by The Ethics committee of Peking Union Medical College Hospital. Written informed consent to participate in this study was provided by the participants/participants' legal guardian/next of kin.

AUTHOR CONTRIBUTIONS

MP participated in the study design, patient enrollment, data collection and analysis and manuscript drafting. MZ participated in the study design, patient enrollment, data collection and analysis, manuscript drafting, and coordination of experimental work. XL participated in the data interpretation and analysis. PY, CZ, and FG participated in the patient enrollment. MP, YQ, AL, and JX carried out the experimental work. All authors contributed to the article and approved the submitted version.

ACKNOWLEDGMENTS

We would like to thank all the patients and controls who participated in this study and thank Prof. Zhi Zheng and Jun Zhou for help in carrying out the experimental work.

REFERENCES

1. Kurokawa MS, Yoshikawa H, Suzuki N. Behcet's disease. *Semin Respir Crit Care Med* (2004) 25:557–68. doi: 10.1055/s-2004-836147
2. Deuter CM, Kotter I, Wallace GR, Murray PI, Stubiger N, Zierhut M. Behcet's disease: ocular effects and treatment. *Prog Retin Eye Res* (2008) 27:111–36. doi: 10.1016/j.preteyeres.2007.09.002
3. Akman A, Sallakci N, Coskun M, Bacanli A, Yavuzer U, Alpsoy E, et al. TNF-alpha gene 1031 T/C polymorphism in Turkish patients with Behcet's disease. *Br J Dermatol* (2006) 155:350–6. doi: 10.1111/j.1365-2133.2006.07348.x
4. Hisanaga K. [The etiology, diagnosis, and treatment of neurological complications in Behcet disease and its related disorder Sweet disease]. *Rinsho Shinkeigaku* (2019) 59:1–12. doi: 10.5692/clinicalneurol.cn-001238
5. Krause I, Rosen Y, Kaplan I, Milo G, Guedj D, Molad Y, et al. Recurrent aphthous stomatitis in Behcet's disease: clinical features and correlation with systemic disease expression and severity. *J Oral Pathol Med* (1999) 28:193–6. doi: 10.1111/j.1600-0714.1999.tb02023.x
6. Akman A, Ekinci NC, Kacaroglu H, Yavuzer U, Alpsoy E, Yegin O. Relationship between periodontal findings and specific polymorphisms of interleukin-1alpha and -1beta in Turkish patients with Behcet's disease. *Arch Dermatol Res* (2008) 300:19–26. doi: 10.1007/s00403-007-0794-1
7. Gabriel S, Ziaugra L, Tabbaa D. SNP genotyping using the Sequenom MassARRAY iPLEX platform. *Curr Protoc Hum Genet* (2009) Chapter 2: 2–12. doi: 10.1002/0471142905.hg0212s60
8. Alpsoy E, Kodelja V, Goerdt S, Orfanos CE, Zouboulis C. Serum of patients with Behcet's disease induces classical (pro-inflammatory) activation of human macrophages in vitro. *Dermatology* (2003) 206:225–32. doi: 10.1159/000068888
9. Zhou ZY, Chen SL, Shen N, Lu Y. Cytokines and Behcet's disease. *AUTOIMMUN Rev* (2012) 11:699–704. doi: 10.1016/j.autrev.2011.12.005
10. Mochizuki M. Immunotherapy for Behcet's disease. *Int Rev Immunol* (1997) 14:49–66. doi: 10.3109/08830189709116844
11. Molofsky AB, Savage AK, Locksley RM. Interleukin-33 in Tissue Homeostasis, Injury, and Inflammation. *Immunity* (2015) 42:1005–19. doi: 10.1016/j.immuni.2015.06.006
12. Pei C, Barbour M, Fairlie-Clarke KJ, Allan D, Mu R, Jiang HR. Emerging role of interleukin-33 in autoimmune diseases. *Immunology* (2014) 141:9–17. doi: 10.1111/imm.12174
13. Yang Z, Liang Y, Xi W, Li C, Zhong R. Association of increased serum IL-33 levels with clinical and laboratory characteristics of systemic lupus erythematosus in Chinese population. *Clin Exp Med* (2011) 11:75–80. doi: 10.1007/s10238-010-0115-4
14. Yagami A, Orihara K, Morita H, Futamura K, Hashimoto N, Matsumoto K, et al. IL-33 mediates inflammatory responses in human lung tissue cells. *J Immunol* (2010) 185:5743–50. doi: 10.4049/jimmunol.0903818
15. Wei ZH, Li YY, Huang SQ, Tan ZQ. Genetic variants in IL-33/ST2 pathway with the susceptibility to hepatocellular carcinoma in a Chinese population. *Cytokine* (2019) 118:124–9. doi: 10.1016/j.cyto.2018.03.036
16. Wu F, Li L, Wen Q, Yang J, Chen Z, Wu P, et al. A functional variant in ST2 gene is associated with risk of hypertension via interfering MiR-202-3p. *J Cell Mol Med* (2017) 21:1292–9. doi: 10.1111/jcmm.13058
17. Tu X, Nie S, Liao Y, Zhang H, Fan Q, Xu C, et al. The IL-33-ST2L pathway is associated with coronary artery disease in a Chinese Han population. *Am J Hum Genet* (2013) 93:652–60. doi: 10.1016/j.ajhg.2013.08.009
18. Hong YS, Moon SJ, Joo YB, Jeon CH, Cho ML, Ju JH, et al. Measurement of interleukin-33 (IL-33) and IL-33 receptors (sST2 and ST2L) in patients with rheumatoid arthritis. *J Korean Med Sci* (2011) 26:1132–9. doi: 10.3346/jkms.2011.26.9.1132
19. Kim DJ, Baek SY, Park MK, Park KS, Lee JH, Park SH, et al. Serum level of interleukin-33 and soluble ST2 and their association with disease activity in patients with Behcet's disease. *J Korean Med Sci* (2013) 28:1145–53. doi: 10.3346/jkms.2013.28.8.1145
20. Li C, Mu R, Guo J, Wu X, Tu X, Liu X, et al. Genetic variant in *IL33* is associated with susceptibility to rheumatoid arthritis. *Arthritis Res Ther* (2014) 16:R105. doi: 10.1186/ar4554
21. Koca SS, Pehlivan Y, Kara M, Alibaz-Oner F, Oztuzcu S, Yilmaz N, et al. The IL-33 gene is related to increased susceptibility to systemic sclerosis. *RHEUMATOL Int* (2016) 36:579–84. doi: 10.1007/s00296-015-3417-8
22. Koca SS, Kara M, Deniz F, Ozgen M, Demir CF, Ilhan N, et al. Serum IL-33 level and IL-33 gene polymorphisms in Behcet's disease. *Rheumatol Int* (2015) 35:471–7. doi: 10.1007/s00296-014-3111-2
23. Ioannidis JP, Ntzani EE, Trikalinos TA. 'Racial' differences in genetic effects for complex diseases. *Nat Genet* (2004) 36:1312–8. doi: 10.1038/ng1474
24. Ermann J, Fathman CG. Autoimmune diseases: genes, bugs and failed regulation. *Nat Immunol* (2001) 2:759–61. doi: 10.1038/ni0901-759
25. Anaya JM. Common mechanisms of autoimmune diseases (the autoimmune tautology). *Autoimmun Rev* (2012) 11:781–4. doi: 10.1016/j.autrev.2012.02.002
26. Latiano A, Palmieri O, Pastorelli L, Vecchi M, Pizarro TT, Bossa F, et al. Associations between genetic polymorphisms in IL-33, IL1R1 and risk for inflammatory bowel disease. *PloS One* (2013) 8:e62144. doi: 10.1371/journal.pone.0062144

27. Fan D, Ding N, Yang T, Wu S, Liu S, Liu L, et al. Single nucleotide polymorphisms of the interleukin-33 (IL-33) gene are associated with ankylosing spondylitis in Chinese individuals: a case-control pilot study. *Scand J Rheumatol* (2014) 43:374–9. doi: 10.3109/03009742.2014.882408
28. Koca SS, Pehlivan Y, Kara M, Oner FA, Yilmaz N, Cetin GY, et al. AB0152 The rs11792633-t allele of il-33 gene is associated with systemic sclerosis. *Ann RHEUM Dis* (2013) 72:A832. doi: 10.1136/annrheumdis-2013-eular.2475
29. Sfikakis PP. Behcet's disease: a new target for anti-tumour necrosis factor treatment. *Ann Rheum Dis* (2002) 61(Suppl 2):i51–3. doi: 10.1136/ard.61.suppl_2.ii51

10

HLA-A29 and Birdshot Uveitis: Further Down the Rabbit Hole

Jonas J. W. Kuiper[1,2*] *and Wouter J. Venema*[1,2]

[1] *Department of Ophthalmology, University Medical Center Utrecht, University of Utrecht, Utrecht, Netherlands,* [2] *Center for Translational Immunology, University Medical Center Utrecht, University of Utrecht, Utrecht, Netherlands*

Correspondence:
Jonas J. W. Kuiper
J.J.W.Kuiper@umcutrecht.nl

HLA class I alleles constitute established risk factors for non-infectious uveitis and preemptive genotyping of HLA class I alleles is standard practice in the diagnostic work-up. The HLA-A29 serotype is indispensable to Birdshot Uveitis (BU) and renders this enigmatic eye condition a unique model to better understand how the antigen processing and presentation machinery contributes to non-infectious uveitis or chronic inflammatory conditions in general. This review will discuss salient points regarding the protein structure of HLA-A29 and how key amino acid positions impact the peptide binding preference and interaction with T cells. We discuss to what extent the risk genes *ERAP1* and *ERAP2* uniquely affect HLA-A29 and how the discovery of a HLA-A29-specific submotif may impact autoantigen discovery. We further provide a compelling argument to solve the long-standing question why BU only affects HLA-A29-positive individuals from Western-European ancestry by exploiting data from the 1000 Genomes Project. We combine novel insights from structural and immunopeptidomic studies and discuss the functional implications of genetic associations across the HLA class I antigen presentation pathway to refine the etiological basis of Birdshot Uveitis.

Keywords: birdshot, HLA-A29, antigen presentation, uveitis, peptide

INTRODUCTION INTO BIRDSHOT UVEITIS

Birdshot Uveitis (also known as *Birdshot chorioretinopathy* or *Birdshot retinochoroidopathy*) is a well-characterized form of autoimmune uveitis (inflammation of the uveal layer of the eye) mostly known for its ovoid light lesions, which appear 'shotgun pattern'-like distributed along the vascular arcades in the back of the eye (i.e., the 'fundus' of the eye where these lesions are visible by photography) (1). Inflammation and extensive depigmentation of the choroid, macular edema, peripheral ischemia (2), degeneration of the retina, and the progressive formation of thin layer of scar tissue on the retina ("epiretinal membrane") (3, 4), progressively impair vision in a substantial proportion of patients. BU is unusual in the young (5) and typically affects patients over 50 years of age of Western-European ancestry, with more women than men affected (6). Long-term systemic corticosteroid-sparing immunomodulatory therapy is the mainstay of treatment (7, 8), but a fraction of patients may exhibit a more benign disease course that does not require systemic therapy (9). Histopathology studies of eye tissues and modern imaging technologies show that early lesions are located deep inside the vascular layer of the eye (the "choroid") between the retina and the white outer layer of the eyeball (sclera). In the choroid, the large-vessel layer (choroidal stroma)—densely populated with pigmented "melanocyte" cells—shows abnormalities before the characteristic fundus lesions are visible (10, 11). Because BU shows early inflammation of the choroidal stroma (12), Herbort and associates proposed to classify BU as a primary *stromal choroiditis*, together with *Vogt-Koyanagi-Harada* (VKH) disease. VKH is a condition characterized by chronic inflammation toward melanocytes that affect multiple parts of the body, including the choroidal stroma and the larger choroidal vessels (11, 13). In VKH no retinal involvement at early stages of disease are noticeable. In contrast, retinal inflammation (e.g., leakage of vessels) is an early clinical characteristic of BU (14), which suggests that retina involvement is not merely the result of inflammation spilling over from the choroid. However, the cause and interdependence of the retinal and choroidal inflammation are unknown, which is reflected in the use of multiple terms to define the eye condition; birdshot retinitis, birdshot *chorioretinopathy*, or birdshot *retinochoroidopathy*. For lack of understanding the disease pathology, here the broader term "birdshot uveitis" was chosen.

Microscopic anatomy studies (or *histological* studies) of eye tissue of patients with BU are scarce because of the rarity of the condition (estimated 1 to 5 cases per 500,000) (6, 15). The most recent histological study by Sohn and coworkers (16) in a patient with end-stage BU showed extensive degeneration of the retina and near complete loss of choroidal layers and the retinal pigment epithelium, a highly specialized cell layer critical to the homeostasis photoreceptors of the retina. Changes in retinal pigment epithelium are also evident by retinal imaging in patients with established disease (17). Each of the histological studies show massive infiltration of blood leukocytes into the choroid and retina layers; mostly T lymphocytes not only express the glycoproteins CD4 ("T helper" cells) and CD8 ("Cytotoxic" T cells) (16, 18, 19) but also relatively increased numbers of other immune cells, such as myeloid cells and B lymphocytes. The cases in two of these studies were remarkable for a history of malignant melanoma, but evidence that directly links melanoma to BU is lacking. At most, the evidence is circumstantial, such as "Birdshot-like disease" in melanoma cancer patients that develop autoimmune uveitis due to checkpoint inhibitor therapy (a treatment setting T cells free to kill tumor, but also normal tissue) (20) or the presence of blood antibodies that can bind to proteins in melanoma tumor cell lines (21). These phenomena may be explained by the fact the proteins involved in immunity toward melanoma are also expressed in normal melanocytes (22) and may actually support that choroidal melanocytes are among target cells deliberately attacked by the derailed immune system in BU.

THE GENETIC ASSOCIATION WITH HLA-A29

Short after BU was first described in 1980 (23), the unusually strong genetic association of the *Human-Leukocyte Antigen A*29* (*HLA-A*29*) with BU was discovered in 1982 by Nussenblatt and coworkers (24). HLA-A29-positive testing is now widely considered critical to diagnosis and led key opinion leaders in the field propose to rename the condition to "HLA-A29 uveitis" (25). *HLA-A*29* is one of the hundreds of variants of the *HLA-A* gene that together with different versions of *HLA-B* and *HLA-C* genes form the *HLA class I complex* of functionally related proteins in humans. The *HLA-A* gene encodes slightly different versions of a the cell-surface protein HLA-A. Like other HLA class I proteins, HLA-A plays a central role in the immune system by instructing immune cells (e.g., cytotoxic T cells) if a cell must be destroyed because it is infected by foreign invaders (e.g., a virus) or when a cell has become cancerous after mutation of the DNA (26). In most cells of the body, HLA-A achieves this by constant sampling of protein fragments from foreign invaders or self-proteins (termed "antigenic" peptides, or antigens in short) from the inside of the cell and "presenting" these peptides on the outside of the cell for scrutiny by surveilling immune cells (26, 27). This "antigen presenting pathway" is critical to monitor cellular integrity and is based on differentiating "self" from "non-self" (pathogen) or "altered-self" (cancer) (26). Aberrant function of this pathway can result in persistent infection, cancer or autoimmune disease (27).

Because all patients with BU carry a copy of the HLA-A29 *allele* (the term for "gene variant"), it is considered to be critically involved in the unidentified disease mechanisms (1). This is supported by rare familiar cases of BU that show that all cases with the eye phenotype are also HLA-A29-positive (28). Also, the allele frequency of HLA-A29 is high in Western-European countries (29), where also the vast majority of BU patients are reported in Europe, while BU is anecdotally reported in populations with low occurrence of HLA-A29 (30, 31). How exactly HLA-A29 contributes to eye inflammation is unknown, but several unique properties of HLA-A29 distinguish this allele from others *HLA-A* alleles in the population; A gel electrophoresis study from 1992 indicated that HLA-A29 in cases is identical to unaffected controls that carry HLA-A29 (~5–10% of the Western-European populations) (32), which is supported by small DNA sequencing studies (29). In two genome-wide association studies (33, 34), we used detailed genetic analysis of HLA alleles in BU cases that revealed that the main risk allele for BU is *HLA-A*29:02*, the most common HLA-A29 allele in Europe. These studies further ascertained that other associations in the *MHC* locus (the DNA region where HLA genes are embedded) are a result of positive linkage disequilibrium (LD) with HLA-A29. In other words, near-by gene variants such as for example the *HLA-B*44* allele are often (yet not always) inherited together with HLA-A29 but most likely not relevant for the disease. One study of a murine model in which a copy of HLA-A29 DNA from a BU patient was genetically expressed initially showed an eye disease similar to BU (35), but in a later underappreciated study, the mice strain used for the BU model was found to harbor a wide-spread and previously unnoticed genetic mutation that causes retinal degenerative disease (not uveitis) that also affected the control mice (36). This supports that the HLA-A29 allele itself is not sufficient and that the susceptibility to BU is mediated by additional etiological triggers. This also fits the observation that HLA-A29 is a common allele (~10% of the Western-European population is HLA-A29-positive), but BU is a rare condition (~250 cases in the Netherlands at 17 Mill. citizens as of June 2020). Also, *HLA-A*29:02* is also very common among specific ethnic groups of non-European ancestry where BU has not been reported, such as the South African Zulu (37) or the Luhya in Webuye of Kenya in Africa (~10% HLA-A*29:02-positive individuals) (38, 39).

THE HLA-A29 PROTEIN STRUCTURE

In 2020, the *immuno polymorphism database* (40) contains >200 reported HLA-A29 alleles, but only the most common alleles—*HLA-A*29:02, HLA-A*29:01*, and *HLA-A*29:10*—have been reported in cases with birdshot (41). Structurally, HLA-A*29:01 (D102H) and HLA-A*29:10 (E177K) differ from HLA-A*29:02 at single amino acids positions in the external alpha 2 domain of HLA-A29 (**Figure 1A**), but these positions do not influence the expression, conformation, or interaction of the HLA-A complex with T cells (46–48). In other words, these alleles can be considered functionally similar. The most relevant amino acid positions in HLA-A29 for disease risk were statistically linked to amino acids at positions 62 and 63 in the protein sequence (33). As shown in **Figure 2**, the amino acids *Leucine* at position 62 (62-L) and *Glutamine* at position 63 (63-Q) distinguish HLA-A29 from other *HLA-A* alleles. This is of interest because computational modelling of HLA-A by changing amino acids at indicated positions (or amino acid substitution modelling) revealed that position 63 has the largest effect on the ability to bind antigenic peptides over all polymorphic positions in the peptide-binding "groove" of HLA-A *allotypes* (the term for "protein variants") (49). Specific mutation of the positions 62-63 can completely abrogate HLA-peptide recognition by T cells (50). Most other *HLA-A* alleles encode the amino acids *asparagine* (N) or *glutamic acid* (E) at amino acid position 63 (**Figure 2**). Despite the degree of similarity of the chemical characteristics of the side chains of the amino acids, the effects of Q and N on the local structure of protein are different (51) and changing the chemically related glutamine (Q) to glutamic acid (E) at single amino acid position in the HLA-A molecule can modulate the interaction with CD8 of T cells (52). Indeed, amino acid substitution modelling of position 62 and 63 in HLA-A29 demonstrates that the strength of binding of peptides (i.e., the binding "affinity") into the peptide-binding groove of HLA-A29 is decreased if the amino acids at these positions are changed to any of the other other naturally occurring combinations of amino acids at positions 62-63 in HLA-A (**Figure 1B**). Curiously, substituting position 62 is predicted to have a larger effect than substitutions on position 63. Also, the 'theoretical' motif 62-L 63-E (which does not occur in any known *HLA-A* alleles) provides a globally similar binding capacity for peptides compared to the 62-L 63-Q of HLA-A29. Phylogenetically related alleles of HLA-A29 (i.e., *HLA-Aw19* complex) (53) encode 62-Q 63-E and would require changing 'only' position 62 to achieve a globally similar functionality. However, as mentioned, the local structural effects of the chemically related E and Q can be quite distinct and functional analysis is required to better understand the hierarchy of impact of these positions on defining the HLA-A29 peptidome. Also, these amino acids do not completely account for the peptide specificity of HLA-A29. In fact, 62-L 63-Q is detected in some other alleles such as *HLA-A*43:01, HLA-A*11:11*, and *HLA-A*68:130* [allele frequency of *HLA-A*43:01 and HLA-A*11:11* in the European population >15,000 times less than *HLA-A*29:02* (54), and *HLA-A*68:130* is not well documented (40)]. However, these alleles differ from HLA-A29 alleles on various other key positions that influence peptide binding in the peptide-binding groove, including amino acid position 9 (55), 70, 76, 77, or positions 97 or 152, which influence the interaction with T cells (56, 57). Notwithstanding these exceptional alleles, the amino acid motif 62-L 63-Q near exclusively accounts for HLA-A29 in the European population (54). Amino acid residues 62 and 63 are positioned at the edge of the peptide-binding groove (**Figure 1A**) in a cavity that directly interacts with the side chain of the amino acid at position 2 (P2) of the displayed antigenic peptide (58). Therefore, the 62-63 motif may influence the flexibility to accommodate antigenic peptides with distinct P2 residues, a feature most likely relevant to autoantigen discovery for BU.

THE HLA-A29 PEPTIDE MOTIF

The peptide binding motif—or the 'conserved' positional residue preference considering the amino acid sequences of all "presented" peptides—of HLA-A29 is relatively flexible on condition of a C-terminal (the last amino acid in a peptide) *Tyrosine* (Y) or less frequently a *Phenylalanine* (F) (45). Peptides with a C-terminal Y also make up a significant proportion of the peptides presented on other HLA-A alleles, including HLA-A*01:01, HLA-A*03:01, and HLA-A*30:02 (45) (but also HLA-A*43:01 and HLA-A*68:130). This includes peptides that are detected in the binding groove of more than one HLA-A allotype (demonstrated by mass-spectrometry studies of single-HLA-expressing cell lines), a phenomenon termed peptide 'promiscuity' (59). We and others have studied the complete set of antigenic peptides (termed the 'immunopeptidome') bound by HLA-A29 and used multidimensional scaling (a visual representation of the immunopeptidome where all peptides are positioned in a graph based on their relative similarity or difference in amino acid sequence) to cluster the peptides into subdominant binding motifs (or "submotifs") (43, 45, 60). This approach facilitates the identification of clusters of antigenic peptides (submotifs) that are shared with other HLA class allotypes or that are unique to HLA-A29. These studies revealed patterns of submotif preferences easy to miss in conventional studies when considering the immunopeptidome as a whole. In short, HLA-A29 presents a palette of submotifs mostly defined by distinct amino acids at position 2 (P2) and 7 (P7) in the antigenic peptide sequence. As discussed, a fraction of peptides presented by HLA-A29 is also found in the binding groove of other HLA-A alleles and consequently some submotifs of HLA-A29 were also detected in immunopeptidome data of other HLA allotypes. This helped to

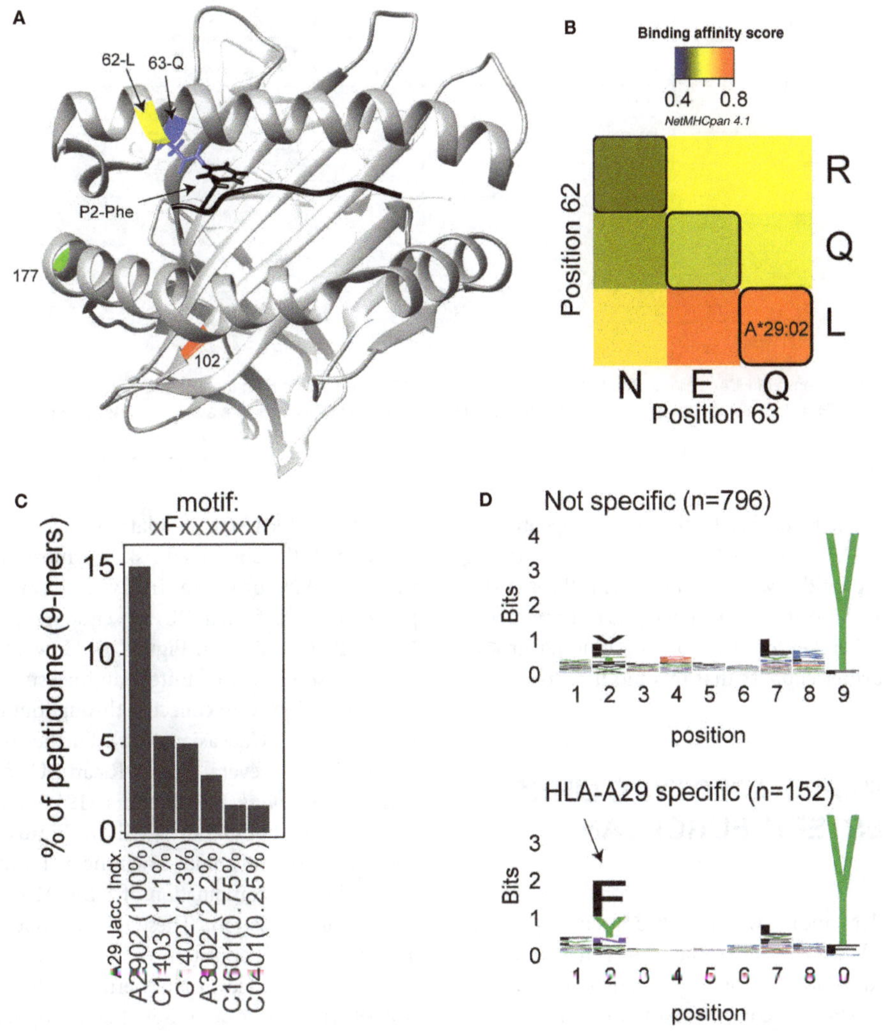

FIGURE 1 | Structure and function of amino acid positions 62 and 63 in HLA-A29. **(A)** View into the peptide-binding groove of a three-dimensional ribbon model for HLA-A29 (Based on Protein Data Bank entry: 6J1W modelling using UCSF Chimera (42). The amino acids Leucine (L in yellow) at position 62 and Glutamine (Q in blue) at position 63 defining HLA-A29 are indicated. The binding peptide is shown in black with phenylalanine at position 2 (P2-Phe) interacting with position 63-Q (with energy-minimized positions of side chains). Polymorphic amino acid positions associated with the alleles *HLA-A29:01* (pos 102 in red) and *HLA-A29:10* (position 177 in green) are also shown. **(B)** The effect of amino acid substitutions for position 62 and 63 on predicted binding affinity for HLA-A29-presented peptides. The average binding scores of 9-mers (n = 948) detected by mass-spectrometry analysis of HLA-A29 reported by Venema et al. (43). Replacement of position 62 and 63 with the most commonly occurring amino acids at that position encoded by *HLA-A* alleles was done in netMHCpan 4.1 server (44). Naturally occurring motifs are indicated with black lines, other motifs (e.g., QN) do not occur in human HLA-A allotypes. **(C)** The percentage of 9-mer peptides with P2-Phe and P9-Tyr detected in immunopeptidomes of HLA class I alleles as reported by Sarkizova et al. (45). The top 5 (of 95 alleles tested) class I alleles other than HLA-A29 are shown. The jaccard similarity index for the HLA-A*29:02 peptidome (overlap in presented peptides) and each allele is indicated (in %). Peptidome data were derived from Sarkizova et al. (45). **(D)** Sequence logos of 9-mers (n = 948) from HLA-A29 [the same peptides as in **(C)**] stratified into non-specific for HLA-A29 [with binding score MSi > 0.6 for HLA-A*43:01 or HLA-A*68:130 according to the *HLAthena* server (45)] or specific for HLA-A29 (MSi < 0.6 for HLA-A*43:01 and HLA-A*68:130). The arrow indicates the aromatic P2 in the binding motif specific for HLA-A29.

narrow down a submotif that is specific to HLA-A29 (43), which is characterized by the amino acids F or Y at P2 in conjunction with the HLA-A29-characteristic C-terminal (PC) Y (F/Y-P2 + Y-PC motif). This motif makes up ~15% of the HLA-A29 immunopeptidome (**Figure 1C**). Peptides with this motif are substantially less frequently presented on other HLA allotypes and those that do are uncommon in the Western-European population and/or display very low similarity in the immunopeptidome composition with HLA-A29 (<3% of the peptides are shared, **Figure 1C**). Note that 'just' P2-F and P2-Y (so without PC-Y) is not uncommon in the immunopeptidomes of other HLA-A allotypes, such as HLA-A24 [see supplemental data of Sarkizova et al. (45)], but the amino acids that occupy the pocket accommodating P2 of binding peptides is completely different from

```
AA Pos.                  10         20         30         40         50         60         70         80         90        100
A*01:01:01:01    GSHSMRYFFT SVSRPGRGEP RFIAVGYVDD TQFVRFDSDA ASQKMEPRAP WIEQEGPEYW DQETRNMKAH SQTDRANLGT LRGYYNQSED GSHTIQIMYG
A*02:01:01:01    ---------- ---------- ---------- ---------- ---R------ ---------- -G---KV--- ---H-VD--- ---------A ----V-R---
A*03:01:01:01    ---------- ---------- ---------- ---------- ---R------ ---------- ------V--Q -----VD--- ---------A ----------
A*11:01:01:01    --------Y- ---------- ---------- ---------- ---R------ ---------- ------V--Q -----VD--- ---------- ----------
A*23:01:01:01    --------S- ---------- ---------- ---------- ---R------ ---------- -E--GKV--- -----E--RI ALR------A ----L-M-F-
A*24:02:01:01    --------S- ---------- ---------- ---------- ---R------ ---------- -E--GKV--- -----E--RI ALR------A ----L-M-F-
A*26:01:01:01    --------Y- ---------- ---------- ---------- ---R------ ---------- -RN---V--- ---------- ---------- ------R---
A*29:01:01:01    --------T- ---------- ---------- ---------- ---R------ ---------- -LQ---V--Q ---------- ---------A ------M---
A*29:02:01:01    --------T- ---------- ---------- ---------- ---R------ ---------- -LQ---V--Q ---------- ---------A ------M---
A*29:10:01       --------T- ---------- ---------- ---------- ---R------ ---------- -LQ---V--Q ---------- ---------A ------M---
A*30:01:01:01    --------S- ------S--- ---------- ---------- ---R------ -----R---- ------V--Q -----VD--- ---------A ----------
A*31:01:02:01    --------T- ---------- ---------- ---------- ---R------ -----R---- ------V--- --I--VD--- ---------A ------M---
A*32:01:01:01    ---------- ---------- ---------- ---------- ---R------ ---------- ------V--- -----ES-RI ALR------A ------M---
A*33:01:01:01    --------T- ---------- ---------- ---------- ---R------ ---------- -RN---V--- --I--VD--- ---------A ------M---
A*43:01          --------Y- ---------- ---------- ---------- ---R------ ---------- -LQ---V--- ---------- ---------- ------R---
A*66:01:01:01    --------Y- ---------- ---------- ---------- ---R------ ---------- -RN---V--Q -----VD--- ---------- ------R---
A*68:01:01:01    --------Y- ---------- ---------- ---------- ---R------ ---------- -RN---V--Q -----VD--- ---------A ------M---
A*74:01:01:01    ---------- ---------- ---------- ---------- ---R------ ---------- ------V--- -----VD--- ---------A ------M---
A*80:01:01:01    ---------- ---------- ---------- S---Q----- ---R------ -----E---- -E----V--- ---N------ ---------- ----------
```

FIGURE 2 | The amino acid sequence of HLA-A alleles. The first 100 amino acids for 19 HLA-A alleles from the IPD-IMGT/HLA Database (40). The amino acids at positions 62 and 63 distinguish HLA-A29 alleles, with the exception of the rare HLA-A43 (± 15,000 times lower allele frequency compared to *HLA-A29:02* in the European population).

HLA-A29. Although we were unable to find immunopeptidome studies of the HLA-A*43:01 and HLA-A*68:130 alleles, binding prediction shows that peptides with the motif F/Y-P2 + Y-PC are poorly presented by these alleles, most likely as a consequence of the differences in other key positions in the binding groove (**Figure 1D**), which further support that this motif is specific to HLA-A29.

THE ERAP1-ERAP2 HAPLOTYPE LINKS BU TO THE WESTERN-EUROPEAN ANCESTRY

Key to progress in understanding why merely a fraction of HLA-A29-positive individuals develop BU came from genetic studies, including work from our lab. We identified that beyond HLA-A29, genetic polymorphisms (or common variations in the DNA sequence among individuals) at chromosome *5q15* confer strong disease risk (34, 61). The signal on chromosome 5 covers the endoplasmic reticulum aminopeptidase (*ERAP*)-1 and *ERAP2* genes, and *LNPEP*, all enzymes involved in trimming the peptide fragments before they are bound by HLA class I (e.g., HLA-A29). Importantly, the combination of two polymorphisms functionally linked to *ERAP1* (rs2287987) and *ERAP2* (rs10044354), conferred a risk for BU that was significantly larger than the risk from either one the two polymorphisms individually (61). Analysis of patients and HLA-A29-positive controls showed that the combined polymorphisms linked to *ERAP1* and *ERAP2* also showed the largest disease risk (detected in 50% of 130 cases and 25% of 439 HLA-A29-positive controls). This indicates that the genetic changes affecting both ERAP1 and ERAP2 in tandem increase the risk in the HLA-A29-positive population (61). Indeed, if we look at publicly available data from the 1000 genomes project, the risk-variant linked to *ERAP2* (rs10044354-T) or the risk variant linked to *ERAP1* (rs2287987-C) are also observed in HLA-A29-positive individuals of non-European ancestry (**Figure 4**). For example, most of the HLA-A29-positive cases in the Luhya in Webuye (LWT in **Figure 3**) of Kenya also carry the BU risk-variant near *ERAP2*, a population where no BU has been reported. In contrast, the combined risk polymorphisms are only observed in HLA-A29-positive individuals in Western-European populations in which BU is "endemic", with the exception of Puerto Ricans (PUR in **Figure 4**). However, the majority (>60%) of Puerto Ricans is of European ancestry and the samples from this population were collected throughout the entire country (i.e., predominantly Caucasian) (64). Furthermore, BU is reported in Puerto Ricans (several Puerto Rican BU cases are reported in the *Retina Image Bank;* file numbers 6191 and 6178) (65). In contrast, the Tuscany population (TSI in **Figure 4**) includes samples collected from a small town near Florence in Italy. In this population the combination of HLA-A29 and the ERAP1-ERAP2 polymorphisms is rare. These data do not necessarily represent all individuals of a population of a country that is of mixed ancestry [e.g., BU is reported in Northern Italy (66)], but serves to explain why BU is very rare or non-existing in populations where the genetic combination associated with BU risk is exceptional.

This also implies that the ERAP1, ERAP2, and HLA-A29 collectively drive the pathogenesis of BU. We do like to emphasize that the number of individuals "burdened" with the "birdshot-genotype" still exceeds the estimated cases in each population (~1% of people from Western-European ancestry, of which about 1 in 500 develop BU as a rough estimate). Here, it is good to consider that the cause of HLA-A29-dependent BU is most likely heterogenous and in some patients may be mediated by genetic susceptibility imprinted in *ERAP* genes, while in others ERAPs may be dysregulated by alternative mechanisms. For example, ERAP1 is tightly regulated by TNF-alpha, a pro-inflammatory cytokine that is increased in concentration in eye fluids of BU patients and blocking TNF-alpha by anti-TNF therapy alleviates severe symptoms of BU (67–70). Polymorphisms linked to *ERAP1* and *ERAP2* genes are also associated with other HLA class I associated conditions that manifest with non-infectious uveitis, including HLA-B27-associated anterior uveitis and ankylosing spondylitis, or HLA-B51-associated Behcet's disease (71–73). This supports the interdependence of ERAPs and HLA class I in the pathophysiology of non-infectious uveitis.

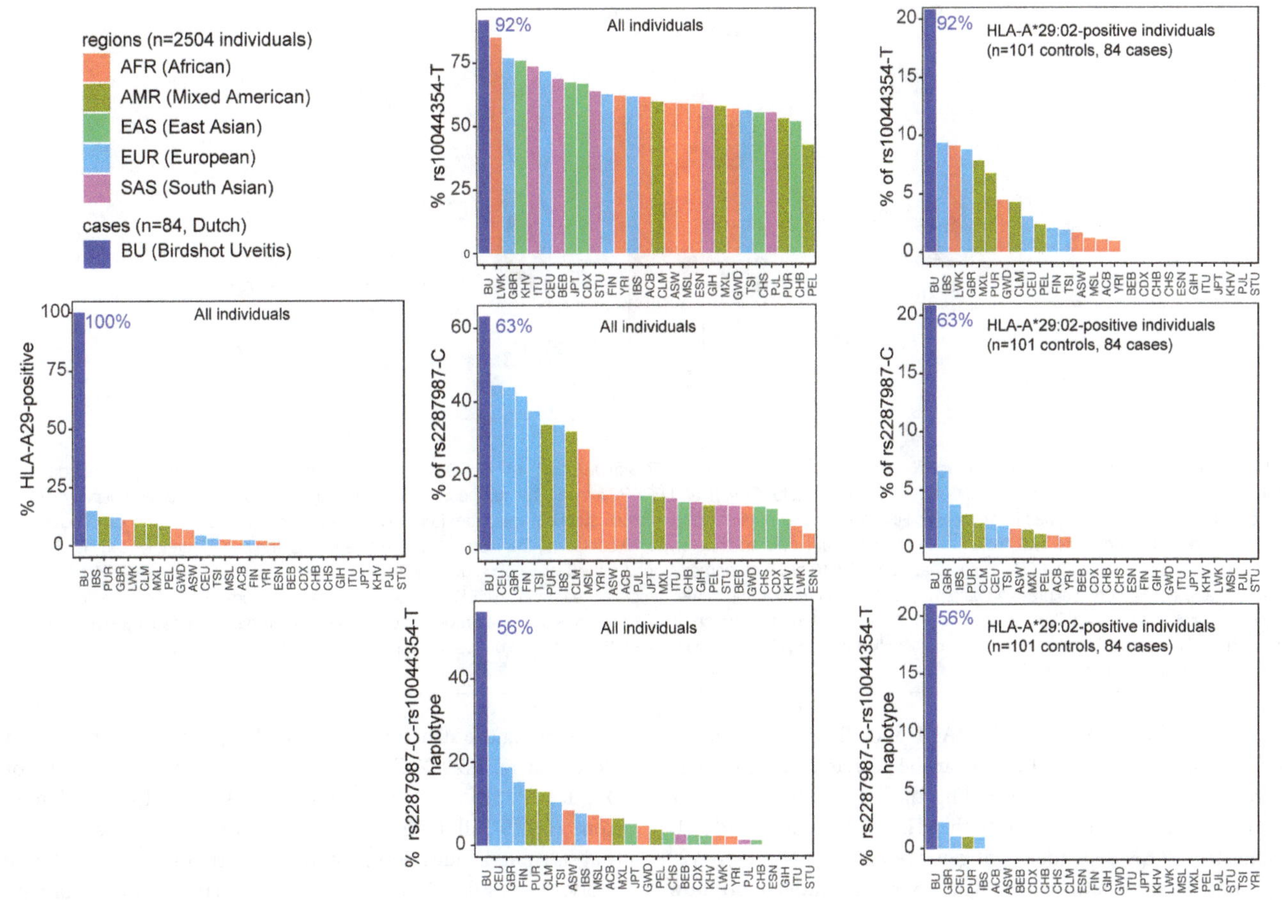

FIGURE 3 | The combined risk factors HLA-A29 and the ERAP1-ERAP2 haplotype are restricted to populations of Western-European ancestry. The percentage of individuals that carry a copy of *HLA-A*29:02*, the C allele of the polymorphism rs2287987 (in *ERAP1*), and the T allele of rs10044354 (near *ERAP2*) in 84 BU patients and the 2504 individuals of 26 ethnic populations of the 1000 Genomes Project. Data from BU patients was derived from (61). The graphs in the middle are the data for all 2504 individuals of the 1000 Genomes. The graphs on the right are the genotype data limited to HLA-A*29:02-positive individuals. This data demonstrates that the combined risk haplotype of rs2287987-rs10044354 in HLA-A29 is rare or absent in populations of non-Western-European ancestry. HLA data was obtained from (39) and genotype data for rs10044354 and rs22878987 from the 1000 Genomes project (63). The regions and populations are indicated using the following abbreviations: CHB, Han Chinese in Beijing; JPT, Japanese in Tokyo; CHS, Southern Han Chinese; CDX, Chinese Dai in Xishuangbanna; KHV, Kinh in Ho Chi Minh City; CEU, Utah Residents (CEPH) with Northern and Western European Ancestry; TSI, Tuscans in Italy; FIN, Finnish in Finland; GBR, British in England and Scotland; IBS, Iberian Population in Spain; YRI, Yoruba in Ibadan; LWK, Luhya in Webuye; GWD, Gambian in Western Divisions in the Gambia; MSL, Mende in Sierra Leone; ESN, Esan in Nigeria; ASW, Americans of African Ancestry in SW USA; ACB, African Caribbeans in Barbados; MXL, Mexican Ancestry from Los Angeles USA; PUR, Puerto Ricans from Puerto Rico; CLM, Colombians from Medellin; PEL, Peruvians from Lima; GIH, Gujarati Indian from Houston; PJL, Punjabi from Lahore; BEB, Bengali from Bangladesh; STU, Sri Lankan Tamil from the UK; ITU, Indian Telugu from the UK.

ERAP1 AND ERAP2 IN THE ANTIGEN PRESENTATION PATHWAY

The antigen presenting pathway for HLA(-A) starts with the degradation of cellular proteins (proteolysis) by the proteasome, a continuous and normal process to eliminate dysfunctional or mature proteins into shorter peptides (26, 27). A selection of peptides up to 20 amino acids long are transported into the endoplasmic reticulum (ER) by the *Transporter associated with antigen processing* (or TAP) and trimmed to generally 8-10 amino acid long peptides by ERAP1 and ERAP2 (26, 27, 74). ERAP1 and ERAP2 are specialized aminopeptidases that reside in ER (hence their name) where they each trim a proportion of the antigenic peptide pool before the peptides bind to HLA class I molecules for presentation at the cell surface (74). Structural studies have shown that the trimming process involves sequestering the entire peptide sequence inside the enzyme's cavity after which the N-terminal (first amino acid in the peptide sequence) is trimmed off (75, 76), which indicates that the majority of peptides are trimmed before binding (77) to HLA class I (e.g. HLA-A29). Some HLA class II alleles lack protection of their peptide-binding groove when exposed to peptides in the endoplasmic reticulum and bind these peptides before their transportation to the cell surface (78). It's not unlikely that ERAPs may influence the peptide cargo presented by a selective group of these 'unprotected' HLA class II alleles, but

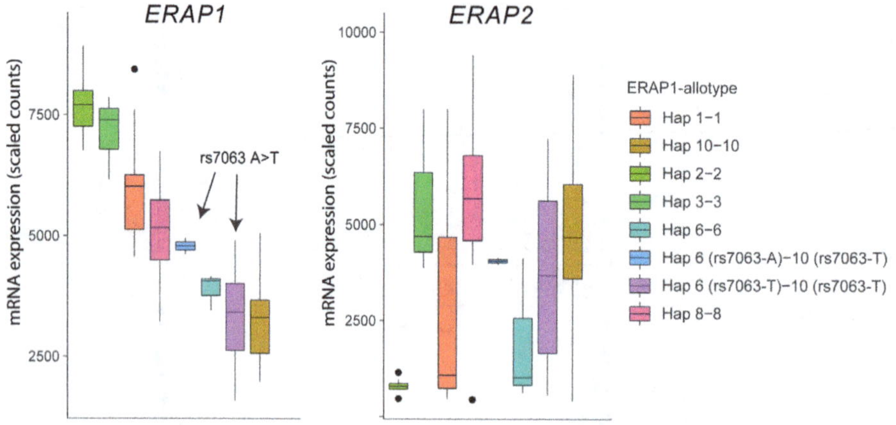

FIGURE 4 | The splice associated variant rs7063 associated with haplotype 6 (97% of all *Hap6*) and 10 (99% of all Hap10) of *ERAP1* mediates low expression of these haplotypes in lymphoblastoid cells. Gene expression data for *ERAP1* and *ERAP2* from 85 homozygous or heterozygous cell lines with indicated haplotypes (and rs7063 allele) were obtained from available RNA-sequencing data of 358 lymphoblastoid cell lines from European ancestry of the GEUVADIS cohort (loaded using the *recount* R package) (62). Note that in cell lines that harbor the haplotype 10 containing the T allele of rs7063 genotype, the rs7063 genotype in Hap6 governs the expression of total *ERAP1* and that Hap6/Hap10 cell lines homozygous for the T allele of rs7063 show similar low expression compared to Hap10/ Hap10 cell lines. The gene expression pattern for *ERAP2* (left plot) in the same samples does not mimic ERAP1 gene expression patterns, but reflect the non-random distribution of the ERAP2-protein coding haplotype across common *ERAP1* haplotypes, as we previously described (61). In particular haplotype 2 (Hap2; encoding *allotype 2*) is found infrequently in conjunction with ERAP2 haplotype A and, thus, shows low overall expression for ERAP2 in the *Hap2* homozygous cell lines in this example (n = 9).

this is unexplored. Also, 'free' ERAP1 and ERAP2 is found in body fluids and blood (79), and can be secreted by stimulated immune cells (80). Notwithstanding these other functions, the strong genetic association with HLA-A29-associated BU implicates ERAP-dependent antigen presentation by HLA-A29 as a key disease pathway in BU. To better understand how ERAP1 and ERAP2 modulate HLA-A29, let's first detail the genetic associations mapped to these genes.

ERAP1 AND BIRDSHOT

The *ERAP1* gene encodes various distinct ERAP1 haplotypes (a group of polymorphisms inherited together) that encode functionally different protein variants (which are termed "allotypes") with markedly different capacity to cut antigen peptides in terms of speed and specificity (61, 81). Genetics studies showed that the C allele of the polymorphism rs2287987 was more frequently seen in patients with BU (61). The rs2287987-C is found almost exclusively in the haplotype (named *Hap10*) that encodes *Allotype 10* (61). Detailed description of ERAP1 polymorphisms and their effects on functions of ERAP1 can be found elsewhere (74, 82). Briefly, the minor C allele of rs2287987 located in exon 6 of ERAP1 results in the change of Methionine to Valine at amino acid position 349 in ERAP1. This amino acid change occurs in the active site of ERAP1 next to the hallmark zinc-binding motif of the family of M1 zinc metallopeptidases (H-E-X-X-H-(X)18-E motif) and affects the enzymatic activity of the enzyme. However, the rs2287987 bearing allotype 10 contains additional polymorphisms that indirectly affect the specificity or activity by changing the structural conformation of the enzyme (83, 84). Note that rs2287987-C is also common in African populations (**Figure 3**) but it often resides in ERAP1 haplotypes different from Hap10. Allotype 10 is characterized by enzymatic activity that is magnitudes lower compared to other characterized allotypes of ERAP1, but also shows relatively low expression (61). The latter feature is caused by moderate LD between the C allele of rs2287987 and a splice interfering variant [T allele of rs7036 (85)] located upstream in an untranslated region of *ERAP1* [rs7063 is present in >90% of *Hap10* and typically <5–10% of other common haplotypes of *ERAP1* (61)]. Although low expression and low enzymatic activity of *Hap10* is often mentioned in the same breath in discussions of its pathogenic contribution to disease, rs2287987 is associated with BU independently from rs7063, thus, the BU risk linked to rs2287987 represents more likely the diminished enzymatic activity of ERAP1 (61). In fact, rs7063-T is also found in >90% of another common haplotype of ERAP1 named Hap6 (61).

Because the vast majority of Hap6 shares the T allele of rs7063 with Hap10 (61), gene expression data from the 1000 Genomes project shows that consequently the expression of the two haplotypes is comparably low (**Figure 4**). Although the ERAP1 expression levels have been shown to influence the immunopeptidome of HLA-A29 (86), the low expressed Hap6 is not associated with BU (61) and makes it more plausible that the highly distinct enzymatic features of Hap10 contribute to the susceptibility to BU. This is further supported by the fact that the highly active ERAP1 allotype encoded by *Hap2*, the functional "antagonist" of Hap10, is protective against BU (61). Because of these differences in trimming capacity, the lack of destruction of a uveitogenic epitope is a plausible mechanism for disease.

ERAP2 AND BIRDSHOT

Of the two common haplotypes (A and B) of *ERAP2* detected in the population, *haplotype A* (HapA) encodes the canonical full-length ERAP2 protein (87), but is consists of many polymorphisms that are located also far outside *ERAP2* and deep into the *LNPEP* gene. The polymorphisms of *HapA* outside *ERAP2* are located in the intragenic regions of the *LNPEP* gene and are not encoded into the *LNPEP* gene products. Haplotype B (HapB) contains a polymorphism (the G allele of rs2248734) that changes a splice region and facilitates intronic read-through until a stop codon, which under steady state conditions targets the transcript for destruction and results in barely detectable levels of the full-length ERAP2 protein (87). However, HapB has been shown to produce a truncated ERAP2 protein in response to infection by various microbial pathogens, interferon alpha or bacterial lipopolysaccharides (88–90). The strongest association at *5q15* is linked to the polymorphisms in HapA (tagged by rs10044354 in an intragenic location of *LNPEP*). We showed that this signal did not influence the splicing or expression of the *LNPEP* gene, but showed that high ERAP2 expression controlled by this genetic signal embedded in HapA is a risk factor for BU (34, 61). Here we note that the polymorphism rs10044354 (and variants in LD) is independently associated with BU from the polymorphism rs2248374 that governs splicing of *ERAP2* into its main haplotypes (61). Data from the *The Genotype-Tissue Expression (GTEx) project* supports that rs10044354 is strongly associated with the expression of *ERAP2* and mildly impacts the expression of *LNPEP* across various tissues (91). However, the effect sizes of rs10044354 on the expression of other nearby genes *ERAP1* and *CAST* are in the same range as for *LNPEP* and of unknown biological significance. In summary, high ERAP2 expression is a significant risk factor for BU in HLA-A29-positive individuals. The generation of *uveitogenic* peptides by ERAP2, which hypoactive ERAP1 fails to destroy, is a plausible disease mechanism for BU.

ERAP1 AND ERAP2 SHAPE THE HLA-A29 IMMUNOPEPTIDOME

Both ERAP1 and ERAP2 have been shown to affect the HLA-A29 peptidome of cell model systems (86, 92), which has been reviewed in detail elsewhere (74). In short, by global assessment of the immunopeptidome, active ERAP1 allotypes (e.g. *Hap2*) decrease the length of peptides of 10 amino acids or longer (10-mers), with a net increase of 9-mers (86). In the presence of active ERAP1 allotypes, the number of peptides with phenylalanine (F) and tyrosine (Y) at the first two amino acids of the peptide sequence (the N-terminal position 1 [P1] or 2 [P2]) of the binding peptides was slightly increased (86). ERAP2 shapes the HLA-A29 immunopeptidome predominantly by destruction of peptides with a P1 amino acid that are preferred substrates for ERAP2, predominantly Lysine (K), Arginine (R), and Alanine (A) (93). Large aromatic amino acids F and Y are poor substrates for ERAP2. Because ERAP2 destroys competing peptides that harbor optimal residues (K, R, or A at P1) for ERAP2, peptides that contain F or Y at P1 consequently make up a relatively larger proportion of the available antigen peptides to bind HLA-A29 and become "over-represented" in the presence of ERAP2 (43, 92). Other studies from the López de Castro group also demonstrated these ERAP2 effects on the immunopeptidome of risk HLA allotypes of other types of uveitis, such as HLA-B27 (94). In a recent study, we demonstrated that the effect of ERAP2 on P1 is actually a common feature of ERAP2 observable in the immunopeptidomes of all HLA class I alleles expressed by the cell (43). Intriguingly, Abelin and coworkers showed that peptides presented by HLA class I allotypes show a depletion for K, R and A residues at P1, which we believe can be attributed to the fact that their studied cell line expresses ERAP2 (60). So perhaps ERAP2 is evolutionary designed to destroy epitopes with these characteristics as a means to lower the immunogenicity of the presented immunopeptidome. This hypothesis comes from the observation that cancer patients with high ERAP2 expression showed worse overall survival after checkpoint inhibitor therapy (allowing T cells to kill cancer cells), relative to those with low ERAP2 expression (95). In other words, when T cells are "licensed" to attack tumors unrestrictedly, immune responses are more dependent on the level of antigen presentation to T cells. Here, ERAP2 may influence the HLA class I immunopeptidome so it provides less T cell epitopes to destroy tumors (and perhaps normal tissue, but this was not evaluated). This may in part be explained by the fact that the side chains of the amino acids at P1 influence the spatial configuration of amino acid position 167 in HLA-A, which has been shown to tune the peptide recognition by T cells and affect the peptide binding repertoire (49, 96). Here, the amino acids K and R induce a similar configuration of position 167 that is distinct from the configuration the alpha domain adapts at this position if P1 contains a F or Y (96) which functionally parallels the preference for trimming these amino acids by ERAP2. Beyond the universal effects on P1, peptides that are destroyed by ERAP2 may also share additional characteristics. For example, ERAP2 also showed preference for amino acids at position 3 and 7 in the antigenic peptide (43), which matches the pockets of ERAP2 that would interact with the sidechain of these residues (75). Similar to the effects of P1, as mentioned, the destruction of HLA-A29 epitopes by ERAP2 most likely represents a canonical function of ERAP2.

THE ERAP1-ERAP2 RISK HAPLOTYPE EXHIBITS HLA-A29-SPECIFIC EFFECTS

In contrast to the shared effects of ERAP2 across HLA class I immunopeptidomes, in patient derived cell lines homozygous for the risk ERAP1 allotype *Hap10*, ERAP2 facilitated the increased presentation of peptides with F or Y at P2 specifically for HLA-A29 (43, 92). Because this is the same submotif that distinguishes HLA-A29 from other HLA class I alleles, this observation provides a possible explanation for the association of these genes with BU. These submotif-specific effects of ERAP2 were also detected in different source data regarding immunopeptidomics of HLA-A29 (43). This indicates these effects of ERAP2 on HLA-A29 are generalizable, but may also help narrow down the putative disease modifying effects of the antigen presentation pathway. Recall that active ERAP1 allotypes (other than *Hap10* and in ERAP2-deficient cells) also showed a moderate increase of F at P2 in the HLA-A29 immunopeptidome (86). However, submotif analysis of this data revealed that ERAP1 did not bias the immunopeptidome in favor of the HLA-A29-specific submotif like ERAP (43). This may be because the pocket in which the side chain of P2 binds in ERAP2 has limited space which doesn't allow bulky aromatic residues (75), while the analogous pocket in which P2 would bind in ERAP1 is more open and could accommodate bulky residues to some degree (i.e., F or Y) (76). Furthermore, considering individual peptides, there is low correlation between the effects of ERAP1 and ERAP2 on HLA-A29 (43), which indicates context specificity and possible non-redundant pathogenic contributions to antigen presentation by HLA-A29 that increase the risk for BU. Such independent pathogenic contributions by ERAP1 and ERAP2 are supported by the genetic studies (61) of BU as discussed.

HLA-A29 AND AUTOANTIGEN PRESENTATION

Given that HLA-A29 is prerequisite for the development of BU, we hypothesize that disease mechanisms associated with antigen presentation are most likely driven by a limited set of epitopes (or single peptide) because of promiscuity of peptides across HLA class I (59). Based on the submotif that is specific to HLA-A29 and supported by ERAP2, we hypothesize that 'uveitogenic' HLA-A29-restricted peptides may more likely harbor a F or Y at P2 (and a Y at PC). The importance of P2 in HLA-A29-restricted peptides is in line with the fact that the amino acids at position 62-63—which define HLA-A29—directly interact with P2 of the binding peptide (**Figure 1**). The hypoactive ERAP1 allotype strongly linked to BU predominantly may prevent the destruction of 9-mers or longer peptides (43, 73, 92). There are examples of HLA-A29-presented 10-mers that cause strong T cell-mediated responses in humans, such as AELLNIPFLY encoded by *UGT2B17* (97, 98).

Curiously, the *HLA-A*29* alleles are among the lowest expressed *HLA-A* alleles (99). However, the amount of peptides presented by HLA class I only weakly correlates with HLA levels at the cell surface, plus immunopeptidome studies support that HLA-A29 is potent in presentation of peptides at the cell surface (43, 45, 92). Of interest, HLA class I is generally low expressed in the retina (100), while HLA class I expression is relatively high around endothelial cells of large vessels of the choroid (101), the presumed epicenter of inflammation in BU (12). Choroid melanocytes are densely located around these endothelial cells and have been proposed as an autoantigen-source in BU etiology (1). Perhaps BU is driven by HLA-A29-presented ERAP-dependent melanocyte-derived peptides (1, 61). This also fits the "*autoimmune surveillance of hypersecreting mutants*" (ASHM) theory, which predicts that autoantigens involved in organ-specific autoimmunity (the eye) should be linked to secreting cells such as melanocytes (102), where autoimmunity is considered a natural tradeoff to prevent lethal disease mediated by hypersecreting mutants. Besides their more commonly known role in pigment production, choroid melanocytes have also been shown to contribute to the maintenance of the normal vasculature structure of the choroid (103). Of interest, melanocytes can produce powerful angiogenic factors upon suppression of tyrosinase activity, the key enzyme in pigment production (104). It is conceivable that proteins highly expressed in choroidal melanocytes are closely monitored by surveilling self-reactive T cells (following the ASHM theory), because of the potential devastating effects of hypersecreting mutants, at the cost of autoimmunity. The autoimmune conditions VKH, *vitiligo*, and *psoriasis* are a proof of principle that melanocytes harbour autoantigens that are targets for autoreactive T cells (105–108). Gene expression or proteomic studies comparing cutaneous and choroid melanocytes are warranted to understand their potential differences to better understand the restriction of BU inflammation to the eye. Of interest, the ERAP2-promoted HLA-A29-specific peptide motif (P2-F + PC-Y) is observed in the amino acid sequence of key proteins of melanogenesis that are expressed in the eye (43). These include a number of putative candidate peptides from melanocyte proteins, such as CFVALFVRY (SLC45A2), CFPLLRLLY (OCA2), or SFSKLLLPY (PLXNC1) (43). Of course, functional experiments are required to validate if any of these 'potential' peptides are actually presented by HLA-A29. As mentioned, the circumstantial association with melanoma (i.e., a 'hyper' anti-melanoma response) has sparked interest for this theory, but lacks evidence for any causal relation (109). Remarkably, although HLA-A29 can effectively present melanoma epitopes (1), HLA-A29 is associated with worse survival compared to HLA-A29-negative melanoma patients (110). This could indicate that perhaps similar to the effects of ERAP2, in general, HLA-A29 and ERAP2 may 'lower' the immunogenic peptide cargo presented to T cells, but only increase the expression of a very limited (perhaps single) antigen under specific conditions that cause BU. Alternatively, the loss of choroidal melanocytes may be collateral damage from dysfunction in the choroidal endothelium. More specifically, the disruption of a *Hedgehog*-signaling axis from choroidal endothelial cells to choroidal stromal cells (i.e., perivascular mesenchymal stem cell-like cells that suppress T cell function) resulted in the loss of choroid melanocytes and illustrates a key role for the choroidal endothelium for the maintenance of choroidal immune homeostasis (111).

The retinal S-antigen has long been considered as a major autoantigen for BU, because S-antigen causes a birdshot-like phenotype in primate models (112, 113) and T cells from patients proliferate after stimulation with S-antigen (24, 114). However, S-antigen immune reactivity is widespread among clinically distinct phenotypes of uveitis and linked to T helper cell responses (linked to HLA class II), which suggests it plays a role in BU independent of HLA-A29, perhaps at later stages of the disease. This is in line with the retinal lesions observed in BU patients and suggests the retinal S-antigen may have a role at the clinical stage. However, also other retinal proteins contain peptides that may be presented by HLA-A29 (109). Previous *in vitro* studies determined that peptides derived from the S-antigen can bind to HLA-A29 (115), but further research using immunopeptidomics of cells expressing S-antigen are required to define the HLA-A29 presented epitopes of S-antigen. We recently identified that a naturally HLA-A29-presented peptide of S-antigen is VTLTCAFRY and currently assess if this peptide is also recognized by T cells of patients (43).

THE MICROBIOME, TH17 CELLS, AND HLA-A29

The *commensal microbiome* is a fast universe of diverse and mostly uncharacterized microbial species which inhabit tissues such as the skin and gastrointestinal tract where they collectively influence the functions of the immune system (116). For example, CD8+ T cells are primed by microbial derived metabolites and MHC-I presented microbial derived peptides to cross-react with cancer antigens as a means to facilitate anti-tumor immunity (117, 118). Gut microbiome dysbiosis is observed in patients with inflammatory conditions and considered to cause disturbance of systemic immune homeostasis in uveitis (119). In animal models, gut commensals have been shown to directly activate T helper 17 (Th17) cells to trigger uveitis (120).

This is of interest, because BU patients show increased numbers of blood Th17 cells and elevated levels of Th17-cytokines (68, 121–123). Of interest, Th17 cells induced by infection such as the fungal commensal *C. Albicans* may persist and aggravate autoimmune disease of the kidney (124). Protective anti-*C. albicans* responses by Th17 cells have also paradoxically been shown to result in inflammatory lung disease or inflammatory bowel disease in some individuals (125). Although *C. albicans* infection can affect the choroid and retina in a small percentage of patients (126), this shows a very different clinical phenotype. Regardless, the Th17-signature in BU could be related to changes in the microbiome. Studies of the microbiome of patients with BU are not yet conducted, the first study of HLA-A29-positive individuals as a whole show show a distinct intestinal microbiome composition (127) as demonstrated for HLA-B27-positive or HLA-DRB1-positive controls (128). In fact, microbiome similarity is observed in individuals who shared HLA alleles (129), which suggests that HLA influences the composition of the gut microbiome in part as a canonical feature of the immune homeostasis. The interaction of the microbiome in antigen-presentation *via* HLA-A29 in the disease mechanisms of BU requires further investigation, ideally by integrating the novel insights from studies of ERAP1 and ERAP2. Of interest, HLA class I bound by *Killer immunoglobulin-Like Receptors* (KIRs) on T cells promotes the expansion of Th17 cells in patients with HLA-B27 pathologies (130). Furthermore, specific modulation of ERAP1 has been shown to influence Th17 expansion (131). Therefore, it would be interesting to determine if similar biological mechanisms are linking HLA-A29 to Th17 responses in BU.

KIR RECEPTORS AND BIRDSHOT

BU may be driven by additional inflammatory genes since its genetic profile displayed shared genetic contributions with other inflammatory conditions, including *systemic lupus erythema* and *Neuromyelitis optica*, that both involve the eye (132). Among these may also be additional factors of the antigen presentation pathway, including the autophagy gene *TECPR2* previously reported (34) or *Killer immunoglobulin-Like Receptor* (KIR) (KIRs) genes (133). KIR genes have been associated with BU, however, the allele frequencies of controls used in a study of BU patients may not be representative for European populations and stringent correction for multiple testing is required to avoid false-positives, which may influence the outcomes of *KIR* associations in BU (133, 134). Regardless, KIRs are important receptors for T cells, but also *Natural Killer* (NK) *cells*, an understudied immune cell in the context of non-infectious uveitis that is decreased in the circulation of BU patients (135). Curiously, immunosuppression therapy restores the number of NK cells in patients with uveitis (136). The role of KIRs in BU also merits further functional investigation because NK cells have been shown to get activated by HLA class I by altering the presented peptide (137). It will be interesting to explore the role of the *ERAP1-ERAP2* haplotype in peptide presentation by HLA-A29 and NK cell responses in patients. However, in HLA-B27-associated ankylosing spondylitis, the strong genetic interaction of *ERAP1* with *HLA-B*27* was independent from genetic associations with *KIR* genes, suggesting that the disease mechanisms of ERAP and HLA class I may be mostly distinct from interaction of KIRs with HLA class I (138), and perhaps represent complementary mechanisms such as shown for free heavy chain expression by HLA-B27 and KIR interaction (131), while ERAP may mediated antigen-specific T cell responses. Indeed, T cell receptor (TCR) analysis of CD8+ T cells in patients with AS suggest differential antigen exposure (139) and similar studies of TCR repertoires of BU are currently underway.

CONCLUDING REMARKS

In this review, we discussed how key features of the antigen presentation pathway predispose to eye-specific autoimmunity in BU. The prerequisite for HLA-A29 and the enrichment for functional polymorphisms that affect the function of antigen processing enzymes ERAP1 and ERAP2 point toward a key contribution for the antigen presentation pathway in the etiology of BU. Using functional studies, we are beginning to understand how ERAPs shape the immunopeptidome of HLA-A29 and a growing body of evidence is closing in on their disease modifying effects. This will help to better predict the outcome of pharmacological interference of ERAPs activity using newly available small molecule inhibitors (140) that may soon be applied as a high precision medicine to halt autoimmunity and restore eye health in patients, while leaving immunity toward pathogens and cancerous tissues intact.

AUTHOR CONTRIBUTIONS

All authors contributed to the article and approved the submitted version.

REFERENCES

1. Kuiper J, Rothova A, de Boer J, Radstake T. The immunopathogenesis of birdshot chorioretinopathy; a bird of many feathers. *Prog Retin Eye Res* (2015) 44:99–110. doi: 10.1016/j.preteyeres.2014.11.003
2. Testi I, Ajamil-Rodanes S, AlBloushi AF, Pavesio C. Peripheral Capillary Non-perfusion in Birdshot Retinochoroiditis: A Novel Finding on Ultra-widefield Fluorescein Angiography. *Ocul Immunol Inflamm* (2020) 1–4. doi: 10.1080/09273948.2020.1758157

3. Papadia M, Jeannin B, Herbort CP. OCT findings in birdshot chorioretinitis: a glimpse into retinal disease evolution. Ophthalmic surgery, lasers imaging. *Off J Int Soc Imaging Eye* (2012) 43:S25–31. doi: 10.3928/15428877-20120816-01
4. Elahi S, Lages V, Jeannin B, Herbort CP. Advanced Cases of Birdshot HLA-A29 Retinochoroiditis: Prevalence and Characteristics. *Klin Monbl Augenheilkd* (2020) 237:431–40. doi: 10.1055/a-1081-1683
5. Lee J, Smith WM, Goldstein DA. Birdshot chorioretinopathy presenting in a teenager. *Am J Ophthalmol Case Rep* (2020) 19:100807. doi: 10.1016/j.ajoc.2020.100807
6. Minos E, Barry RJ, Southworth S, Folkard A, Murray PI, Duker JS, et al. Birdshot chorioretinopathy: Current knowledge and new concepts in pathophysiology, diagnosis, monitoring and treatment. *Orphanet J Rare Dis* (2016) 11:1–17. doi: 10.1186/s13023-016-0429-8
7. Kiss S, Ahmed M, Letko E, Foster CS. Long-term follow-up of patients with birdshot retinochoroidopathy treated with corticosteroid-sparing systemic immunomodulatory therapy. *Ophthalmology* (2005) 112:1066–71. doi: 10.1016/j.ophtha.2004.12.036
8. You C, Lasave AF, Kubaisi B, Syeda S, Ma L, Wai KCK, et al. Long-term outcomes of systemic corticosteroid-sparingimmunomodulatory therapy for Birdshot Retinochoroidopathy. *Ocul Immunol Inflamm* (2020) 28 (6):966–74. doi: 10.1080/09273948.2019.1641610
9. Lages V, Skvortsova N, Jeannin B, Gasc A, Herbort CP. Low-grade 'benign' birdshot retinochoroiditis: prevalence and characteristics. *Int Ophthalmol* (2019) 39:2111—2120. doi: 10.1007/s10792-018-1050-8
10. Pepple KL, Chu Z, Weinstein J, Munk MR, Van Gelder RN, Wang RK, et al. Use of En Face Swept-Source Optical Coherence Tomography Angiography in Identifying Choroidal Flow Voids in 3 Patients With Birdshot Chorioretinopathy. *JAMA Ophthalmol* (2018) 136:1288–92. doi: 10.1001/jamaophthalmol.2018.3474
11. Elahi S, Herbort CPJ. Vogt-Koyanagi-Harada Disease and Birdshot Retinochoroidopathy, Similarities and Differences: A Glimpse into the Clinicopathology of Stromal Choroiditis, a Perspective and a Review. *Klin Monbl Augenheilkd* (2019) 236:492–510. doi: 10.1055/a-0829-6763
12. Böni C, Thorne JE, Spaide RF, Ostheimer TA, Sarraf D, Levinson RD, et al. Choroidal Findings in Eyes With Birdshot Chorioretinitis Using Enhanced-Depth Optical Coherence Tomography. *Invest Ophthalmol Vis Sci* (2016) 57: OCT591–9. doi: 10.1167/iovs.15-18832
13. Balci O, Jeannin B, Herbort CPJ. Contribution of dual fluorescein and indocyanine green angiography to the appraisal of posterior involvement in birdshot retinochoroiditis and Vogt-Koyanagi-Harada disease. *Int Ophthalmol* (2018) 38:527–39. doi: 10.1007/s10792-017-0487-5
14. Papadia M, Herbort CP. New concepts in the appraisal and management of birdshot retinochoroiditis, a global perspective. *Int Ophthalmol* (2015) 35:287–301. doi: 10.1007/s10792-015-0046-x
15. Shah KH, Levinson RD, Yu F, Goldhardt R, Gordon LK, Gonzales CR, et al. Birdshot chorioretinopathy. *Surv Ophthalmol* (2005) 50:519–41. doi: 10.1016/j.survophthal.2005.08.004
16. Sohn EH, Chirco KR, Folk JC, Mullins RF. Clinicopathological Correlation In A Patient With Previously Treated Birdshot Chorioretinopathy. *Retin cases Brief Rep* (2017) 11:344–7. doi: 10.1097/ICB.0000000000000367
17. Böni C, Thorne JE, Spaide RF, Ostheimer TA, Sarraf D, Levinson RD, et al. Fundus Autofluorescence Findings in Eyes With Birdshot Chorioretinitis. *Invest Ophthalmol Vis Sci* (2017) 58:4015–25. doi: 10.1167/iovs.17-21897
18. Pulido JS, Canal I, Salomão D, Kravitz D, Bradley E, Vile R. Histological findings of birdshot chorioretinopathy in an eye with ciliochoroidal melanoma. *Eye* (2012) 26:862–5. doi: 10.1038/eye.2012.10
19. Gaudio PA, Kaye DB, Crawford JB. Histopathology of birdshot retinochoroidopathy. *Br J Ophthalmol* (2002) 86:1439–41. doi: 10.1136/bjo.86.12.1439
20. Acaba-Berrocal LA, Lucio-Alvarez JA, Mashayekhi A, Ho AC, Dunn JP, Shields LA, et al. Birdshot like Chorioretinopathy Associated With Pembrolizumab Treatment. *JAMA Ophthalmol* (2018) 136:1205–7. doi: 10.1001/jamaophthalmol.2018.1851
21. Hassman L, Warren M, Huxlin KR, Chung MM, xu l. Evidence of melanoma immunoreactivity in patients with Birdshot retinochoroidopathy. *Invest Ophthalmol Vis Sci* (2017) 58:5745.
22. Naveh HP, Rao UNM, Butterfield LH. Melanoma-associated leukoderma - immunology in black and white? *Pigment Cell Melanoma Res* (2013) 26:796–804. doi: 10.1111/pcmr.12161
23. Ryan SJ, Maumenee AE. Birdshot retinochoroidopathy. *Am J Ophthalmol* (1980) 89:31–45. doi: 10.1016/0002-9394(80)90226-3
24. Nussenblatt RB, Mittal KK, Ryan S, Richard Green W, Edward Maumenee A. Birdshot Retinochoroidopathy Associated with Hla-A29 Antigen and Immune Responsiveness to Retinal S-Antigen. *Am J Ophthalmol* (1982) 94:147–58. doi: 10.1016/0002-9394(82)90069-1
25. Herbort CP, Pavésio C, LeHoang P, Bodaghi B, Fardeau C, Kestelyn P, et al. Why birdshot retinochoroiditis should rather be called 'HLA-A29 uveitis'? *Br J Ophthalmol* (2017) 101:851–5. doi: 10.1136/bjophthalmol-2016-309764
26. Rock KL, Reits E, Neefjes J. Present Yourself! By MHC Class I and MHC Class II Molecules. *Trends Immunol* (2016) 37:724–37. doi: 10.1016/j.it.2016.08.010
27. Neefjes J, Ovaa H. A peptide's perspective on antigen presentation to the immune system. *Nat Chem Biol* (2013) 9:769–75. doi: 10.1038/nchembio.1391
28. Tsui E, Takhar JS, Joye A, Ahmad TR, Acharya NR, Gonzales JA. High Resolution DNA Typing of Human Leukocyte Antigen A29 in Familial Birdshot Chorioretinopathy. *Ocul Immunol Inflamm* (2019) 1–4. doi: 10.1080/09273948.2019.1682173
29. Arnaiz-Villena A, Gomez-Casado E, Martinez-Laso J. Population genetic relationships between Mediterranean populations determined by HLA allele distribution and a historic perspective. *Tissue Antigens* (2002) 60:111–21. doi: 10.1034/j.1399-0039.2002.600201.x
30. Knezevic A, Munk MR, Pappas F, Merrill PT, Goldstein DA. HLA-A29-Positive Birdshot Chorioretinopathy In An African American Patient. *Retin cases Brief Rep* (2016) 10:201–4. doi: 10.1097/ICB.0000000000000224
31. Baddar D, Goldstein DA. HLA-A29-positive Birdshot Chorioretinopathy in a Hispanic Patient. *Ocular Immunol Inflammation* (2016) 24:110–2. doi: 10.3109/09273948.2014.928733
32. LeHoang P, Ozdemir N, Benhamou A, Tabary T, Edelson C, Betuel H, et al. HLA-A29.2 subtype associated with birdshot retinochoroidopathy. *Am J Ophthalmol* (1992) 113:33–5. doi: 10.1016/S0002-9394(14)75749-6
33. Márquez A, ,Cordero-Coma M, Martın-Villa JM, Gorroño-Echebarrıa MB, Blanco R, Dıaz Valle D, et al. New insights into the genetic component of non-infectious uveitis through an Immunochip strategy. *J Med Genet* (2017) 54:38–46. doi: 10.1136/jmedgenet-2016-104144
34. Kuiper JJW, Van Setten J, Ripke S, Van 'T Slot R, Mulder F, Missotten T, et al. A genome-wide association study identifies a functional ERAP2 haplotype associated with birdshot chorioretinopathy. *Hum Mol Genet* (2014) 23:6081–7. doi: 10.1093/hmg/ddu307
35. Szpak Y, Vieville JC, Tabary T, Naud MC, Chopin M, Edelson C, et al. Spontaneous retinopathy in HLA-A29 transgenic mice. *Proc Natl Acad Sci USA* (2001) 98:2572–6. doi: 10.1073/pnas.051595998
36. Mattapallil MJ, Wawrousek EF, Chan CC, Zhao H, Roychoudhury J, Ferguson TA, et al. The Rd8 mutation of the Crb1 gene is present in vendor lines of C57BL/6N mice and embryonic stem cells, and confounds ocular induced mutant phenotypes. *Invest Ophthalmol Vis Sci* (2012) 53:2921–7. doi: 10.1167/iovs.12-9662
37. Middleton D, Williams F, Meenagh A, Daar AS, Gorodezky C, Hammond M, et al. Analysis of the distribution of HLA-A alleles in populations from five continents. *Hum Immunol* (2000) 61:1048–52. doi: 10.1016/S0198-8859(00)00178-6
38. Luo M, Embree J, Ramdahin S, Ndinya-Achola J, Njenga S, Bwayo JB, et al. HLA-A and HLA-B in Kenya, Africa: allele frequencies and identification of HLA-B*1567 and HLA-B*4426. *Tissue Antigens* (2002) 59:370–80. doi: 10.1034/j.1399-0039.2002.590503.x
39. Abi-Rached L, Gouret P, Yeh J-H, Di Cristofaro J, Pontarotti P, Picard C, et al. Immune diversity sheds light on missing variation in worldwide genetic diversity panels. *PloS One* (2018) 13:e0206512. doi: 10.1371/journal.pone.0206512
40. Robinson J, Barker DJ, Georgiou X, Cooper MA, Flicek P, Marsh SGE. IPD-IMGT/HLA Database. *Nucleic Acids Res* (2020) 48:D948–55. doi: 10.1093/nar/gkz950

41. Donvito B, Monnet D, Tabary T, Delair E, Vittier M, Réveil B, et al. A new HLA extended haplotype containing the A*2910 allele in birdshot retinochoroidopathy: susceptibility narrowed to the HLA molecule itself. *Invest Ophthalmol Vis Sci* (2010) 51:2525–8. doi: 10.1167/iovs.09-4329
42. Pettersen EF, Goddard TD, Huang CC, Couch GS, Greenblatt DM, Meng EC, et al. UCSF Chimera–a visualization system for exploratory research and analysis. *J Comput Chem* (2004) 25:1605–12. doi: 10.1002/jcc.20084
43. Venema WJ, Hiddingh S, de Boer JH, Claas FHJ, Mulder A, Den Hollander AI, et al. ERAP2 facilitates a subpeptidome of Birdshot Uveitis-associated HLA-A29. *bioRxiv* (2020) 2020.08.14.250654. doi: 10.1101/2020.08.14.250654
44. Reynisson B, Alvarez B, Paul S, Peters B, Nielsen M. NetMHCpan-4.1 and NetMHCIIpan-4.0: improved predictions of MHC antigen presentation by concurrent motif deconvolution and integration of MS MHC eluted ligand data. *Nucleic Acids Res* (2020) 48:W449–54. doi: 10.1093/nar/gkaa379
45. Sarkizova S, Klaeger S, Le PM, Li LW, Oliveira G, Keshishian H, et al. A large peptidome dataset improves HLA class I epitope predictionacross most of the human population. *Nat Biotechnol* (2020) 38:199–209. doi: 10.1038/s41587-019-0322-9
46. Dellgren C, Ekwelum VAC, Ormhøj M, Pallesen N, Knudsen J, Nehlin JO, et al. Low Constitutive Cell Surface Expression of HLA-B Is Caused by a Posttranslational Mechanism Involving Glu180 and Arg239. *J Immunol* (2016) 197:4807–16. doi: 10.4049/jimmunol.1502546
47. Moots RJ, Matsui M, Pazmany L, McMichael AJ, Frelinger JA. A cluster of mutations in HLA-A2 alpha 2 helix abolishes peptide recognition by T cells. *Immunogenetics* (1991) 34:141–8. doi: 10.1007/BF00205816
48. Serçinoğlu O, Ozbek P. Sequence-structure-function relationships in class I MHC: A local frustration perspective. *PloS One* (2020) 15:e0232849. doi: 10.1371/journal.pone.0232849
49. van Deutekom HWM, Keşmir C. Zooming into the binding groove of HLA molecules: which positions and which substitutions change peptide binding most? *Immunogenetics* (2015) 67:425–36. doi: 10.1007/s00251-015-0849-y
50. McMichael AJ, Gotch FM, Santos-Aguado J, Strominger JL. Effect of mutations and variations of HLA-A2 on recognition of a virus peptide epitope by cytotoxic T lymphocytes. *Proc Natl Acad Sci USA* (1988) 85:9194–8. doi: 10.1073/pnas.85.23.9194
51. Vasudev PG, Banerjee M, Ramakrishnan C, Balaram P. Asparagine and glutamine differ in their propensities to form specific side chain-backbone hydrogen bonded motifs in proteins. *Proteins* (2012) 80:991–1002. doi: 10.1002/prot.24001
52. Wooldridge L, van den Berg HA, Glick M, Gostick E, Laugel B, Hutchinson SL, et al. Interaction between the CD8 coreceptor and major histocompatibility complex class I stabilizes T cell receptor-antigen complexes at the cell surface. *J Biol Chem* (2005) 280:27491–501. doi: 10.1074/jbc.M500555200
53. McKenzie LM, Pecon-Slattery J, Carrington M, O'Brien SJ. Taxonomic hierarchy of HLA class I allele sequences. *Genes Immun* (1999) 1:120–9. doi: 10.1038/sj.gene.6363648
54. Hurley CK, Kempenich J, Wadsworth K, Sauter J, Hofmann JA, Schefzyk D, et al. Common, intermediate and well-documented HLA alleles in world populations: CIWD version 3.0.0. *HLA* (2020) 95:516–31. doi: 10.1111/tan.13811
55. Binkowski TA, Marino SR, Joachimiak A. Predicting HLA class I non-permissive amino acid residues substitutions. *PloS One* (2012) 7:e41710. doi: 10.1371/journal.pone.0041710
56. Maeurer MJ, Chan HW, Karbach J, Salter RD, Knuth A, Lotze MT, et al. Amino acid substitutions at position 97 in HLA-A2 segregate cytolysis from cytokine release in MART-1/Melan-A peptide AAGIGILTV-specific cytotoxic T lymphocytes. *Eur J Immunol* (1996) 26:2613–23. doi: 10.1002/eji.1830261112
57. Hogan KT, Clayberger C, Bernhard EJ, Walk SF, Ridge JP, Parham P, et al. A panel of unique HLA-A2 mutant molecules define epitopes recognized by HLA-A2-specific antibodies and cytotoxic T lymphocytes. *J Immunol* (1989) 142:2097–104.
58. Doytchinova IA, Guan P, Flower DR. Identifiying human MHC supertypes using bioinformatic methods. *J Immunol* (2004) 172:4314–23. doi: 10.4049/jimmunol.172.7.4314
59. Rao X, Hoof I, Costa AII, van Baarle D, Kesmir C. HLA class I allele promiscuity revisited. *Immunogenetics* (2011) 63:691–701. doi: 10.1007/s00251-011-0552-6
60. Abelin JG, Keskin DB, Sarkizova S, Hartigan CR, Zhang W, Sidney J, et al. Mass Spectrometry Profiling of HLA-Associated Peptidomes in Mono-allelic Cells Enables More Accurate Epitope Prediction. *Immunity* (2017) 46:315–26. doi: 10.1016/j.immuni.2017.02.007
61. Kuiper JJW, Van Setten J, Devall M, Cretu-Stancu M, Hiddingh S, Ophoff RA, et al. Functionally distinct ERAP1 and ERAP2 are a hallmark of HLA-A29-(Birdshot) Uveitis. *Hum Mol Genet* (2018) 27:4333–43. doi: 10.1101/338228
62. Lappalainen T, Sammeth M, Friedländer MR, 't Hoen PAC, Monlong J, Rivas MA, et al. Transcriptome and genome sequencing uncovers functional variation in humans. *Nature* (2013) 501:506–11. doi: 10.1038/nature12531
63. Auton A, Brooks LD, Durbin RM, Garrison EP, Kang HM, Korbel JO, et al. A global reference for human genetic variation. *Nature* (2015) 526:68–74. doi: 10.1038/nature15393
64. Pérez-Mayoral J, Soto-Salgado M, Shah E, Kittles R, Stern MC, Olivera MI, et al. Association of genetic ancestry with colorectal tumor location in Puerto Rican Latinos. *Hum Genomics* (2019) 13:12. doi: 10.1186/s40246-019-0196-4
65. Marrero FM, De Jesus E, Alvarez S, Mendez Bermudez IJ, Vila M, Marrero FM, Santos C, et al. Characteristics, Upon Presentation, of a Cohort of Hispanic Patientswith Birdshot Retinochoroidopathy. *P R Health Sci J* (2020) 39(3):249–53. doi: 10.1007/s10792-016-0434-x
66. Cimino L, Aldigeri R, Marchi S, Mastrofilippo V, Viscogliosi F, Coassin M, et al. Changes in patterns of uveitis at a tertiary referral center in Northern Italy: analysis of 990 consecutive cases. *Int Ophthalmol* (2018) 38:133–42. doi: 10.1007/s10792-016-0434-x
67. Garancher A, Suzuki H, Haricharan S, Chau LQ, Masihi MB, Rusert JM, et al. Tumor necrosis factor overcomes immune evasion in p53-mutant medulloblastoma. *Nat Neurosci* (2020) 23:842–53. doi: 10.1038/s41593-020-0628-4
68. Kuiper JJW, Mutis T, de Jager W, de Groot-Mijnes JDF, Rothova A. Intraocular interleukin-17 and proinflammatory cytokines in HLA-A29-associated birdshot chorioretinopathy. *Am J Ophthalmol* (2011) 152:177–82.e1. doi: 10.1016/j.ajo.2011.01.031
69. Huis in het Veld PI, van Asten F, Kuijpers RWAM, Rothova A, De Jong EK, Hoyng CB. Adalimumab Therapy For Refractory Birdshot Chorioretinopathy. *Retina* (2019) 39:2189–97. doi: 10.1097/IAE.0000000000002281
70. Steeples LR, Spry P, Lee RWJ, Carreño E. Adalimumab in refractory cystoid macular edema associated with birdshot chorioretinopathy. *Int Ophthalmol* (2018) 38:1357–62. doi: 10.1007/s10792-017-0592-5
71. Kirino Y, Bertsias G, Ishigatsubo Y, Mizuki N, Tugal-Tutkun I, Seyahi E, et al. Genome-wide association analysis identifies new susceptibility locifor Behcet's disease and epistasis between HLA-B*51 and ERAP1. *NatGenet* (2013) 45:202–7. doi: 10.1038/ng.2520
72. Evans DM, Spencer CCA, Pointon JJ, Su Z, Harvey D, Kochan G, et al. Interaction between ERAP1 and HLA-B27 in ankylosing spondylitis implicates peptide handling in the mechanism for HLA-B27 in disease susceptibility. *Nat Genet* (2011) 43:761–7. doi: 10.1038/ng0911-919a
73. Huang X-F, Li Z, De Guzman E, Robinson P, Gensler L, Ward MM, et al. Genomewide Association Study of Acute Anterior Uveitis Identifies New Susceptibility Loci. *Invest Ophthalmol Vis Sci* (2020) 61:3. doi: 10.1167/iovs.61.6.3
74. López de Castro JA. How ERAP1 and ERAP2 Shape the Peptidomes of Disease-Associated MHC-I Proteins. *Front Immunol* (2018) 9:2463. doi: 10.3389/fimmu.2018.02463
75. Mpakali A, Giastas P, Mathioudakis N, Mavridis IM, Saridakis E, Stratikos E. Structural basis for antigenic peptide recognition and processing by Endoplasmic reticulum (ER) aminopeptidase 2. *J Biol Chem* (2015) 290:26021–32. doi: 10.1074/jbc.M115.685909
76. Giastas P, Mpakali A, Papakyriakou A, Lelis A, Kokkala P, Neu M, et al. Mechanism for antigenic peptide selection by endoplasmic reticulum aminopeptidase 1. *Proc Natl Acad Sci* (2019) 116:26709–16. doi: 10.1073/pnas.1912070116

77. Mavridis G, Arya R, Domnick A, Zoidakis J, Makridakis M, Vlahou A, et al. A systematic re-examination of processing of MHCI-bound antigenic peptide precursors by endoplasmic reticulum aminopeptidase 1. *J Biol Chem* (2020) 295:7193–210. doi: 10.1074/jbc.RA120.012976
78. Yamashita Y, Anczurowski M, Nakatsugawa M, Tanaka M, Kagoya Y, Sinha A, et al. HLA-DP(84Gly) constitutively presents endogenous peptides generated by the class I antigen processing pathway. *Nat Commun* (2017) 8:15244. doi: 10.1038/ncomms15244
79. Suhre K, Arnold M, Bhagwat AM, Cotton RJ, Engelke R, Raffler J, et al. Connecting genetic risk to disease end points through the human blood plasma proteome. *Nat Commun* (2017) 8:14357. doi: 10.1038/ncomms15345
80. Goto Y, Ogawa K, Nakamura TJ, Hattori A, Tsujimoto M. TLR-mediated secretion of endoplasmic reticulum aminopeptidase 1 from macrophages. *J Immunol* (2014) 192:4443–52. doi: 10.4049/jimmunol.1300935
81. Ombrello MJ, Kastner DL, Remmers EF. Endoplasmic reticulum-associated amino-peptidase 1 and rheumatic disease: Genetics. *Curr Opin Rheumatol* (2015) 27:349–56. doi: 10.1097/BOR.0000000000000189
82. Reeves E, James E. The role of polymorphic ERAP1 in autoinflammatory disease. *Biosci Rep* (2018) 38(4):BSR20171503. doi: 10.1042/BSR20171503
83. Harvey D, Pointon JJ, Evans DM, Karaderi T, Farrar C, Appleton LH, et al. Investigating the genetic association between ERAP1 and ankylosing spondylitis. *Hum Mol Genet* (2009) 18(21):4204–12. doi: 10.1093/hmg/ddp371
84. Nguyen TT, Chang SC, Evnouchidou I, York IA, Zikos C, Rock KL, et al. Structural basis for antigenic peptide precursor processing by the endoplasmic reticulum aminopeptidase ERAP1. *Nat Struct Mol Biol* (2011) 18(5):604–13. doi: 10.1038/nsmb.2021
85. Hanson AL, Cuddihy T, Haynes K, Loo D, Morton CJ, Oppermann U, et al. Genetic Variants in ERAP1 and ERAP2 Associated With Immune-Mediated Diseases Influence Protein Expression and the Isoform Profile. *Arthritis Rheumatol* (2018) 70:255–65. doi: 10.1002/art.40369
86. Alvarez-Navarro C, Martín-Esteban A, Barnea E, Admon A, López De Castro JA. Endoplasmic reticulum aminopeptidase 1 (ERAP1) polymorphism relevant to inflammatory disease shapes the peptidome of the birdshot chorioretinopathy-associated HLA-A*29:02 Antigen. *Mol Cell Proteomics* (2015) 14:1770–80. doi: 10.1074/mcp.M115.048959
87. Andrés AM, Dennis MY, Kretzschmar WW, Cannons JL, Lee-Lin S-Q, Hurle B, et al. Balancing selection maintains a form of ERAP2 that undergoes nonsense-mediated decay and affects antigen presentation. *PloS Genet* (2010) 6:e1001157. doi: 10.1371/journal.pgen.1001157
88. Tanioka T, Hattori A, Masuda S, Nomura Y, Nakayama H, Mizutani S, et al. Human leukocyte-derived arginine aminopeptidase. The third member of the oxytocinase subfamily of aminopeptidases. *J Biol Chem* (2003) 278:32275–83. doi: 10.1074/jbc.M305076200
89. Ye CJ, Chen J, Villani AC, Gate RE, Subramaniam M, Bhangale T, et al. Genetic analysis of isoform usage in the human anti-viral response reveals influenza-specific regulation of ERAP2 transcripts under balancing selection. *Genome Res* (2018) 28:1812–25. doi: 10.1101/gr.240390.118
90. Saulle I, Vanetti C, Goglia S, Vicentini C, Tombetti E, Garziano M, et al. A New ERAP2/Iso3 Isoform Expression Is Triggered by Different Microbial Stimuli in Human Cells. Could It Play a Role in the Modulation of SARS-CoV-2 Infection? *Cells* (2020) 9:1951. doi: 10.3390/cells9091951
91. GTEx Consortium. The Genotype-Tissue Expression (GTEx) project.*Nat Genet* (2013)45:580–5. doi: 10.1038/ng.2653
92. Sanz-Bravo A, Martín-Esteban A, Kuiper JJW, García-Peydro M, Barnea E, Admon A, et al. Allele-specific alterations in the peptidome underlie the joint association of HLA-A*29:02 and endoplasmic reticulum aminopeptidase 2 (ERAP2) with birdshot chorioretinopathy. *Mol Cell Proteomics* (2018) 17:1564–77. doi: 10.1074/mcp.RA118.000778
93. López de Castro JA, Alvarez-Navarro C, Brito A, Guasp P, Martín-Esteban A, Sanz-Bravo A, et al. Molecular and pathogenic effects of endoplasmic reticulum aminopeptidases ERAP1 and ERAP2 in MHC-I-associated inflammatory disorders: Towards a unifying view. *Mol Immunol* (2016) 77:193–204. doi: 10.1016/j.molimm.2016.08.005
94. Martín-Esteban A, Guasp P, Barnea E, Admon A, López de Castro JA. Functional Interaction of the Ankylosing Spondylitis-Associated Endoplasmic Reticulum Aminopeptidase 2 With the HLA-B*27 Peptidome in Human Cells. *Arthritis Rheumatol (Hoboken NJ)* (2016) 68:2466–75. doi: 10.1002/art.39734
95. Lim YW, Chen-Harris H, Mayba O, Lianoglou S, Wuster A, Bhangale T, et al. Germline genetic polymorphisms influence tumor gene expression and immune cell infiltration. *Proc Natl Acad Sci USA* (2018) 115:E11701–10. doi: 10.1073/pnas.1804506115
96. Coles CH, McMurran C, Lloyd A, Hock M, Hibbert L, Raman MCC, et al. T Cell Receptor interactions with Human Leukocyte Antigen governindirect peptide selectivity for the cancer testis antigen MAGE-A4. *J BiolChem* (2020) 295:11486–94. doi: 10.1074/jbc.RA120.014016
97. Terakura S, Murata M, Warren EH, Sette A, Sidney J, Naoe T, et al. A single minor histocompatibility antigen encoded by UGT2B17 and presented by human leukocyte antigen-A*2902 and -B*4403. *Transplantation* (2007) 83:1242–8. doi: 10.1097/01.tp.0000259931.72622.d1
98. Koziel MJ, Dudley D, Wong JT, Dienstag J, Houghton M, Ralston R, et al. Intrahepatic cytotoxic T lymphocytes specific for hepatitis C virus in persons with chronic hepatitis. *J Immunol* (1992) 149:3339–44.
99. René C, Lozano C, Villalba M, Eliaou J-F. 5' and 3' untranslated regions contribute to the differential expression of specific HLA-A alleles. *Eur J Immunol* (2015) 45:3454–63. doi: 10.1002/eji.201545927
100. Boegel S, Löwer M, Bukur T, Sorn P, Castle JC, Sahin U, et al. HLA and proteasome expression body map. *BMC Med Genomics* (2018) 11:36. doi: 10.1186/s12920-018-0354-x
101. Goverdhan SV, Howell MW, Mullins RF, Osmond C, Hodgkins PR, Self J, et al. Association of HLA class I and class II polymorphisms with age-related macular degeneration. *Invest Ophthalmol Vis Sci* (2005) 46:1726–34. doi: 10.1167/iovs.04-0928
102. Korem Kohanim Y, Tendler A, Mayo A, Friedman N, Alon U. Endocrine Autoimmune Disease as a Fragility of Immune Surveillance against Hypersecreting Mutants. *Immunity* (2020) 52:872–84.e5. doi: 10.1016/j.immuni.2020.04.022
103. Shibuya H, Watanabe R, Maeno A, Ichimura K, Tamura M, Wakana S, et al. Melanocytes contribute to the vasculature of the choroid. *Genes Genet Syst* (2018) 93:51–8. doi: 10.1266/ggs.17-00058
104. Adini I, Ghosh K, Adini A, Chi Z-L, Yoshimura T, Benny O, et al. Melanocyte-secreted fibromodulin promotes an angiogenic microenvironment. *J Clin Invest* (2014) 124:425–36. doi: 10.1172/JCI69404
105. Sugita S, Takase H, Taguchi C, Imai Y, Kamoi K, Kawaguchi T, et al. Ocular infiltrating CD4+ T cells from patients with Vogt-Koyanagi-Harada disease recognize human melanocyte antigens. *Invest Ophthalmol Vis Sci* (2006) 47:2547–54. doi: 10.1167/iovs.05-1547
106. Otani S, Sakurai T, Yamamoto K, Fujita T, Matsuzaki Y, Goto Y, et al. Frequent immune response to a melanocyte specific protein KU-MEL-1 in patients with Vogt-Koyanagi-Harada disease. *Br J Ophthalmol* (2006) 90:773–7. doi: 10.1136/bjo.2005.086520
107. Frączek A, Owczarczyk-Saczonek A, Placek W. The Role of T(RM) Cells in the Pathogenesis of Vitiligo-A Review ofthe Current State-Of-The-Art. *Int J Mol Sci* (2020) 21(10):3552. doi: 10.3390/ijms21103552
108. Arakawa A, Siewert K, Stöhr J, Besgen P, Kim S-M, Rühl G, et al. Melanocyte antigen triggers autoimmunity in human psoriasis. *J Exp Med* (2015) 212:2203–12. doi: 10.1084/jem.20151093
109. Kuiper JJW, Rothova A, Schellekens PAW, Ossewaarde-van Norel A, Bloem AC, Mutis T. Detection of choroid- and retina-antigen reactive CD8+ and CD4+ T lymphocytes in the vitreous fluid of patients with birdshot chorioretinopathy. *Hum Immunol* (2014) 75:570–7. doi: 10.1016/j.humimm.2014.02.012
110. Dhall A, Patiyal S, Kaur H, Bhalla S, Arora C, Raghava GPS. Computing Skin Cutaneous Melanoma Outcome From the HLA-Alleles and Clinical Characteristics. *Front Genet* (2020) 11:221. doi: 10.3389/fgene.2020.00221
111. Lehmann G, Hanke-Gogokhia C, Hu Y, Bareja R, Salfati Z, Ginsberg M, et al. Single-cell profiling reveals an endothelium-mediated immunomodulatory pathway in the eye choroid. *J Exp Med* (2020) 217(6):e20190730. doi: 10.1084/jem.20190730
112. Nussenblatt RB, Kuwabara T, de Monasterio FM, Wacker WB. S-antigen uveitis in primates. A new model for human disease. *Arch Ophthalmol (Chicago Ill 1960)* (1981) 99:1090–2. doi: 10.1001/archopht.1981.03930011090021
113. Faure JP, Phuc LH, Takano S, Sterkers M, Thillaye B, De Kozak Y. [Experimental uveoretinitis induced in monkeys by retinal S antigen. Induction, histopathology (author's transl)]. *J Fr Ophtalmol* (1981) 4:465–72.

114. Nussenblatt RB, Gery I, Ballintine EJ, Wacker WB. Cellular immune responsiveness of uveitis patients to retinal S-antigen. *Am J Ophthalmol* (1980) 89:173–179. doi: 10.1016/0002-9394(80)90108-7
115. Boisgerault F, Khalil I, Tieng V, Connan F, Tabary T, Cohen JH, et al. Definition of the HLA-A29 peptide ligand motif allows prediction of potential T-cell epitopes from the retinal soluble antigen, a candidate autoantigen in birdshot retinopathy. *Proc Natl Acad Sci U S A* (1996) 93:3466–3470. doi: 10.1073/pnas.93.8.3466
116. Yadava K, Pattaroni C, Sichelstiel AK, Trompette A, Gollwitzer ES, Salami O, et al. Microbiota Promotes Chronic Pulmonary Inflammation by Enhancing IL-17A and Autoantibodies. *Am J Respir Crit Care Med* (2016) 193:975–87. doi: 10.1164/rccm.201504-0779OC
117. Fluckiger A, Daillère R, Sassi M, Sixt BS, Liu P, Loos F, et al. Cross-reactivity between tumor MHC class I-restricted antigens and an enterococcal bacteriophage. *Science* (2020) 369:936–42 doi: 10.1126/science.aax0701
118. Mager LF, Burkhard R, Pett N, Cooke NCA, Brown K, Ramay H, et al. Microbiome-derived inosine modulates response to checkpoint inhibitor immunotherapy. *Science* (2020). doi: 10.1126/science.abc3421
119. Fu X, Chen Y, Chen D. The Role of Gut Microbiome in Autoimmune Uveitis. *Ophthalmic Res* (2020). doi: 10.1159/000510212
120. Horai R, Caspi RR. Microbiome and Autoimmune Uveitis. *Front Immunol* (2019) 10:232. doi: 10.3389/fimmu.2019.00232
121. Daien V, Mura F, Martin G, Audo R, Rivière S, Konate A, et al. Th17 and regulatory T cells are increased in blood of patients with birdshot chorioretinopathy. *Acta Ophthalmol* (2017) 95:e161–3. doi: 10.1111/aos.12949
122. Molins B, Mesquida M, Llorenç V, de la Maza M, Adán A. Elevated Serum Immune Mediators and Subclinical Inflammation in HLA-A29-associated Birdshot Chorioretinopathy. *Ocul Immunol Inflamm* (2016) 24:647–52. doi: 10.3109/09273948.2015.1057601
123. Yang P, Foster CS. Interleukin 21, interleukin 23, and transforming growth factor β1 in HLA-A29-associated birdshot retinochoroidopathy. *Am J Ophthalmol* (2013) 156:400–6.e2. doi: 10.1016/j.ajo.2013.03.004
124. Krebs CF, Reimers D, Zhao Y, Paust H-J, Bartsch P, Nuñez S, et al. Pathogen-induced tissue-resident memory T(H)17 (T(RM)17) cells amplify autoimmune kidney disease. *Immunol* (2020) 5:eaba4163 doi: 10.1126/sciimmunol.aba4163
125. Bacher P, Hohnstein T, Beerbaum E, Röcker M, Blango MG, Kaufmann S, et al. Human Anti-fungal Th17 Immunity and Pathology Rely on Cross-Reactivity against Candida albicans. *Cell* (2019) 176:1340–55.e15. doi: 10.1016/j.cell.2019.01.041
126. Donahue SP, Greven CM, Zuravleff JJ, Eller AW, Nguyen MH, Peacock JEJ, et al. Intraocular candidiasis in patients with candidemia. Clinical implications derived from a prospective multicenter study. *Ophthalmology* (1994) 101:1302–9. doi: 10.1016/S0161-6420(94)31175-4
127. Sternes PR, Martin TM, Paley M, Diamond S, Asquith MJ, Brown MA, et al. HLA-A alleles including HLA-A29 affect the composition of the gutmicrobiome: a potential clue to the pathogenesis of birdshot retinochoroidopathy *Sci Rep* (2020) 10(1):17636. doi: 10.1038/s41598-020-74751-0.
128. Asquith M, Sternes PR, Costello M-E, Karstens L, Diamond S, Martin TM, et al. HLA Alleles Associated With Risk of Ankylosing Spondylitis and Rheumatoid Arthritis Influence the Gut Microbiome. *Arthritis Rheumatol (Hoboken NJ)* (2019) 71:1642–50. doi: 10.1002/art.40917
129. Andeweg SP, Keşmir C, Dutilh BE. Quantifying the impact of Human Leukocyte Antigen on the human gut microbiome. *bioRxiv* (2020). doi: 10.1101/2020.01.14.907196 2020.01.14.907196.
130. Ridley A, Hatano H, Wong-Baeza I, Shaw J, Matthews KK, Al-Mossawi H, et al. Activation-Induced Killer Cell Immunoglobulin-like Receptor 3DL2 Binding to HLA-B27 Licenses Pathogenic T Cell Differentiation in Spondyloarthritis. *Arthritis Rheumatol (Hoboken NJ)* (2016) 68:901–14. doi: 10.1002/art.39515
131. Chen L, Ridley A, Hammitzsch A, Al-Mossawi MH, Bunting H, Georgiadis D, et al. Silencing or inhibition of endoplasmic reticulum aminopeptidase 1 (ERAP1) suppresses free heavy chain expression and Th17 responses in ankylosing spondylitis. *Ann Rheumatol Dis* (2016) 75:916–23. doi: 10.1136/annrheumdis-2014-206996
132. Burren OS, Reales G, Wong L, Bowes J, Lee JC, Barton A, et al. Informed dimension reduction of clinically-related genome-wide association summary data characterises cross-trait axes of genetic risk. *bioRxiv* (2020). doi: 10.1101/2020.01.14.905869 2020.01.14.905869.
133. Levinson RD, Du Z, Luo L, Monnet D, Tabary T, Brezin AP, et al. Combination of KIR and HLA gene variants augments the risk of developing birdshot chorioretinopathy in HLA-A*29-positive individuals. *Genes Immun* (2008) 9:249–58. doi: 10.1038/gene.2008.13
134. Singh KM, Phung YT, Kohla MS, Lan BY-A, Chan S, Suen DL, et al. KIR genotypic diversity can track ancestries in heterogeneous populations: a potential confounder for disease association studies. *Immunogenetics* (2012) 64:97–109. doi: 10.1007/s00251-011-0569-x
135. Verhagen FH, Hiddingh S, Rijken R, Pandit A, Leijten E, Olde Nordkamp M, et al. High-Dimensional Profiling Reveals Heterogeneity of the Th17 Subset and Its Association With Systemic Immunomodulatory Treatment in Non-infectious Uveitis. *Front Immunol* (2018) 9:2519. doi: 10.3389/fimmu.2018.02519
136. Li Z, Lim WK, Mahesh SP, Liu B, Nussenblatt RB. Cutting edge: in vivo blockade of human IL-2 receptor induces expansion of CD56(bright) regulatory NK cells in patients with active uveitis. *J Immunol* (2005) 174:5187–91. doi: 10.4049/jimmunol.174.9.5187
137. Mbiribindi B, Mukherjee S, Wellington D, Das J, Khakoo SII. Spatial Clustering of Receptors and Signaling Molecules Regulates NK Cell Response to Peptide Repertoire Changes. *Front Immunol* (2019) 10:605. doi: 10.3389/fimmu.2019.00605
138. Hanson AL, Vukcevic D, Leslie S, Harris J, Lê Cao K-A, Kenna TJ, et al. Epistatic interactions between killer immunoglobulin-like receptors and human leukocyte antigen ligands are associated with ankylosing spondylitis. *PloS Genet* (2020) 16:e1008906. doi: 10.1371/journal.pgen.1008906
139. Hanson AL, Nel HJ, Bradbury L, Phipps J, Thomas R, Lê Cao K-A, et al. Altered Repertoire Diversity and Disease-Associated Clonal Expansions Revealed by T Cell Receptor Immunosequencing in Ankylosing Spondylitis Patients. *Arthritis Rheumatol (Hoboken NJ)* (2020) 72(8):1289–302. doi: 10.1002/art.41252
140. Georgiadis D, Mpakali A, Koumantou D, Stratikos E. Inhibitors of ER Aminopeptidase 1 and 2: From Design to Clinical Application. *Curr Med Chem* (2019) 26:2715–29. doi: 10.2174/0929867325666180214111849

11

Recent Developments in HLA B27 Anterior Uveitis

Denis Wakefield[1,2], Daniel Clarke[3] and Peter McCluskey[4,5]*

[1] Faculty of Medicine, University of NSW Sydney, Kensington, NSW, Australia, [2] NSW Health Pathology and South Eastern Sydney, LHD, Sydney, NSW, Australia, [3] Department of Medicine, South Eastern Sydney, LHD, Sydney, NSW, Australia, [4] Save Sight Institute, The University of Sydney, Sydney, NSW, Australia, [5] Discipline of Clinical Ophthalmology and Eye Health, Faculty of Medicine and Health, The University of Sydney, Sydney, NSW, Australia

***Correspondence:**
Peter McCluskey
peter.mccluskey@sydney.edu.au

There has been steady progress in understanding the pathogenesis, clinical features, and effective treatment of acute anterior uveitis (AU) over the past 5 years. Large gene wide association studies have confirmed that AU is a polygenic disease, with overlaps with the seronegative arthropathies and inflammatory bowel diseases, associations that have been repeatedly confirmed in clinical studies. The role of the microbiome in AU has received increased research attention, with recent evidence indicating that human leukocyte antigen B27 (HLA B27) may influence the composition of the gut microbiome in experimental animals. Extensive clinical investigations have confirmed the typical features of acute AU (AAU) and its response to topical, regional and systemic immunosuppressive treatment. Increased understanding of the role of cytokines has resulted in studies confirming the value of anti-cytokine therapy [anti–tumor necrosis factor (anti-TNF) and interleukin 6 (IL-6) therapy] in severe and recurrent cases of AAU, particularly in subjects with an associated spondyloarthopathy (SpA) and in juvenile idiopathic arthritis (JIA)–associated AAU.

Keywords: acute anterior uveitis, HLA B27, pathogenesis, microbiome, review

INTRODUCTION

Uveitis is a common vision threatening inflammatory eye disease with a reported annual incidence of between 17 and 52 per 100,000 and prevalence of between 38 and 370 per 100,000 of the population (1–4). The disease is most common in children, young and middle-aged adults. Uveitis and its complications account for up to 10% of those with severe vision impairment and blindness (5). Anterior uveitis (AU) is present in up to 90% of cases of uveitis and approximately 50% of all patients with acute AU (AAU) are human leukocyte antigen B27 (HLA B27) positive. HLA B27 is also strongly associated with ankylosing spondylitis (AS), reactive arthritis (ReA), and other spondyloarthropathies (SpA) (6). These associations are among the strongest of any HLA antigen to a human disease, although the pathogenetic mechanism(s) involved remain unknown (7). There has been relatively little research devoted to the immunopathogenesis of HLA B27 AAU, compared with the numerous studies of the immunopathogenesis of the SpA's.

Evidence that HLA B27 is directly involved in the pathogenesis of this group of diseases is supported by the fact that HLA B27 is associated with AAU and SpA in many populations and ethnic groups, in the context of over 140 haplotypes (the HLA B2705 subtype is the most common in Caucasians). Secondly, some HLA B27 subtypes are not associated to AAU or SpA, suggesting that subtype polymorphism modulate disease susceptibility, and thirdly, HLA B27 transgenic rats and mice develop a disease that strongly resembles human SpA, although these animals do not spontaneously develop AAU (8).

CLINICAL FEATURES OF HLA B27 ANTERIOR UVEITIS

In a large study of over 2000 patients with axial SpA from 83 rheumatology centers in the United Kingdom 23.5% of the patients in the cohort reported at least 1 episode of AAU. The mean age of patients was 51 years with a male to female ratio of 2:1. The factors associated with increased prevalence of AAU in this cohort were HLA B27 positivity, university education, age, and the presence and duration of axial spondylo-arthritis (9). There is a well-defined clinical phenotype for patients with AAU associated with spondyloarthritis which was confirmed in a study by Peizeng et al. in a large Chinese population (10). Typical symptoms include: acute onset of blurred vision, ocular redness, pain and photophobia. Important clinical descriptors include: unilateral episodes, alternation between eyes, sudden onset and limited duration. HLA B27 AAU is non-granulomatous and characterized by flare and cells in the anterior chamber that commonly spills over into the anterior vitreous. Other clinical features such as hypopyon and posterior synechiae may occur. HLA B27 associated uveitis is nearly always confined to the anterior uvea as AAU, although uncommonly there can be prominent intermediate uveitis and involvement of the posterior segment (11). A Chinese study also found that asymptomatic previously unrecognized, retinal vascular involvement often involving the peripheral retina is not uncommon (10). HLA B27 associated AAU is further characterized by recurrences, which are more frequent early in the course of the disease and become less frequent with the duration of disease (12).

Severe and/or recurrent episodes of AAU may result in structural complications such as cataract, elevated intraocular pressure, glaucoma and cystoid macular oedema, which become increasingly common with multiple episodes of uveitis (13). Some patients develop chronic AU following very severe attacks or frequent recurrences. D'Ambrosia and colleagues performed a literature-based meta-analysis to characterize the clinical features and complications associated with HLA B27 AU. The results confirmed the strong association of AU with AS, increased male prevalence, unilateral alternating episodes of uveitis often characterized by a fibrinous inflammatory reaction with or without hypopyon, and occasionally optic disc swelling. The prevalence of raised intraocular pressure and glaucoma were more common in the HLA B27 negative cases of AAU. Interestingly, they concluded that there is no significant difference between HLA B27 positive and HLA B27 negative AAU with regard to final visual acuity and structural complications, such as posterior synechiae, cataract, and macular oedema (14).

GENETICS AND ANTERIOR UVEITIS

The heritability of HLA B27 AAU has a strong association with the major histocombatibility complex (MHC) type 1 allele which over 50% of those with primary AAU possess (7). In an examination of 152 first degree relatives of 42 randomly selected HLA B27 AAU patients, 6% were found to develop the condition (15). The same Dutch study also identified that there may be other genetic factors influencing inheritance, with higher rates of proband first degree relatives developing AAU than in the normal HLA B27 population (15). Recent genotyping studies have supported this observation with several non MHC loci demonstrating genome wide association significance. In one study comparing AAU subjects to healthy controls using the Illumina Immunochip, associations were established with ERAP1, IL23R, and the intergenic region 2p15 (16).

The first genome wide association study (GWAS) of patients with AAU with or without AS identified new susceptibility genes and confirmed the strong association of HLA B27 AAU with SpA (17). Gene associations were observed for 11 loci, including the previously reported ERAP1 and NOS2. Associations were also found at previously unrecognized sites for AS and AU including MERTK, KIFAP3, CLCN 7, ACAA2, and five intergenic loci (17). A number of genetic factors critical to the immune response to microorganisms, such as IL10, IL18R1-IL1R1, IL6R, and KIF21B, were previously reported in a GWAS study of patients with AS and AAU (16).

Despite the association of the ERAP1 gene with HLA B27 SpA and AAU the role of this gene in peptide selection and processing in the pathogenesis of these diseases has not been defined. Barnea et al. examined the effect of ERAP1 deletion in HLA B27 transgenic rats. The male HLA B27 transgenic rats develop a spondylo-arthritic type of disease, but not AU, and have been used as a model of spondylo-arthritis. Deletion of the ERAP1 gene did not affect the development of SpA (18). Interestingly, examination of the peptidomes of rats susceptible to arthritis was similar to those of non-susceptible rats and no peptides were found to be uniquely associated with arthritis.

Using next generation sequencing to identify T-cell receptor beta motifs and amino acid sequences specific to HLA B27 positive patients with AS. Faham et al. recently reported sequences specific to AS, indicating that specific antigens possibly related to the pathogenesis of AS may be identifiable using such an approach (19). Such studies have not been reported in patients with HLA B27 associated AAU but could yield results strengthening the argument that CD8 positive T cells are pivotal in the pathogenesis of this disease.

INFECTION AND HLA B27 AAU

There is considerable epidemiological, clinical, and experimental evidence in patients with AU implicating the role of microbial infections as part of the molecular mimicry or arthritogenic peptide hypothesis. In particular, infection with *Chlamydia Trachomatis* and gram negative bacteria including *Klebsiella*,

Salmonella, Yersinia, Shigella species, and *Campylobacter jejuni*, has been reported to trigger AU and SpA (20–22). Furthermore, there is compelling evidence implicating *Chlamydia trachomatis* in the pathogenesis of ReA and undifferentiated spondylarthroses (19, 20, 22–24). More recently, epidemiological evidence has emerged implicating *Ureaplasma Urealyticum* (25) and a yet to be identified fungus (26) with the occurrence of uveitis. We have previously provided evidence for the role of microbial triggers in the pathogenesis of HLA B27 AAU, by demonstrating humoral and cellular immune responses to *C. trachomatis* and *Yersinia* (26, 27).

Schofield et al. have delineated potential inciting peptide sequences common between enteric bacteria capsules and the third hypervariable region of the HLA B27 molecule (28). Further studies in this vein have found that *Klebsiella* nitrogenase shares six consecutive amino-acids with HLA B27 (29) and surface proteins of *Salmonella, Yersinia,* and *Shigella* have homologous sequences (30). Investigating mice models of disease Horai and colleagues demonstrated that the presence of enteric bacteria triggers retinal specific auto reactive T cells and subsequently spontaneous uveitis (31). Unfortunately, attempts to further localize the effect to self-peptides or self-antigens have thus far failed.

Schittenhelm and colleagues have searched for the existence of disease inducing peptides, the so-called arthrogenic or uveitic peptide(s) proposed to be important in the pathogenesis of HLA B27 related diseases (32). Using sophisticated Mass Spectroscopy they examined 1,500 epitopes across several different HLA class I allotypes (HLA B27:02- HLA B27:09). Analysis of this large data set identified 26 peptides, which were present in lower abundance by non-disease-related HLA B27 allotypes compared with the disease associated HLA B27 subtypes. It is yet to be ascertained whether these peptides represent the arthrogenic peptide proposed to cause SpA's. The high amount of overlap found in the absolute peptide binding preferences of the HLA B27 allotypes (:02 to :09) has shifted the focus of the arthritogenic peptide hypothesis to quantitative analysis of peptide binding conformation, self-peptide presentation and T cell activation (33). It would be of great interest to use similar technology to identify potential peptides related to HLA B27 AU.

THE ROLE OF THE MICROBIOME

There is considerable recent interest in the role of the microbiome in influencing immune responses and susceptibility to diseases such as Crohn's disease, ulcerative colitis, SpA's, and uveitis (34–36). Studies in HLA B27 transgenic rats demonstrate an altered microbiome compared to non-transgenic animals (37). The mechanisms by which the microbiome may influence immune responses are poorly understood. One theory is that gut microbes or their products may alter the permeability of the gut wall allowing translocation of bacteria and/or microbial products to regional lymph nodes, which generate a systemic immune response. Such increased gut permeability has been described in patients with AS and inflammatory bowel disease. Patient with ReA have had microbial antigens detected in joint fluid and subsequently been shown to have a clinical response to antibiotic therapy (38). Additionally, endotoxin, which is a component of Gram negative bacteria cell-walls has been shown in experimental animals to induce AU when injected into the foot pad of rodents (39). Similarly, we have shown that patients with active AU have increased expression of Toll like receptors 4 (which binds endotoxin) in the peripheral blood during acute attacks of AU (40). An alternative theory holds that there is molecular mimicry between microbial and self-antigens. Such micro-organisms and their associated antigens may generate an immune response whereby antibodies or T cells cross-reacts with self-antigens as is known to occur in diseases such as rheumatic fever and post-infection Gilliam Barré syndrome (41). Thirdly, it has been shown that the microbiome may affect the immune response by influencing T cells to synthesize increased amounts of IL-17 and the number of regulatory T cells that express the transcription factor fox P3 (42). Furthermore, it has been shown that a large number of microbial peptides bind the HLA B27 molecule and such microbial peptides may induce an immune response in certain target organs such as the eye and joint (43). We have recently shown, for example, that peptides derived from Chlamydia trachomatis bind the HLA B27 molecule and when such peptides are injected with adjuvant into experimental animals they induce an arthritis and less frequently AU (27).

An immune response to peptides derived from gut microorganisms (microbiome) could cross-react with endogenous peptides leading to the development of AU (34). This concept is strengthened by the results of the recent studies indicating that a large number of peptides derived from microorganisms bind to the HLA B27 molecule as well as our studies showing increased affinity of chlamydia and derived peptides for the HLA B27 molecule (27, 28, 44–46). We have also shown that immunizing rats with chlamydia derived peptides leads to a polyarthritis and occasional uveitis in these animals (47). Furthermore, a peptide (C34) derived from type VI collagen was shown to be recognized by $CD8^+$ T cells from patients with AS (48). Additionally, cross-reactivity between *chlamydial* peptides and homologous peptides from the heart muscle-specific protein -myosin was shown to be involved in the pathogenesis of autoimmune myocarditis in mice (49).

The microbiome of the aqueous humor has not been examined in patients with acute and recurrent AU. The anterior chamber of the eye is usually considered to be sterile, although a recent study indicated that in fact the aqueous humor may have a microbiome that was previously unrecognized (50). Examination of the aqueous humor for evidence of microorganisms during acute attacks of AU could reveal valuable information with regard to the microbial and immunological mechanisms underlying this common inflammatory disease. If the gut microbiome does play a key role in diseases induction, a variety of therapeutic strategies could be developed to alter the microbiome or the immune response to particular microorganisms implicated to prevent or ameliorate the development of immune mediated diseases such as AAU and SpAs.

IMMUNE MECHANISMS AND ANTERIOR UVEITIS

Immune mechanisms involved in the pathogenesis of AU have been investigated in human and animal studies. It was recently reported that in patients with HLA B27 AAU the aqueous humor concentration of CC chemokines, including CCL8, CCL13, and CCL20, were upregulated, compared with patients with granulomatous uveitis and control subjects (51). Such chemokines play a key role in attracting inflammatory cells to the eye during attacks of uveitis and may represent potential therapeutic targets.

The pro-inflammatory cytokine IL-6 has previously been shown to be produced by ocular parenchymal cells and to promote the differentiation of B cells to plasma cells (52). Recently Kumar et al. demonstrated that tear levels of IL-6 and IL-10 are elevated during acute and multiple episodes of uveitis (53) building on previous work identifying elevated IL-6 levels in human aqueous (54), vitreous and monocyte culture supernatant (55). In a study examining cytokine profiles of specific uveitic entities Abu El-Asrar et al. discovered elevated GM-CSF, IL-11, and IL-35 levels in HLA B27 AAU (56). IL-11 is classed within the IL-6 family, based on its shared use of the glycoprotein-130 receptor β-subunit (57) and in the study had a particularly strong association with disease activity. The coupled elevation of inhibitory cytokines IL-35 and IL-10 with IL-6 and IL-ll may represent an immunoregulatory response in uveitis (53, 56).

A recent study by Zhao et al. reported increased levels of IL37 mRNA and protein expression by peripheral blood mononuclear cells from patients with active AAU compared with control (58). There was no difference between HLA B27 positive and negative patients with AAU. Interestingly IL37 was shown to inhibit the production of pro-inflammatory cytokines, including IL-1, IL-6, IL-10, IL-21, IL-23, TNF, and gamma interferon in the supernatant of dendritic cells (58). Thus, IL37 may inhibit pro-inflammatory cytokines in patients with AAU and may be a new therapeutic approach to treating this disease.

It has previously been demonstrated that HLA B27 homodimers on the surface of T-cells, monocytes and natural killer cells may trigger innate immune mechanisms through binding to killer immunoglobulin-like receptors (KIR) (59). Specifically, KIR3DL2 receptor expression has been found to be increased on NK cells in the peripheral blood of patients with HLA B27 AAU, associated with higher active numbers and increased cytotoxicity (60). Using flow cytometric methods Huang et al. have now also implicated mucosa associated innate lymphoid (MAIT) cells, which in the study produced more IL-17A than controls (61), an important proinflammatory cytokine seen in HLA B27 AAU (62, 63).

In a comparison of peripheral monocytes in patients with idiopathic uveitis against those with HLA B27 AAU using ELISA methods, increased expression of S100A8/A9 was found in patients with HLA B27 AAU outside of uveitis episodes accompanied by heightened numbers and activity of monocytes and T cells (64).

NEW DEVELOPMENTS IN THE TREATMENT OF HLA B27 ANTERIOR UVEITIS

A better understanding of the pathogenesis of AAU will provide new avenues for management of uveitis with the possibility of specific therapy that can alter the natural history or even cure uveitis. At present, treatment options consist of local or systemic anti-inflammatory or immunosuppressive drugs, which may be associated with treatment limiting side effects.

Current first line therapy for acute episodes of HLA B27 AAU is a cycloplegic, typically atropine 1%, and very frequent administration of potent topical corticosteroids (1–2 hourly) which are then slowly tapered over 8–10 weeks (65). The so called "steroid response" leads to elevated intraocular pressure in up to 30% of patients using topical corticosteroids, often requiring the addition of pressure lowering medication and requiring cessation of topical corticosteroid therapy in some patients. Corticosteroid therapy is also associated with increased rates of posterior subcapsular cataract (66). Although a large randomized clinical trial of 193 subjects failed to achieve non-inferiority of iontophoresis as a method to increase anterior chamber corticosteroid levels compared to topical therapy, there was a promising signal that should be tested using larger data sets (67).

In patients with vision threatening uveitis, periocular corticosteroid injections are safe and efficacious, either alone or as adjuncts to systemic therapies (68). Peri- and intra-ocular injections reduce macular oedema which is the major inflammatory mediated cause of visual loss in uveitis patients (69). Regional corticosteroid therapies have a relatively short duration of effect necessitating 3 to 6 monthly injections. The development of both bioerodible (Iluvien) and non-biodegradable (Retisert) intravitreal implants of polymers allow the controlled release of fluocinolone acetate into the vitreous for up to 3 years. Both the multicenter uveitis steroid treatment (MUST) study and a recent Cochrane review that compared Retisert implants to systemic combination immunosuppressive therapy, showed that systemic therapy resulted in superior visual outcomes and lower rates of raised intraocular pressure, cataract formation, retinal detachment and endophthalmitis (70). There was no difference in systemic side effects such as weight gain, diabetes and hypertension in the two groups and the only significant adverse outcome was increased use of antibiotics for infections in those on systemic therapy (71). Nearly two thirds of the patients in the systemic therapy arm of the MUST study required intermittent local corticosteroids.

The systemic treatment for eye diseases (SITE) cohort study retrospectively examined the efficacy of systemic therapies in 7,957 patients across five centers from 1979 to 2005 who had non-infectious ocular inflammatory disease. For patients with AU corticosteroid sparing success (tapering to 10 mg or less) was achieved over a 6-month period in 47.2% with mycophenolate mofetil, 16.6% with azathioprine, 28.5% with cyclosporine, and 46.1% with methotrexate (72–75). The role of disease modifying agents (DMARDS) have now been examined specifically in HLA B27 AAU with methotrexate and sulfasalazine both shown to reduce relapse rates and methotrexate additionally proven to reduce AU related macular oedema (76).

There is significant evidence that anti-TNF alpha therapy is of benefit in patients with HLA B27 uveitis (77–80). In a retrospective analysis of 717 patients with SpA those who were treated with either infliximab or etanercept had 6.8 AAU recurrences per hundred patient years versus 15.6 in the placebo group (81). Data from the use of adalimumab in another cohort of 1,250 patients with SpA demonstrated an overall 51% reduction in uveitis recurrence rate (82). Further analysis of these cohorts showed that of the anti-TNF therapies available, anti-TNF antibodies appear to have greater efficacy than soluble TNF receptor blockers (83). Adding weight to this preference is a collection of case reports and new data from a large Swedish rheumatology study suggesting that in AS etanercept may induce new uveitis (84, 85). Prospective studies of anti-TNF antibodies have now been performed on small cohorts of patients with frequent and/or refractory AAU. The use of infliximab led to the complete resolution of HLA B27 AAU in 6 of 7 patients following an average of 8 days (86). The new anti-TNF alpha agent golimumab induced the remission of uveitis in 12 of 15 eyes with significant improvements in visual acuity (87). Certolizumab pegol has been used in AAU cases refractory to even previous biologic therapy and achieved quiescence in 5 of 7 patients (88).

The success of the antibiotic sulfasalazine as a DMARD in HLA B27 AAU adds weight to the prospect of targeting the microbiome for disease control. Clinical studies are currently underway evaluating faecal microbial transplants in AS and it will be interesting to see whether this influences rates of uveitis in these patients (89). If the gut microbiome does play a key role in diseases induction, a variety of therapeutic strategies could be developed to alter the microbiome or the immune response to particular microorganisms implicated to prevent or ameliorate the development of immune mediated diseases such as AAU and SpA's.

ADVANTAGES IN STUDYING HLA B27 ACUTE ANTERIOR UVEITIS

There are significant advantages in studying the immuno-pathogenesis of AAU as a pathophysiological model for HLA B27 related disease. AAU is well defined disorder, that is readily and reliably diagnosed clinically by slit lamp bio-microscopy. Importantly there are agreed objective grading systems to determine the severity and changes in the grade of the protein exudation and cellular infiltration in the anterior chamber that characterize AU (90). Additionally, aqueous humor can be easily sampled for analysis. The natural history of AAU has been extensively studied and has a recurrent, relapsing and remitting course. Importantly, there is a group of subjects with a similar clinical phenotype, who are HLA B27 negative and form a relevant critical disease control group. The recurrent nature of the disease also has advantages for investigators studying environmental factors, such as the gut microbiome, that may trigger relapses of uveitis. There is a large number of patients with recurrent AAU, not on systemic therapy or immunosuppressive medication, which can influence immunological and bio-molecular investigations. As 50%–70% with HLA B27 AU have an associated systemic disease, usually a SpA or inflammatory bowel disease, subjects without confounding systemic disease can be studied and compared with subjects with systemic disease (91, 92).

CONCLUSION

AU is a relatively common polygenic disease, strongly associated with HLA B27 and a number of other inflammatory diseases that share a common gene pool. The function of HLA B27 and the other recently described genes predisposing to AAU is poorly understood. The role of infection and in particular the microbiome remain active areas of research, as does the importance of innate immunity in the pathogenesis of this disease. New insights into genetic, microbial, and immune mechanisms has the potential to lead to more effective preventative and suppressive forms of therapy.

AUTHOR CONTRIBUTIONS

All authors contributed to writing, editing, and reviewing the manuscript. All authors contributed to the article and approved the submitted version.

REFERENCES

1. Baarsma GS. The epidemiology and genetics of endogenous uveitis: a review. *Curr Eye Res* (1992) 11 Suppl:1–9. doi: 10.3109/02713689208999505
2. Wakefield D, Chang JH. Epidemiology of Uveitis. *Int Ophthalmol Clin* (2005) 45:1–13. doi: 10.1097/01.iio.0000155938.83083.94
3. González MM, Solano MM, Porco TC, Oldenburg CE, Acharya NR, Lin SC, et al. Epidemiology of uveitis in a US population-based study. *J Ophthalmic Inflammation Infect* (2018) 8:6. doi: 10.1186/s12348-018-0148-5
4. Kopplin LJ, Mount G, Suhler EB. Review for Disease of the Year: Epidemiology of HLA-B27 Associated Ocular Disorders. *Ocul Immunol Inflammation* (2016) 24:470–5. doi: 10.1080/09273948.2016.1175642
5. Suttorp-Schulten MS, Rothova A. The possible impact of uveitis in blindness: a literature survey. *Br J Ophthalmol* (1996) 80:844–8. doi: 10.1136/bjo.80.9.844
6. Khan MA. HLA-B27 and its pathogenic role. *J Clin Rheumatol* (2008) 14:50–2. doi: 10.1097/RHU.0b013e3181637a38
7. Martin TM, Rosenbaum JT. An update on the genetics of HLA-B27 associated acute anterior uveitis. *Ocul Immunol Inflammation* (2011) 19:108–14. doi: 10.3109/09273948.2011.559302
8. Braun J, Sieper J. Ankylosing spondylitis. *Lancet* (2007) 369:1379–90. doi: 10.1016/s0140-6736(07)60635-7
9. Derakhshan MH, Dean L, Jones GT, Macfarlane GJ, Siebert S, Gaffney K. Op0262 Factors Associated with Acute Anterior Uveitis in Patients with Axial Spondyloarthritis: Analysis of the Bsrbr-as Register Database. *Ann Rheum Dis* (2019) 78:212–2. doi: 10.1136/annrheumdis-2019-eular.2859
10. Yang P, Wan W, Du L, Zhou Q, Qi J, Liang L, et al. Clinical features of HLA-B27-positive acute anterior uveitis with or without ankylosing spondylitis in a Chinese cohort. *Br J Ophthalmol* (2018) 102:215. doi: 10.1136/bjophthalmol-2016-309499

11. Dodds EM, Lowder CY, Meisler DM. Posterior segment inflammation in HLA-B27+ acute anterior uveitis: clinical characteristics. *Ocul Immunol Inflammation* (1999) 7:85–92. doi: 10.1076/ocii.7.2.85.4015
12. Rothova A, van Veenedaal WG, Linssen A, Glasius E, Kijlstra A, de Jong PT. Clinical features of acute anterior uveitis. *Am J Ophthalmol* (1987) 103:137–45. doi: 10.1016/s0002-9394(14)74218-7
13. Gritz DC, Schwaber EJ, Wong IG. Complications of Uveitis: The Northern California Epidemiology of Uveitis Study. *Ocul Immunol Inflammation* (2018) 26:584–94. doi: 10.1080/09273948.2016.1247174
14. D'Ambrosio EM, La Cava M, Tortorella P, Gharbiya M, Campanella M, Iannetti L. Clinical Features and Complications of the HLA-B27-associated Acute Anterior Uveitis: A Metanalysis. *Semin Ophthalmol* (2017) 32:689–701. doi: 10.3109/08820538.2016.1170158
15. Derhaag PJ, Linssen A, Broekema N, de Waal LP, Feltkamp TE. A familial study of the inheritance of HLA-B27-positive acute anterior uveitis. *Am J Ophthalmol* (1988) 105:603–6. doi: 10.1016/0002-9394(88)90051-7
16. Robinson PC, Claushuis TA, Cortes A, Martin TM, Evans DM, Leo P, et al. Genetic dissection of acute anterior uveitis reveals similarities and differences in associations observed with ankylosing spondylitis. *Arthritis Rheumatol* (2015) 67:140–51. doi: 10.1002/art.38873
17. Huang X-F, Li Z, De Guzman E, Robinson P, Gensler L, Ward MM, et al. Genomewide Association Study of Acute Anterior Uveitis Identifies New Susceptibility Loci. *Invest Ophthalmol Vis Sci* (2020) 61. doi: 10.1167/iovs.61.6.3
18. Barnea E, Melamed Kadosh D, Haimovich Y, Satumtira N, Dorris ML, Nguyen MT, et al. The Human Leukocyte Antigen (HLA)-B27 Peptidome in Vivo, in Spondyloarthritis-susceptible HLA-B27 Transgenic Rats and the Effect of Erap1 Deletion. *Mol Cell Proteomics MCP* (2017) 16:642–62. doi: 10.1074/mcp.M116.066241
19. Faham M, Carlton V, Moorhead M, Zheng J, Klinger M, Pepin F, et al. Discovery of T Cell Receptor beta Motifs Specific to HLA-B27-Positive Ankylosing Spondylitis by Deep Repertoire Sequence Analysis. *Arthritis Rheumatol* (2017) 69:774–84. doi: 10.1002/art.40028
20. Savolainen E, Kettunen A, Narvanen A, Kautiainen H, Karkkainen U, Luosujarvi R, et al. Prevalence of antibodies against Chlamydia trachomatis and incidence of C. trachomatis-induced reactive arthritis in an early arthritis series in Finland in 2000. *Scand J Rheumatol* (2009) 38:353–6. doi: 10.1080/03009740902769559
21. Carter JD, Gerard HC, Espinoza LR, Ricca LR, Valeriano J, Snelgrove J, et al. Chlamydiae as etiologic agents in chronic undifferentiated spondylarthritis. *Arthritis Rheum* (2009) 60:1311–6. doi: 10.1002/art.24431
22. Girschick HJ, Guilherme L, Inman RD, Latsch K, Rihl M, Sherer Y, et al. Bacterial triggers and autoimmune rheumatic diseases. *Clin Exp Rheumatol* (2008) 26:S12–7.
23. Siala M, Gdoura R, Younes M, Fourati H, Cheour I, Meddeb N, et al. Detection and frequency of Chlamydia trachomatis DNA in synovial samples from Tunisian patients with reactive arthritis and undifferentiated oligoarthritis. *FEMS Immunol Med Microbiol* (2009) 55:178–86. doi: 10.1111/j.1574-695X.2008.00524.x
24. Kuipers JG, Sibilia J, Bas S, Gaston H, Granfors K, Vischer TL, et al. Reactive and undifferentiated arthritis in North Africa: use of PCR for detection of Chlamydia trachomatis. *Clin Rheumatol* (2009) 28:11–6. doi: 10.1007/s10067-008-0968-z
25. Banicioiu-Covei S, Vreju AF, Ciurea PL. Correlations between infection patterns and eye damage in reactive arthritis. *Rom J Morphol Embryol* (2019) 60:601–4.
26. Maillet J, Ottaviani S, Tubach F, Roy C, Nicaise-Rolland P, Palazzo E, et al. Anti-Saccharomyces cerevisiae antibodies (ASCA) in spondyloarthritis: Prevalence and associated phenotype. *Joint Bone Spine* (2016) 83:665–8. doi: 10.1016/j.jbspin.2015.10.011
27. Wakefield D, Easter J, Robinson P, Graham D, Penny R. Chlamydial antibody crossreactivity with peripheral blood mononuclear cells of patients with ankylosing spondylitis: the role of HLA B27. *Clin Exp Immunol* (1986) 63:49–57.
28. Scofield RH, Kurien B, Gross T, Warren WL, Harley JB. HLA-B27 binding of peptide from its own sequence and similar peptides from bacteria: implications for spondyloarthropathies. *Lancet* (1995) 345:1542–4. doi: 10.1016/s0140-6736(95)91089-1
29. Schwimmbeck PL, Oldstone MB. Molecular mimicry between human leukocyte antigen B27 and Klebsiella. Consequences for spondyloarthropathies. *Am J Med* (1988) 85:51–3. doi: 10.1016/0002-9343(88)90385-3
30. Lahesmaa R, Skurnik M, Vaara M, Leirisalo-Repo M, Nissila M, Granfors K, et al. Molecular mimickry between HLA B27 and Yersinia, Salmonella, Shigella and Klebsiella within the same region of HLA alpha 1-helix. *Clin Exp Immunol* (1991) 86:399–404. doi: 10.1111/j.1365-2249.1991.tb02944.x
31. Horai R, Zárate-Bladés CR, Dillenburg-Pilla P, Chen J, Kielczewski JL, Silver PB, et al. Microbiota-Dependent Activation of an Autoreactive T Cell Receptor Provokes Autoimmunity in an Immunologically Privileged Site. *Immunity* (2015) 43:343–53. doi: 10.1016/j.immuni.2015.07.014
32. Schittenhelm RB, Sivaneswaran S, Lim Kam Sian TCC, Croft NP, Purcell AW. Human Leukocyte Antigen (HLA) B27 Allotype-Specific Binding and Candidate Arthritogenic Peptides Revealed through Heuristic Clustering of Data-independent Acquisition Mass Spectrometry (DIA-MS) Data. *Mol Cell Proteomics MCP* (2016) 15:1867–76. doi: 10.1074/mcp.M115.056358
33. Schittenhelm RB, Sian TC, Wilmann PG, Dudek NL, Purcell AW. Revisiting the arthritogenic peptide theory: quantitative not qualitative changes in the peptide repertoire of HLA-B27 allotypes. *Arthritis Rheumatol* (2015) 67:702–13. doi: 10.1002/art.38963
34. Rosenbaum JT, Asquith M. The Microbiome and HLA B27-associated acute anterior uveitis. *Nat Rev Rheumatol* (2018) 14:704–13. doi: 10.1038/s41584-018-0097-2
35. Clemente JC, Manasson J, Scher JU. The role of the gut microbiome in systemic inflammatory disease. *BMJ* (2018) 360. doi: 10.1136/bmj.j5145
36. Rosenbaum JT, Lin P, Asquith M. Does the microbiome cause B27-related acute anterior uveitis? *Ocul Immunol Inflammation* (2016) 24:440–4. doi: 10.3109/09273948.2016.1142574
37. Lin P, Bach M, Asquith M, Lee AY, Akileswaran L, Stauffer P, et al. HLA-B27 and Human β2-Microglobulin Affect the Gut Microbiota of Transgenic Rats. *PloS One* (2014) 9. doi: 10.1371/journal.pone.0105684
38. Colmegna I, Cuchacovich R, Espinoza LR. HLA-B27-Associated Reactive Arthritis: Pathogenetic and Clinical Considerations. *Clin Microbiol Rev* (2004) 17:348–69. doi: 10.1128/CMR.17.2.348-369.2004
39. Hoekzema R, Verhagen C, van HM, Kijlstra A. Endotoxin-induced uveitis in the rat. The significance of intraocular interleukin-6. *Invest Ophthalmol Vis Sci* (1992) 33:532–9.
40. Chang JH, Hampartzoumian T, Everett B, Lloyd A, McCluskey PJ, Wakefield D. Changes in Toll-like Receptor (TLR)-2 and TLR4 Expression and Function but Not Polymorphisms Are Associated with Acute Anterior Uveitis. *Invest Ophthalmol Vis Sci* (2007) 48:1711–7. doi: 10.1167/iovs.06-0807
41. Cusick MF, Libbey JE, Fujinami RS. Molecular Mimicry as a Mechanism of Autoimmune Disease. *Clin Rev Allergy Immunol* (2012) 42:102–11. doi: 10.1007/s12016-011-8294-7
42. Luo A, Leach ST, Barres R, Hesson LB, Grimm MC, Simar D. The Microbiota and Epigenetic Regulation of T Helper 17/Regulatory T Cells: In Search of a Balanced Immune System. *Front Immunol* (2017) 8:417. doi: 10.3389/fimmu.2017.00417
43. Bodis G, Toth V, Schwarting A. Role of Human Leukocyte Antigens (HLA) in Autoimmune Diseases. *Rheumatol Ther* (2018) 5:5–20. doi: 10.1007/s40744-018-0100-z
44. Wakefield D, Stahlberg TH, Toivanen A, Granfors K, Tennant C. Serologic evidence of Yersinia infection in patients with anterior uveitis. *Arch Ophthalmol* (1990) 108:219–21. doi: 10.1001/archopht.1990.01070040071033
45. Geczy AF, Alexander K, Bashir HV, Edmonds J. A factor(s) in Klebsiella culture filtrates specifically modifies an HLA-B27 associated cell-surface component. *Nature* (1980) 283:782–4. doi: 10.1038/283782a0
46. Scofield RH, Warren WL, Koelsch G, Harley JB. A hypothesis for the HLA-B27 immune dysregulation in spondyloarthropathy: contributions from enteric organisms, B27 structure, peptides bound by B27, and convergent evolution. *Proc Natl Acad Sci USA* (1993) 90:9330–4. doi: 10.1073/pnas.90.20.9330
47. Amjadi S, Robertson P, McCluskey P, Wakefield D. The role of Chlamydia in HLA-B27 Acute Anterior Uveitis and Seronegative Arthritis Amjadi S, Robertson P, McCluskey PJ, Wakefield D. *Invest Ophthalmol Vis Sci* (2015) 56:1847.
48. Kuon W, Kuhne M, Busch DH, Atagunduz P, Seipel M, Wu P, et al. Identification of novel human aggrecan T cell epitopes in HLA-B27 transgenic mice associated with spondyloarthropathy. *J Immunol* (2004) 173:4859–66. doi: 10.4049/jimmunol.173.8.4859

49. Tsuchiya N, Williams Jr.RC. Molecular mimicry–hypothesis or reality? *West J Med* (1992) 157:133–8.
50. Wen X, Hu X, Miao L, Ge X, Deng Y, Bible PW, et al. Epigenetics, microbiota, and intraocular inflammation: New paradigms of immune regulation in the eye. *Prog Retin Eye Res* (2018) 64:84–95. doi: 10.1016/j.preteyeres.2018.01.001
51. Abu El-Asrar AM, Berghmans N, Al-Obeidan SA, Gikandi PW, Opdenakker G, Van Damme J, et al. The CC chemokines CCL8, CCL13 and CCL20 are local inflammatory biomarkers of HLA-B27-associated uveitis. *Acta Ophthalmol (Copenh)* (2019) 97:e122–8. doi: 10.1111/aos.13835
52. Horai R, Caspi RR. Cytokines in autoimmune uveitis. *J Interferon Cytokine Res* (2011) 31:733–44. doi: 10.1089/jir.2011.0042
53. Kumar A, Sharma SP, Agarwal A, Gupta V, Katoch D, Sehgal S, et al. Tear IL-6 and IL-10 levels in HLA-B27-Associated Uveitis and Its clinical Implications. *Ocul Immunol Inflammation* (2020) 28:1–7. doi: 10.1080/09273948.2019.1704022
54. Abu El-Asrar AM, Berghmans N, Al-Obeidan SA, Mousa A, Opdenakker G, Van Damme J, et al. The Cytokine Interleukin-6 and the Chemokines CCL20 and CXCL13 Are Novel Biomarkers of Specific Endogenous Uveitic Entities. *Invest Ophthalmol Vis Sci* (2016) 57:4606–13. doi: 10.1167/iovs.16-19758
55. Perez VL, Papaliodis GN, Chu D, Anzaar F, Christen W, Foster CS. Elevated levels of interleukin 6 in the vitreous fluid of patients with pars planitis and posterior uveitis: the Massachusetts eye & ear experience and review of previous studies. *Ocul Immunol Inflammation* (2004) 12:193–201. doi: 10.1080/092739490500282
56. Abu El-Asrar AM, Berghmans N, Al-Obeidan SA, Gikandi PW, Opdenakker G, Van Damme J, et al. Local Cytokine Expression Profiling in Patients with Specific Autoimmune Uveitic Entities. *Ocul Immunol Inflammation* (2019) 27:1–10. doi: 10.1080/09273948.2019.1604974
57. Murakami M, Kamimura D, Hirano T. New IL-6 (gp130) family cytokine members, CLC/NNT1/BSF3 and IL-27. *Growth Factors* (2004) 22:75–7. doi: 10.1080/08977190410001715181
58. Zhao B, Zhang S, Chen W, Zhang R, Jiang R, Zhang R, et al. Elevated Interleukin 37 Expression Associated With Disease Activity in HLA-B27 Associated Anterior Uveitis and Idiopathic Anterior Uveitis. *Curr Mol Med* (2018) 17:460–7. doi: 10.2174/1566524018666180207152941
59. Kuon W, Holzhutter HG, Appel H, Grolms M, Kollnberger S, Traeder A, et al. Identification of HLA-B27-restricted peptides from the Chlamydia trachomatis proteome with possible relevance to HLA-B27-associated diseases. *J Immunol* (2001) 167:4738–46. doi: 10.4049/jimmunol.167.8.4738
60. Chan AT, Kollnberger SD, Wedderburn LR, Bowness P. Expansion and enhanced survival of natural killer cells expressing the killer immunoglobulin-like receptor KIR3DL2 in spondylarthritis. *Arthritis Rheum* (2005) 52:3586–95. doi: 10.1002/art.21395
61. Huang JC-C, Schleisman M, Choi D, Mitchell C, Watson L, Asquith M, et al. Preliminary Report on Interleukin-22, GM-CSF, and IL-17F in the Pathogenesis of Acute Anterior Uveitis. *Ocul Immunol Inflammation* (2019) 27:1–8. doi: 10.1080/09273948.2019.1686156
62. Zou W, Wu Z, Xiang X, Sun S, Zhang J. The expression and significance of T helper cell subsets and regulatory T cells CD(4)(+) CD(2)(5)(+) in peripheral blood of patients with human leukocyte antigen B27-positive acute anterior uveitis. *Graefes Arch Clin Exp Ophthalmol* (2014) 252:665–72. doi: 10.1007/s00417-014-2567-9
63. El-Asrar AM, Struyf S, Kangave D, Al-Obeidan SS, Opdenakker G, Geboes K, et al. Cytokine profiles in aqueous humor of patients with different clinical entities of endogenous uveitis. *Clin Immunol* (2011) 139:177–84. doi: 10.1016/j.clim.2011.01.014
64. Kasper M, Walscheid K, Laffer B, Bauer D, Busch M, Wildschütz L, et al. The Phenotype of Monocytes in Anterior Uveitis Depends on the HLA-B27 Status. *Front Immunol* (2018) 9:1773. doi: 10.3389/fimmu.2018.01773
65. Dunn JP. Review of immunosuppressive drug therapy in uveitis. *Curr Opin Ophthalmol* (2004) 15:293–8. doi: 10.1097/00055735-200408000-00003
66. Tripathi RC, Parapuram SK, Tripathi BJ, Zhong Y, Chalam KV. Corticosteroids and glaucoma risk. *Drugs Aging* (1999) 15:439–50. doi: 10.2165/00002512-199915060-00004
67. Sheppard J, Garg S, Lievens C, Brandano L, Wirostko B, Korenfeld M, et al. Iontophoretic Dexamethasone Phosphate Compared to Topical Prednisolone Acetate 1% for Noninfectious Anterior Segment Uveitis. *Am J Ophthalmol* (2020) 211:76–86. doi: 10.1016/j.ajo.2019.10.032
68. Thorne JE, Sugar EA, Holbrook JT, Burke AE, Altaweel MM, Vitale AT, et al. Multicenter Uveitis Steroid Treatment Trial Research Group. Periocular Triamcinolone vs. Intravitreal Triamcinolone vs. Intravitreal Dexamethasone Implant for the Treatment of Uveitic Macular Edema: The PeriOcular vs. INTravitreal corticosteroids for uveitic macular edema (POINT) Trial. *Ophthalmology* (2019) 126:283–95. doi: 10.1016/j.ophtha.2018.08.021
69. Rothova A, Suttorp-van Schulten MS, Frits Treffers W, Kijlstra A. Causes and frequency of blindness in patients with intraocular inflammatory disease. *Br J Ophthalmol* (1996) 80:332–6. doi: 10.1136/bjo.80.4.332
70. Brady CJ, Villanti AC, Law HA, Rahimy E, Reddy R, Sieving PC, et al. Corticosteroid implants for chronic non-infectious uveitis. *Cochrane Database Syst Rev* (2016) 2016(2). doi: 10.1002/14651858.CD010469.pub2
71. Kempen JH, Altaweel MM, Holbrook JT, Sugar EA, Thorne JE, Jabs DA. Association Between Long-Lasting Intravitreous Fluocinolone Acetonide Implant vs Systemic Anti-inflammatory Therapy and Visual Acuity at 7 Years Among Patients With Intermediate, Posterior, or Panuveitis. *JAMA* (2017) 317:1993–2005. doi: 10.1001/jama.2017.5103
72. Gangaputra S, Newcomb CW, Liesegang TL, Kaçmaz RO, Jabs DA, Levy-Clarke GA, et al. Methotrexate for ocular inflammatory diseases. *Ophthalmology* (2009) 116:2188–98.e1. doi: 10.1016/j.ophtha.2009.04.020
73. Daniel E, Thorne JE, Newcomb CW, Pujari SS, Kaçmaz RO, Levy-Clarke GA, et al. Mycophenolate Mofetil for Ocular Inflammation. *Am J Ophthalmol* (2010) 149:423–32. doi: 10.1016/j.ajo.2009.09.026
74. Kaçmaz RO, Kempen JH, Newcomb C, Daniel E, Gangaputra S, Nussenblatt RB, et al. Cyclosporine for Ocular Inflammatory Diseases. *Ophthalmology* (2010) 117:576–84. doi: 10.1016/j.ophtha.2009.08.010
75. Pasadhika S, Kempen JH, Newcomb C, Liesegang TL, Pujari SS, Rosenbaum JT, et al. Azathioprine for Ocular Inflammatory Diseases. *Am J Ophthalmol* (2009) 148:500–9.e2. doi: 10.1016/j.ajo.2009.05.008
76. zu Hoerste MM, Walscheid K, Tappeiner C, Zurek-Imhoff B, Heinz C, Heiligenhaus A. The effect of methotrexate and sulfasalazine on the course of HLA-B27-positive anterior uveitis: results from a retrospective cohort study. *Graefes Arch Clin Exp Ophthalmol* (2018) 256:1985–92. doi: 10.1007/s00417-018-4082-x
77. Dick AD, Duncan L, Hale G, Waldmann H, Isaacs J. Neutralizing TNF-alpha activity modulates T-cell phenotype and function in experimental autoimmune uveoretinitis. *J Autoimmun* (1998) 11:255–64. doi: 10.1006/jaut.1998.0197
78. Dick AD, Forrester JV, Liversidge J, Cope AP. The role of tumour necrosis factor (TNF-alpha) in experimental autoimmune uveoretinitis (EAU). *Prog Retin Eye Res* (2004) 23:617–37. doi: 10.1016/j.preteyeres.2004.06.005
79. Khera TK, Dick AD, Nicholson LB. Mechanisms of TNFα regulation in uveitis: focus on RNA-binding proteins. *Prog Retin Eye Res* (2010) 29:610–21. doi: 10.1016/j.preteyeres.2010.08.003
80. Giraudo E, Primo L, Audero E, Gerber HP, Koolwijk P, Soker S, et al. Tumor necrosis factor-alpha regulates expression of vascular endothelial growth factor receptor-2 and of its co-receptor neuropilin-1 in human vascular endothelial cells. *J Biol Chem* (1998) 273:22128–35. doi: 10.1074/jbc.273.34.22128
81. Braun J, Baraliakos X, Listing J, Sieper J. Decreased incidence of anterior uveitis in patients with ankylosing spondylitis treated with the anti-tumor necrosis factor agents infliximab and etanercept. *Arthritis Rheum* (2005) 52:2447–51. doi: 10.1002/art.21197
82. Rudwaleit M, Rødevand E, Holck P, Vanhoof J, Kron M, Kary S, et al. Adalimumab effectively reduces the rate of anterior uveitis flares in patients with active ankylosing spondylitis: results of a prospective open-label study. *Ann Rheum Dis* (2008) 68:696–701. doi: 10.1136/ard.2008.092585
83. Guignard S, Gossec L, Salliot C, Ruyssen-Witrand A, Luc M, Duclos M, et al. Efficacy of tumour necrosis factor blockers in reducing uveitis flares in patients with spondylarthropathy: a retrospective study. *Ann Rheum Dis* (2006) 65:1631–4. doi: 10.1136/ard.2006.052092
84. Reddy AR, Backhouse OC. Does etanercept induce uveitis? *Br J Ophthalmol* (2003) 87:925. doi: 10.1136/bjo.87.7.925
85. Lie E, Lindström U, Zverkova-Sandström T, Olsen IC, Forsblad-d'Elia H, Askling J, et al. Tumour necrosis factor inhibitor treatment and occurrence of anterior uveitis in ankylosing spondylitis: results from the Swedish biologics register. *Ann Rheum Dis* (2017) 76:1515–21. doi: 10.1136/annrheumdis-2016-210931
86. El-Shabrawi Y, Hermann J. Anti-tumor necrosis factor-alpha therapy with infliximab as an alternative to corticosteroids in the treatment of human

leukocyte antigen B27-associated acute anterior uveitis. *Ophthalmology* (2002) 109:2342–6. doi: 10.1016/s0161-6420(02)01292-7

87. Yazgan S, Celik U, Işık M, Yeşil NK, Baki AE, Şahin H, et al. Efficacy of golimumab on recurrent uveitis in HLA-B27-positive ankylosing spondylitis. *Int Ophthalmol* (2017) 37:139–45. doi: 10.1007/s10792-016-0239-y
88. Llorenç V, Mesquida M, de la Maza MS, Blanco R, Calvo V, Maíz O, et al. Certolizumab Pegol, a New Anti-TNF-α in the Armamentarium against Ocular Inflammation. *Ocul Immunol Inflammation* (2016) 24:167–72. doi: 10.3109/09273948.2014.967779
89. Hiltunen J. *The Role of Gut Microbiota in the Pathogenesis of Ankylosing Spondylitis (AS), and the Effect of Fecal Microbiota Transplantation on Gut Microbiota, Gut Wall Inflammation and Clinical Activity of AS. clinicaltrials.gov* (2019). Available at: https://clinicaltrials.gov/ct2/show/NCT03726645 (Accessed November 5, 2020).
90. Jabs DA, Nussenblatt RB, Rosenbaum JT. Standardization of Uveitis Nomenclature (SUN) Working Group. Standardization of uveitis nomenclature for reporting clinical data. Results of the First International Workshop. *Am J Ophthalmol* (2005) 140:509–16. doi: 10.1016/j.ajo.2005.03.057
91. Park SC, Ham D-I. Clinical Features and Prognosis of HLA-B27 Positive and Negative Anterior Uveitis in a Korean Population. *J Korean Med Sci* (2009) 24:722–8. doi: 10.3346/jkms.2009.24.4.722
92. Barisani-Asenbauer T, Maca SM, Mejdoubi L, Emminger W, Machold K, Auer H. Uveitis- a rare disease often associated with systemic diseases and infections- a systematic review of 2619 patients. *Orphanet J Rare Dis* (2012) 7:57. doi: 10.1186/1750-1172-7-57

12

Molecular Mimicry and Uveitis

*Gerhild Wildner** *and Maria Diedrichs-Möhring*

Section of Immunobiology, Department of Ophthalmology, University Hospital, LMU Munich, München, Germany

Correspondence:
Gerhild Wildner
gerhild.wildner@med.uni-muenchen.de

Molecular or antigenic mimicry is a term for the similarity of different antigens, which can be confused by the immune system. Antigen recognition by antibodies and T cell receptors is specific, but not restricted to a single antigen. Both types of receptors specifically recognize antigens and are expressed with a very high but still restricted variability compared to the number of different antigens they potentially could bind. T cell receptors only can bind to antigen peptides presented on certain self-MHC-molecules by screening only some amino acid side chains on both the presented peptides and the MHC molecule. The other amino acids of the peptide are not directly perceived by the T cell, offering the opportunity for a single T cell to recognize a variety of different antigens with the same receptor, which significantly increases the immune repertoire. The immune system is usually tolerant to autoantigens, especially to those of immune privileged sites, like the eye. Therefore, autoimmune diseases targeting these organs were hard to explain, unless a T cell is activated by an environmental peptide (e.g. pathogen) that is similar, but not necessarily identical with an autoantigen. Here we describe antigenic mimicry of retinal autoantigens with a variety of non-ocular antigens resulting in the induction of intraocular inflammation. T cells that are activated by mimotopes outside of the eye can pass the blood-retina barrier and enter ocular tissues. When reactivated in the eye by crossreaction with autoantigens they induce uveitis by recruiting inflammatory cells.

Keywords: autoimmune disease, T cells, HLA, tolerance, nutritional antigens, microbiome, intraocular inflammation, pathogens

INTRODUCTION

The inner eye as an immune privileged site is rarely affected by inflammation. Autoimmune uveitis with a frequency of 0.2% is an uncommon autoimmune diseases. The immune privilege is usually maintained by a number of mechanisms including anterior chamber-associated immune deviation, protective surfaces of intraocular cells, suppressive factors and the blood-retina-barrier (BRB) (1). The latter is impermeable for large molecules such as antibodies and non-activated lymphocytes, sequestering unique intraocular autoantigens from the immune system (2). Therefore, autoimmunity to intraocular antigens was initially hard to explain. Only previously activated lymphocytes are able to pass tissue barriers to screen tissues for potential hidden pathogens and tumor cells. An activation of lymphocytes to retinal autoantigens is only possible in the case of ocular trauma destroying the protective vascular barriers, the premise for the pathogenesis of sympathetic ophthalmia (3). In this condition injury to one eye allows local activation of T cells, which are then enabled to enter the partner eye to initiate a destructive autoimmune response. This is a very rare event. Usually intraocular inflammation occurs without any injury to the eye.

Therefore, autoimmunity to intraocular antigens must be initiated by activated T cells, which had their primary antigen contact outside of the eye. This antigen is not an intraocular, but rather a similar, crossreactive extraocular or environmental antigen. This phenomenon of "antigenic mimicry" is postulated to be the initiating event of most autoimmune diseases, and we and others have described a series of molecules and epitopes from pathogens (bacteria, viruses, fungi, parasites) and some harmless nutritional molecules (bovine milk casein) that can serve as primary activating antigens for subsequent induction of uveitis (4–7). Antigenic mimicry leading to crossreactive T cell recognition is based on the manner of antigen peptide recognition by T cell receptors: the receptor molecule does not screen each amino acid side chains of a peptide but only a few amino acids, therefore many different peptides with similar amino acids at a certain position are sufficient for the activation of the receptor (**Figure 1**) (8, 9). This is a pivotal way to increase the repertoire of antigen recognition with a restricted number of receptors, which is desirable for the defense against pathogens, but less

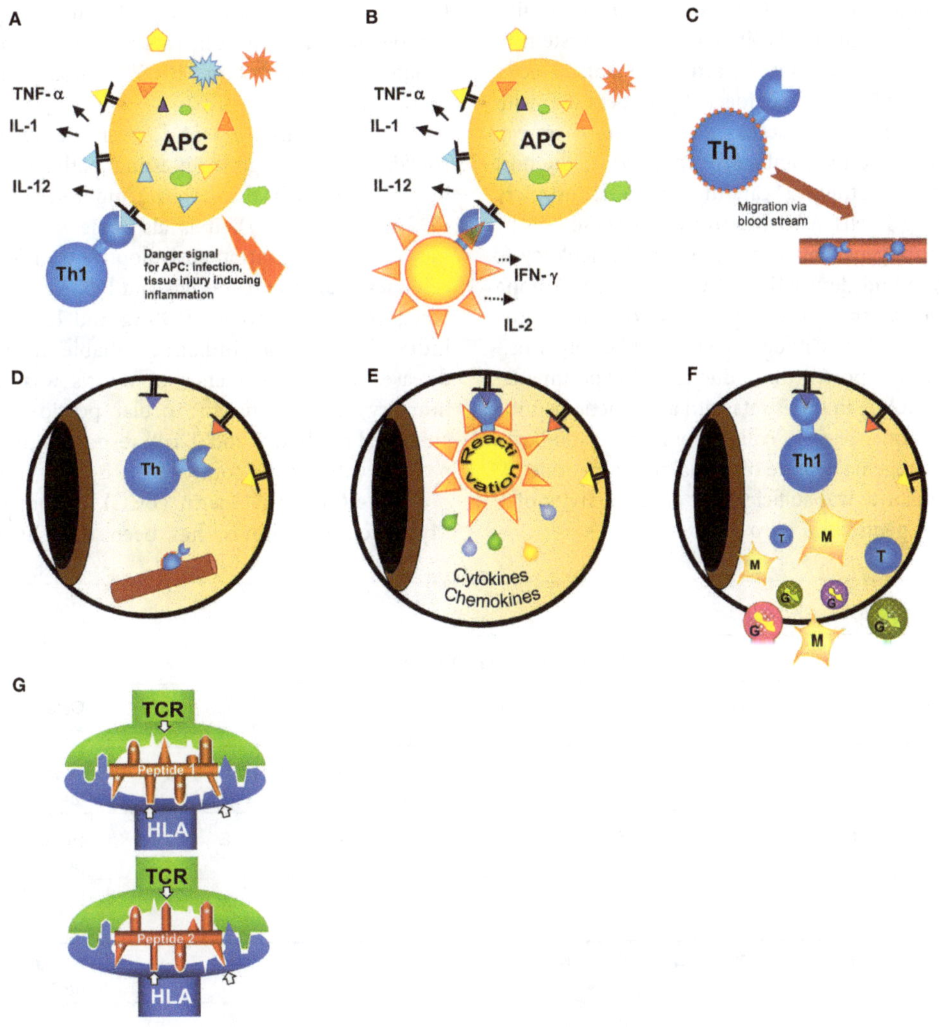

FIGURE 1 | Hypothesis of the induction of a T cell mimicry response leading to ocular autoimmunity. **(A)** Outside of the eye in the body (gut)?: A naive T cell has first contact with a non-eye-related antigen. In case of a concomitant danger signal (injury of the tissue, infection) innate antigen-presenting cells (APCs) are activated to induce effector T cell responses. **(B)** The antigen recognized by the T cell can either be from a pathogen [from infection or a food antigen, see **(A)**]. If the T cell recognizes harmless food antigen and erroneously receives concomitant activation signals from the APC alerted by danger signals the T cell gets activated and differentiates into a T helper (e.g. here: Th1) cell. **(C)** Activated T cells migrate in the blood circulation. In search of their antigen they can leave the blood vessels and enter even immune privileged organs like the eye. **(D)** The triangles represent retinal autoantigen peptides presented on MHC class II. The precise signals of attracting a T cell to a certain organ at a certain site (blood vessel) are still unknown. **(E)** When the T cell has screened the eye and found an antigen binding to its receptor, it gets reactivated and secretes cytokines and chemokines to recruit inflammatory cells. The intraocular antigen is different to the antigen of the original T cell priming outside of the eye. **(F)** Innate cells (monocytes/macrophages and/or granulocytes) recruited from the circulation are causing inflammation and tissue destruction resulting in uveitis. **(G)** Two different peptides presented and recognized by the same HLA molecule and T cell receptor (TCR), despite their restricted homologies. Only the core sequence of 8 amino acids presented in the groove is shown. Identical amino acid side chains are marked by white asterisks, the arrows point to similar side chains representing different amino acids also anchoring to the presenting HLA-molecule or being bound by the TCR.

appreciated when antigens from pathogens and autoantigens are confused. Antigenic mimicry exists for T cell as well as antibody recognition (10), here we are focusing on mimicry and T cell responses.

MIMOTOPES OF RETINAL AUTOANTIGENS

Environmental Pathogens and Harmless Microbes

In contrast to autoantigens, infections with pathogens, like viruses or bacteria, alert cells of the innate immune system to initiate an adaptive immune response by activating B and T cells. If these pathogens accidentally provide antigen peptides with similarity to autoantigens, crossreactive immune responses can lead to an attack focused on self-antigens expressed by the host tissue. Molecules from pathogens can thus serve as mimicry molecules and activate T cells. After reactivation of these cells by crossreactive ocular antigens they recruit non-specific leukocytes causing inflammation and destruction of ocular tissue. Among these microbial mimicry candidates are proteins from microbiota like E. coli or yeast as well as pathogenic viruses like rotavirus.

In 1989 Singh et al. reported the induction of experimental autoimmune uveitis (EAU) in Lewis rats with a synthetic peptide corresponding to a sequence of E. coli protein and a similarity with 6 aa from a uveitogenic peptide of retinal S-Ag (peptide M, aa303-320). This similarity was sufficient for crossreactivity of T lymphocytes to these peptides *in vitro* (11).

A synthetic peptide from yeast Histone 3 with a sequence homology of 5 N-terminal amino acids with peptide M was also uveitogenic in rats in a dose-dependent manner and induced similar ocular damage/inflammation as the retinal autoantigen S-Ag or its Peptide M. This mimicry was confirmed by the adoptive transfer of T cells specific for the yeast histone 3 peptide that induced EAU as well (4, 5, 12).

In the follow up a series of peptides were identified with homology to retinal S-Ag, including peptides from Hepatitis B virus, Baboon virus, murine leukemia virus, murine sarcoma virus or potato proteinase IIa. They all induced signs of EAU in Lewis rats upon immunization, but in some cases very high doses (up to 2 mg/rat) were needed. These peptides, defined as pathogenic mimotopes in rats were also capable of inducing a proliferating response in PBMC isolated from S-Ag-immunized monkeys (13).

We showed that a peptide from the outer capsid protein of rotavirus (Rota), a gastrointestinal pathogen, shares amino acid homologies with the uveitogenic retinal S-antigen peptide PDSAg (aa 341-354). It is also able to induce EAU in Lewis rats after immunization and adoptive transfer of Rota-specific T cell lines (**Table 1**) (6). Rota- and PDSAg-specific rat T cell lines recognize both peptides, PDSAg and Rota, respectively. Rota-induced EAU was indistinguishable from PDSAg-induced disease, but the incidence of uveitis was reduced. Antigenic mimicry of rotavirus and ocular peptide was also shown by enhanced antibody- and T cell responses to both antigens from patients with uveitis compared to healthy individuals (6).

Bacille-Calmette-Guérin (BCG), a nonpathogenic strain of Mycobacterium bovis, has been used as a vaccine against

TABLE 1 | Mimotopes of retinal autoantigen in uveitis.

Source	Amino acid sequence of peptide/epitope															Protein
Rotavirus				W	T	E	V	S	E	V	A	T	E	V		Outer capsid protein aa 591-601 (peptide Rota)
Bovine milk				S	E	E	S	A	E	V	A	T	E	E	V	Bovine αs2-casein aa 73-84 (peptide Cas)
Retinal autoantigen	**F**	**L**	**G**	**E**	**L**	**T**	**S**	**S**	**E**	**V**	**A**	**T**	**E**	**V**		**Human retinal S-Ag, peptide PDSAg aa 341-354**
HLA-B	A	L	N	E	D	L	S	S	W	T	A	A	**D**	T		HLA-B, α1 domain aa 125-138 (peptide B27PD)
Retinal autoantigen	**V**	**T**	**I**	**Y**	**L**	**G**	**N**									**Human retinal S-Ag aa 26-32**
M. bovis (BCG)	V	T	I	Y	L	G	N									Invasion protein aa 433-439
Retinal autoantigen	**V**	**G**	**T**	**P**	**A**	**E**	**Q**	**A**								**Human IRBP aa 304-311**
M. bovis (BCG)	V	G	T	P	A	E	V	A								MabA protein aa 231-238
Retinal autoantigen	**D**	**G**	**S**	**S**	**W**	**E**	**G**									**Human IRBP, peptide R14 aa 1200-1206**
M. bovis (BCG)	D	G	S	S	W	D	G									Membrane acyltransferase aa 173-179
Retinal autoantigen	**D**	**S**	**L**	**S**	**P**	**E**	**A**									**Human CRALBP aa 129-135**
M. bovis (BCG)	D	S	L	S	P	E	A									Polyketide synthase aa 997-1003

S-Ag, retinal soluble antigen; IRBP, interphotoreceptor retinoid-binding protein; CRALBP, cellular retinaldehyde-binding protein, M. bovis, Mycobacterium bovis. Amino acids identical with the sequence of the retinal autoantigen are marked by grey fields.

tuberculosis and as treatment for bladder carcinoma. Uveitis is a known, but rare potential side effect, although BCG does not infect the eye. We therefore postulated antigenic mimicry of BCG proteins with ocular autoantigens to explain ocular inflammation, since we could show that peripheral blood lymphocytes (PBL) from a 70 year old patient, who developed uveitis for the first time after the third cycle of BCG-treatment within 3 years for bladder carcinoma, responded to PPD (purified protein derivative of M. tuberculosis) as well as various ocular proteins and peptides with proliferation and secretion of cytokines including IFN-γ, IL-6, IL-8, TNF-α and MCP-1. T cells clones to directly test crossreactivity were not available from this patient. A data base search identified sequence homologies of several potential epitopes of M. tuberculosis proteins with retinal autoantigens like S-Ag, interphotoreceptor retinoid-binding protein (IRBP) and cellular retinal-binding-protein (cRALBP), suggesting antigenic mimicry (**Table 1**) (7).

In transgenic as well as in "classic" murine EAU models Horai et al. have demonstrated that commensal bacteria in the gut may contribute to ocular autoimmunity through a molecular mimicry mechanism. Alteration of the gut microbiota may contribute to ocular autoimmunity at several stages: (1) innate microbial stimuli, (2) loss of distinct microbiota producing anti-inflammatory stimuli, (3) presence of pathogenic bacteria disturbing the intestinal barrier and secreting inflammatory mediators, (4) and mimicry of microbiota proteins with autoantigens (14–17). Antigenic mimicry of heat shock proteins (hsp) from gut microbiota and hsp expressed by retinal ganglion cells and axons as a stress response to elevated intraocular pressure has recently been described as a potential cause of chronic progressive destruction of neuronal cells in normal tension glaucoma. The pathogenesis of chronic, low-grade autoreactive T cell responses initiated in the gut and finally acting in the eye is similar to that postulated for autoimmune uveitis (18).

In addition, antigenic mimicry between ocular antigens and antigens derived from (commensal) bacteria, yeast, viruses and parasites might lead to the activation of pathogenic autoreactive immune responses. Subsequent ocular inflammation after infection with Onchocerca volvulus has been proposed as antigenic mimicry between worm proteins and ocular autoantigens; immunization of Lewis rats with recombinant protein (Ov39) from Onchocerca volvulus caused ocular inflammation, and T cells from Ov39-immunized rats responded to an ocular protein (hr44) *in vitro*. The pathogenicity of Ov39-specific T cells was confirmed by adoptive transfer experiments (19).

Mimicry of Food Antigens

Like the eye, the gut is a tissue with a strong ability to induce tolerance. Soluble protein antigens, for example from food, without providing PAMPs (pathogen-associated molecular pattern) to activate TLR (Toll like receptors) or inflammasomes, usually induce tolerance when they get access to cells of the immune system in submucosal tissues. This phenomenon is called "mucosal tolerance" or "oral tolerance" (20, 21). Oral tolerance is effective systemically. Regulatory T cells induced in the gut are screening the body systemically and prevent activation of effector cells to nutritional antigen. This is necessary, because food proteins are foreign molecules that might not be completely digested to the level of amino acids before being absorbed. As entire intact proteins they could induce adverse systemic immune reactions. Failure of oral tolerance induction could result in food allergies, but in general this mechanism is very reliable and therefore immune reactions to nutritional proteins are rare events, also when the food proteins are mimicking antigens from pathogens or autoantigens. Antigenic mimicry of food antigens and antigens from infectious agents has been described for antibody binding, Vodjani for example demonstrated antibody crossreactivities between Borrelia burgdorferi, Epstein-Barr-virus and rotavirus and a variety of different food antigens, likely induced by the pathogens, but without clinical consequences (22).

We had previously shown antigenic mimicry of a peptide from bovine milk casein (Cas) and peptide PDSAg from retinal S-Antigen (6) (**Table 1**). We found increased antibody responses to Cas and PDSAg in sera of patients with uveitis compared to healthy individuals, as well as increased T cell responses among PBL of such patients. However, mimicry could not be proven on the level of a single TCR recognizing both mimotopes on the same MHC molecule. Moreover, we could induce experimental uveitis in Lewis rats after immunization with peptide Cas and also transfer disease by Cas-specific T cells. The primary natural contact of the immune system with Cas, as well as with the peptide from Rotavirus (see above), would be in the gut, therefore we have tried to induce uveitis by oral antigen application together with Cholera toxin as Th1-shifting gastrointestinal adjuvant (6). In contrast to the peptides, only the casein protein or bovine milk was able to induce uveitis *via* the oral challenge. Cas-specific rat T cell lines recognize peptide PDSAg and also the peptide from Rotavirus, and Cas is recognized by PDSAg- as well as Rota-specific T cells.

Normally, a nutritional protein like bovine milk casein should not induce an adverse immune reaction, unless it is accidentally presented in an inflammatory environment, such as during a gastrointestinal infection breaking oral tolerance. On the other hand, bovine milk casein is the typical nutrition of a calf, which has no oral tolerance mechanisms and is a food allergen for human infants, probably having some characteristics to induce immune defense and effector rather than regulatory T cells in humans. Moreover, we have failed to induce oral tolerance with peptide Cas and also with peptide Rota from rotavirus to prevent PDSAg-induced uveitis, while the autoantigen PDSAg itself is a very strong oral tolerogen (6, 23).

Self-Antigens Mimicking Autoantigens

Since antigenic mimicry is only dependent on similar antigenic peptides to induce crossreactive immune responses also the body's own antigens can mimic each other. Self-antigens usually do not provide "danger" signals to initiate innate and immune effector responses, so they should induce tolerance. We have shown antigenic mimicry of the retinal S-Antigen peptide PDSAg (human S-Ag, aa341-352, FLGELTSSEVATEV) and an oligomorphic peptide from the first domain of HLA-B antigens (B27PD, aa125-138, ALNEDLSSWTAADT) (**Table 1**). This peptide was originally thought to be specific for the amino acid sequence of HLA-B27 and thus regarded as an explanation for the strong HLA-class I-B27-association with anterior uveitis, despite the dominant role of HLA-class II-restricted T-helper cells in uveitis (24). Later it turned out that the sequence represented by peptide B27PD is found in the first domain of most HLA-B-molecules and thus not specific for HLA-B27. The consequence was that most patients with uveitis bear at least one HLA-B molecule with the sequence of B27PD. Therefore, we hypothesized that this peptide could represent a key mimotope for most types of uveitis. In fact, lymph node cells from PDSAg-immunized Lewis rats as well as lymphocytes from patients with uveitis showed crossreactivity to both, PDSAg and B27PD, in proliferation assays *in vitro*. However, the HLA-peptide B27PD was only marginally pathogenic after immunization in rat EAU. In contrast, the HLA-peptide B27PD was highly tolerogenic when applied orally to rats prior to induction of uveitis with S-Ag or peptide PDSAg (oral tolerance).

Surprisingly, in rat EAU the oral tolerance-inducing mimotopes were recognized by $\gamma\delta^+$T cell receptors and not by $\alpha\beta^+$T cells that induce the disease (25). We have shown this by adoptive transfer of tolerance to PDSAg-induced EAU with $CD8^+\gamma\delta^+$T cells from rats fed with either peptide PDSAg itself or with the mimotope B27PD. Moreover, we have demonstrated the *in vitro*-proliferation of orally induced $\gamma\delta^+$T cells in response to their tolerogen or the respective mimicry peptide. In this case, the $\alpha\beta^+TCR^+$ effector T cells served as antigen-presenting cells, and the proliferation of the $CD8^+TCR\text{-}\gamma\delta^+$ cells was impeded by the addition of antibodies blocking the peptide-restricted MHC class II-molecule as well as by antibodies blocking CD8 (25, 26).

These findings favored a new hypothesis for natural self-tolerance in the gut, maintained by constant shedding and processing of HLA-molecules from intestinal epithelial cells (e.g. HLA-B molecules with the sequence of B27PD) and inducing mucosal tolerance to self-HLA molecules. This tolerance might be promoted and specified by additional oral application of the peptide B27PD with crossreactivity to the retinal autoantigen, thus leading to therapeutic tolerance in uveitis (27, 28).

Peptides from any self protein, including HLA, can be presented on HLA-molecules and might serve as a constant trigger of self-tolerance for the immune system. Immunomodulatory properties of peptides derived from the sequence of HLA-molecules have also been described by others (29). Due to its high tolerogenic potency and a lack of pathogenicity the peptide B27PD was successfully used as an oral tolerogen for patients with uveitis in a phase 1 therapeutic trial (30–32). However, a following placebo-controlled phase I/II trial with this oral peptide did lack efficacy and was completed early (clinicaltrials.gov-identifier NCT01195948, September 7, 2020).

DISCUSSION

Low-affinity self-reactive T cells are found in the body where these autoreactive T cells are normally controlled. These pre-existing, self-reactive T cells can be activated in response to similar antigens from environmental microbes and/or food and become pathogenic under certain circumstances.

Molecular mimicry of environmental antigens in conjunction with the ability of T cells to escape immune tolerance has been suggested as a potential mechanism for the pathogenesis not only of autoimmune uveitis but also of other autoimmune diseases, including: multiple sclerosis, diabetes mellitus and spondylarthropathies (10).

Retinal autoantigens are sequestered behind the BRB (1, 2) and therefore normally invisible for naïve T cells. Since only activated T-lymphocytes can pass the BRB and enter the eye their primary activation must be extraocular.

The activation of pattern recognition receptors (PRR) by pathogens is a prerequisite for the initiation of an immune response, however, this is lacking for usually tolerizing food proteins. In that situation we proposed a concomitant infection with the presentation of the food antigen (33), leading to an erroneous bystander activation of effector T cells instead of (oral) tolerance induction. For example to orally induce EAU with milk casein we used Cholera toxin for the activation of PRR in the gut-associated lymphoid tissue (GALT) (34).

Interestingly, in addition to peripheral activation, which enables the T cells to pass the BRB, the barrier itself and the passage of the T cells through the barrier seemed to be essential for the pathogenicity of the T cells, since intravitreal injection of autoreactive T cells does not cause inflammation (35).

Autoimmune uveitis is mediated by $CD4^+$Th cells which recognized peptide presented on MHC class II molecules. For an antigen recognition the minimum prerequisite is the binding of the antigen peptide to the presenting MHC molecule and the subsequent recognition of this complex by a TCR. Crossreactivity of antigen peptides could be observed either with partially overlapping consecutive amino acid sequences, identities between ocular antigens and viral or bacterial proteins (4, 5, 11–13, 36) or by discontinuous sequence homologies with amino acids at respective positions to anchor the peptide to the MHC and also to bind to the TCR (6) (**Figure 1**). The interactions between antigen peptides, presenting MHC and TCR are based on charges of amino acid side chains, hydrogen bonds and complementary structures. Even a peptide with structural homology but not sharing identical/similar amino acids can be sufficient for antigenic mimicry (10, 37), thus complicating the search and definition of mimotopes.

While Wucherpfennig and Strominger could demonstrate antigenic mimicry with similar peptides at the clonal level of T cells (38), a certain T cell might also express a second T cell receptor, one recognizing a foreign peptide and the other a self peptide (39, 40). We have shown a cross-reactivity on the T cell population level (41), but we could not prove the use of a certain single T cell receptor to crossreact with peptides PDSAg, Rota and Cas (unpublished). In that case, we might not have a single T cell receptor recognizing all three peptides, but perhaps several T cells crossreacting with two of the mimotopes, finally resulting in crossreactivity to all three peptides on the population level of T cell lines.

Most peptide mimics were defined for retinal S-Ag in animal models and in humans (5, 6, 11–13, 24, 36). We have demonstrated the proliferative response and cytokine secretion to several ocular autoantigens (IRBP, S-Ag, cRALBP) of PBL from a patient experiencing uveitis as an adverse event after BCG-treatment. Whether this rarely observed recognition of multiple retinal autoantigens is due to mimicry of multiple mycobacterial antigens and several autoantigens or just a broad autoimmune response developing over time by epitope spreading cannot be ascertained (7). Both, intramolecular as well as intermolecular epitope spreading has been described in experimental models of uveitis (42–44).

Autoreactive lymphocytes are not only found in the peripheral blood of patients with autoimmune diseases but also in healthy people (45, 46), indicating that further conditions are required for pathogenicity. We assume that in addition to the presence of autoreactive T cells the target organ itself contributes to the initiation and maintenance of uveitis. In the eye the autoantigen must be expressed and properly processed and presented by local antigen-presenting cells to reactivate immigrating T cells with a corresponding receptor followed by the recuitment of inflammatory cells that finally cause destruction of ocular tissues (18, 47).

AUTHOR CONTRIBUTIONS

GW: Writing the manuscript, design of the figure MD-M: writing the manuscript. All authors contributed to the article and approved the submitted version.

ACKNOWLEDGMENTS

We thank Denis Wakefield and Stephan Thurau for critically reading the manuscript.

REFERENCES

1. Streilein JW. Ocular immune privilege: the eye takes a dim but practical view of immunity and inflammation. *J Leukocyte Biol* (2003) 74(2):179–85. doi: 10.1189/jlb.1102574
2. Shechter R, London A, Schwartz M. Orchestrated leukocyte recruitment to immune-privileged sites: absolute barriers versus educational gates. *Nat Rev Immunol* (2013) 13(3):206–18. doi: 10.1038/nri3391
3. Chu XK, Chan C-C. Sympathetic ophthalmia: to the twenty-first century and beyond. *J Ophthalmic Inflammation Infect* (2013) 3(1):49–. doi: 10.1186/1869-5760-3-49
4. Shinohara T, Singh VK, Tsuda M, Yamaki K, Abe T, Suzuki S. S-antigen: from gene to autoimmune uveitis. *Exp Eye Res* (1990) 50(6):751–7. doi: 10.1016/0014-4835(90)90125-E
5. Shinohara T, Singh VK, Yamaki K, Abe T, Tsuda M, Suzuki S. S-antigen: molecular mimicry may play a role in autoimmune uveitis. *Prog Clin Biol Res* (1991) 362:163–90. Issn: 0361-7742. doi: 10.1002/eji.1830241103
6. Wildner G, Diedrichs-Möhring M. Autoimmune uveitis induced by molecular mimicry of peptides from rotavirus, bovine casein and retinal S-antigen. *Eur J Immunol* (2003) 33(9):2577–87. doi: 10.1002/eji.200324058
7. Garip A, Diedrichs-Mohring M, Thurau SR, Deeg CA, Wildner G. Uveitis in a patient treated with Bacille-Calmette-Guerin: possible antigenic mimicry of mycobacterial and retinal antigens. *Ophthalmology* (2009) 116(12):2457–62.e1-2. doi: 10.1016/j.ophtha.2009.05.021
8. Daniel C, Horvath S, Allen PM. A Basis for Alloreactivity: MHC Helical Residues Broaden Peptide Recognition by the TCR. *Immunity* (1998) 8 (5):543–52. doi: 10.1016/S1074-7613(00)80559-2
9. Sundberg EJ, Deng L, Mariuzza RA. TCR recognition of peptide/MHC class II complexes and superantigens. *Semin Immunol* (2007) 19(4):262–71. doi: 10.1016/j.smim.2007.04.006
10. Oldstone MBA. Molecular mimicry and immune-mediated diseases. *FASEB J* (1998) 12(13):1255–65. doi: 10.1096/fasebj.12.13.1255
11. Singh VK, Yamaki K, Abe T, Shinohara T. Molecular mimicry between uveitopathogenic site of retinal S-antigen and Escherichia coli protein: induction of experimental autoimmune uveitis and lymphocyte cross-reaction. *Cell Immunol* (1989) 122(1):262–73. doi: 10.1016/0008-8749(89)90166-4
12. Singh VK, Yamaki K, Donoso LA, Shinohara T. Sequence homology between yeast histone H3 and uveitopathogenic site of S-antigen: lymphocyte cross-reaction and adoptive transfer of the disease. *Cell Immunol* (1989) 119(1):211–21. doi: 10.1016/0008-8749(89)90237-2
13. Singh VK, Kalra HK, Yamaki K, Abe T, Donoso LA, Shinohara T. Molecular mimicry between a uveitopathogenic site of S-antigen and viral peptides. Induction of experimental autoimmune uveitis in Lewis rats. *J Immunol (Baltimore Md 1950)* (1990) 144(4):1282–7.
14. Horai R, Zárate-Bladés CR, Dillenburg-Pilla P, Chen J, Kielczewski JL, Silver PB, et al. Microbiota-dependent activation of an autoreactive T cell receptor provokes autoimmunity in an immunologically privileged site. *Immunity* (2015) 43(2):343–53. doi: 10.1016/j.immuni.2015.07.014
15. Zárate-Bladés CR, Horai R, Caspi RR. Regulation of Autoimmunity by the Microbiome. *DNA Cell Biol* (2016) 35(9):455–8. doi: 10.1089/dna.2016.3432
16. Zárate-Bladés CR, Horai R, Mattapallil MJ, Ajami NJ, Wong M, Petrosino JF, et al. Gut microbiota as a source of a surrogate antigen that triggers autoimmunity in an immune privileged site. *Gut Microbes* (2017) 8(1):59–66. doi: 10.1080/19490976.2016.1273996
17. Horai R, Sen HN, Caspi RR. Commensal microbiota as a potential trigger of autoimmune uveitis. *Expert Rev Clin Immunol* (2017) 13(4):291–3. doi: 10.1080/1744666X.2017.1288098
18. Chen H, Cho K-S, Vu THK, Shen C-H, Kaur M, Chen G, et al. Commensal microflora-induced T cell responses mediate progressive neurodegeneration in glaucoma. *Nat Commun* (2018) 9(1):3209. doi: 10.1038/s41467-018-06428-2
19. McKechnie NM, Gurr W, Yamada H, Copland D, Braun G. Antigenic mimicry: Onchocerca volvulus antigen-specific T cells and ocular inflammation. *Invest Ophthalmol Visual Sci* (2002) 43(2):411–8.
20. von Boehmer H. Oral tolerance: is it all retinoic acid? *J Exp Med* (2007) 204 (8):1737–9. doi: 10.1084/jem.20071251
21. Weiner HL, da Cunha AP, Quintana F, Wu H. Oral tolerance. *Immunol Rev* (2011) 241(1):241–59. doi: 10.1111/j.1600-065X.2011.01017.x
22. Vodjani A. Reaction of Monoclonal and Polyclonal Antibodies Made against Infectious Agents with Various Food Antigens. *J Clin Cell Immunol* (2015) 6:359. doi: 10.4172/2155-9899.1000359
23. Wildner G, Diedrichs-Möhring M. Autoimmune uveitis and antigenic mimicry of environmental antigens. *Autoimmun Rev* (2004) 3(5):383–7. doi: 10.1016/j.autrev.2004.01.002
24. Wildner G, Thurau SR. Cross-reactivity between an HLA-B27-derived peptide and a retinal autoantigen peptide: a clue to major histocompatibility complex association with autoimmune disease. *Eur J Immunol* (1994) 24(11):2579–85. doi: 10.1002/eji.1830241103
25. Wildner G, Hunig T, Thurau SR. Orally induced, peptide-specific gamma/delta TCR+ cells suppress experimental autoimmune uveitis. *Eur J Immunol* (1996) 26(9):2140–8. doi: 10.1002/eji.1830260927
26. Wildner G, Thurau SR, Diedrichs-Möhring M. Gamma-delta T cells as orally induced suppressor cells in rats: in vitro characterization. *Ann New Y Acad Sci* (2004) 1029:416–21. doi: 10.1196/annals.1309.050
27. Thurau SR, Wildner G. An HLA-peptide mimics organ-specific antigen in autoimmune uveitis: its role in pathogenesis and therapeutic induction of oral tolerance. *Autoimmun Rev* (2003) 2(4):171–6. doi: 10.1016/S1568-9972(03)00011-9
28. Mannie MD, DeOca KB, Bastian AG, Moorman CD. Tolerogenic vaccines: Targeting the antigenic and cytokine niches of FOXP3+ regulatory T cells. *Cell Immunol* (2020) 355:104173. doi: 10.1016/j.cellimm.2020.104173
29. Clayberger C, Krensky AM. Immunosuppressive peptides corresponding to MHC class I sequences. *Curr Opin Immunol* (1995) 7(5):644–8. doi: 10.1016/0952-7915(95)80071-9

30. Thurau SR, Diedrichs Mohring M, Fricke H, Burchardi C, Wildner G. Oral tolerance with an HLA-peptide mimicking retinal autoantigen as a treatment of autoimmune uveitis. *Immunol Lett* (1999) 68(2-3):205–12. doi: 10.1016/S0165-2478(99)00071-1
31. Thurau SR, Diedrichs-Möhring M, Fricke H, Arbogast S, Wildner G. Molecular mimicry as a therapeutic approach for an autoimmune disease: oral treatment of uveitis-patients with an MHC-peptide crossreactive with autoantigen–first results. *Immunol Lett* (1997) 57(1-3):193–201. doi: 10.1016/S0165-2478(97)00058-8
32. Thurau SR, Fricke H, Burchardi C, Diedrichs-Mohring M, Wildner G. Long-term follow-up of oral tolerance induction with HLA-peptide B27PD in patients with uveitis. *Ann New Y Acad Sci* (2004) 1029:408–12. doi: 10.1196/annals.1309.048
33. Voigt V, Wikstrom ME, Kezic JM, Schuster IS, Fleming P, Makinen K, et al. Ocular antigen does not cause disease unless presented in the context of inflammation. *Sci Rep* (2017) 7(1):14226. doi: 10.1038/s41598-017-14618-z
34. Wilson AD, Bailey M, Williams NA, Stokes CR. The in vitro production of cytokines by mucosal lymphocytes immunized by oral administration of keyhole limpet hemocyanin using cholera toxin as an adjuvant. *Eur J Immunol* (1991) 21(10):2333–9. doi: 10.1002/eji.1830211007
35. Mochizuki M, Kuwabara T, McAllister C, Nussenblatt RB, Gery I. Adoptive transfer of experimental autoimmune uveoretinitis in rats. Immunopathogenic mechanisms and histologic features. *Invest Ophthalmol Vis Sci* (1985) 26(1):1–9.
36. Singh VK, Yamaki K, Donoso LA, Shinohara T. Molecular mimicry. Yeast histone H3-induced experimental autoimmune uveitis. *J Immunol (Baltimore Md 1950)* (1989) 142(5):1512–7.
37. Quaratino S, Thorpe CJ, Travers PJ, Londei M. Similar antigenic surfaces, rather than sequence homology, dictate T-cell epitope molecular mimicry. *Proc Natl Acad Sci* (1995) 92(22):10398. doi: 10.1073/pnas.92.22.10398
38. Wucherpfennig KW, Strominger JL. Molecular mimicry in T cell-mediated autoimmunity: viral peptides activate human T cell clones specific for myelin basic protein. *Cell* (1995) 80(5):695–705. doi: 10.1016/0092-8674(95)90348-8
39. Schuldt NJ, Binstadt BA. Dual TCR T Cells: Identity Crisis or Multitaskers? *J Immunol* (2019) 202(3):637. doi: 10.4049/jimmunol.1800904
40. Elliott JI, Altmann DM. Dual T cell receptor alpha chain T cells in autoimmunity. *J Exp Med* (1995) 182(4):953–9. doi: 10.1084/jem.182.4.953
41. Mason D. A very high level of crossreactivity is an essential feature of the T-cell receptor. *Immunol Today* (1998) 19(9):395–404. doi: 10.1016/S0167-5699(98)01299-7
42. Deeg CA, Thurau SR, Gerhards H, Ehrenhofer M, Wildner G, Kaspers B. Uveitis in horses induced by interphotoreceptor retinoid-binding protein is similar to the spontaneous disease. *Eur J Immunol* (2002) 32(9):2598–606. doi: 10.1002/1521-4141(200209)32:9<2598::AID-IMMU2598>3.0.CO;2-#
43. Boldison J, Khera TK, Copland DA, Stimpson ML, Crawford GL, Dick AD, et al. A novel pathogenic RBP-3 peptide reveals epitope spreading in persistent experimental autoimmune uveoretinitis. *Immunology* (2015) 146(2):301–11. doi: 10.1111/imm.12503
44. Diedrichs-Mohring M, Hoffmann C, Wildner G. Antigen-dependent monophasic or recurrent autoimmune uveitis in rats. *Int Immunol* (2008) 20(3):365–74. doi: 10.1093/intimm/dxm148
45. Goebels N, Hofstetter H, Schmidt S, Brunner C, Wekerle H, Hohlfeld R. Repertoire dynamics of autoreactive T cells in multiple sclerosis patients and healthy subjects: Epitope spreading versus clonal persistence. *Brain* (2000) 123 (3):508–18. doi: 10.1093/brain/123.3.508
46. Danke NA, Koelle DM, Yee C, Beheray S, Kwok WW. Autoreactive T Cells in Healthy Individuals. *J Immunol* (2004) 172(10):5967. doi: 10.4049/jimmunol.172.10.5967
47. Thurau SR, Mempel TR, Flugel A, Diedrichs Mohring M, Krombach F, Kawakami N, et al. The fate of autoreactive, GFP+ T cells in rat models of uveitis analyzed by intravital fluorescence microscopy and FACS. *Int Immunol* (2004) 16(11):1573–82. doi: 10.1093/intimm/dxh158

13

Quantitative Assessment of Experimental Ocular Inflammatory Disease

Lydia J. Bradley[1], *Amy Ward*[1], *Madeleine C. Y. Hsue*[1], *Jian Liu*[2], *David A. Copland*[2], *Andrew D. Dick*[1,2,3] *and Lindsay B. Nicholson*[1*]

[1] School of Cellular and Molecular Medicine, University of Bristol, Bristol, United Kingdom, [2] Academic Unit of Ophthalmology, Translational Health Sciences, University of Bristol, Bristol, United Kingdom, [3] University College London, Institute of Ophthalmology, London, United Kingdom

***Correspondence:**
Lindsay B. Nicholson
l.nicholson@bristol.ac.uk

Ocular inflammation imposes a high medical burden on patients and substantial costs on the health-care systems that mange these often chronic and debilitating diseases. Many clinical phenotypes are recognized and classifying the severity of inflammation in an eye with uveitis is an ongoing challenge. With the widespread application of optical coherence tomography in the clinic has come the impetus for more robust methods to compare disease between different patients and different treatment centers. Models can recapitulate many of the features seen in the clinic, but until recently the quality of imaging available has lagged that applied in humans. In the model experimental autoimmune uveitis (EAU), we highlight three linked clinical states that produce retinal vulnerability to inflammation, all different from healthy tissue, but distinct from each other. Deploying longitudinal, multimodal imaging approaches can be coupled to analysis in the tissue of changes in architecture, cell content and function. This can enrich our understanding of pathology, increase the sensitivity with which the impacts of therapeutic interventions are assessed and address questions of tissue regeneration and repair. Modern image processing, including the application of artificial intelligence, in the context of such models of disease can lay a foundation for new approaches to monitoring tissue health.

Keywords: uveitis, EAU, OCT, image processing, automated analysis

INTRODUCTION

Ocular inflammation is an important medical concern with a wide range of manifestations from the easily treatable to sight threatening. It arises both as an ocular specific condition and in association with systemic disease and it manifests as more than 30 defined uveitic phenotypes. The pathogenesis is complex and multifactorial and there is a lively debate as to the relative contribution of subclinical infection, autoinflammation and autoimmunity (1, 2). Conventional approaches to imaging do not distinguish between these different causes.

Animal models of uveitis are often autoimmune (e.g. experimental autoimmune uveitis; EAU), inspired in the mouse by early work identifying susceptible strains (3, 4) and used widely to probe important aspects of immune function including tolerance (5, 6), regulation (7, 8), microbiome (9), lymphocyte dynamics (10) and macrophage/monocyte function (11). But other models of ocular inflammation are also important, including endotoxin induced uveitis (EIU) (12–14) and primed mycobacterial uveitis (PMU) (15). Ocular infectious disease can also be studied and has proven to be an informative model of inflammation (16–18).

Over the last 15 years, techniques for imaging the mouse retina have advanced substantially, first with fundal photography, acquired by topical endoscopic fundal imaging (TEFI) (19–21) facilitating clinical grading by individuals blinded to the origin of the images. Then followed by adaptation of clinical tools (12) and development of the Micron system for imaging rodent eyes (Phoenix technologies, CA). These advances have made acquisition of experimental image data more accessible and routine (12, 22–24). The application of optical coherence tomography (OCT) to the mouse eye adds new information on changes deep in the tissue. The eye offers unique advantages for imaging studies of the autoimmune process in a target tissue, permitting serial assessment, and sophisticated quantification of different parameters of inflammation that go beyond more general clinical scores used in models such as experimental autoimmune encephalomyelitis.

Advances in image processing that have been developed in patient populations can also find application in experimental studies. There is potential for automatic segmentation of structures (in which the boundaries between, for example, different layers of the retina are identified in an unsupervised process), quantification of infiltration and disease classification by machine learning, which can be used to support unsupervised clinical assessment (25, 26). This is seen in the recent application of deep learning to EAU (27). Alternative powerful technologies are also available; using bioluminescent reporters, can delineate sequential cell population specific patterns of infiltration (28, 29), and multi-optical imaging approaches can produce data on phenotype and the spatial relationship between different cell types (30). Objective measurements, that provide a more granular multi-modal analysis of the state of the tissue, can then form the basis for quantifying the impact of treatment on ocular disease not limited to a single time-point but integrated across a longer disease course.

OCULAR TISSUE AND INFLAMMATION

EAU is often studied with a focus on the acute inflammation that occurs with the explosive influx of immune cells that flood into the tissue in the first wave of clinical disease. But it has been apparent for a number of years (31, 32) that it can also be used to develop insights into the processes of persistent disease and tissue remodeling. For example, memory cells that reside in the bone marrow are implicated in chronic retinal degeneration (33) and persistent inflammation can lead to retinal angiogenesis (34). In both mouse (35) and human (36), chronic disease can drive the development of ectopic lymphoid like structures and is accompanied by changes in the other lymphocyte populations and vascular remodeling (10, 34). The ocular tissue can therefore exist in a minimum of four well demarcated states (**Figure 1**).

Healthy tissue resists insult and maintains normal visual function. In the EAU model, there are a minimum of three non-healthy states, which correlate with changes in immune cell content and vascular function (31). Vulnerable tissue may be in the prodromal phase of EAU, at peak of disease, with active infiltration by many different leukocytes, or vulnerable but to a greater or lesser extent recovered, which state is described as post-peak. It is possible to observe experimentally that the pre-peak state can resolve to a state of health, or progress to peak disease. Tissue can reach peak disease from either the pre-peak state or as a relapse from the post-peak state (37). But it is unknown whether from peak or post-peak, tissue can ever return to a healthy state. In the broader context, a useful framework for these changes is found in the extensive literature describing the development and resolution of inflammation, but here too, the question of active resolution in the tissue and the mechanisms by which it occurs remains controversial (38). While this review focuses studies in the eye, it is evident that other diseases and disease models, such as arthritis, can be fitted into a similar framework (39).

One essential tool for advancing understanding of these different tissue states is a rigorous method of clinical assessment that separates healthy tissue from the vulnerable and that also distinguishes between different states of the vulnerable tissue. Such a scheme could then complement studies describing gene expression in different forms of ocular inflammation (13, 40). Recent advances in the range and quality of techniques that can be applied to quantify ocular inflammatory disease make such objective and transferrable assessments increasingly feasible.

ASSESSMENT OF OCULAR INFLAMMATION

The measurement of inflammatory activity is a core objective for clinical studies of uveitis and has inspired work that seeks to improve its ability to discriminate between lower levels of disease as well as improving its sensitivity (41). Progress in this area can also inform animal studies.

Clinical Scoring

In human eye disease, improvements in imaging have driven diagnostic sensitivity and specificity (42, 43). Scoring systems serve as tools for categorizing disease activity into ordinal groups and as a convenient measure of clinical outcome and directional change. The first aqueous and vitreous inflammation scoring systems based on ophthalmic observation of cell counts in patients were published in 1959 (44, 45), but consensus

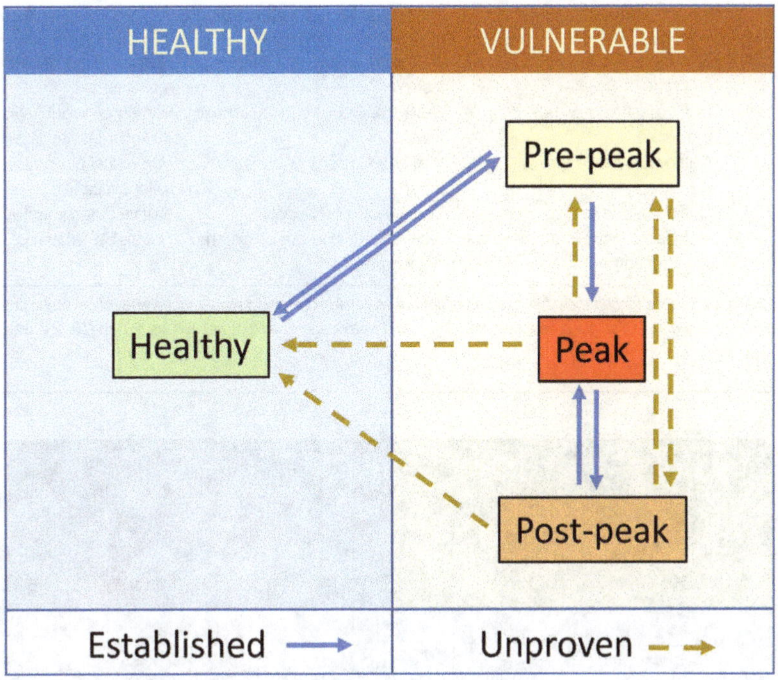

FIGURE 1 | Tissue states in ocular inflammation. Healthy ocular tissue is 'immune-privileged' and under low-level immunosurveillance. Specific (ocular antigen driven) and non-specific (extra-ocular inflammation) stimuli disturb this homeostasis and increase interactions across the blood retinal barrier making the tissue more vulnerable to the development of disease. In uveitis following active immunization, this starts with the prodrome (8), which can resolve back to the healthy state. When the prodrome progresses to clinical EAU in immunocompetent animals, there is an influx of cells to a maximum (peak) followed by a reduction in immune cell content, which does not return to base line. The post-peak (in EAU described as secondary regulation) is distinguished from the pre-peak by changes in the relative proportion of different lymphocyte populations (CD4 T regulatory cells, CD8 T resident memory cells). There is currently no evidence that disease proceeds directly from pre-peak to post-peak, nor that eyes that have reached peak disease ever return to the normal healthy state.

recommendations did not emerge until 2005, under the umbrella of the Standardization of Uveitis Nomenclature (SUN) workshop (46). For some diseases, for example Behçet's disease, specific scoring systems have proven useful is assessing treatment response (47). It is a recognized concern with scoring systems that there is a tension between precision and simplicity. Levels of interobserver agreement remain modest and non-linearity in the scaling can lead to poor resolution of differences in disease especially at lower levels of inflammation (48–50). The use of digital images, where biological data is quantified as pixel values, expands the possibilities for analysis by computer imaging (25) for example for automated grading of vitreous haze (51). Scoring of clinical disease in EAU has evolved from early approaches using slit-lamp aided visualization and semi-quantitative histological scoring to more sophisticated scoring approaches based on blinded assessment of fundal photographs (20, 21, 23, 52, 53) and most recently using machine learning. Scoring can be on a simple ordinal scale (0–4) or can categorize disease into three indicators of inflammation and one of structural damage with inflammation and structural damage reported independently or as a summary score (0–5) calculated as the total or average score for the eye (10, 21, 54) (**Table 1**). When applied as a summary score, this approach can be insensitive to differences in aspects of the underlying pathology, for example in **Figure 2**, the two images, although clearly different, received the same summary clinical score.

Complementing photography is optical coherence tomography (OCT). Developed in the 1990s (55, 56) it has rapidly become the state of the art for non-invasive retinal imaging. OCT is an interferometric technique providing depth resolved cross sectional images of the retina, known as B-scans. In normal eyes the vitreous is optically transparent, retinal layers show different degrees of backscatter, and in humans the RPE is one of the most hyper-reflective layers. Modern OCT in humans can also go some way to visualizing the choroid beneath the RPE (57). OCT can resolve retinal substructure and its vasculature, can be important in the diagnosis and image guided management of human uveitis and can capture changes in the state of the tissue through time in EAU (12, 24, 58, 59).

Ocular Tissue Analysis

In contrast to the wealth of sophisticated imaging that can be directed at the human eye in uveitis, access to human tissue is severely limited. Enucleation of the globe in uveitis is rare and is usually from individuals with long-standing disease (36). But in the EAU model, histology was the first accepted standard for disease assessment (60–62). Immunohistochemistry and immunofluorescence of retinal tissue revealed the profound

TABLE 1 | Scheme for scoring clinical ocular inflammation.

Score	Optic disc	Retinal vessels	Retinal tissue infiltration	Structural damage
1	Minimal inflammation	Cuffing: 1–4 mild	1–4 small lesions or 1 linear lesion	Retinal lesions or retinal atrophy involving 1/4 to 3/4 of retinal area
2	Mild inflammation	Cuffing: >4 mild or 1–3 moderate	5–10 small lesions or 2–3 linear lesions	Panretinal atrophy with multiple small lesions (scars) or ≤3 linear lesions (scars)
3	Moderate inflammation	Cuffing: >3 moderate	>10 small lesions or >3 linear lesions	Pan-retinal atrophy with >3 linear lesions or confluent lesions (scars)
4	Severe inflammation	Cuffing: >1 severe	Linear lesion confluent	Retinal detachment with folding
5	Not visible (white-out or extreme detachment)	Not visible (white-out or extreme detachment)	Not visible (white-out or extreme detachment)	Not visible (white-out or extreme detachment)

A blinded observer assigns scores to retinal photographs for changes that relate to inflammation of the optic disc, retinal vessels and retinal tissue and a score for structural damage. These scores can then be summed independently (score of 0-20) or given as a summary score of the average of all features (score of 0-5) (10, 21, 54).

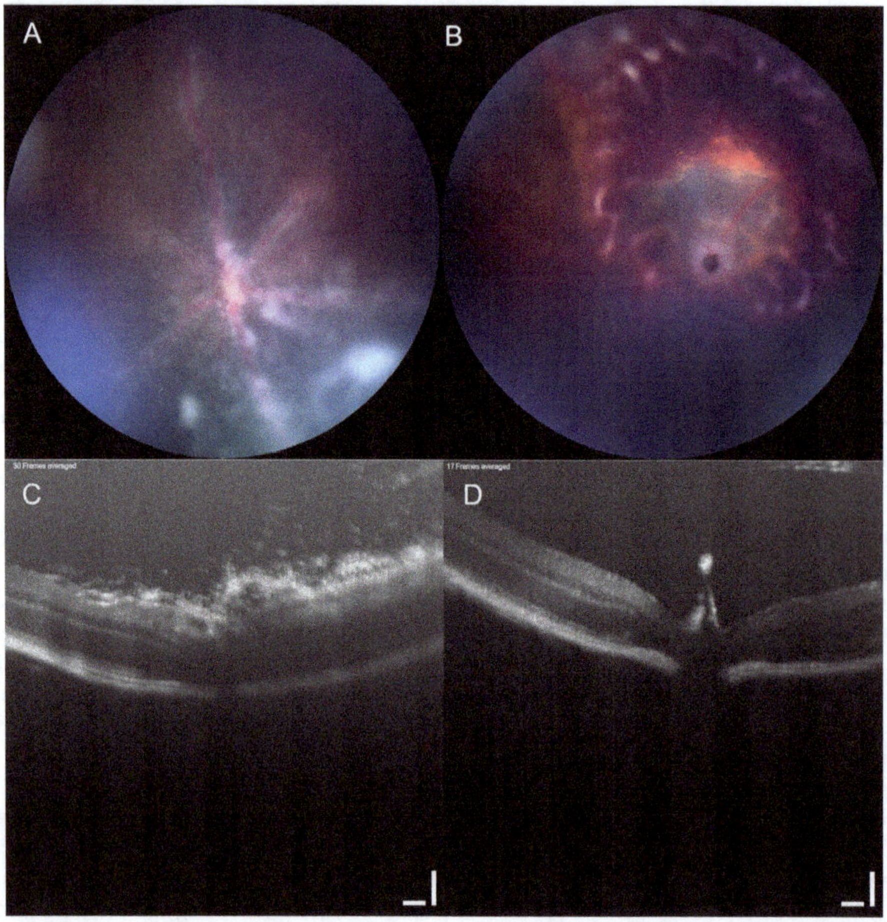

FIGURE 2 | Clinical score can be insensitive to underlying pathology. Mouse eyes imaged using Micron IV with OCT (Phoenix technology group, CA). Two mouse eyes **(A, C)** and **(B, D)** imaged using Micron IV (Phoenix technology group, CA) and assessed by fundal photography **(A, B)** and OCT **(C, D)**. Retinal photographs scored in a set of images by an observer blinded to the treatment groups, both received the same summary clinical score. Scale bar 100 μm.

structural disruption that accompanies acute inflammation, and was used, for example, to show how macrophages reciprocally alter their expression of CD68 and arginase-1 during the persistent (post-peak) phase of uveitis (34). For higher dimensional analysis of cell infiltrate, investigators have used multiparameter flow cytometry which can quantify many different cell populations (8, 63, 64). Sampling the cell infiltrate at different time points has been instrumental in demonstrating important changes in the relative frequencies of CD4 T regulatory cells (65) and CD8 cells (10). In EAU this is strong evidence that at the cellular level as well as in serial imaging studies, the tissue and the immune infiltrate change and adapt through time. Developing improved quantitative methods to assess tissue health in EAU offers more sensitive and specific approaches to analyze the impact of therapies for autoimmunity and inflammation.

Quantitative Assessment of EAU

Using formal criteria, EAU can be assessed semi-quantitatively, but interobserver disagreement and subjectivity limits the usefulness of direct comparison between results from different labs and even individual researchers (21). As with human clinical graders, experience is required to achieve the highest levels of interobserver agreement (66). Employing contemporary technology has the capacity to improve on these limitations. In addition, in EAU as in other medical images, these can be annotated, with the results of end point tissue analysis added to the meta-data associated with the image. This enriches their interpretation and provides a resource that can be applied to other studies. Pooling data from animal cohorts at selected timepoints runs the risk of obscuring subtle patterns, and overweighting the importance of the certain trends. This can be countered by the use of analysis that exploits modern image processing, with its scope for a higher degree of quantitation (66–68). A critical element of complementary analysis is therefore the use of non-invasive techniques and computational means to maximize information retrieved from the data.

Fundus photography, for example obtained by TEFI, correlates well with disease scores from histopathological analysis (20) but the images produce a 2D projection of 3D semi-transparent biological tissue. Spatial information is only available in two dimensions and artifacts are introduced by flattening depth information onto a plane. More accurate measures of infiltrate, oedema and structural changes, that are important manifestations of disease, can be obtained with OCT (24, 59). Because OCT produces a depth profile of different features, it can be more sensitive than 2D fundus imaging in monitoring the appearance and development of pathological changes. In particular, cross sectional images are more sensitive to early disease because they can visualize small amounts of infiltrate around the optic nerve, and measure changes in optic nerve diameter and retinal thickness due to inflammatory oedema (23, 59, 66, 68).

Aqueous and Vitreous Assessment

A defining characteristic of uveitis is cellular infiltrate, and grading is an important quantitative metric in preclinical animal model research. In human disease, anterior uveitis produces 'flare' which can be categorized by laser flare photometry and which correlates well with conventional clinical grading (69, 70) while in the vitreous, 'haze' is an accepted and clinically validated proxy for inflammatory status in patients (51). Moreover, these changes have a marked impact on visual acuity in humans and so are biologically and clinically relevant outcome measures (50).

In OCT, cells in either chamber appear as hyperreflective dots, whose profile is a function of many variables (71–73). Cells and exudate incrementally reduce the optical transparency of the ocular media leading to the aqueous and vitreous becoming inhomogeneous as disease severity increases. These changes reduce the contrast of object boundaries and the results of qualitative or quantitative image analysis lose precision.

Because of difficulty in imaging the anterior chamber of small eyes, literature for OCT based cell counting in these models is relatively sparse (74). However, automated counts of absolute cell numbers have been obtained with excellent correspondence to manual image counts. This approach has been developed into a fully automated pipeline for cell counting in volumetric OCT images, achieving 98% congruence to manual slit lamp counts. Importantly, the subjective manual element of the segmentation step was eliminated. The automated segmentation step involved removal of anatomical structures connected to image boundaries (75). Compared with counts from histological sections, OCT tended to undercount, which was attributed to insensitivity to cell clumps, sediments and exclusion of the extremities of the iris interface (74). It may also be contributory that histology is unaffected by overlying opacities, whereas OCT is vulnerable to signal degradation. However, histology introduces artifacts and postmortem changes that themselves affect tissue measurement (74).

Loss of precision becomes more evident when imaging the vitreous, where the optical pathway traverses deeper through affected media. Further complicating the analysis of the rodent vitreous, is the anatomical vestige of the hyaloid artery (71, 76), protruding upwards from the optic disc towards the lens. It confuses the vitreoretinal boundary and can appear somewhat discontinuous, with hyperreflective regions that are subjectively indistinguishable from cell clusters.

Automated counting algorithms usually require a preceding segmentation step, that defines a boundary for the area or volume of interest. Variations in signal quality and the ambiguity of discontinuous image features frustrate the development of accurate, fully automated methods of rodent image segmentation and analysis. Quantification of changes in the vitreous has largely been restricted to human images, and global signal parameters, as opposed to absolute cell counts.

To account for signal strength variations in human OCT images, the average intensity of the segmented vitreous compartment can be indexed relative to a hyperreflective reference layer such as the RPE, providing a relative intensity ratio. These ratios correlate moderately with clinical vitreous haze scores, along with other surrogates of disease such as retinal thickness (72, 77). This process has been fully automated using rule-based algorithms for segmentation, reducing subjectivity. The same operation was also performed using a textural descriptor of the vitreous, which was marginally better correlated to clinical scores than vitreous intensity (73). These operations were performed on 2D datasets, obtaining an averaged intensity ratio based on several B-scans and data analyzed in 3D may potentially offer further improvements.

Since the scan region is much smaller than the ocular globe, one consideration is the selection of a representative and informative region of interest (ROI) that must be equivalent between scans and subjects. Within human images, landmarks such as the macula can be located automatically and used as a central anchor point for region boundary positioning (73).

In rodents, the optic disc is an obvious landmark choice, but the presence of the hyaloid remnant, particularly in severely diseased eyes warrants additional steps to remove its influence. Recently, an automated method of quantifying vitreous inflammation in clinical fundus photographs has been suggested (50, 51).

Retinal Layers

OCT of the healthy retina produces good definition of the different layers of light sensitive tissue. In uveitis it can resolve and localize lesions and pathologies, and identify vasodilation and perivascular exudate (24, 59). Standard clinical OCT has an axial resolution of less than 4 microns, which can produce images with near histological detail. Thickness is ascertained from OCT images by measuring the distance between two boundaries of choice (**Figure 3**). Before measurements can be taken, the layers must be defined.

Techniques for segmentation to define different retinal layers have progressed through manual, semi-automated and fully automated protocols, with work on human data leading rodent OCT imaging. Both rule-based algorithms and learner-based approaches have been applied to the problem and new approaches are under active investigation. Retinal thickness can be measured by OCT absolutely, using assumptions such as an average tissue refractive index (78), or by fold change compared to pre-disease measurements (66). Both are in high agreement with histological measurements (24, 59, 66, 78, 79). Several schemes exist for displaying changes in thickness. One that is commonly used shows thickness at different distances from the optic nerve head (**Supplementary Figure 1**).

Rule-based methods execute a pre-programmed set of instructions, designed with the expected properties of the image and the desired features in mind. Many image properties can be analyzed, including intensity variation, geometric contours and texture (80–84). The number of segmented layers defined varies between four and nine, and depends on the approach, with the most successful techniques to date being learner models (26, 80, 85–88)

OCT offers the potential of assessing layer deformation without the artefacts that can be introduced by tissue fixation, sectioning and staining (89). Mechanical deformation can also introduce ambiguous artifacts, with likeness to retinal detachments (78), and congenital abnormalities in the retina may also confound the definition of anatomical normality (90). The literature pertaining to automated quantitation of retinal structure is more extensive than that related to infiltrate, because retinal layer changes are associated with a wide variety of ocular diseases (91, 92). The laminated reflectance profile of the retina's architecture also lends itself to image segmentation and the measurement of quantitative indices such as layer thickness and geometric descriptors. Protocols for automatic layer segmentation developed for human studies have been tested in different mouse strains. These performed well when assessing the inner retinal layers, but were less successful in defining the murine RPE, whose location displaced distally into the sclera (68).

Longitudinal studies of retinal thickness have revealed details about the kinetics of disease progression, with respect to other important manifestations of pathology (59, 66). In the pre-peak to peak phase of disease, retinal thickness increases rapidly due to inflammatory oedema, correlating with inflammatory infiltrate, measured longitudinally by OCT and confirmed by histology (66, 78). In the post-peak resolution phase, the clearance of exudate reveals features on OCT with greater clarity, such as infiltrate, photoreceptor atrophy, retinal folds and choroiditis (59). Photoreceptor damage persists beyond the peak phase of disease as retinal oedema is slower to resolve than inflammatory infiltrate. When the swelling does subside, the retina thins to below pre-disease levels because of photoreceptor loss.

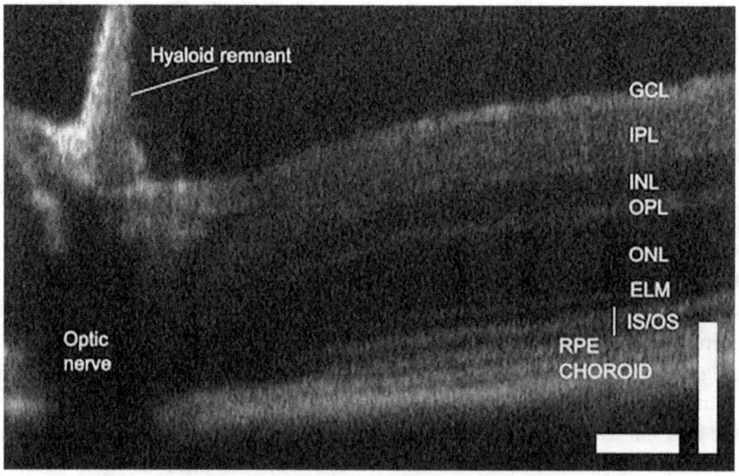

FIGURE 3 | OCT of the normal mouse retina delineates layers and allows retinal dimensions to be quantified. Scale bars are 100 microns and illustrate differences in axial and lateral resolution. GCL, ganglion cell layer; IPL, inner plexiform layer; INL, inner nuclear layer; OPL, outer plexiform layer; ONL, outer nuclear layer; ELM, external limiting membrane; IS/OS, inner and outer segments; RPE, retinal pigment epithelium (68).

OCT confirms that neither infiltrate or retinal thickness returns to baseline in late disease or even after resolution is complete (20, 59, 78). Therefore, quantitative directional changes and relative rates of change between retinal thickness and inflammatory infiltrate can provide an additional metric for disease activity.

In severe uveitis, retinal layers are obscured by opacification of the vitreous and aqueous due to infiltrate and proteinaceous exudate (59) which presents a challenge for scoring systems, that must be robust to substantial signal variation and may need to incorporate metrics of opacity into the model as proxies of inflammation.

Vasculature

Important changes in the vasculature occur in uveitis, including ischemia, neovascularization and retinal/choroidal vasculitis (93). In disease models these are assessed less commonly than structural changes, but as in humans they are often interrogated by angiography. Confocal scanning laser ophthalmoscopy (SLO) can be coupled to fundus fluorescein angiography (FFA) to quantify vessel diameter and leakage in EAU. When average vascular dilation was measured immediately prior to sacrifice and histology, major vessel diameter was well correlated with retina-choroid thickness and with clinical and histological scores. This indicated that inflammatory vasodilation of superficial vasculature was a novel measure of EAU severity (66). Complementary to dye-based angiography are OCT based methodologies. Vascular dilation and perivascular exudate attributed to retinal vasculitis can be localized to specific retinal layers during the course of EAU (23, 59) and OCT has been used for imaging vasculature disturbances, such as choroiditis and retinal vasculitis (43). Blood flow can be visualized and depth resolved (94) using OCT angiography (OCTA) and this has been used to assess retinal microvascular changes (95, 96).

Many methods of segmenting retinal blood vessels from fundus photographs have been published (97). A much smaller number of approaches have been successfully devised using OCT images, which include the use of multimodal imaging (corresponding fundus photographs) and learner models (98, 99). In humans, segmentation of fine capillary networks has been achieved in OCTA enface images (100) while in mice segmentation of retinal vasculature using OCTA has been reported for longitudinal monitoring of angiogenesis (101). Current advances applying deep learning to vessel segmentation continue to improve the performance of these methods and this has been helped by the public access to data sets (102).

Functional

As EAU progresses, electroretinogram (ERG) amplitudes change. There is a dramatic reduction in function (a and b wave), that accompanies early disease (103), presenting before morphologic changes. These findings indicate that functional loss could be mediated by inflammation rather than just physical damage, and that retinal function is potentially a sensitive early indicator (59, 66). However, photoreceptor damage continues while inflammation is receding and in the post-peak phase, ERG amplitudes are correlated with OCT measures of retinal thickness. As swelling diminishes, photoreceptor atrophy becomes apparent and results in an overall retinal thinning compared to baseline. Neither retinal thickness nor functionality ever fully recover (59, 103).

Taken together, multimodal quantitative measures can provide information on perceptually subtle, but biologically significant changes whose quantification would aid clinical grading and pre-clinical research.

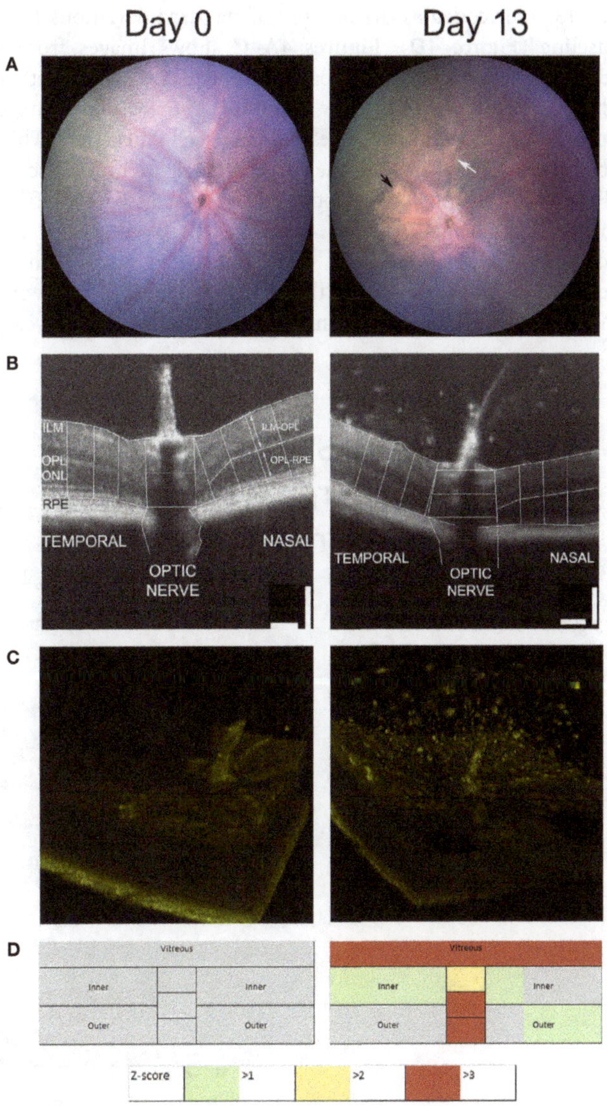

FIGURE 4 | Multimodal analysis of EAU. Mouse eyes were imaged at day 0 and day 13 after the induction of EAU and one representative image of the same eye is shown **(A–C)**. Clinical disease can be assessed by photography **(A)**, measurements of retinal thickness and optic nerve diameter at three points from the temporal, nasal and optic nerve regions of the OCT B-scans **(B)**, 3D-reconstuction of retinal infiltrate **(C)** and summary data of retinal scores from all groups **(D)**. Summary scores are assembled from unsupervised quantitative assessment of vitreal involvement, manual segmentation and measurement of inner and outer layer thickness and optic nerve diameter transformed and represented as Z-scores.

EXAMPLES OF MULTIMODAL MEASUREMENT

A multimodal approach to assessing uveitis is outlined in **Figure 4**. EAU was induced by the transfer of pathogenic autoantigen reactive T cells. Sequential imaging of all eyes was carried out by fundal photography and OCT. B-scans were segmented manually and measured by an observer blinded to treatment conditions. Measurements of retinal thickness were made at baseline from all eyes (n=11) and these were compared as a Z-score expressing the magnitude of change in thickness on day 13 color coded as the number of standard deviations from baseline (**Figure 4D**). **Figures 4A–C** shows images from a representative single eye at baseline and day 13. The retinal photographs (**Figure 4A**) show that at day 13 there is an enlarged optic nerve, sheathing of the vessels due to cell infiltration (white arrow) and infiltrates in the tissue (black arrow). B-scans (**Figure 4B**) through the optic nerve, were assembled from multiple averaged frames and are displayed with the accompanying 100 micron scale bars that were used to generate measurements of the retinal thickness following manual segmentation using ImageJ (104). At day 13 it is easy to see objects in the vitreous around the optic nerve. The 3D image (**Figure 4C**) is prepared from 512 sequential B scans, processed using code in MATLAB (Natick, Massachusetts: The MathWorks Inc) and ImageJ (26) adapted for use with murine images and rendered using ImageJ (1.53 3D viewer plugin). These pictures give a better appreciation of the spatial distribution of the vitreal infiltrate and can be used to make a semi-quantitative estimate of the degree of vitreal infiltration.

Following changes in disease scores through time, it is useful to display the aggregate data from the multiple images, and this has been used to produce a color-coded map of the retina, with changes normalized to baseline scans (usually on day 0) and scaled by Z-score. Retinal maps are also useful when comparing the pattern of pathological change between different disease models. For example, compare **Figure 4D**, which shows that at day 13 the major impact of uveitis is found in the vitreous and the optic nerve with **Figure 5** which shows the does dependent effect of intra-vitreal instillation of paraquat, a model of oxidative stress, in C57BL/6 mice. This induces neuronal degeneration which varies with stain (105) and in this case particularly impacts the inner retina, seen as a negative Z-score increasing in magnitude with dose. But quantitative analysis also reveals that

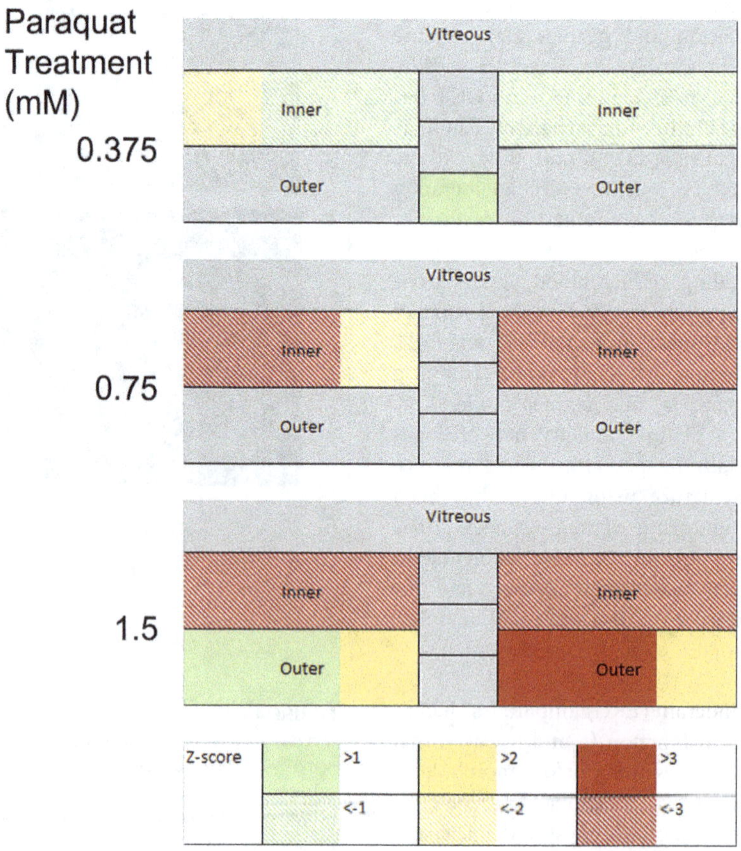

FIGURE 5 | Changes in retinal thickness in mouse eyes following intra-vitreal paraquat instillation were measured on day 10. Images were visualized by OCT, manually segmented, and measured at three points in the temporal, nasal, and optic nerve regions. Measurements are expressed as positive and negative Z-scores relative to a PBS injected control group. Changes in the inner and outer layers are decoupled.

at higher concentrations of paraquat, this is accompanied by an expansion of the outer segments, due to inflammation. This finding, using multimodal analysis is in agreement with a previous report showing more pronounced TUNEL-positive cells in the inner retina than in the outer retina of C57BL/6 mice treated intravitreally with paraquat (105).

Opportunities for Automation

Machine learning has made an impact in human clinical care in recent years because of its ability to reach expert-level diagnosis. The automated analysis of ocular disease has led the way in carrying these methodologies into the clinic, but they have been less extensively utilized in disease models (106, 107).

Images are inherently data rich because in theory each pixel can be regarded as a separate input parameter (106). This offers opportunities for uncovering novel aspects of pathological processes but also challenges, especially in assembling well annotated data sets that are large enough to avoid overparameterization when they are used to train classification algorithms in a machine learning framework. Advances in predictive statistical methods may in time alleviate the need for such extensive input data. One helpful approach, applied in OCT, is decoupling the methods for segmentation from artificial intelligence driven disease classification (108). This moves practice towards device-independent representation of the disease process, which may aid in comparison between studies carried out by different investigators.

Recently the field has advanced with the application of a deep learning model to analyze photographs of the retinas of mice with EAU. Using a data set of images that was extended by data augmentation, disease images were divided into three categories and by applying deep learning methods (convolutional neural networks) the overall performance assessed by area under the receiver operating characteristic curve (AUC) when the model was applied to an external dataset of 33 images was approximately 0.90 (27).

Another area of opportunity in multi-modal ocular imaging is the fusion of information from different modalities such as fundal photography and OCT (109, 110). Image fusion aims to yield a more complete, accurate and efficient account of an object by combining different visualizations together. Integrating this methodology into the assessment of experimental clinical disease will inform our ability to distinguish between different states of tissue health (**Figure 1**).

CONCLUSION

Persistent ocular inflammation is a significant and challenging clinical entity that is associated with long term changes in the retina and serious sight threatening complications (111). Experimental models of non-infectious and infectious ocular inflammation have been widely and successfully deployed. But fundamental insights regarding how tissue homeostasis is perturbed and how it might be restored are still needed (112). Such concerns are important in a much broader context than uveitis. Restoring complex tissues, damaged by persistent inflammation, to normal physiological function will have wide application. Multimodal and quantitative imaging of the eye, in an experimental context, has potential to advance our understanding of the kinetics, cell biology, transcriptomic and proteomic architecture of how this multifactorial process is regulated. By providing non-invasive techniques to probe the underlaying nature of the tissue, there is an opportunity for a more precise and comprehensive discrimination between different states that can be used to stratify information gleaned from detailed examination of the transcriptome and microbiome, multiparameter flow cytometry and proteomics.

AUTHOR CONTRIBUTIONS

Literature survey and drafting of original manuscript and figures (LB, AW, LN). Preparation and provision of data (AW, MH, JL, DC). All authors contributed to the article and approved the submitted version.

ACKNOWLEDGMENTS

The authors gratefully acknowledge support of the National Eye Research Centre, Fight for Sight (5077/5078) and the Underwood Trust to research carried out in their laboratories.

REFERENCES

1. Forrester JV, Kuffova L, Dick AD. Autoimmunity, Autoinflammation, and Infection in Uveitis. *Am J Ophthalmol* (2018) 189:77–85. doi: 10.1016/j.ajo.2018.02.019
2. Lee RWJ, Nicholson LB, Sen HN, Chan CC, Wei L, Nussenblatt RB, et al. Autoimmune and Autoinflammatory Mechanisms in Uveitis. *Semin Immunopathol* (2014) 36:581–94. doi: 10.1007/s00281-014-0433-9
3. Caspi RR, Roberge FG, Chan CC, Wiggert B, Chader GJ, Rozenszajn LA, et al. A New Model of Autoimmune Disease. Experimental Autoimmune Uveoretinitis Induced in Mice With Two Different Retinal Antigens. *J Immunol* (1988) 140(5):1490–5.
4. Caspi RR. A Look at Autoimmunity and Inflammation in the Eye. *J Clin Invest* (2010) 120(9):3073–83. doi: 10.1172/JCI42440
5. Lin HH, Faunce DE, Stacey M, Terajewicz A, Nakamura T, Zhang-Hoover J, et al. The Macrophage F4/80 Receptor Is Required for the Induction of Antigen-Specific Efferent Regulatory T Cells in Peripheral Tolerance. *J Exp Med* (2005) 201(10):1615–25. doi: 10.1084/jem.20042307
6. Lee DJ, Taylor AW. Recovery From Experimental Autoimmune Uveitis Promotes Induction of Antiuveitic Inducible Tregs. *J Leukocyte Biol* (2015) 97(6):1101–9. doi: 10.1189/jlb.3A1014-466RR
7. Wang R-X, Yu C-R, Dambuza IM, Mahdi RM, Dolinska M, Sergeey YV, et al. Interleukin-35 Induces Regulatory B Cells That Suppress Autoimmune Disease. *Nat Med* (2014) 20(6):633–41. doi: 10.1038/nm.3554
8. Kerr EC, Raveney BJE, Copland DA, Dick AD, Nicholson LB. Analysis of Retinal Cellular Infiltrate in Experimental Autoimmune Uveoretinitis Reveals Multiple Regulatory Cell Populations. *J Autoimmun* (2008) 31:354–61. doi: 10.1016/j.jaut.2008.08.006
9. Horai R, Zárate-Bladés CR, Dillenburg-Pilla P, Chen J, Kielczewski JL, Silver Phyllis B, et al. Microbiota-Dependent Activation of an Autoreactive T Cell Receptor Provokes Autoimmunity in an Immunologically Privileged Site. *Immunity* (2015) 43(2):343–53. doi: 10.1016/j.immuni.2015.07.014

10. Boldison J, Chu CJ, Copland DA, Lait PJP, Khera TK, Dick AD, et al. Tissue-Resident Exhausted Effector Memory CD8+ T Cells Accumulate in the Retina During Chronic Experimental Autoimmune Uveoretinitis. *J Immunol* (2014) 192:4541–50. doi: 10.4049/jimmunol.1301390
11. Raveney BJE, Copland DA, Dick AD, Nicholson LB. Tnfr1-Dependent Regulation of Myeloid Cell Function in Experimental Autoimmune Uveoretinitis. *J Immunol* (2009) 183:2321–9. doi: 10.4049/jimmunol.0901340
12. Chu CJ, Gardner PJ, Copland DA, Liyanage SE, Gonzalez-Cordero A, kleine Holthaus S-M, et al. Multimodal Analysis of Ocular Inflammation Using the Endotoxin-Induced Uveitis Mouse Model. *Dis Models Mech* (2016) 9 (4):473–81. doi: 10.1242/dmm.022475
13. Bell OH, Copland DA, Ward A, Nicholson LB, Lange CAK, Chu CJ, et al. Single Eye mRNA-Seq Reveals Normalisation of the Retinal Microglial Transcriptome Following Acute Inflammation. *Front Immunol* (2020) 10:3033. doi: 10.3389/fimmu.2019.03033
14. Forrester JV, Worgul BV, Merriam GRJr. Endotoxin-Induced Uveitis in the Rat. *Albrecht Von Graefes Archiv fur Klinische und Experimentelle Ophthalmologie* (1980) 213(4):221–33. doi: 10.1007/BF00417543
15. Pepple KL, Rotkis L, Van Grol J, Wilson L, Sandt A, Lam DL, et al. Primed Mycobacterial Uveitis (PMU): Histologic and Cytokine Characterization of a Model of Uveitis in Rats. *Invest Ophthalmol Vis Sci* (2015) 56(13):8438–48. doi: 10.1167/iovs.15-17523
16. Zinkernagel MS, Bolinger B, Krebs P, Onder L, Miller S, Ludewig B. Immunopathological Basis of Lymphocytic Choriomeningitis Virus-Induced Chorioretinitis and Keratitis. *J Virol* (2009) 83(1):159–66. doi: 10.1128/jvi.01211-08
17. Zinkernagel MS, Chinnery HR, Ong ML, Petitjean C, Voigt V, McLenachan S, et al. Interferon γ-Dependent Migration of Microglial Cells in the Retina After Systemic Cytomegalovirus Infection. *Am J Pathol* (2013) 182(3):875–85. doi: 10.1016/j.ajpath.2012.11.031
18. Zinkernagel MS, Petitjean C, Wikstrom ME, Degli-Esposti MA. Kinetics of Ocular and Systemic Antigen-Specific T-Cell Responses Elicited During Murine Cytomegalovirus Retinitis. *Immunol Cell Biol* (2012) 90(3):330–6. doi: 10.1038/icb.2011.43
19. Paques M, Guyomard JL, Simonutti M, Roux MJ, Picaud S, LeGargasson JF, et al. Panretinal, High-Resolution Color Photography of the Mouse Fundus. *Invest Ophthalmol Vis Sci* (2007) 48(6):2769–74. doi: 10.1167/iovs.06-1099
20. Copland DA, Wertheim MS, Raveney BJE, Armitage WJ, Nicholson LB, Dick AD. The Clinical Time-Course of Experimental Autoimmune Uveoretinitis Using Topical Endoscopic Fundal Imaging With Histological and Cellular Infiltrate Correlation. *Invest Ophthalmol Vis Sci* (2008) 49:5458–65. doi: 10.1167/iovs.08-2348
21. Xu HP, Koch P, Chen M, Lau A, Reid DM, Forrester JV. A Clinical Grading System for Retinal Inflammation in the Chronic Model of Experimental Autoimmune Uveoretinitis Using Digital Fundus Images. *Exp Eye Res* (2008) 87(4):319–26. doi: 10.1016/j.exer.2008.06.012
22. Zhong X, Aredo B, Ding Y, Zhang K, Zhao CX, Ufret-Vincenty RL. Fundus Camera-Delivered Light-Induced Retinal Degeneration in Mice With the RPE65 Leu450met Variant Is Associated With Oxidative Stress and Apoptosis. *Invest Ophthalmol Vis Sci* (2016) 57(13):5558–67. doi: 10.1167/iovs.16-19965
23. Chen J, Caspi RR. Clinical and Functional Evaluation of Ocular Inflammatory Disease Using the Model of Experimental Autoimmune Uveitis. In: AS Boyd, editor. *Immunological Tolerance: Methods and Protocols*. New York, NY: Springer New York (2019). p. 211–27.
24. Chu CJ, Herrmann P, Carvalho LS, Liyanage SE, Bainbridge JWB, Ali RR, et al. Assessment and *In Vivo* Scoring of Murine Experimental Autoimmune Uveoretinitis Using Optical Coherence Tomography. *PloS One* (2013) 8(5): e63002. doi: 10.1371/journal.pone.0063002
25. Abramoff MD, Garvin MK, Sonka M. Retinal Imaging and Image Analysis. *IEEE Rev Biomed Eng* (2010) 3:169–208. doi: 10.1109/rbme.2010.2084567
26. Anantrasirichai N, Nicholson LB, Morgan JE, Erchova I, Mortlock K, North RV, et al. Adaptive-Weighted Bilateral Filtering and Other Pre-Processing Techniques for Optical Coherence Tomography. *Computerized Med Imaging Graphics* (2014) 38(6):526–39. doi: 10.1016/j.compmedimag.2014.06.012
27. Sun J, Huang X, Egwuagu C, Badr Y, Dryden SC, Fowler BT, et al. Identifying Mouse Autoimmune Uveitis From Fundus Photographs Using Deep Learning. *Trans Vision Sci Technol* (2020) 9(2):59–. doi: 10.1167/tvst.9.2.59
28. Gutowski MB, Wilson L, Van Gelder RN, Pepple KL. In Vivo Bioluminescence Imaging for Longitudinal Monitoring of Inflammation in Animal Models of Uveitis. *Invest Ophthalmol Vis Sci* (2017) 58(3):1521–8. doi: 10.1167/iovs.16-20824
29. John S, Rolnick K, Wilson L, Wong S, Van Gelder RN, Pepple KL. Bioluminescence for *In Vivo* Detection of Cell-Type-Specific Inflammation in a Mouse Model of Uveitis. *Sci Rep* (2020) 10(1):11377. doi: 10.1038/s41598-020-68227-4
30. Radtke AJ, Kandov E, Lowekamp B, Speranza E, Chu CJ, Gola A, et al. Ibex: A Versatile Multiplex Optical Imaging Approach for Deep Phenotyping and Spatial Analysis of Cells in Complex Tissues. *Proc Natl Acad Sci USA* (2020) 117(52):33455–65. doi: 10.1073/pnas.2018488117
31. Kerr EC, Copland DA, Dick AD, Nicholson LB. The Dynamics of Leukocyte Infiltration in Experimental Autoimmune Uveoretinitis. *Prog Retin Eye Res* (2008) 27:527–35. doi: 10.1016/j.preteyeres.2008.07.001
32. Shao H, Liao T, Ke Y, Shi H, Kaplan HJ, Sun D. Severe Chronic Experimental Autoimmune Uveitis (EAU) of the C57BL/6 Mouse Induced by Adoptive Transfer of IRBP1–20-Specific T Cells. *Exp Eye Res* (2006) 82 (2):323–31. doi: 10.1016/j.exer.2005.07.008
33. Oh H-M, Yu C-R, Lee Y, Chan C-C, Maminishkis A, Egwuagu CE. Autoreactive Memory CD4+ T Lymphocytes That Mediate Chronic Uveitis Reside in the Bone Marrow Through STAT3-Dependent Mechanisms. *J Immunol* (2011) 187(6):3338–46. doi: 10.4049/jimmunol.1004019
34. Chen M, Copland DA, Zhao J, Liu J, Forrester JV, Dick AD, et al. Persistent Inflammation Subverts Thrombospondin-1–Induced Regulation of Retinal Angiogenesis and Is Driven by CCR2 Ligation. *Am J Pathol* (2012) 180 (1):235–45. doi: 10.1016/j.ajpath.2011.09.020
35. Kielczewski JL, Horai R, Jittayasothorn Y, Chan C-C, Caspi RR. Tertiary Lymphoid Tissue Forms in Retinas of Mice With Spontaneous Autoimmune Uveitis and Has Consequences on Visual Function. *J Immunol* (2016) 196 (3):1013–25. doi: 10.4049/jimmunol.1501570
36. Epps SJ, Coplin N, Luthert PJ, Dick AD, Coupland SE, Nicholson LB. Features of Ectopic Lymphoid-Like Structures in Human Uveitis. *Exp Eye Res* (2020) 191:1–9. doi: 10.1016/j.exer.2019.107901
37. Diedrichs-Möhring M, Kaufmann U, Wildner G. The Immunopathogenesis of Chronic and Relapsing Autoimmune Uveitis – Lessons From Experimental Rat Models. *Prog Retin Eye Res* (2018) 65:107–26. doi: 10.1016/j.preteyeres.2018.02.003
38. Weavers H, Martin P. The Cell Biology of Inflammation: From Common Traits to Remarkable Immunological Adaptations. *J Cell Biol* (2020) 219 (7):1–14. doi: 10.1083/jcb.202004003
39. Jones GW, Hill DG, Jones SA. Understanding Immune Cells in Tertiary Lymphoid Organ Development: It Is All Starting to Come Together. *Front Immunol* (2016) 7:401. doi: 10.3389/fimmu.2016.00401
40. Heng JS, Hackett SF, Stein-O'Brien GL, Winer BL, Williams J, Goff LA, et al. Comprehensive Analysis of a Mouse Model of Spontaneous Uveoretinitis Using Single-Cell RNA Sequencing. *Proc Natl Acad Sci USA* (2019), 201915571. doi: 10.1073/pnas.1915571116
41. Montesano G, Way CM, Ometto G, Ibrahim H, Jones PR, Carmichael R, et al. Optimizing OCT Acquisition Parameters for Assessments of Vitreous Haze for Application in Uveitis. *Sci Rep* (2018) 8:1–7. doi: 10.1038/s41598-018-20092-y
42. Ravin JG. Sesquicentennial of the Ophthalmoscope. *Arch Ophthalmol* (1999) 117(12):1634–8. doi: 10.1001/archopht.117.12.1634
43. Marchese A, Agarwal A, Moretti AG, Handa S, Modorati G, Querques G, et al. Advances in Imaging of Uveitis. *Ther Adv Ophthalmol* (2020) 12:2515841420917781. doi: 10.1177/2515841420917781
44. Kimura SJ, Thygeson P, Hogan MJ. Signs and Symptoms of Uveitis. II. Classification of the Posterior Manifestations of Uveitis. *Am J Ophthalmol* (1959) 47(5 Pt 2):171–6. doi: 10.1016/s0002-9394(14)78240-6
45. Hogan MJ, Kimura SJ, Thygeson P. Signs and Symptoms of Uveitis. I. Anterior Uveitis. *Am J Ophthalmol* (1959) 47(5 Pt 2):155–70. doi: 10.1016/s0002-9394(14)78239-x

46. Trusko B, Thorne J, Jabs D, Belfort R, Dick A, Gangaputra S, et al. The Standardization of Uveitis Nomenclature (SUN) Project Development of a Clinical Evidence Base Utilizing Informatics Tools and Techniques. *Methods Inf Med* (2013) 52(3):259–65. doi: 10.3414/me12-01-0063
47. Kaburaki T, Namba K, Sonoda K-H, Kezuka T, Keino H, Fukuhara T, et al. Behçet's Disease Ocular Attack Score 24: Evaluation of Ocular Disease Activity Before and After Initiation of Infliximab. *Japanese J Ophthalmol* (2014) 58(2):120–30. doi: 10.1007/s10384-013-0294-0
48. Denniston AK, Keane PA, Srivastava SK. Biomarkers and Surrogate Endpoints in Uveitis: The Impact of Quantitative Imaging. *Invest Ophthalmol Vis Sci* (2017) 58(6):BIO131–BIO40. doi: 10.1167/iovs.17-21788
49. Hornbeak DM, Payal A, Pistilli M, Biswas J, Ganesh SK, Gupta V, et al. Interobserver Agreement in Clinical Grading of Vitreous Haze Using Alternative Grading Scales. *Ophthalmology* (2014) 121(8):1643–8. doi: 10.1016/j.ophtha.2014.02.018
50. Davis JL, Madow B, Cornett J, Stratton R, Hess D, Porciatti V, et al. Scale for Photographic Grading of Vitreous Haze in Uveitis. *Am J Ophthalmol* (2010) 150(5):637–41. doi: 10.1016/j.ajo.2010.05.036
51. Passaglia CL, Arvaneh T, Greenberg E, Richards D, Madow B. Automated Method of Grading Vitreous Haze in Patients With Uveitis for Clinical Trials. *Transl Vis Sci Technol* (2018) 7(2):10. doi: 10.1167/tvst.7.2.10
52. Agarwal RK, Caspi RR. Rodent Models of Experimental Autoimmune Uveitis. *Methods Mol Med* (2004) 102:395–419. doi: 10.1385/1-59259-805-6:395
53. Agarwal RK, Silver PB, Caspi RR. Rodent Models of Experimental Autoimmune Uveitis. *Methods Mol Biol* (2012) 900:443–69. doi: 10.1007/978-1-60761-720-4_22
54. Copland DA, Liu J, Schewitz-Bowers LP, Brinkmann V, Anderson K, Nicholson LB, et al. Therapeutic Dosing of Fingolimod (FTY720) Prevents Cell Infiltration, Rapidly Suppresses Ocular Inflammation, and Maintains the Blood-Ocular Barrier. *Am J Pathol* (2012) 180:672–81. doi: 10.1016/j.ajpath.2011.10.008
55. Huang D, Swanson E, Lin C, Schuman J, Stinson W, Chang W, et al. Optical Coherence Tomography. *Science* (1991) 254(5035):1178–81. doi: 10.1126/science.1957169
56. Drexler W, Liu MY, Kumar A, Kamali T, Unterhuber A, Leitgeb RA. Optical Coherence Tomography Today: Speed, Contrast, and Multimodality. *J Biomed Optics* (2014) 19(7):1–34. doi: 10.1117/1.jbo.19.7.071412
57. Mrejen S, Spaide RF. Optical Coherence Tomography: Imaging of the Choroid and Beyond. *Survey Ophthalmol* (2013) 58(5):387–429. doi: 10.1016/j.survophthal.2012.12.001
58. Yu C-R, Kim S-H, Mahdi RM, Egwuagu CE. SOCS3 Deletion in T Lymphocytes Suppresses Development of Chronic Ocular Inflammation *Via* Upregulation of CTLA-4 and Expansion of Regulatory T Cells. *J Immunol* (2013) 191(10):5036–43. doi: 10.4049/jimmunol.1301132
59. Chen J, Qian H, Horai R, Chan CC, Caspi RR. Use of Optical Coherence Tomography and Electroretinography to Evaluate Retinal Pathology in a Mouse Model of Autoimmune Uveitis. *PloS One* (2013) 8(5):e63904. doi: 10.1371/journal.pone.0063904
60. Nussenblatt RB, Gery I, Wacker WB. Experimental Autoimmune Uveitis - Cellular Immune Responsiveness. *Invest Ophthalmol Vis Sci* (1980) 19 (6):686–90.
61. Kozak YD, Sakai J, Thillaye B, Faure JP. S Antigen-Induced Experimental Autoimmune Uveo-Retinitis in Rats. *Curr Eye Res* (1981) 1(6):327–37. doi: 10.3109/02713688108998359
62. Mochizuki M, Kuwabara T, McAllister C, Nussenblatt RB, Gery I. Adoptive Transfer of Experimental Autoimmune Uveoretinitis in Rats. Immunopathogenic Mechanisms and Histologic Features. *Invest Ophthalmol Vis Sci* (1985) 26(1):1–9.
63. Thurau SR, Mempel TR, Flugel A, Edrichs-Mohring M, Krombach F, Kawakami N, et al. The Fate of Autoreactive, GFP+ T Cells in Rat Models of Uveitis Analyzed by Intravital Fluorescence Microscopy and FACS. *Int Immunol* (2004) 16(11):1573–82. doi: 10.1093/intimm/dxh158
64. Luger D, Silver PB, Tang J, Cua D, Chen Z, Iwakura Y, et al. Either a Th17 or a Th1 Effector Response can Drive Autoimmunity: Conditions of Disease Induction Affect Dominant Effector Category. *J Exp Med* (2008) 205(4):799–810. doi: 10.1084/jem.20071258
65. Silver PB, Horai R, Chen J, Jittayasothorn Y, Chan C-C, Villasmil R, et al. Retina-Specific T Regulatory Cells Bring About Resolution and Maintain Remission of Autoimmune Uveitis. *J Immunol* (2015) 194(7):3011–9. doi: 10.4049/jimmunol.1402650
66. Li J, Ren J, Yip YWY, Zhang X, Chu KO, Ng TK, et al. Quantitative Characterization of Autoimmune Uveoretinitis in an Experimental Mouse Model. *Invest Ophthalmol Vis Sci* (2017) 58(10):4193–200. doi: 10.1167/iovs.17-22436
67. Choi WJ, Pepple KL, Wang RK. Automated Three-Dimensional Cell Counting Method for Grading Uveitis of Rodent Eye *In Vivo* With Optical Coherence Tomography. *J Biophotonics* (2018) 11(9):e201800140. doi: 10.1002/jbio.201800140
68. Dysli C, Enzmann V, Sznitman R, Zinkernagel MS. Quantitative Analysis of Mouse Retinal Layers Using Automated Segmentation of Spectral Domain Optical Coherence Tomography Images. *Trans Vision Sci Technol* (2015) 4 (4):9. doi: 10.1167/tvst.4.4.9
69. Holland GN. A Reconsideration of Anterior Chamber Flare and its Clinical Relevance for Children With Chronic Anterior Uveitis (An American Ophthalmological Society Thesis). *Trans Am Ophthalmological Soc* (2007) 105:344–64.
70. Agrawal R, Keane PA, Singh J, Saihan Z, Kontos A, Pavesio CE. Classification of Semi-Automated Flare Readings Using the Kowa FM 700 Laser Cell Flare Meter in Patients With Uveitis. *Acta Ophthalmologica* (2016) 94(2):e135–e41. doi: 10.1111/aos.12833
71. Ruggeri M, Wehbe H, Jiao S, Gregori G, Jockovich ME, Hackam A, et al. In Vivo Three-Dimensional High-Resolution Imaging of Rodent Retina With Spectral-Domain Optical Coherence Tomography. *Invest Ophthalmol Vis Sci* (2007) 48(4):1808–14. doi: 10.1167/iovs.06-0815
72. Zarranz-Ventura J, Keane PA, Sim DA, Llorens V, Tufail A, Sadda SR, et al. Evaluation of Objective Vitritis Grading Method Using Optical Coherence Tomography: Influence of Phakic Status and Previous Vitrectomy. *Am J Ophthalmol* (2016) 161:172–80.e1-4. doi: 10.1016/j.ajo.2015.10.009
73. Keane PA, Balaskas K, Sim DA, Aman K, Denniston AK, Aslam T, et al. Automated Analysis of Vitreous Inflammation Using Spectral-Domain Optical Coherence Tomography. *Trans Vision Sci Technol* (2015) 4(5):1–10. doi: 10.1167/tvst.4.5.4
74. Pepple KL, Choi WJ, Wilson L, Van Gelder RN, Wang RK. Quantitative Assessment of Anterior Segment Inflammation in a Rat Model of Uveitis Using Spectral-Domain Optical Coherence Tomography. *Invest Ophthalmol Vis Sci* (2016) 57(8):3567–75. doi: 10.1167/iovs.16-19276
75. Choi WJ, Pepple KL, Wang RK. Automated Three-Dimensional Cell Counting Method for Grading Uveitis of Rodent Eye. In: Vivo Optical Coherence Tomography. *J Biophotonics* (2018) 11(9):e201800140. doi: 10.1002/jbio.201800140
76. Smith RS, John SWM, Nishina PM, Sundberg JP. *Systematic Evaluation of the Mouse Eye: Anatomy, Pathology, and Biomethods*. Boca Raton, FL: CRC Press (2002).
77. Keane PA, Karampelas M, Sim DA, Sadda SR, Tufail A, Sen HN, et al. Objective Measurement of Vitreous Inflammation Using Optical Coherence Tomography. *Ophthalmology* (2014) 121(9):1706–14. doi: 10.1016/j.ophtha.2014.03.006
78. Gadjanski I, Williams SK, Hein K, Sattler MB, Bahr M, Diem R. Correlation of Optical Coherence Tomography With Clinical and Histopathological Findings in Experimental Autoimmune Uveoretinitis. *Exp Eye Res* (2011) 93 (1):82–90. doi: 10.1016/j.exer.2011.04.012
79. Berger A, Cavallero S, Dominguez E, Barbe P, Simonutti M, Sahel JA, et al. Spectral-Domain Optical Coherence Tomography of the Rodent Eye: Highlighting Layers of the Outer Retina Using Signal Averaging and Comparison With Histology. *PloS One* (2014) 9(5):e96494. doi: 10.1371/journal.pone.0096494
80. Kajic V, Povazay B, Hermann B, Hofer B, Marshall D, Rosin PL, et al. Robust Segmentation of Intraretinal Layers in the Normal Human Fovea Using a Novel Statistical Model Based on Texture and Shape Analysis. *Opt Express* (2010) 18(14):14730–44. doi: 10.1364/OE.18.014730
81. Ishikawa H, Stein DM, Wollstein G, Beaton S, Fujimoto JG, Schuman JS. Macular Segmentation With Optical Coherence Tomography. *Invest Ophthalmol Vis Sci* (2005) 46(6):2012–7. doi: 10.1167/iovs.04-0335

82. Mishra A, Wong A, Bizheva K, Clausi DA. Intra-Retinal Layer Segmentation in Optical Coherence Tomography Images. *Opt Express* (2009) 17 (26):23719–28. doi: 10.1364/OE.17.023719
83. Mujat M, Chan R, Cense B, Park B, Joo C, Akkin T, et al. Retinal Nerve Fiber Layer Thickness Map Determined From Optical Coherence Tomography Images. *Opt Express* (2005) 13(23):9480–91. doi: 10.1364/opex.13.009480
84. Gonzalez-Lopez A, de Moura J, Novo J, Ortega M, Penedo MG. Robust Segmentation of Retinal Layers in Optical Coherence Tomography Images Based on a Multistage Active Contour Model. *Heliyon* (2019) 5(2):e01271. doi: 10.1016/j.heliyon.2019.e01271
85. Venhuizen FG, van Ginneken B, Liefers B, van Grinsven M, Fauser S, Hoyng C, et al. Robust Total Retina Thickness Segmentation in Optical Coherence Tomography Images Using Convolutional Neural Networks. *BioMed Opt Express* (2017) 8(7):3292–316. doi: 10.1364/BOE.8.003292
86. Garvin MK, Abramoff MD, Wu X, Russell SR, Burns TL, Sonka M. Automated 3-D Intraretinal Layer Segmentation of Macular Spectral-Domain Optical Coherence Tomography Images. *IEEE Trans Med Imaging* (2009) 28(9):1436–47. doi: 10.1109/TMI.2009.2016958
87. Lang A, Carass A, Hauser M, Sotirchos ES, Calabresi PA, Ying HS, et al. Retinal Layer Segmentation of Macular OCT Images Using Boundary Classification. *BioMed Opt Express* (2013) 4(7):1133–52. doi: 10.1364/BOE.4.001133
88. Kajic V, Esmaeelpour M, Povazay B, Marshall D, Rosin PL, Drexler W. Automated Choroidal Segmentation of 1060 Nm OCT in Healthy and Pathologic Eyes Using a Statistical Model. *BioMed Opt Express* (2012) 3 (1):86–103. doi: 10.1364/BOE.3.000086
89. Spaide RF, Curcio CA. Anatomical Correlates to the Bands Seen in the Outer Retina by Optical Coherence Tomography: Literature Review and Model. *Retina* (2011) 31(8):1609–19. doi: 10.1097/IAE.0b013e3182247535
90. Mattapallil MJ, Wawrousek EF, Chan C-C, Zhao H, Roychoudhury J, Ferguson TA, et al. The rd8 Mutation of the Crb1 Gene is Present in Vendor Lines of C57BL/6N Mice and Embryonic Stem Cells, and Confounds Ocular Induced Mutant Phenotypes. *Invest Ophthalmol Vis Sci* (2012) 53 (6):2921–7. doi: 10.1167/iovs.12-9662
91. Fischer MD, Huber G, Beck SC, Tanimoto N, Muehlfriedel R, Fahl E, et al. Noninvasive, In Vivo Assessment of Mouse Retinal Structure Using Optical Coherence Tomography. *PloS One* (2009) 4(10):1–7. doi: 10.1371/journal.pone.0007507
92. Srinivasan VJ, Ko TH, Wojtkowski M, Carvalho M, Clermont A, Bursell SE, et al. Noninvasive Volumetric Imaging and Morphometry of the Rodent Retina With High-Speed, Ultrahigh-Resolution Optical Coherence Tomography. *Invest Ophthalmol Vis Sci* (2006) 47(12):5522–8. doi: 10.1167/iovs.06-0195
93. Dingerkus VLS, Munk MR, Brinkmann MP, Freiberg FJ, Heussen FMA, Kinzl S, et al. Optical Coherence Tomography Angiography (OCTA) as a New Diagnostic Tool in Uveitis. *J Ophthalmic Inflammation Infect* (2019) 9 (1):10. doi: 10.1186/s12348-019-0176-9
94. Alnawaiseh M, Rosentreter A, Hillmann A, Alex AF, Niekamper D, Heiduschka P, et al. OCT Angiography in the Mouse: A Novel Evaluation Method for Vascular Pathologies of the Mouse Retina. *Exp Eye Res* (2016) 145:417–23. doi: 10.1016/j.exer.2016.02.012
95. Kim AY, Rodger DC, Shahidzadeh A, Chu Z, Koulisis N, Burkemper B, et al. Quantifying Retinal Microvascular Changes in Uveitis Using Spectral-Domain Optical Coherence Tomography Angiography. *Am J Ophthalmol* (2016) 171:101–12. doi: 10.1016/j.ajo.2016.08.035
96. Chu Z, Lin J, Gao C, Xin C, Zhang Q, Chen CL, et al. Quantitative Assessment of the Retinal Microvasculature Using Optical Coherence Tomography Angiography. *J BioMed Opt* (2016) 21(6):66008. doi: 10.1117/1.JBO.21.6.066008
97. Moccia S, De Momi E, El Hadji S, Mattos LS. Blood Vessel Segmentation Algorithms - Review of Methods, Datasets and Evaluation Metrics. *Comput Methods Programs BioMed* (2018) 158:71–91. doi: 10.1016/j.cmpb.2018.02.001
98. Hu Z, Niemeijer M, Abramoff MD, Garvin MK. Multimodal Retinal Vessel Segmentation From Spectral-Domain Optical Coherence Tomography and Fundus Photography. *IEEE Trans Med Imaging* (2012) 31(10):1900–11. doi: 10.1109/TMI.2012.2206822
99. Rodrigues P, Guimaraes P, Santos T, Simao S, Miranda T, Serranho P, et al. Two-Dimensional Segmentation of the Retinal Vascular Network From Optical Coherence Tomography. *J BioMed Opt* (2013) 18(12):126011. doi: 10.1117/1.JBO.18.12.126011
100. Zhu Q, Xing X, Zhu M, Xiao H, Ma L, Chen L, et al. A New Approach for the Segmentation of Three Distinct Retinal Capillary Plexuses Using Optical Coherence Tomography Angiography. *Transl Vis Sci Technol* (2019) 8(3):57. doi: 10.1167/tvst.8.3.57
101. Li A, You J, Du C, Pan Y. Automated Segmentation and Quantification of OCT Angiography for Tracking Angiogenesis Progression. *BioMed Opt Express* (2017) 8(12):5604–16. doi: 10.1364/BOE.8.005604
102. Ma Y, Hao H, Xie J, Fu H, Zhang J, Yang J, et al. Rose: A Retinal OCT-Angiography Vessel Segmentation Dataset and New Model. *IEEE Trans Med Imaging* (2021) 40(3):928–39. doi: 10.1109/TMI.2020.3042802
103. Chen J, Caspi RR. Clinical and Functional Evaluation of Ocular Inflammatory Disease Using the Model of Experimental Autoimmune Uveitis. *Methods Mol Biol* (2019) 1899:211–27. doi: 10.1007/978-1-4939-8938-6_15
104. Schneider CA, Rasband WS, Eliceiri KW. NIH Image to ImageJ: 25 Years of Image Analysis. *Nat Methods* (2012) 9(7):671–5. doi: 10.1038/nmeth.2089
105. Cingolani C, Rogers B, Lu L, Kachi S, Shen J, Campochiaro PA. Retinal Degeneration From Oxidative Damage. *Free Radical Biol Med* (2006) 40 (4):660–9. doi: 10.1016/j.freeradbiomed.2005.09.032
106. Faes L, Liu X, Wagner SK, Fu DJ, Balaskas K, Sim DA, et al. A Clinician's Guide to Artificial Intelligence: How to Critically Appraise Machine Learning Studies. *Trans Vision Sci Technol* (2020) 9(2):7–. doi: 10.1167/tvst.9.2.7
107. Liu XX, Faes L, Kale AU, Wagner SK, Fu DJ, Bruynseels A, et al. A Comparison of Deep Learning Performance Against Health-Care Professionals in Detecting Diseases From Medical Imaging: A Systematic Review and Meta-Analysis. *Lancet Digital Health* (2019) 1(6):E271–E97. doi: 10.1016/s2589-7500(19)30123-2
108. De Fauw J, Ledsam JR, Romera-Paredes B, Nikolov S, Tomasev N, Blackwell S, et al. Clinically Applicable Deep Learning for Diagnosis and Referral in Retinal Disease. *Nat Med* (2018) 24(9):1342–50. doi: 10.1038/s41591-018-0107-6
109. Dogra A, Goyal B, Agrawal S, Ahuja CK. Efficient Fusion of Osseous and Vascular Details in Wavelet Domain. *Pattern Recognit Lett* (2017) 94:189–93. doi: 10.1016/j.patrec.2017.03.002
110. Mitchell HB. *Image Fusion: Theories, Techniques and Applications.* Berlin Heidelberg: Springer (2010) p. 1–247 p.
111. Dick AD, Tundia N, Sorg R, Zhao C, Chao JD, Joshi A, et al. Risk of Ocular Complications in Patients With Noninfectious Intermediate Uveitis, Posterior Uveitis, or Panuveitis. *Ophthalmology* (2016) 123(3):655–62. doi: 10.1016/j.ophtha.2015.10.028
112. Epps SJ, Boldison J, Stimpson ML, Khera TK, Lait PJP, Copland DA, et al. Re-Programming Immunosurveillance in Persistent Non-Infectious Ocular Inflammation. *Prog Retin Eye Res* (2018) 65:93–106. doi: 10.1016/j.preteyeres.2018.03.001

14

Zika Virus Infection of Human Iris Pigment Epithelial Cells

Feargal J. Ryan[1†], Jillian M. Carr[2†], João M. Furtado[3†], Yuefang Ma[2], Liam M. Ashander[2], Milena Simões[3], Genevieve F. Oliver[2], G. Bracho Granado[2], Abby C. Dawson[2], Michael Z. Michael[2], Binoy Appukuttan[2], David J. Lynn[1,2‡] and Justine R. Smith[1,2*‡]

[1] Precision Medicine Theme, South Australian Health & Medical Research Institute, Adelaide, SA, Australia, [2] Flinders University College of Medicine and Public Health, Bedford Park, SA, Australia, [3] Ophthalmology Division, Ribeirão Preto Medical School, University of São Paulo, Ribeirão Preto, Brazil

***Correspondence:**
Justine R. Smith
justine.smith@flinders.edu.au

†These authors have contributed equally to this work and share first authorship

‡These authors have contributed equally to this work and share senior authorship

During recent Zika epidemics, adults infected with Zika virus (ZIKV) have developed organ-specific inflammatory complications. The most serious Zika-associated inflammatory eye disease is uveitis, which is commonly anterior in type, affecting both eyes and responding to corticosteroid eye drops. Mechanisms of Zika-associated anterior uveitis are unknown, but ZIKV has been identified in the aqueous humor of affected individuals. The iris pigment epithelium is a target cell population in viral anterior uveitis, and it acts to maintain immune privilege within the anterior eye. Interactions between ZIKV and human iris pigment epithelial cells were investigated with infectivity assays and RNA-sequencing. Primary cell isolates were prepared from eyes of 20 cadaveric donors, and infected for 24 hours with PRVABC59 strain ZIKV or incubated uninfected as control. Cytoimmunofluorescence, RT-qPCR on total cellular RNA, and focus-forming assays of culture supernatant showed cell isolates were permissive to infection, and supported replication and release of infectious ZIKV. To explore molecular responses of cell isolates to ZIKV infection at the whole transcriptome level, RNA was sequenced on the Illumina NextSeq 500 platform, and results were aligned to the human GRCh38 genome. Multidimensional scaling showed clear separation between transcriptomes of infected and uninfected cell isolates. Differential expression analysis indicated a vigorous molecular response of the cell to ZIKV: 7,935 genes were differentially expressed between ZIKV-infected and uninfected cells (FDR < 0.05), and 99% of 613 genes that changed at least two-fold were up-regulated. Reactome and KEGG pathway and Gene Ontology enrichment analyses indicated strong activation of viral recognition and defense, in addition to biosynthesis processes. A CHAT network included 6275 molecular nodes and 24 contextual hubs in the cell response to ZIKV infection. Receptor-interacting serine/threonine kinase 1 (RIPK1) was the most significantly connected contextual hub. Correlation of gene expression with read counts assigned to the ZIKV genome identified a negative correlation between interferon signaling and viral load across isolates. This work represents the first investigation of mechanisms of Zika-associated anterior uveitis using an *in vitro* human cell model. The results suggest the iris pigment epithelium mounts a molecular response that limits intraocular pathology in most individuals.

Keywords: Zika, virus, ZIKV, human, eye, iris, epithelium, pigment epithelial cell

INTRODUCTION

Zika virus (ZIKV) is a single-stranded RNA flavivirus, which was first isolated from non-human primates in Uganda in 1947, and from humans in the same country in the early 1950s (1). Zika virus disease is generally considered to pose little risk to human health unless it is contracted *in utero*. In recent epidemics from 2013 to 2014 in French Polynesia, and from 2015 to 2016 in Brazil and other American nations, women who were infected while pregnant delivered infants with a spectrum of developmental abnormalities (2, 3), now referred to as congenital Zika syndrome (4). Characteristic abnormalities in this disease include severe microcephaly, thinned cerebral cortex with subcortical calcification, extrapyramidal motor disturbances and contractures. In addition, approximately 70% of babies with congenital Zika syndrome develop ocular abnormalities, including retinal dystrophic lesions that show a preference for the macula, and therefore cause blindness (5). However, in some adults, infection with ZIKV results in serious inflammatory conditions (1).

Uveitis –or intraocular inflammation– represents a diverse spectrum of diseases, classified according to anatomical localization within the eye and by specific phenotype (6). Different types of uveitis have been reported in adult patients infected with ZIKV (7). The most common form is anterior uveitis –based in the iris and ciliary body– which occurs in approximately 50% of patients who present with "red eyes" in the context of Zika fever (8). This uveitis is typically bilateral, may impact the visual acuity, and often is accompanied by an elevation of intraocular pressure, as we (9) and others (8, 10, 11) have documented (**Table 1**). In one of the first reports of Zika-associated anterior uveitis, aqueous humor was collected from the eye of a patient treated with corticosteroid eye drops alone; ZIKV RNA was recovered from fluid taken at 8 days after the onset of systemic symptoms, but not at 16 days (9). This implies that Zika-associated anterior uveitis is associated with the presence of ZIKV inside the eye.

Several independently conducted studies have explored the pathogenic mechanisms of congenital Zika syndrome in mouse models (12–15), and human retinal cells or cell lines (16–19). However, the pathogenic mechanisms that are responsible for Zika-associated anterior uveitis have not been investigated previously. In the anterior eye, iris pigment epithelial cells play a major role in controlling the immune microenvironment (20). In herpes viral anterior uveitis, which is the most studied viral anterior uveitis, pathological changes involving these cells result in a variety of gross ocular changes, including tissue defects that may impact iris appearance (21). To address the important knowledge gap around the pathogenesis of Zika-associated anterior uveitis, we investigated interactions between ZIKV and primary human iris pigment epithelial cells using infectivity assays and next generation sequencing of cellular RNA content (RNA-Seq).

METHODS

Human Iris Pigment Epithelial Cells

Iris pigment epithelial cell isolates were prepared from paired human cadaver donor eyes, using methods that were adapted from the technique published by Mai et al. (22). Irises were carefully dissected from the two posterior eyecups, digested in 0.25% trypsin (Thermo Fisher Scientific-Gibco, Grand Island, NY) for 45 minutes at 37°C, and transferred to phosphate buffered saline (PBS) with 2% fetal bovine serum (FBS; Bovogen Biologicals, Keilor East, Australia) at room temperature. Pigment epithelial cells were gently brushed from the tissue using the bent tip of a Pasteur pipette. The cell suspension was pelleted at 10 x g for 5 minutes at room temperature, washed with PBS with 2% FBS, and re-suspended in Epithelial Cell Medium (ScienCell Research Laboratories, Carlsbad, CA; catalog number 4101, consisting of basal medium, 2% FBS, Epithelial Cell Growth Supplement and a penicillin-streptomycin solution). Cells were expanded at 37°C and 5% CO_2 in air, with medium refreshed twice a week, initially in a 6 cm diameter dish, subsequently trypsin-passaged and transferred to a T75 flask, and finally stored frozen in liquid nitrogen on reaching confluence. Cell phenotype was confirmed for all cell isolates by immunocytochemical detection of cytokeratin-8 indicating epithelial lineage and absence of α-smooth muscle actin, which is expressed during mesenchymal differentiation (see *Cytoimmunofluorescence*). All cell isolates were demonstrated to be free of *Mycoplasma* species contamination by quantitative real-time polymerase chain reaction (qPCR) of DNA extracted from culture supernatant.

Zika Virus

Zika virus (strain PRVABC59: National Center for Biotechnology Information Nucleotide (GenBank) Accession Number, KU501215; originally isolated from human serum in Puerto Rico in 2015) was propagated in C6/36 mosquito cells (American Type Culture Collection [ATCC], Gaithersburg, MA) that were grown in Eagle's basal medium, 1 mM sodium pyruvate, 1x MEM Non-Essential Amino Acids Solution, 2 mM L-glutamine and 10% FBS (all from Thermo Fisher

TABLE 1 | Clinical features of ZIKV-associated anterior uveitis diagnosed in patients presenting to the Ophthalmology Clinic of Ribeirão Preto General Hospital, Ribeirão Preto, São Paulo or reported in the medical literature.

Location; Demographics (Reference if applicable)*	Clinical features	Basis for diagnosis	Treatment and course
Ribeirão Preto, Brazil; M, 40 years (9)	OD/OS; VA=20/20 OD, 20/60 OS; AC cell=0.5+ OD, 2+ OS; IOP=16mmHg OD, 15mmHg OS; other=punctate keratitis	Epidemiology; Systemic features; Serology; Aqueous and blood RT-PCR	Topical glucocorticoid; Remission of uveitis with improvement of VA
Ribeirão Preto, Brazil; F, 55 years	OD/OS; VA=20/30 OD, 20/25 OS; AC cell=3+ OD, 2+ OS; IOP=34mmHg OD, 17mmHg OS	Epidemiology; Systemic features; Aqueous and blood RT-PCR	Topical glucocorticoid and hypotensive; Remission of uveitis with improvement of VA
Ribeirão Preto, Brazil; F, 41 years	OD; VA=20/100 OD, 20/20 OS (unrelated corneal dystrophy OD); AC cell=3+ OD, 0+ OS; IOP=17mmHg OD, 16mmHg OS	Epidemiology; Systemic features; Negative work-up for other causes	Topical glucocorticoid; Remission of uveitis with no change in VA
Ribeirão Preto, Brazil; F, 40 years	OS; VA=20/100 OD, 20/30 OS (unrelated toxoplasmic retinal scar OD); AC cell=0+ OD, 1+ OS; IOP=16mmHg OD, 16mmHg OS	Epidemiology; Systemic features; Negative work-up for other causes	Topical glucocorticoid; Remission of uveitis with improvement of VA
Ribeirão Preto, Brazil; F, 66 years	OD; VA=20/40 OD, 20/30 OS; (unrelated macular hole OD); AC cell=2+ OD, 0+ OS; IOP=14mmHg OD, 14mmHg OS	Epidemiology; Systemic features; Negative work-up for other causes	Topical glucocorticoid; Remission of uveitis with no change in VA
Rio de Janeiro, Brazil; M, 39 years (10)	OD/OS; VA=20/40 OD, 20/40 OS; AC cell=1+ OD, 1+ OS; IOP=40mmHg OD, 28mmHg OS	Epidemiology; Systemic features; Negative work-up for other causes	Topical glucocorticoid and hypotensive; Remission of uveitis with improvement of VA and lowering of IOP
Martinique, France; W, 50s (11)	OD/OS; VA=20/25 OD, 20/20 OS; AC cell present (grade NS); IOP=36mmHg OD, 26mmHg OS	Epidemiology; Systemic features; Urine RT-PCR; Negative work-up for other causes	Topical hypotensive; Remission of uveitis and lowering of IOP#
Martinique, France; W, 60s (11)	OD/OS; VA=20/40 OD, 20/20 OS; AC cell present (grade NS); IOP=58mmHg OD, 32mmHg OS; other=corneal edema	Epidemiology; Systemic features; Aqueous and urine RT-PCR; Negative work-up for other causes	Topical hypotensive; Remission of uveitis and lowering of IOP
Guadeloupe, France; F, adult (age NS) (8)	OD/OS; VA=20/20 OD, 20/25 OS; AC cell=0.5+ OD, 1+ OS; IOP normal (value NS)	Epidemiology; Systemic features; Aqueous RT-PCR; Negative work-up for other causes	Topical glucocorticoid; Remission of uveitis and recovery of VA
Guadeloupe, France; M, adult (age NS) (8)	OD/OS; VA=20/20 OD, 20/25 OS; AC cell=0 OD, 0.5+ OS; IOP=16mmHg OD, 28mmHg OS	Epidemiology; Systemic features; Aqueous RT-PCR; Negative work-up for other causes	Topical glucocorticoid and hypotensive; Remission of uveitis; Persistent elevation of IOP
Guadeloupe, France; Gender NS, adult (Age NS) (8)	OD/OS; VA=20/32 OD, 20/20 OS; AC cell=0 OD, 1+ OS; IOP=25mmHg OD, 16mmHg OS	Epidemiology; Systemic features; Aqueous RT-PCR; Negative work-up for other causes	Topical glucocorticoid and hypotensive; Remission of uveitis; Persistent elevation of IOP
Guadeloupe, France; Gender NS, adult (Age NS) (8)	OD/OS; VA=20/20 OD, 20/40 OS; AC cell=0 OD, 1+ OS; IOP=16mmHg OD, 30mmHg OS	Epidemiology; Systemic features; Aqueous RT-PCR; Negative work-up for other causes	Topical glucocorticoid and hypotensive; Remission of uveitis; Persistent elevation of IOP

AC, anterior chamber; F, female; IOP, intraocular pressure; M, male; NS, not specified; OD, right eye; OS, left eye; RT-PCR, reverse transcription-polymerase reaction; VA, visual acuity.
**Reference 8 reports an observational study of 62 patients that included case histories from 4 patients whose diagnoses were based on aqueous RT-PCR plus other tests for Zika. Results of other tests were not specified. Visual acuity outcome was not stated for 3 of the 4 cases.*

Scientific-Gibco), and transferred to a medium modified by the removal of the amino acid supplement and reduction of FBS to 7.5%, and with the addition of 10 mM HEPES, ahead of infection. Virus stocks were titered by plaque assay on Vero cells, with plaques detected by neutral red overlay and expressed as plaque forming units/mL, as previously published (23).

Viral Infection of Human Iris Pigment Epithelial Cells

Human iris pigment epithelial cells were rapidly thawed and plated in 10 cm diameter tissue culture dishes in Epithelial Cell Medium with 2% FBS. After cells reached confluence, they were subcultured to 6 cm dishes (2 x 10^6 cells/dish) or 6-well plates, including wells with coverslips (2 x 10^5 cells/well), and rested overnight. Subconfluent monolayers of iris epithelial cells were infected with ZIKV at multiplicity of infection (MOI) of 1 or 5, or mock-infected, in a minimum amount of FBS-free Dulbecco's Modified Eagle Medium (DMEM, Thermo Fisher Scientific-Gibco; catalog number 11965). After 90 minutes, the inoculum was removed, and the infected cultures were returned to incubation in fresh Epithelial Cell Medium for a total of 24 hours, when cells were either lyzed with TRIzol Reagent (Thermo Fisher Scientific-Invitrogen, Carlsbad, CA) and stored at -80°C ahead of RNA extraction, or fixed with 2% paraformaldehyde for 30 minutes and stored in 70% ethanol at 4°C for cytoimmunofluorescence. Culture supernatant was snap-frozen at -80°C. A 24-hour time interval was selected to obtain a comprehensive picture of the host cell response to replicating virus. All work with live virus was conducted in a Physical Containment Level 2 Facility, under a Microbiological Dealing issued by the Flinders University Institutional Biosafety Committee (dealing number: 2016-07.1).

Focus Forming Assay

Supernatants from ZIKV-infected and uninfected human iris pigment epithelial cell monolayers were tested for infectious virus with a high throughput plaque assay performed on an Operetta High-Content Analysis System (PerkinElmer, Waltham, MA), modifying a previously reported method (24). In brief, Vero cells were seeded at 1 x 10^4 cell/well in 96-well plates and rested overnight, subsequently exposed in triplicate to serially diluted supernatant –or medium only control or ZIKV (3 x 10^6 pfu/mL) positive control– for 90 minutes, and finally incubated in fresh medium for 24 hours. Cell monolayers were fixed with 2% paraformaldehyde, permeabilized with 0.05% IGEPAL CA-630, and labeled with mouse anti-flavivirus envelope protein (ENV) antibody (ATCC HB-112TM hybridoma [clone 4G2] culture supernatant diluted 1:10, applied overnight at 4 °C), followed by Alexa Fluor 488-tagged donkey anti-mouse immunoglobulin antibody (Thermo Fisher Scientific-Molecular Probes, Eugene, OR; catalog number A21202; working concentration, 10 µg/mL, applied for 1 hour at room temperature) with Hoechst 33342 (2'-[4-ethoxyphenyl]-5-[4-methyl-1-piperazinyl]-2,5'-bi-1H-benzimidazole trihydrochloride trihydrate) counterstain. Wells were imaged using the Operetta High-Content Analysis System (11 fields/well, 100x magnification), and images were analyzed using the Columbus Image Data Storage and Analysis v2.7 (PerkinElmer) to quantify the number of labeled infected cell clusters per well. Data was processed in Vortex v2014.03.71496.59-s (Dotmatics, Bishops Stortford, UK), including calculation of focus forming units/mL for each supernatant sample and dilution.

Cytoimmunofluorescence

Human iris pigment epithelial cell monolayers were fixed with 2% or 4% paraformaldehyde in preparation for cytoimmunofluorescence labeling. For cell phenotyping, monolayers were labeled overnight at 4°C with one of following rabbit polyclonal antibodies diluted in 0.05% Triton X-100 and 2% bovine serum albumin in PBS: anti-human cytokeratin 8 (Abcam, Cambridge, United Kingdom; catalog number ab53280; working dilution, 1:250, equivalent to 0.132 µg/mL), α-smooth muscle actin (Abcam, catalog number ab5694; working dilution, 1:100, equivalent to 2 µg/mL) and rabbit immunoglobulin (Vector Laboratories, Burlingame, CA; catalog number I-1000, working concentration, 2 µg/mL). Cell monolayers were incubated with Alexa Fluor 488-tagged donkey anti-rabbit immunoglobulin antibody (Thermo Fisher Scientific-Molecular Probes; catalog number A11008; working concentration, 1 µg/mL) for 1 hour at room temperature, counterstained with DAPI (4',6-diamidino-2-phenylindole) for 2 minutes, and imaged by fluorescence microscopy at 200x magnification. For demonstration of viral infection, ZIKV-infected and uninfected cell monolayers were labeled for 1 hour at room temperature with mouse anti-flavivirus envelope protein antibody, used as hybridoma culture supernatant diluted 1:10 in Hanks' balanced salt solution with 2% goat serum. Cell monolayers were incubated with Alexa Fluor 488-tagged goat anti-mouse immunoglobulin antibody (Thermo Fisher Scientific-Molecular Probes; catalog number A11001; working concentration, 13 µg/mL) for 30 minutes at room temperature, counterstained with Hoechst 33342 for 10 minutes, and imaged by confocal microscopy at 100x magnification.

RNA Extraction

Total RNA was recovered from ZIKV-infected and uninfected iris pigment epithelial cells by phenol/chloroform extraction using Trizol Reagent, according to the manufacturer's protocol. RNase-free glycogen was added to all samples during precipitation to maximize RNA yields. RNA was frozen at -80°C prior to use for RNA-Seq and reverse transcription (RT)-qPCR. Nucleic acid concentrations were determined using the Qubit 2.0 Fluorometer (Thermo Fisher Scientific-Life Technologies, Carlsbad, CA).

Reverse Transcription-Polymerase Chain Reaction

Reverse transcription was carried out using iScript Reverse Transcription Supermix for RT-qPCR (Bio-Rad, Hercules, CA). Total RNA input was 500 ng per reaction, yielding 20 µl of cDNA which was diluted 10-fold ahead of use in qPCR.

Quantitative real-time PCR was performed using the CFX Connect Real Time PCR Detection System (Bio-Rad), and a reaction mix consisting of 4 µL of iQ Sybr Green Supermix or SsoAdvanced SYBR Green Supermix (Bio-Rad), 1.5 µL each of 20 µM forward and reverse primer, 11 µL of nuclease-free water and 2 µL of diluted cDNA. Primer sequences (and expected product sizes) were as follows: ZIKV ENV forward 5'-GCTGGDGCRGACACHGGRACT-3', reverse 5'-RTCYACYGCCATYTGGRCTG-3' (304 bp); interferon-β (IFN-β) forward 5'-AAACTCATGAGCAGTCTGCA-3', reverse 5'-AGGAGATCTTCAGTTTCGGAGG-3' (168 bp); peptidylprolyl isomerase A (PPIA) forward 5'-GAGCACTGGAGAGAAAGGATTT-3', reverse 5'-GGTGATCTTCTTGCTGGTCTT-3' (355 bp); and ribosomal protein lateral stalk subunit P0 (RPLP0) forward 5'-GCAGCATCTACAACCCTGAA-3', reverse 5'-GCAGATGGATCAGCCAAGAA-3' (235 bp). Primer efficiency for all primer sets was greater than 85.0% except in the case of ZIKV ENV, for which efficiency was 76.5%. Melting curves were included in each RT-qPCR run to confirm a single peak was produced, and amplicon sizes for all primers were confirmed by agarose gel electrophoresis.

Absolute quantification of viral genome equivalents was carried out by generating a standard curve for ZIKV ENV using purified PCR product serially diluted 10-fold from an initial concentration of 10 pg/µL. Starting quantity in ng (SQ) was determined for ZIKV-infected and uninfected samples using CFX Manager software v3.1 (Bio-Rad). Viral genome equivalent number was calculated using the equation ([SQ/10^9]/[bp molecular mass x product size]) x 6.02214 x 10^{23}. Relative expression of IFN-β was determined by the Pfaffl method (25) and normalized to two reference genes –PPIA and RPLP0– which were stable as indicated by CV-value less than 0.25 and M-value less than 0.5.

RNA Sequencing

An RNA integrity number of at least 8 was confirmed on the LabChip GX Touch 24 Nucleic Acid Analyzer (Perkin Elmer, Hopkinton, MA). The cDNA libraries were prepared with the TruSeq Stranded Total RNA Kit (Illumina, San Diego, CA), strictly in accordance with the manufacturer's instructions. Pooled libraries were sequenced on the NextSeq 500, with the High-Output Kit for 2 x 75 cycles of sequencing, and aiming for an average depth of 50 x 10^6 reads per sample. The PhiX Control v3 library (Illumina) was used as a sequencing control.

Processing and Analysis of RNA Sequencing Data

Quality of the data obtained by RNA sequencing was assessed with FastQC v0.11.3 (26). Sequences were trimmed with Trimmomatic v0.38 (27) for minimum and maximum lengths of 50 and 75 nucleotides, respectively, and a 4-nucleotide sliding window with an average Phred score of 25. Reads passing quality control were aligned to the GRCh38 human genome using HiSAT2 v2.1.0 (28) set to default parameters. FeatureCounts v1.5.0-p2 (29) was employed to count reads aligning to genes, as annotated in Ensembl v93, and counts of those genes uniquely mapped to the human genome were taken forward in the analysis. To investigate samples for contamination with non-human organisms, sequence reads were classified against the NCBI RefSeq database of bacterial, archaeal, viral and eukaryotic microbial genomes, as well as the human genome, using Kraken2 (30).

Further statistical analyses and visualization were performed in R v3.5.0 (31). The EdgeR v3.22.3 (32) package from Bioconductor was used to perform library size normalization (with the trimmed mean of M-values [TMM] method), multi-dimensional scaling, and differential expression analyses (with the glmQFit function). Variation in the data from unknown sources was examined using svaseq (33), and differential expression analysis was performed in a genewise negative binomial generalized linear model in EdgeR that controlled for donor effect (see *Data Availability Statement* for link to BitBucket data repository). Differentially expressed genes were defined by two-fold or greater change, and a Benjamini and Hochberg corrected p-value or false discovery rate (FDR) (34) less than 0.05. Pathway and Gene Ontology enrichment analyses were performed in InnateDB (35). To identify differentially expressed genes associated with estimated viral load, host gene expression was correlated with read counts per million assigned to the ZIKV genome in each sample by Kraken2 (Spearman correlation, p-value less than 0.05). Transcription factor binding site analysis was performed using the findMotifs.pl program in HOMER v4.10 (36), with the human promoter set. A network of molecular interactions between differentially expressed genes, products encoded by those genes and/or their first neighbor interactors was constructed using the Contextual Hub Analysis Tool (CHAT) (37) in Cytoscape v3.8.1 (38), with annotations by Interferome v2.0 (39) and InnateDB (35). This tool identifies "nodes" in the network that are more highly connected to differentially expressed genes than is expected by chance alone (FDR less than 0.05).

RESULTS

Iris pigment epithelial cells were sourced from 12 men and 8 women cadaveric donors, whose ages at death ranged from 44 to 78 years (median = 61.5 years). Time from death to processing of the human eyecups ranged from 7 to 23 hours (median = 12.5 hours), and iris pigment epithelial cells were isolated over a period of 13 to 19 days (median = 16 days). The cells presented as rounded bodies, with some spindle morphology when plated subconfluent ahead of infection (**Figure 1A**). Across all 20 isolates, cytoimmunofluorescence on cells from the same passage as used for subsequent infections indicated homogeneous expression of cytokeratin-8 and complete absence of α-smooth muscle actin, indicating highly pure epithelial cell isolates with no evidence of mesenchymal differentiation (**Figure 1B**).

To investigate the susceptibility of human iris pigment epithelial cells to infection with ZIKV, subconfluent cell monolayers were exposed to the PRVABC59 strain for 24 hours at an MOI of 1. Cytoimmunofluorescent labeling of cell monolayers for the flavivirus ENV identified ZIKV in all 20 isolates following exposure, with viral antigen detected in between 4.4% and 43.2% (median = 14.3%) of cells across the isolates (**Figure 1C**). The RT-qPCR analysis of cellular RNA and focus forming assay of culture supernatant also indicated productive infection of cells at 24 hours, with obvious variation in susceptibility between the 20 isolates, and this result was replicated at an MOI of 5 (**Figure 1D**). For an initial assessment of the type I IFN response of human iris pigment epithelial cell to infection with ZIKV, IFN-β was measured by RT-qPCR in isolates infected at an MOI of 5. This indicated substantial, but variable, increase in cellular IFN-β transcript following infection (**Figure 1E**). These results demonstrated that human iris pigment epithelial cells were moderately susceptible to ZIKV infection, and suggested that this cell population mounted a strong anti-viral response. The results also indicated considerable variation in these parameters across cells isolated from eyes of different individuals.

To explore the molecular response of human iris pigment epithelial cells to infection with ZIKV at a whole transcriptome level, RNA-Seq was performed on total RNA extracted from the 20 primary cell isolates 24 hours following infection with the PRVABC59 strain at an MOI of 5. Across the samples from uninfected isolates, there were 33.6 x 10^6 mean paired reads, with 33.4 x 10^6 (99.5%) of reads aligned to the human genome, and 25.0 x 10^6 (74.5%) mean paired reads assigned to annotated genes. After correction for library size differences, reads aligned to the flavivirus genome in samples infected with ZIKV averaged 9.9% (range = 2.0-24.9%) (**Supplementary Figure 1**). Comparison with a RefSeq database of bacterial, archaeal, viral and eukaryotic genomes indicated negligible contamination with

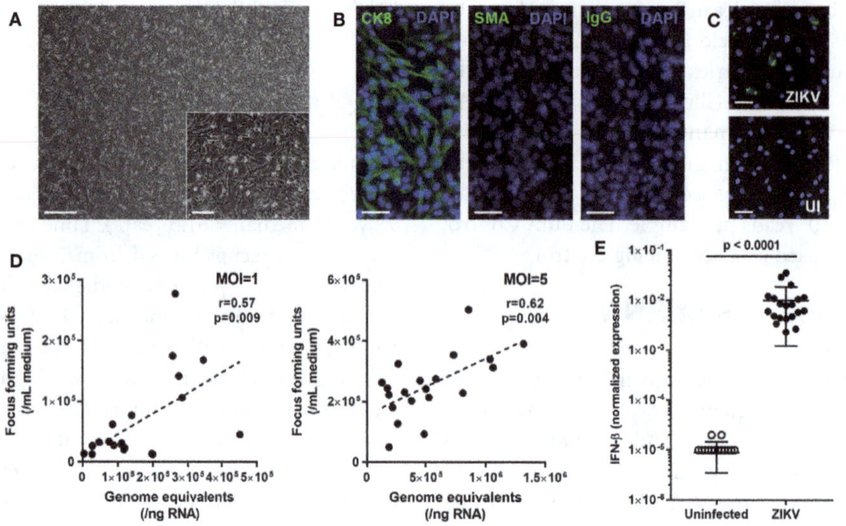

FIGURE 1 | **(A)** Light photomicrograph of human iris pigment epithelial cells immediately prior to infection. Original magnifications: 40x (main image) and 100x (inset image); Scale bars: 500 μm (main image) and 200 μm (inset image). **(B)** Fluorescence photomicrographs of human iris pigment epithelial cells immunolabeled to detect presence of cytokeratin 8 (CK8) and absence of alpha-smooth muscle actin (SMA), with negative control labeled with species-matched immunoglobulin (IgG). Alexa Fluor 488 (green) with DAPI nuclear counterstain (blue). Original magnification: 200x; Scale bar: 100 μm. **(C)** Fluorescence photomicrographs of ZIKV-infected and uninfected human iris pigment epithelial cells immunolabeled to detect flavivirus envelope protein. Alexa Fluor 488 (green) with Hoechst 33342 nuclear counterstain (blue). Original magnification: 100x; Scale bar: 100 μm. **(D)** Correlation plots showing cellular viral load in genome equivalents and infectious foci generated from culture supernatant for human iris pigment epithelial cells infected for 24 hours with ZIKV (multiplicity of infection = 1 and 5). Circles represent individual cell isolates from 20 donors. Line indicates trend. Data were analyzed by Pearson correlation coefficient. **(E)** Graph presenting normalized expression of interferon (IFN)-β transcript, calculated relative to peptidylprolyl isomerase A (PPIA) and ribosomal protein lateral stalk subunit P0 (RPLP0), in human iris pigment epithelial cells infected for 24 hours with ZIKV (multiplicity of infection = 5). Circles represent individual cell isolates from 20 donors. Crossbars indicate mean, and error bars indicate standard deviation. Data were analyzed by Wilcoxon signed-rank test.

other organisms, including *Mycoplasma* species. Alignment statistics are presented in **Supplementary Table 1**.

Multidimensional scaling of the gene expression data indicated clear separation of the total RNA transcriptome of ZIKV-infected versus non-infected human iris pigment epithelial cell isolates (**Figure 2A**). Data visualization with svaseq (33) indicated that the largest source of variation in the data related to donor (Kruskal Willis, p = 0.005), but this was not explained on the basis of donor age at death or sex, or time from death to cell isolation, and also was not related to batch. Thus, in order to focus on the common cellular response to ZIKV, differential expression analysis was performed controlling for the impact of donor. A total of 7,935 genes (47% of all annotated genes) were differentially expressed between infected and uninfected cells at FDR less than 0.05, including 606 genes that were increased and 7 genes that were decreased at least two-fold in the infected cells (**Figure 2B**, **Supplementary Table 2**). Heat maps showed obvious separation of the set of all differentially expressed genes between ZIKV-infected and uninfected samples (**Figure 3A**), although the 1,000 most variable genes were less discriminating (**Figure 3B**).

Pathway and Gene Ontology biological process analyses of genes significantly upregulated (ie. two-fold or greater change and FDR less than 0.05) in ZIKV-infected iris pigment epithelial cells compared to uninfected cells revealed a strong transcriptional response to infection, involving over 200 different pathways or processes. Molecules involved in immune functions were highly enriched among differentially expressed genes. More specifically, differentially expressed genes were enriched for groupings that included activation of pathogen recognition systems –with retinoic acid-inducible gene I (RIG-I)-like receptor (RLR) and toll-like receptor (TLR) signaling– and anti-viral and inflammatory cytokine responses –with type I and type II IFN signaling (**Figures 3C, D**, **Supplementary Table 3**). Gene ontology molecular function analysis of differentially expressed genes similarly indicated an active response to the virus. Highly enriched functions included broad terms, such as cytokine and chemokine activities, as well as more specific categories, such as single- and double- stranded RNA binding –signifying viral recognition– and 2′,5′-oligoadenylate synthetase (OAS) activity and tumor necrosis factor (TNF) receptor binding –consistent with anti-viral responses (**Figure 3E**, **Supplementary Table 3**). Transcription factor binding site analysis identified 13 regulatory motifs that were enriched in promoter regions of significantly upregulated genes, including multiple IFN-regulating factors (**Table 2**). No binding sites were enriched in genes with significantly downregulated expression.

A system-level CHAT network (37) was built around genes that were significantly differentially expressed between ZIKV-infected and uninfected human iris pigment epithelial cells, including first-neighbor interactors. This network included 6275 nodes (**Figure 4**, **Supplementary Table 4**). There were 24 contextual hubs that interacted with differentially expressed genes more frequently than predicted by chance alone (**Table 3**).

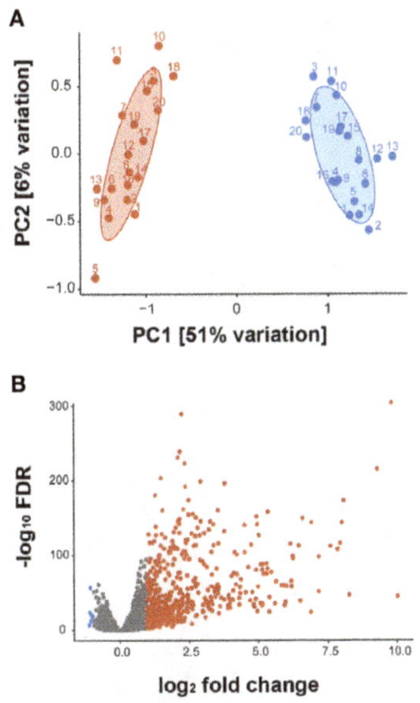

FIGURE 2 | **(A)** Multidimensional scaling plots showing global gene expression in ZIKV-infected (red) and uninfected (blue) human iris pigment epithelial cell isolates. Numbers indicate the 20 individual donors from whose eyes each isolate was generated. PC = principal component. **(B)** Volcano plot displaying differentially expressed genes between ZIKV-infected and uninfected human iris pigment epithelial cells, based on normalized counts per million (false discovery rate < 0.05 and fold change > 2). Red dots indicate significantly upregulated transcripts, and blue dots indicate significantly downregulated transcripts.

The most highly connected contextual hubs -with greater than 15 contextual neighbors and greater than 200 total neighbors- were members of the Janus kinase (JAK)-signal transducer and activator of transcription (STAT), or nuclear factor κ-light-chain-enhancer of activated B cells (NF-κB) intracellular signaling pathways, indicating their involvement in type I IFN anti-viral responses and inflammation. These six hubs included: inhibitor of NF-κB kinase, regulatory subunit γ (IKBKG); rela protooncogene, NF-κB subunit (RELA); TNF receptor-associated factor 6 (TRAF6); STAT1; STAT3; and ubiquitin-like modifier ISG15 (ISG15). Receptor-interacting serine/threonine kinase 1 (RIPK1) was the most significantly connected contextual hub ($p = 5.49 \times 10^{-5}$), with 16 contextual neighbors and 102 total neighbors.

Associations between gene expression by the host cell and intracellular ZIKV load were identified by correlating upregulated genes with normalized read counts assigned to the viral genome in the infected iris pigment epithelial cell isolates across the 20 human donors. This analysis identified 146 upregulated genes that were significantly correlated with read counts assigned to ZIKV, including 122 that were positively correlated and 24 that were negatively correlated (**Supplementary Table 5**). Reactome pathway enrichment analysis of these genes indicated 'IFN signaling' and 'immune system' were negatively correlated with ZIKV read counts, while cell cycle-related pathways were positively correlated (**Figure 5A**). Examples of upregulated IFN-stimulated genes that were negatively correlated with ZIKV load included: adenosine deaminase, RNA-specific (ADAR); IFN-induced protein 44 (ITI44); IFN-induced protein with tetratricopeptide repeats 5 (IFIT5); and OAS1 (**Figure 5B**).

DISCUSSION

Zika virus disease is often asymptomatic or manifest as a mild and self-limited systemic illness in adult patients. However, serious inflammatory complications may occur, and these include anterior uveitis, which has been linked with presence of ZIKV in the anterior eye (8, 9). Our work represents the first research to examine mechanisms of Zika-associated anterior uveitis, focusing on the interactions between the virus and iris pigment epithelial cells, and using the PRVABC59 strain isolated during the American epidemic and primary cells isolated within 24 hours of death from human cadaveric donors. Human iris pigment epithelial cell isolates generated from 20 donors were permissive to ZIKV infection, and supported replication and release of the virus. RNA-Seq indicated a vigorous molecular response of the host cell to ZIKV. Almost 50% of annotated genes were differentially expressed between infected and uninfected cells, and 99% of the 613 genes that changed at least two-fold were up-regulated. Pathway, Gene Ontology and network analyses indicated strong activation of viral recognition and defense, as well as biosynthesis mechanisms consistent with production of virus. Although all iris pigment epithelial cell isolates mounted a type I IFN response, intracellular virus load correlated inversely to overall IFN signaling across the donors.

When uveitis occurs in the context of a systemic infectious disease, the pathology usually represents a combination of tissue damage induced by the microbe and reactive inflammation by the host. Although some forms of infection-associated uveitis are believed to be primarily immune-mediated (40), recent widespread molecular testing of ocular fluids has demonstrated that a broad range of both dangerous and innocuous viruses access the eyes in immunocompetent persons to cause uveitis – for example, cytomegalovirus (CMV), rubella virus and Ebola virus (EBOV) (41–43). ZIKV also has been recovered from the aqueous humor in anterior uveitis (**Table 1**). Studies in mice suggest that ZIKV accesses the eye from the blood stream in myeloid cells that become hypermotile (44, 45), as is also the case for more common ocular pathogens such as *Toxoplasma gondii* (46). Various ocular cell populations are preferred hosts for different organisms, including retinal pigment epithelium for EBOV and *Mycobacterium tuberculosis* (47, 48), and retinal Müller glial cells for CMV and *T. gondii* (49, 50). Given that ZIKV causes serious retinal pathology *in utero*, previous research in the field has focused on cells of the posterior eye, including Müller cells, retinal pigment epithelial cells and retinal vascular endothelial cells (17, 19, 51). Iris pigment epithelial cells are key players in inflammation of the anterior segment of the eye, which defines anterior uveitis. They have a dual role, as key regulators of ocular immune privilege (20), and as the source of an array of

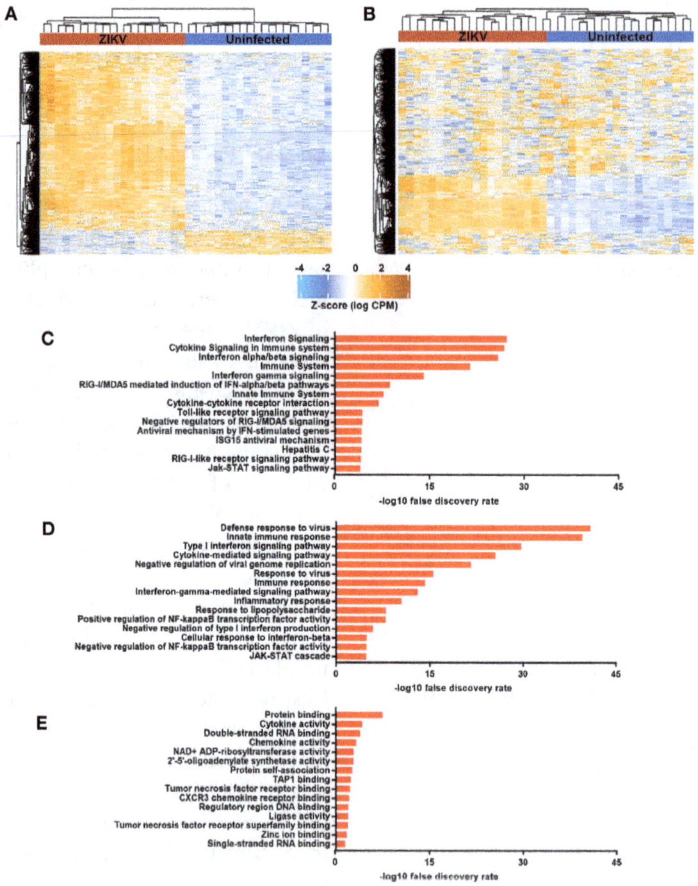

FIGURE 3 | **(A)** and **(B)** Heat maps indicating normalized counts per million from sequencing of total RNA from ZIKV-infected (red) and uninfected (blue) human iris pigment epithelial cells isolated from eyes of 20 individual donors. Z-score is shown for **(A)** all differentially expressed genes and **(B)** the 1,000 most variable genes. Color scale changes from orange to blue, with higher intensity orange representing higher counts for each transcript. **(C–E)** Graphs presenting the 15 most enriched categories –by **(C)** Reactome or KEGG pathways, **(D)** Gene Ontology biological processes and **(E)** Gene Ontology molecular functions– for genes that were upregulated in ZIKV-infected cells, as annotated in InnateDB (35).

TABLE 2 | Transcription factor binding sites that were enriched in promoters of highly up-regulated genes (target sequences) in comparison with all genes (background sequences) in human iris pigment epithelial cells 24 hours following infection with ZIKV.

Motif (Family)	Consensus sequence	Number of target sequences with motif (%)	Number of background sequences with motif (%)	False discovery rate
ISRE (IRF)	AGTTTCASTTTC	67 (9.6)	427.5 (1.0)	<0.0001
IRF1 (IRF)	GAAAGTGAAAGT	85 (12.2)	864.1 (2.0)	<0.0001
IRF2 (IRF)	GAAASYGAAASY	76 (10.9)	759.3 (1.8)	<0.0001
p65/RELA (RHD)	GGAAATTCCC	29 (4.2)	404.1 (1.0)	<0.0001
IRF4 (IRF)	ACTGAAACCA	71 (10.2)	2057.2 (4.8)	<0.0001
T1ISRE (IRF)	ACTTTCGTTTCT	10 (1.4)	42.6 (0.1)	<0.0001
bZIP-IRF (bZIP, IRF)	NAGTTTCABTHTGACTNW	61 (8.7)	1706.1 (4.0)	<0.0001
p65/RELA (RHD)	WGGGGATTTCCC	95 (13.6)	3490.7 (8.2)	<0.0001
PU.1-IRF (ETS, IRF)	MGGAAGTGAAAC	194 (27.8)	8745 (20.5)	0.0001
PRDM1 (Zf)	ACTTTCACTTTC	78 (11.2)	2838.8 (6.6)	0.0002
Tbx20 (T-box)	GGTGYTGACAGS	28 (4.0)	885 (2.1)	0.0234
Meis1 (Homeobox)	VGCTGWCAVB	167 (23.9)	8238.7 (19.3)	0.0331

BZIP, basic leucine zipper domain; ETS, erythroblast transformation-specific; IRF, interferon regulatory factor; ISRE, interferon-stimulated response element; Meis1, Meis homeobox 1; NF-kB subunit; PRDM1, PR domain-containing protein 1; PU.1, PU box binding-1; RELA, RelA protooncogene, RHD, rel homology domain; T1ISRE, type I interferon-stimulated response element; Tbx20, T-box transcription factor 20; Zf, zinc finger.

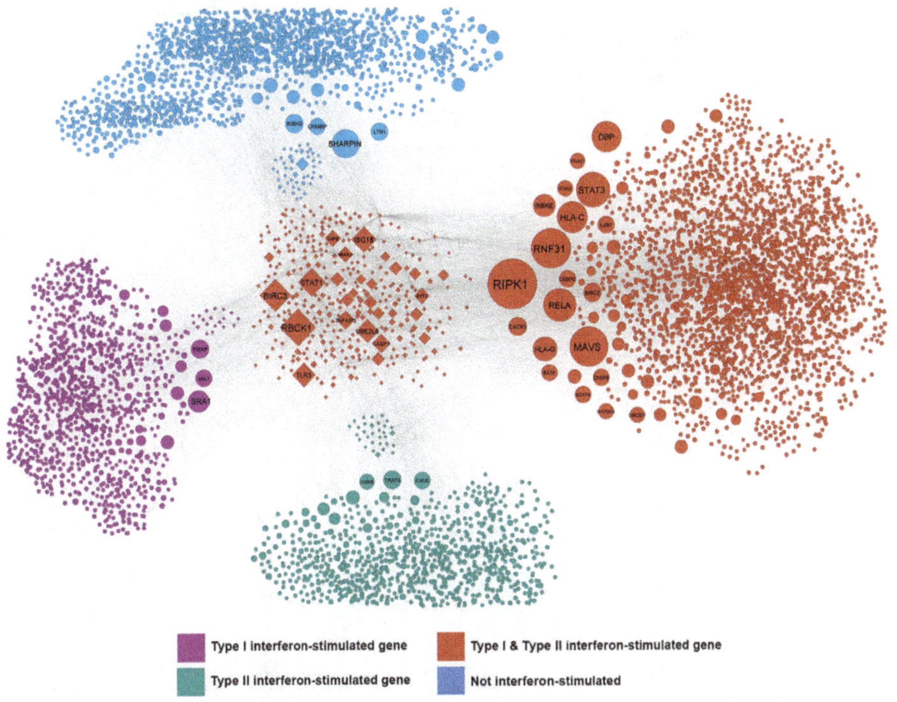

FIGURE 4 | Network of interactions between differentially expressed genes and the first-order interactors of these genes or their encoded products in ZIKV-infected human iris pigment epithelial cell isolates from 20 individual donors. CHAT (37) identified nodes in the network that were connected to differentially expressed genes more than expected by chance. Node size is scaled to -$\log_{10}$ of the false discovery rate where larger nodes are those that were identified as being more statistically significant. Purple nodes are type I interferon (IFN)-stimulated genes (ISGs); green nodes are type II IFN ISGs; red nodes are type I and II IFN ISGs; blue nodes are not IFN-responsive, as annotated by Interferome v2.0 (39). Diamond-shaped nodes represent differentially expressed genes (false discovery rate < 0.05 and fold-change > 2). Edges between nodes represent molecular interactions, as annotated by InnateDB (35). Type I and II IFN ISGs were statistically over-represented in this network. Hypergeometric test, $p < 0.0001$.

inflammatory cytokines (52). Our data indicate that ZIKV is capable of productively infecting human iris pigment epithelial cells.

While all 20 primary human iris pigment epithelial cell isolates were susceptible to infection with ZIKV, infectivity varied across donors, as demonstrated by RT-qPCR measurement of intracellular viral load and a focus forming assay of supernatant collected from cultures of infected cells. Variation in response to infection, as well as at baseline, is likely to be caused by multiple technical and biological factors. A consistent method of cell isolation and culture was used, but donor eyes were necessarily sourced on different dates. There was also unavoidable variation in time from death to cell isolation and time in culture, although these intervals were minimized to avoid mesenchymal transition of cells. Biological variation relates to individual genetics and epigenetics, as well as health and disease status. In work with other primary human ocular cells - including retinal and choroidal endothelial cells, Müller cells and retinal pigment epithelial cells- we (53–55) and other groups (56–59) have demonstrated variation in gene expression by human donor. This highlights the importance of not relying on results from individual cell isolates in drawing conclusions about pathobiological mechanisms. A major strength of our study is the large number of human donors, affording a comprehensive overview of the gene expression of the human iris pigment epithelium by RNA-Seq, while also identifying inter-individual variations.

Intracellular viral recognition is coordinated by two pattern recognition receptor families: TLRs and RLRs (60). Pathway and Gene Ontology analyses indicated high activation of RIG-I and melanoma differentiation-associated protein 5 (MDA5) signaling; TLR3, which recognizes double-stranded RNA specifically, was identified as a contextual hub by CHAT network analysis. Viral defense relies on IFN responses. IFN-β -the prototype type I IFN- was the most highly differentially expressed transcript in infected human iris pigment epithelial cells, with an approximately 900-fold upregulation across the 20 isolates. Enrichment analyses identified activation of type II IFN signaling, as well as type I. Type III IFNs -including IFN-λ1, IFN-λ2 and IFN-λ3- also were substantially increased following infection. The IFNλ receptor is a heterodimer of IL10RB, which is ubiquitously expressed, and IFNLR1, which has considerably restricted expression, but was identified in this cell population by RNA-Seq. The type III IFN system protects barriers (61), including the female reproductive tract in Zika (62). Recent work has identified Type III IFN signaling on the ocular surface, with corneal epithelium also expressing both subunits of IFNλR1 (63). Expression of type III IFNs and IFNR1λ is consistent with

TABLE 3 | Contextual hubs (highly connected molecular nodes) that were found to interact with differentially expressed genes more frequently than expected by chance in human iris pigment epithelial cells 24 hours following infection with ZIKV.

Contextual hub	Contextual neighbors	Total neighbors	False discovery rate
RIPK1	16	102	5.49E-05
RNF31	13	83	4.68E-04
MAVS	14	96	4.68E-04
RBCK1	12	75	8.10E-04
STAT3	24	297	0.0013
RELA	25	329	0.0020
BIRC3	12	87	0.0024
HLA-C	11	75	0.0029
DBP	5	11	0.0034
SHARPIN	8	41	0.0052
STAT1	18	207	0.0052
ISG15	18	218	0.0093
HLA-G	5	15	0.0129
TLR3	7	35	0.0129
UBE2L6	8	49	0.0151
IKBKE	11	98	0.0196
SRA1	7	39	0.0219
IKBKG	25	417	0.0377
BIRC2	13	146	0.0400
CASP1	7	44	0.0415
TNFAIP3	10	92	0.0428
TIRAP	7	45	0.0436
CXCR3	3	5	0.0446
TRAF6	21	330	0.0446

BIRC3, baculoviral IAP repeat-containing protein; CASP1, caspase 1, apoptosis-related cysteine protease; CXCR3, chemokine, CXC motif, receptor 3; DBP , d-box-binding PAR bZIP transcription factor; HLA , major histocompatibility complex, class I; IKBK , inhibitor of nuclear factor kappa-B kinase; ISG15, ubiquitin-like modifier ISG15 (a.k.a. interferon-induced protein 15); MAVS, mitochondrial antiviral signaling protein; RBCK1, RANBP-type and C3HC4-type zinc finger-containing 1; RELA, rela protooncogene, NFKB subunit; RIPK1, receptor-interacting serine/threonine kinase 1; RNF31, ring finger protein 31; SHARPIN, shank-associated RH domain interactor; SRA1, steroid receptor RNA activator 1; STAT, signal transducer and activator of transcription; TIRAP, TIR domain-containing adaptor protein; TLR3, toll-like receptor 3; TNFAIP3, tumor necrosis factor-alpha-induced protein 3; TRAF6, TNF receptor-associated factor 6; UBE2L6, ubiquitin-conjugating enzyme E2L 6.

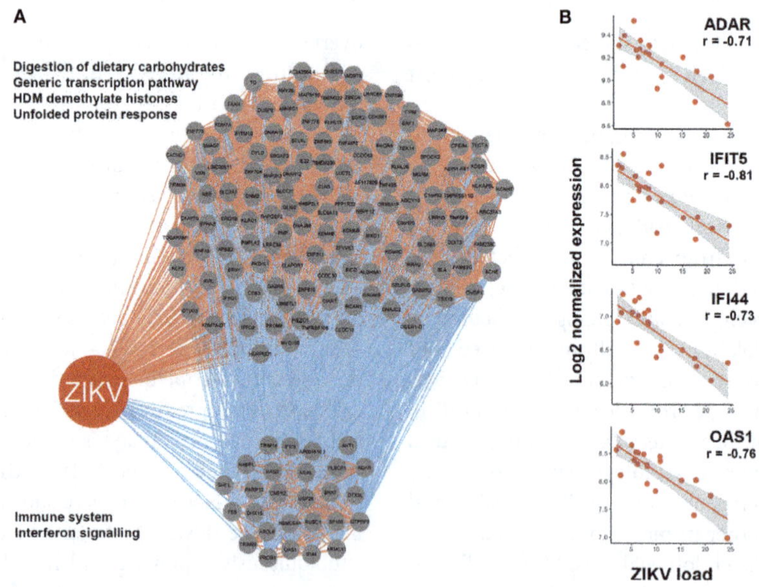

FIGURE 5 | (A) Correlations between genes upregulated in ZIKV-infected human iris pigment epithelial cells and read counts per million assigned to the ZIKV genome (ZIKV load). Spearman correlation, $p < 0.05$. Gray circles indicate upregulated genes. Red lines indicate positive correlations, and blue lines indicate negative correlations. Enriched Reactome pathways achieving false discovery rate < 0.05 are listed left of the relevant grouping, with annotations by InnateDB (35).
(B) Examples of negative correlations between interferon (IFN)-stimulated genes and ZIKV load. Red dots indicate 20 individual donors. Line indicates trend. ADAR, adenosine deaminase, RNA-specific; IFI44, IFN-induced protein 44; IFIT5, IFN-induced protein with tetratricopeptide repeats 5; OAS1, 2'-5'-oligoadenylate synthetase 1.

the role of iris pigment epithelial cells in maintaining ocular immune privilege. The transcription factor analysis also indicated activity in pathways that would increase IFN-stimulated genes. Interestingly, key players in noncanonical NF-κB signaling were upregulated, suggesting the possibility of negatively regulating induction of type I IFNs (64). NF-κB signaling also would be expected to promote inflammatory responses and trigger a breach in immune privilege, consistent with the development of anterior uveitis.

While anti-viral IFN responses were highly upregulated in ZIKV-infected iris pigment epithelial cells, the intracellular viral load correlated inversely with IFN signaling. Consistently, multiple ISGs were upregulated at a relatively low level in heavily infected isolates. This result suggests ZIKV directly interferes with IFN signaling in epithelial cells. The ZIKV polypeptide yields 7 nonstructural (NS) proteins in addition to 3 structural proteins (65). ZIKV NS5 in particular has multiple actions that target IFN signaling. On binding to RIG-I, NS5 represses the ubiquitination that promotes RIG-I-mediated signaling (66). NS5 binds TANK-binding kinase 1 (TBK1), interfering with its ability to phosphorylate and activate IRF3 ahead of nuclear translocation (67); NS5 also binds IRF3 to limit its activity (68). Together with IRF9, STAT1 and STAT2 form the IFN-stimulated gene actor-3 complex (ISGF-3), but NS5 targets STAT2 for proteosomal degradation, by either binding it directly or binding the E3 ubiquitin ligase, seven in absentia homolog 2 (SIAH2), which subsequently binds STAT2 (69, 70). Other nonstructural proteins also may impact IFN production and/or induction of ISGs (68, 71). While NS5 suppresses type I and III IFN signaling, it enhances type II IFN signaling by destabilizing STAT2 and limiting formation of ISGF-3, and promoting formation of STAT1-STAT1 homodimers that bind γ-activated sequence (GAS) elements (72). Thus, increased viral replication could promote anterior uveitis by increasing type II IFN signaling. NS5 also facilitates the assembly of the NLRP3 (NLR family, pyrin domain-containing 3) inflammasome (73).

The "central controller" of cell fate –RIPK1 (74)– was the most significant contextual hub in the molecular network generated from the list of 613 differentially expressed genes in iris pigment epithelial cells following ZIKV infection. While not differentially expressed per our definition of two-fold change and FDR less than 0.05 (**Supplementary Table 2**), RIPK1 increased highly significantly (FDR = 8×10^{-30}) by 1.5-fold post-infection. Originally described as an activator of necroptosis, involvement of RIPK1 in different pathological processes is now known to be multifaceted. The protein has a C-terminal death domain, an N-terminal serine/threonine kinase domain, and an intermediate domain that participates in NF-κB activation (74). In addition to necroptosis, RIPK1 may trigger apoptosis and promote inflammation, and conversely, it may act as a regulator of each of these processes (75–77). The ultimate impact of RIPK1 signaling in ZIKV-infected human iris pigment epithelial cells is thus difficult to predict. Recent work in a mouse central nervous system model of ZIKV infection indicated RIPK1 signaling directed a "metabolic reprogramming" in infected neurons characterized by inhibition of succinate dehydrogenase, which suppressed viral replication (78), suggesting RIPK1-controlled activities might have anti-viral effects.

To interrogate the mechanisms of Zika-associated anterior uveitis as it occurs in the patient, we selected an *in vitro* system with iris pigment epithelial cells isolated from human cadaver eyes. Iris biopsy is not performed in the clinical setting, and thus it is not feasible to conduct such research using tissue from patients diagnosed with this condition. Removing the cells from the local microenvironment and the culture procedure is expected to induce some change in cell phenotype. We used early passage cell isolates, all of which were checked for presence of epithelial and absence of mesenchymal markers. The most common *in vivo* models are induced by systemic inoculation of virus into mice, including animals with deficient type I IFN signaling (12–15). A non-human primate model in the Rhesus macaque has recently been described (79). However, these studies have not involved adult animals. Indeed, in descriptions of several mouse models, Zhao and colleagues (13) commented that wild-type mice infected intraperitoneally with ZIKV lost susceptibility to ocular pathology from one week of age, and A129 mice –with null mutations in the IFN-α/β receptor– showed no ocular disease after 10 weeks. Past works also have focused largely on posterior eye pathology. An interesting new experimental model for investigating anterior uveitis involves injecting ZIKV into the aqueous humor of 1-month-old mice; the animals develop raised intraocular pressure, and pattern recognition receptors and inflammatory chemokines are induced in anterior segment tissues (80).

Zika-associated anterior uveitis occurs when ZIKV accesses the eye during a systemic infection. However, the eye is able to clear the virus, and the inflammation resolves either spontaneously or with the short-term use of corticosteroid eye drops. Our work represents the first observations around basic mechanisms of this emerging form of uveitis in a human-based experimental system. Our results suggest that the iris pigment epithelium is susceptible to ZIKV infection, but also mounts a rigorous pan-IFN response, which when combined with other elements of ocular immune privilege, may limit ocular pathology in the majority of affected individuals. Those persons in whom the virus replicates robustly within the iris pigment epithelium, may generate a stronger inflammatory response and thus be at higher risk of developing anterior uveitis.

ETHICS STATEMENT

Use of human cadaver donor eyes from the Eye Bank of South Australia (Adelaide, Australia) for this work was approved by the Southern Adelaide Clinical Human Research Ethics Committee (protocol number: 175.13). Retrospective collection of the clinical data of individuals diagnosed with ZIKV-associated anterior uveitis at the Ophthalmology Clinic of Ribeirao Preto General Hospital, Ribeirao Preto, Sao Paulo, Brazil, between January 2016 and June 2016, was approved by the Hospital Ethics Committee of Human Research (protocol number: 85195318.0.0000.5540).

AUTHOR CONTRIBUTIONS

JS conceived the study. FR, JC, JF, MM, BA, DL, and JS designed the study. JF and MS collected and synthesized the clinical data. JC, YM, LA, GO, GG, AD, BA and JS performed the laboratory experiments and/or analyzed laboratory data (including contributions to methodology). FR and DL analyzed and interpreted the RNA-Seq data. JS wrote the article including review of the relevant literature. FR and LA contributed substantially to preparation of the figures and/or tables in the article. FR, JC, JF, YM, LA, MS, GO, GG, AD, MM, BA and DL critically reviewed the content of the article. All authors contributed to the article and approved the submitted version.

ACKNOWLEDGMENTS

The authors wish to thank Dr. Renee Smith and Ms. Letitia Pimlott of the Flinders Genomics Facility, and Mr. Mark van der Hoek of the South Australian Health & Medical Research Institute David Gunn Genomics Facility for next generation sequencing services, and Ms. Janet Matthews for administrative support in preparing this manuscript.

REFERENCES

1. Petersen LR, Jamieson DJ, Powers AM, Honein MA. Zika Virus. *N Engl J Med* (2016) 374:1552–63. doi: 10.1056/NEJMra1602113
2. Musso D, Bossin H, Mallet HP, Besnard M, Broult J, Baudouin L, et al. Zika virus in French Polynesia 2013-14: anatomy of a completed outbreak. *Lancet Infect Dis* (2018) 18:e172–82. doi: 10.1016/S1473-3099(17)30446-2
3. de Oliveira WK, de Franca GVA, Carmo EH, Duncan BB, de Souza Kuchenbecker R, Schmidt MI. Infection-related microcephaly after the 2015 and 2016 Zika virus outbreaks in Brazil: a surveillance-based analysis. *Lancet* (2017) 390:861–70. doi: 10.1016/S0140-6736(17)31368-5
4. Moore CA, Staples JE, Dobyns WB, Pessoa A, Ventura CV, Fonseca EB, et al. Characterizing the pattern of anomalies in congenital Zika syndrome for pediatric clinicians. *JAMA Pediatr* (2017) 171:288–95. doi: 10.1001/jamapediatrics.2016.3982
5. de Oliveira Dias JR, Ventura CV, de Paula Freitas B, Prazeres J, Ventura LO, Bravo-Filho V, et al. Zika and the eye: pieces of a puzzle. *Prog Retin Eye Res* (2018) 66:85–106. doi: 10.1016/j.preteyeres.2018.04.004
6. Jabs DA, Nussenblatt RB, Rosenbaum JT. Standardization of Uveitis Nomenclature Working Group. Standardization of uveitis nomenclature for reporting clinical data. Results of the First International Workshop. *Am J Ophthalmol* (2005) 140:509–16. doi: 10.1016/j.ajo.2005.03.057
7. Oliver GF, Carr JM, Smith JR. Emerging infectious uveitis: chikungunya, dengue, Zika and Ebola: a review. *Clin Exp Ophthalmol* (2019) 47:372–80. doi: 10.1111/ceo.13450
8. Troumani Y, Touhami S, Jackson TL, Ventura CV, Stanescu-Segall DM, Errera MH, et al. Association of anterior uveitis with acute Zika virus infection in adults. *JAMA Ophthalmol* (2021) 139:95–102. doi: 10.1001/jamaophthalmol.2020.5131
9. Furtado JM, Esposito DL, Klein TM, Teixeira-Pinto T, da Fonseca BA. Uveitis associated with Zika virus infection. *N Engl J Med* (2016) 375:394–6. doi: 10.1056/NEJMc1603618
10. Fontes BM. Zika virus-related hypertensive iridocyclitis. *Arq Bras Oftalmol* (2016) 79:63. doi: 10.5935/0004-2749.20160020
11. Merle H, Najioullah F, Chassery M, Cesaire R, Hage R. Zika-related bilateral hypertensive anterior acute uveitis. *JAMA Ophthalmol* (2017) 135:284–5. doi: 10.1001/jamaophthalmol.2016.5689
12. Miner JJ, Sene A, Richner JM, Smith AM, Santeford A, Ban N, et al. Zika virus infection in mice causes panuveitis with shedding of virus in tears. *Cell Rep* (2016) 16:3208–18. doi: 10.1016/j.celrep.2016.08.079
13. Zhao Z, Yang M, Azar SR, Soong L, Weaver SC, Sun J, et al. Viral retinopathy in experimental models of Zika infection. *Invest Ophthalmol Vis Sci* (2017) 58:4355–65. doi: 10.1167/iovs.17-22016
14. Manangeeswaran M, Kielczewski JL, Sen HN, Xu BC, Ireland DDC, McWilliams IL, et al. ZIKA virus infection causes persistent chorioretinal lesions. *Emerg Microbes Infect* (2018) 7:96. doi: 10.1038/s41426-018-0096-z
15. Garcia G, Paul S, Beshara S, Ramanujan VK, Ramaiah A, Nielsen-Saines K, et al. Hippo signaling pathway has a critical role in Zika virus replication and in the pathogenesis of neuroinflammation. *Am J Pathol* (2020) 190:844–61. doi: 10.1016/j.ajpath.2019.12.005
16. Chan JF, Yip CC, Tsang JO, Tee KM, Cai JP, Chik KK, et al. Differential cell line susceptibility to the emerging Zika virus: implications for disease pathogenesis, non-vector-borne human transmission and animal reservoirs. *Emerg Microbes Infect* (2016) 5:e93. doi: 10.1038/emi.2016.99
17. Roach T, Alcendor DJ. Zika virus infection of cellular components of the blood-retinal barriers: implications for viral associated congenital ocular disease. *J Neuroinflamm* (2017) 14:43. doi: 10.1186/s12974-017-0824-7
18. Singh PK, Khatri I, Jha A, Pretto CD, Spindler KR, Arumugaswami V, et al. Determination of system level alterations in host transcriptome due to Zika virus (ZIKV) infection in retinal pigment epithelium. *Sci Rep* (2018) 8:11209. doi: 10.1038/s41598-018-29329-2
19. Simonin Y, Erkilic N, Damodar K, Cle M, Desmetz C, Bollore K, et al. Zika virus induces strong inflammatory responses and impairs homeostasis and function of the human retinal pigment epithelium. *EBioMedicine* (2019) 39:315–31. doi: 10.1016/j.ebiom.2018.12.010
20. Mochizuki M, Sugita S, Kamoi K. Immunological homeostasis of the eye. *Prog Retin Eye Res* (2013) 33:10–27. doi: 10.1016/j.preteyeres.2012.10.002
21. Dua HS, Dick AD, Watson NJ. Forrester JV. A spectrum of clinical signs in anterior uveitis. *Eye (Lond)* (1993) 7:68–73. doi: 10.1038/eye.1993.15
22. Mai K, Chui JJ, Di Girolamo N, McCluskey PJ, Wakefield D. Role of toll-like receptors in human iris pigment epithelial cells and their response to pathogen-associated molecular patterns. *J Inflamm* (2014) 11:20. doi: 10.1186/1476-9255-11-20
23. Wati S, Li P, Burrell CJ, Carr JM. Dengue virus (DV) replication in monocyte-derived macrophages is not affected by tumor necrosis factor alpha (TNF-alpha), and DV infection induces altered responsiveness to TNF-alpha stimulation. *J Virol* (2007) 81:10161–71. doi: 10.1128/JVI.00313-07
24. Cabezas S, Bracho G, Aloia AL, Adamson PJ, Bonder CS, Smith JR, et al. Dengue virus induces increased activity of thec Alternative pathway in infected cells. *J Virol* (2018) 92:e00633–18. doi: 10.1128/JVI.00633-18
25. Pfaffl MW. A new mathematical model for relative quantification in real-time RT-PCR. *Nucleic Acids Res* (2001) 29:e45. doi: 10.1093/nar/29.9.e45
26. Andrews S. *FastQC: a quality control tool for high throughput sequence data.* United Kingdom: Babraham Bioinformatics, Babraham Institute, Cambridge (2010).
27. Bolger AM, Lohse M, Usadel B. Trimmomatic: a flexible trimmer for Illumina sequence data. *Bioinformatics* (2014) 30:2114–20. doi: 10.1093/bioinformatics/btu170
28. Kim D, Langmead B, Salzberg SL. HISAT: a fast spliced aligner with low memory requirements. *Nat Methods* (2015) 12:357–60. doi: 10.1038/nmeth.3317
29. Liao Y, Smyth GK, Shi W. featureCounts: an efficient general purpose program for assigning sequence reads to genomic features. *Bioinformatics* (2014) 30:923–30. doi: 10.1093/bioinformatics/btt656
30. Wood DE, Lu J, Langmead B. Improved metagenomic analysis with Kraken 2. *Genome Biol* (2019) 20:257. doi: 10.1186/s13059-019-1891-0
31. R Core Team. *R: a language and environment for statistical computing.* Vienna, Austria: R Foundation for Statistical Computing (2013).
32. Robinson MD, McCarthy DJ, Smyth GK. edgeR: a bioconductor package for differential expression analysis of digital gene expression data. *Bioinformatics* (2010) 26:139–40. doi: 10.1093/bioinformatics/btp616

33. Leek JT. svaseq: removing batch effects and other unwanted noise from sequencing data. *Nucleic Acids Res* (2014) 42:e161. doi: 10.1093/nar/gku864
34. Benjamini YHY. Controlling the false discovery rate: a practical and powerful approach to multiple testing. *J R Stat Soc Ser B Stat Methodol* (1995) 57:289–300. doi: 10.1111/j.2517-6161.1995.tb02031.x
35. Lynn DJ, Winsor GL, Chan C, Richard N, Laird MR, Barsky A, et al. InnateDB: facilitating systems-level analyses of the mammalian innate immune response. *Mol Syst Biol* (2008) 4:218. doi: 10.1038/msb.2008.55
36. Heinz S, Benner C, Spann N, Bertolino E, Lin YC, Laslo P, et al. Simple combinations of lineage-determining transcription factors prime cis-regulatory elements required for macrophage and B cell identities. *Mol Cell* (2010) 38:576–89. doi: 10.1016/j.molcel.2010.05.004
37. Muetze T, Goenawan IH, Wiencko HL, Bernal-Llinares M, Bryan K, Lynn DJ. Contextual Hub Analysis Tool (CHAT): a cytoscape app for identifying contextually relevant hubs in biological networks. *F1000research* (2016) 5:1745. doi: 10.12688/f1000research.9118.1
38. Su G, Morris JH, Demchak B, Bader GD. Biological network exploration with Cytoscape 3. *Curr Protoc Bioinf* (2014) 47:8–13. doi: 10.1002/0471250953.bi0813s47
39. Rusinova I, Forster S, Yu S, Kannan A, Masse M, Cumming H, et al. Interferome v2.0: an updated database of annotated interferon-regulated genes. *Nucleic Acids Res* (2013) 41(Database issue):D1040–6. doi: 10.1093/nar/gks1215
40. Cunningham ET Jr., Forrester JV, Rao NA, Zierhut M. Post-infectious uveitis. *Ocul Immunol Inflamm* (2016) 24:603–6. doi: 10.1080/09273948.2016.1253983
41. Chee SP, Bacsal K, Jap A, Se-Thoe SY, Cheng CL, Tan BH. Clinical features of cytomegalovirus anterior uveitis in immunocompetent patients. *Am J Ophthalmol* (2008) 145:834–40. doi: 10.1016/j.ajo.2007.12.015
42. de Groot-Mijnes JD, de Visser L, Rothova A, Schuller M, van Loon AM, Weersink AJ. Rubella virus is associated with Fuchs heterochromic iridocyclitis. *Am J Ophthalmol* (2006) 141:212–4. doi: 10.1016/j.ajo.2005.07.078
43. Varkey JB, Shantha JG, Crozier I, Kraft CS, Lyon GM, Mehta AK, et al. Persistence of Ebola virus in ocular fluid during convalescence. *N Engl J Med* (2015) 372:2423–7. doi: 10.1056/NEJMoa1500306
44. McDonald EM, Anderson J, Wilusz J, Ebel GD, Brault AC. Zika virus replication in myeloid cells during acute infection is vital to viral dissemination and pathogenesis in a mouse model. *J Virol* (2020) 94: e00838-20. doi: 10.1128/JVI.00838-20
45. Ayala-Nunez NV, Follain G, Delalande F, Hirschler A, Partiot E, Hale GL, et al. Zika virus enhances monocyte adhesion and transmigration favoring viral dissemination to neural cells. *Nat Commun* (2019) 10:4430. doi: 10.1038/s41467-019-12408-x
46. Furtado JM, Bharadwaj AS, Ashander LM, Olivas A, Smith JR. Migration of Toxoplasma gondii-infected dendritic cells across human retinal vascular endothelium. *Invest Ophthalmol Vis Sci* (2012) 53:6856–62. doi: 10.1167/iovs.12-10384
47. Smith JR, Todd S, Ashander LM, Charitou T, Ma Y, Yeh S, et al. Retinal pigment epithelial cells are a potential reservoir for Ebola virus in the human eye. *Transl Vis Sci Technol* (2017) 6:12. doi: 10.1167/tvst.6.4.12
48. Nazari H, Karakousis PC, Rao NA. Replication of Mycobacterium tuberculosis in retinal pigment epithelium. *JAMA Ophthalmol* (2014) 132:724–9. doi: 10.1001/jamaophthalmol.2014.270
49. Rao NA, Zhang J, Ishimoto S. Role of retinal vascular endothelial cells in development of CMV retinitis. *Trans Am Ophthalmol Soc* (1998) 96:111–23.
50. Smith JR, Ashander LM, Arruda SL, Cordeiro CA, Lie S, Rochet E, et al. Pathogenesis of ocular toxoplasmosis. *Prog Retin Eye Res* (2021) 81:100882. doi: 10.1016/j.preteyeres.2020.100882
51. Singh PK, Guest JM, Kanwar M, Boss J, Gao N, Juzych MS, et al. Zika virus infects cells lining the blood-retinal barrier and causes chorioretinal atrophy in mouse eyes. *JCI Insight* (2017) 2:e92340. doi: 10.1172/jci.insight.92340
52. Chui JJ, Li MW, Di Girolamo N, Chang JH, McCluskey PJ, Wakefield D. Iris pigment epithelial cells express a functional lipopolysaccharide receptor complex. *Invest Ophthalmol Vis Sci* (2010) 51:2558–67. doi: 10.1167/iovs.09-3923
53. Smith JR, Choi D, Chipps TJ, Pan Y, Zamora DO, Davies MH, et al. Unique gene expression profiles of donor-matched human retinal and choroidal vascular endothelial cells. *Invest Ophthalmol Vis Sci* (2007) 48:2676–84. doi: 10.1167/iovs.06-0598
54. Rochet E, Appukuttan B, Ma Y, Ashander LM, Smith JR. Expression of long non-coding RNAs by human retinal Muller glial cells infected with clonal and exotic virulent Toxoplasma gondii. *Noncoding RNA* (2019) 5:48. doi: 10.3390/ncrna5040048
55. Lie S, Rochet E, Segerdell E, Ma Y, Ashander LM, Shadforth AMA, et al. Immunological molecular responses of human retinal pigment epithelial cells to infection with Toxoplasma gondii. *Front Immunol* (2019) 10:708. doi: 10.3389/fimmu.2019.00708
56. Browning AC, Halligan EP, Stewart EA, Swan DC, Dove R, Samaranayake GJ, et al. Comparative gene expression profiling of human umbilical vein endothelial cells and ocular vascular endothelial cells. *Br J Ophthalmol* (2012) 96:128–32. doi: 10.1136/bjophthalmol-2011-300572
57. Capozzi ME, Giblin MJ, Penn JS. Palmitic acid induces Muller cell inflammation that is potentiated by co-treatment with glucose. *Sci Rep* (2018) 8:5459. doi: 10.1038/s41598-018-23601-1
58. Cai H, Shin MC, Tezel TH, Kaplan HJ, Del Priore LV. Use of iris pigment epithelium to replace retinal pigment epithelium in age-related macular degeneration: a gene expression analysis. *Arch Ophthalmol* (2006) 124:1276–85. doi: 10.1001/archopht.124.9.1276
59. Munoz-Erazo L, Natoli R, Provis JM, Madigan MC, King NJ. Microarray analysis of gene expression in West Nile virus-infected human retinal pigment epithelium. *Mol Vis* (2012) 18:730–43.
60. Takeuchi O, Akira S. Pattern recognition receptors and inflammation. *Cell* (2010) 140:805–20. doi: 10.1016/j.cell.2010.01.022
61. Zanoni I, Granucci F, Broggi A. Interferon (IFN)-lambda takes the helm: immunomodulatory roles of type III IFNs. *Front Immunol* (2017) 8:1661. doi: 10.3389/fimmu.2017.01661
62. Caine EA, Scheaffer SM, Arora N, Zaitsev K, Artyomov MN, Coyne CB, et al. Interferon lambda protects the female reproductive tract against Zika virus infection. *Nat Commun* (2019) 10:280. doi: 10.1038/s41467-018-07993-2
63. Miner JJ, Platt DJ, Ghaznavi CM, Chandra P, Santeford A, Menos AM, et al. HSV-1 and Zika virus but not SARS-CoV-2 replicate in the human cornea and are restricted by corneal type III interferon. *Cell Rep* (2020) 33:108339. doi: 10.1016/j.celrep.2020.108339
64. Jin J, Hu H, Li HS, Yu J, Xiao Y, Brittain GC, et al. Noncanonical NF-kappaB pathway controls the production of type I interferons in antiviral innate immunity. *Immunity* (2014) 40:342–54. doi: 10.1016/j.immuni.2014.02.006
65. Pierson TC, Diamond MS. The emergence of Zika virus and its new clinical syndromes. *Nature* (2018) 560:573–81. doi: 10.1038/s41586-018-0446-y
66. Li A, Wang W, Wang Y, Chen K, Xiao F, Hu D, et al. NS5 conservative site is required for Zika virus to restrict the RIG-I signaling. *Front Immunol* (2020) 11:51. doi: 10.3389/fimmu.2020.00051
67. Lin S, Yang S, He J, Guest JD, Ma Z, Yang L, et al. Zika virus NS5 protein antagonizes type I interferon production via blocking TBK1 activation. *Virology* (2019) 527:180–7. doi: 10.1016/j.virol.2018.11.009
68. Xia H, Luo H, Shan C, Muruato AE, Nunes BTD, Medeiros DBA, et al. An evolutionary NS1 mutation enhances Zika virus evasion of host interferon induction. *Nat Commun* (2018) 9:414. doi: 10.1038/s41467-017-02816-2
69. Dar HA, Zaheer T, Paracha RZ, Ali A. Structural analysis and insight into Zika virus NS5 mediated interferon inhibition. *Infect Genet Evol* (2017) 51:143–52. doi: 10.1016/j.meegid.2017.03.027
70. Grant A, Ponia SS, Tripathi S, Balasubramaniam V, Miorin L, Sourisseau M, et al. Zika virus targets human STAT2 to inhibit type I interferon signaling. *Cell Host Microbe* (2016) 19:882–90. doi: 10.1016/j.chom.2016.05.009
71. Wu Y, Liu Q, Zhou J, Xie W, Chen C, Wang Z, et al. Zika virus evades interferon-mediated antiviral response through the co-operation of multiple nonstructural proteins in vitro. *Cell Discov* (2017) 3:17006. doi: 10.1038/celldisc.2017.14
72. Chaudhary V, Yuen KS, Chan JF, Chan CP, Wang PH, Cai JP, et al. Selective activation of type II interferon signaling by Zika virus NS5 protein. *J Virol* (2017) 91:e00163–17. doi: 10.1128/JVI.00163-17
73. Wang W, Li G, De W, Luo Z, Pan P, Tian M, et al. Zika virus infection induces host inflammatory responses by facilitating NLRP3 inflammasome assembly and interleukin-1beta secretion. *Nat Commun* (2018) 9:106. doi: 10.1038/s41467-017-02645-3

74. Christofferson DE, Li Y, Yuan J. Control of life-or-death decisions by RIP1 kinase. *Annu Rev Physiol* (2014) 76:129–50. doi: 10.1146/annurev-physiol-021113-170259
75. Degterev A, Ofengeim D, Yuan J. Targeting RIPK1 for the treatment of human diseases. *Proc Natl Acad Sci U S A* (2019) 116:9714–22. doi: 10.1073/pnas.1901179116
76. Lin J, Kumari S, Kim C, Van TM, Wachsmuth L, Polykratis A, et al. RIPK1 counteracts ZBP1-mediated necroptosis to inhibit inflammation. *Nature* (2016) 540:124–8. doi: 10.1038/nature20558
77. Lalaoui N, Boyden SE, Oda H, Wood GM, Stone DL, Chau D, et al. Mutations that prevent caspase cleavage of RIPK1 cause autoinflammatory disease. *Nature* (2020) 577:103–8. doi: 10.1038/s41586-019-1828-5
78. Daniels BP, Kofman SB, Smith JR, Norris GT, Snyder AG, Kolb JP, et al. The nucleotide sensor ZBP1 and Kinase RIPK3 induce the enzyme IRG1 to promote an antiviral metabolic state in neurons. *Immunity* (2019) 50:64–76.e4. doi: 10.1016/j.immuni.2018.11.017
79. Yiu G, Thomasy SM, Casanova MI, Rusakevich AM, Keesler RI, Watanabe J, et al. Evolution of ocular defects in infant macaques following in utero Zika virus infection. *JCI Insight* (2020) 5:143947. doi: 10.1172/jci.insight.143947
80. Singh PK, Kasetti RB, Zode GS, Goyal A, Juzych MS, Kumar A. Zika virus infects trabecular meshwork and causes trabeculitis and glaucomatous pathology in mouse eyes. *mSphere* (2019) 4:e00173–19. doi: 10.1128/mSphere.00173-19

15

Immune Privilege: The Microbiome and Uveitis

Christine Mölzer[1], Jarmila Heissigerova[2], Heather M. Wilson[1], Lucia Kuffova[1,3] and John V. Forrester[1]*

[1] Institute of Medical Sciences, University of Aberdeen, Aberdeen, United Kingdom, [2] Department of Ophthalmology, First Faculty of Medicine, Charles University and General University Hospital in Prague, Prague, Czechia, [3] Eye Clinic, Aberdeen Royal Infirmary, Aberdeen, United Kingdom

***Correspondence:**
John V. Forrester
j.forrester@abdn.ac.uk

Immune privilege (IP), a term introduced to explain the unpredicted acceptance of allogeneic grafts by the eye and the brain, is considered a unique property of these tissues. However, immune responses are modified by the tissue in which they occur, most of which possess IP to some degree. The eye therefore displays a spectrum of IP because it comprises several tissues. IP as originally conceived can only apply to the retina as it contains few tissue-resident bone-marrow derived myeloid cells and is immunologically shielded by a sophisticated barrier – an inner vascular and an outer epithelial barrier at the retinal pigment epithelium. The vascular barrier comprises the vascular endothelium and the glia limitans. Immune cells do not cross the blood-retinal barrier (BRB) despite two-way transport of interstitial fluid, governed by tissue oncotic pressure. The BRB, and the blood-brain barrier (BBB) mature in the neonatal period under signals from the expanding microbiome and by 18 months are fully established. However, the adult eye is susceptible to intraocular inflammation (uveitis; frequency ~200/100,000 population). Uveitis involving the retinal parenchyma (posterior uveitis, PU) breaches IP, while IP is essentially irrelevant in inflammation involving the ocular chambers, uveal tract and ocular coats (anterior/ intermediate uveitis/sclerouveitis, AU). Infections cause ~50% cases of AU and PU but infection may also underlie the pathogenesis of immune-mediated "non-infectious" uveitis. Dysbiosis accompanies the commonest form, HLA-B27–associated AU, while latent infections underlie BRB breakdown in PU. This review considers the pathogenesis of uveitis in the context of IP, infection, environment, and the microbiome.

Keywords: T regulatory cells, folate, probiotics, blood retinal barrier, adjuvant effect, commensals, nutritional metabolites

INTRODUCTION

Immune privilege (IP) was conceived as a protective response to immune challenge by tissues with limited capacity for renewal such as the eye and the brain [reviewed in (1)]. Matzinger and Kamala have suggested that all tissues modulate the immune response including frontline tissues such as skin and mucosa (2). If this is valid, then the eye (and the brain) which are composites of several types of tissue, can be considered to express various levels of "privilege." Thus, the level of IP for each component of the eye and the brain would match the level of IP of corresponding tissues: in the case of the eye, composed as it is of vascular and avascular connective tissues forming a barrier-lined case around neural tissue, several levels of IP probably hold sway, with the retina at the top of the scale (**Figure 1**).

However, it has been observed in several previous reviews that despite high levels of IP, ocular tissues are susceptible to inflammation and infection (1, 4–9). For instance, the long-held reputation for corneal allograft success only truly applies to specific conditions such as keratoconus and certain dystrophies. Once inflamed the cornea loses its IP and becomes "high risk" for rejection with an allograft success rate possibly less than other vascularized solid organs (10). Similarly, the uveal tract and meninges display levels of IP little different from other vascular tissues [reviewed in (11)], and so it is no surprise that the anterior segment is susceptible to inflammation and that anterior uveitis (AU) is the most common brand of uveitis (12). Probably IP in the eye, if it exists as originally conceived, can be applied only to the retina (11). This is not to diminish in any way the unique immunological properties of the retina and the brain parenchyma which are based on physical, cellular, molecular and immunological features setting them apart from other tissues. Nor does it gainsay the influence all tissues have on the immune response (2). Context is everything and a review of these aspects is presented here.

A new facet to immune processes has emerged based on our rapidly evolving appreciation of the influence of the microbiome on development of immunity. The acquisition and maturation of a healthy microbiome during the post-natal period and early infancy shapes the development of the blood-central nervous system (CNS) barrier (13–15) and so the proper establishment of a healthy microbiome is critically linked to the development of a mature immune system which determines susceptibility to CNS infection during this time. This applies not only to the CNS but also to other systems such as the musculoskeletal system. The long-recognized relationship between inflammatory bowel disease (IBD), the spondylo-arthropathies (SpA) and ocular inflammatory disease is now being re-appraised in terms of a dysregulated microbiome (dysbiosis) (16) which in the context of IP raises many questions. This is also discussed.

IMMUNE PRIVILEGE: HOW THE CONCEPT AROSE AND HOW IT HAS BLURRED OUR VISION CONCERNING THE REGULATION OF THE IMMUNE RESPONSE

The concept of IP stems back to the nineteenth century [reviewed in (17)] but the term was coined and popularized by Medawar whose experiments showing acceptance of skin

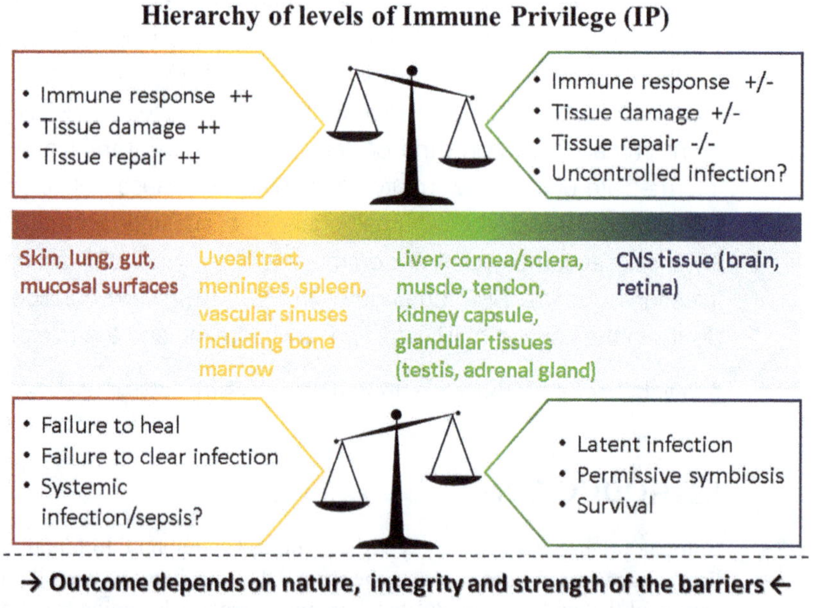

FIGURE 1 | Hierarchy of levels of Immune Privilege (IP). IP may be considered as a property of all tissues with varying degrees of ability to influence the outcome of immune responses played out within their own microenvironment. Thus, tissues such as the skin and mucosal surfaces generate strong immune reactions to pathogens, experience extensive tissue damage and have considerable capacity for repair, while at the other extreme neural tissue (brain parenchyma, retina) temper or even prevent immune responses, induce latency rather than replication in pathogens [reviewed in (3).] but have limited ability for repair if severely damaged. Between these two extremes, different tissues have different levels of "privilege." The outcome of pathogen challenge to any tissue depends on the level of privilege which is determined by the nature, integrity and strength of that tissue's barrier to pathogen invasion. Barriers are complex entities comprising physical, chemical, molecular, cellular, and immunological components and are specific to each tissue. The figure illustrates what happens under normal circumstances in the top panel: here the balance of IP is set toward strong immune and repair processes in the skin at one end of the spectrum but a weak immune response in the CNS at the other end of the spectrum risks uncontrolled infection. In contrast, when this balance is shifted as shown in the lower panel, outcomes tend to reverse: in the skin, a weaker immune response might fail to clear infections or fail to promote repair while in the CNS better control of infection might be possible but still does not clear pathogens, instead promoting latent infections.

allografts in the anterior chamber of the eye supported the notion (18, 19). In essence, IP was considered a special feature of tissues such as the eye and the brain in which the default immune rejection of allografts and alloantigens failed to occur unless the non-rejected tissue developed connecting blood vessels (20). IP has been attributed to sequestration of tissue self-antigens from the immune system behind blood-tissue barriers, due to lack of blood vessels, lack of lymphatic drainage, absence of MHC Class II antigen presenting cells (APC), high concentrations of immunosuppressive tissue immunomodulators, and more recently, the activity of regulatory T cells (Treg) (21). Several reviews of proposed mechanisms underlying IP have been published (5, 7–9, 21–26).

A second phenomenon linked to IP has also been described namely anterior chamber-associated immune deviation (ACAID) (27–29) as has a similar phenomenon in the brain (brain-associated immune deviation, BRAID) (30). Immune deviation is a recognized immunological phenomenon in which antigen-specific immunity, usually in the form of cell-mediated delayed-type hypersensitivity (DTH), is suppressed while being "deviated" toward humoral immunity, usually the generation of IgG2 antibodies. Antigens inoculated into the anterior chamber of experimental animals generated an ACAID response which usually took the form of a reduced DTH response, but an intact complement-fixing IgG2 B cell response, when re-challenged with the same antigen in the skin. As new discoveries in T cell biology were made, ACAID was relabeled to show that the immune deviation was based on a shift from an antigen-specific Th1 response to Th2 (31). However, it was later shown that systemic Th2 responses were also down-regulated after antigen inoculation into the anterior chamber of the eye (32).

How ACAID, and immune deviation more broadly, was induced became a major research focus in the latter half of the twentieth century. Some form of regulatory cell suppressing DTH T effector cells (Teff) had been assumed and $CD4^+$ T cells, $CD4^+$ Treg, natural killer (NK) cells and B cells as well as other thymus-derived cells such as regulatory NK-T cells have all been shown to be involved [reviewed in (11)]. Perhaps the most detailed mechanism described has been the induction of alloantigen specific $CD8^+$ suppressor cells in the spleen through interaction of invariant NK cells with $F4/80^+$ macrophages (7). This is a complex process and the details remain obscure. For instance, it is clear that the spleen is undoubtedly involved since splenectomy abrogates ACAID (33, 34). However, there is a three day window before splenectomy becomes ineffective in preventing ACAID and much has been going on in that interval since signals to immune and trafficking cells are of the order of minutes to hours (35–37). In addition, since there are no lymphatics to the spleen but there are well defined lymphatic channels from the anterior chamber to the eye-draining lymph node (38), the precise trafficking of signals and cells between the anterior chamber, the draining lymph node, the blood circulation, the thymus and eventually the spleen are not clear.

There is no denying that ACAID occurs. However, its physiological relevance is less clear. ACAID is an experimental phenomenon and is often equated with IP, but this is not a safe assumption. IP refers to the reduced or modified immune response by tissues due to the properties of that tissue and, as detailed above, is best exhibited by the retina and parenchymal tissue of the brain. ACAID in contrast is a systemic response involving the induction of suppressor/regulatory cells in the periphery, which is revealed by inoculating antigen into the anterior chamber. There is evidence that this systemic phenomenon may be active during homeostasis. Although it has been suggested that CNS parenchymal and retinal antigens are sequestered behind the blood retinal and blood brain barriers (BRB, BBB) (39), i.e. they are "ignored," recent studies have shown that CNS-specific antigens are recognized by T cells in the periphery but such T cells do not have access to the CNS unless they are activated and do not cause damage except when there is recognition of cognate antigen, e.g. in the context of inflammation with cross-reacting antigens (40, 41). In addition, the BRB (and the BBB) is not only a physical barrier of contiguous endothelial cells bound together by tight junctions, but includes the immunomodulatory pericyte, the resident perivascular macrophage, and the glia limitans composed of the foot processes of glia/Müller cells, with contributions from regulatory microglial cells and neuronal dendrites, all of which comprises the neurovascular unit (NVU) (**Figure 2**). However, the NVU and the BRB/BBB are also presided over by Treg [reviewed in (9, 42)] which theoretically could be the equivalent of ACAID-inducing T suppressor cells and in some sense at least should be specific for CNS antigens, i.e. they should be "educated" by CNS antigen in the way described above.

Whether Treg, which some authors envisage as contributing to the immunological component of the BRB/BBB (43, 44), are physiologically equivalent to the T suppressors and Treg of ACAID may be a question which remains unanswered. More important perhaps is understanding why the BRB and the BBB which normally exclude Teff cells, can be breached if the conditions are right (45). This seems to involve innate immune cells which act as escorts in assisting passage of T cells and further activate T cells when they are *in situ* [reviewed in (46)].

There is considerable evidence that immune protection of the retina (aka IP) involves regulatory immune cells of which there are several types. Treg have a prominent place in overall immune tolerance and are also active in retinal homeostasis. Whether this amounts to a specialized form of immune protection or "privilege" or is a variation on the theme of immunological tolerance (depending on the tissue) may be a fine point. The important issue is to understand how this protection might be lost, particularly if the target of attack is self-antigen. These processes are discussed in the following sections.

IMMUNE DEFENSE, IMMUNE PRIVILEGE, AND TISSUE BARRIERS: INTERNAL AND EXTERNAL BARRIERS

Defense against pathogen/antigen invasion is initially about barriers. Once the barrier is breached defense becomes a question of how quickly and effectively the pathogen can be cleared. The strength of the immune response is then the

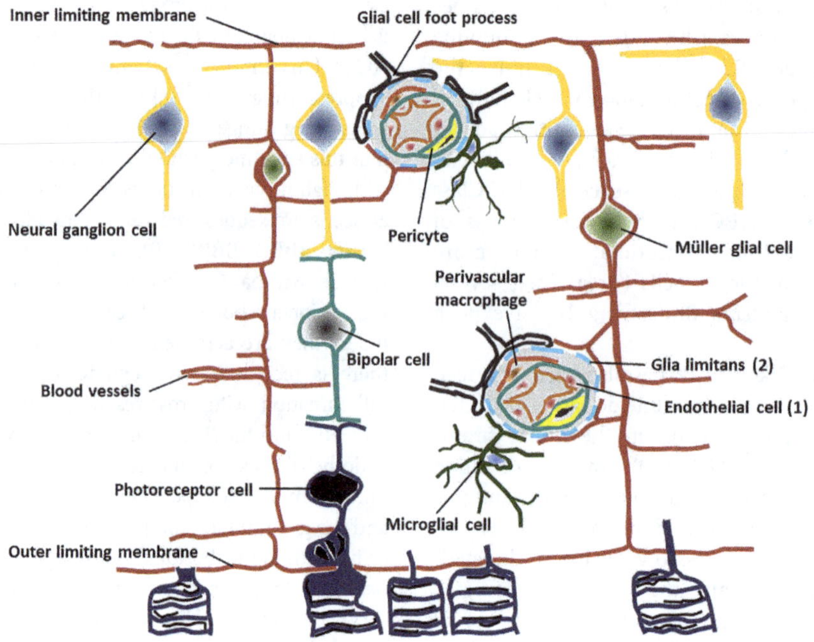

FIGURE 2 | The Retinal Neurovascular Unit. The retinal neurovascular unit (NVU) is the seat of the blood retinal barrier (BRB), situated at the capillary/venous side of the retinal circulation. Two levels of "barrier" exist: a) at the endothelial tight junctions (1), supported by pericytes and under immunological surveillance by perivascular macrophages; and b) at the glia limitans (2), constructed by astrocyte glial cell and Müller glial cell foot processes, with contributions to the continuous membranous structure form microglial cells and neuronal dendritic processes.

deciding factor and can be insufficient, sufficient, or exaggerated. In IP-high tissues, the barrier may be effective initially but under the right conditions, can be broken as in the classic model of experimental autoimmune uveoretinitis (EAU) (47, 48) (**Figures 3** and **4**). Damage can then be extensive and, in the case of the brain, life-threatening. However, many factors modify both the risk of BRB breakdown and the level of damage, particularly genetic factors; for instance, only a restricted number of rodent strains are susceptible to EAU (50, 51). Similar genetic susceptibility to BRB breakdown, as in uveoretinitis, occurs in humans (52, 53) (see below).

The skin and mucosal surfaces are probably the strongest barriers to pathogen invasion. However, these are not simply physical barriers but contain a wide array of immune cells and molecules which can kill or disable pathogens (54, 55). These entities include myeloid cells like Langerhans cells, dendritic cells (DC) and macrophages, a rich variety of T cells such as intraepithelial and dermal/stromal Teff and tissue resident memory (TRM) cells, mucosa-associated invariant T cells (MAIT), Treg, γδT cells, innate lymphocytes (ILC 1, 2, and 3) and NKT cells (56). Immune-modulating molecules include those constitutively present during homeostasis (defensins, neuropeptides, TGFβ, thrombospondin, and connective tissue activating factor/CTAF) (57) and cell associated ligand/receptor pairs such as Fas/FasL, Trail/DR5, CD47/SIRP-α, ICOS/ICOSL, and more (58, 59), as well as inducible molecules such as cytokines and chemokines. These activate resident immune cells as well as initiate a systemic immune response with recruitment of bone marrow derived cells to wall off and insulate against pathogen spread.

These external barriers are strong and display a level of IP whereby they quench potentially damaging immune responses (60). This is particularly important for the skin and mucosal surfaces, specifically the gut mucosa, since they are exposed to a vast panoply (trillions) of commensal microorganisms in the microbiome. This includes bacteria, viruses, fungi, archaea, and protozoa. In the gut, the microbiome actively participates in barrier homeostasis by secreting anti-inflammatory molecules such as short-chain fatty acids (SCFA), small molecules which can pass through the gut barrier into the system and influence immune cell function (61). In this regard, the intestinal and presumably other mucosal barriers share properties with CNS barriers which promote T cell tolerance and the generation of Treg cells (see below) [reviewed in (60)]. The function of the microbiome is not only to suppress settlement of pathogenic entities, but also to harvest and generate nutrients/metabolites (e.g. folate) and energy (e.g. SCFA) from nutritional sources which the host has to provide (62). SCFA have direct stabilizing effects on intestinal integrity (63) as well as priming effects on antigen APC and Treg (64–66) and appear to harness the protective function of gut ILC3 cells through free fatty acid receptor 2 (FFAR2) and the production of IL22 (67).

The skin and mucosal barriers to the external world thus have similarities to the internal barriers between solid organs and the blood. These barriers are variably complete, being easily permeated in tissues with "leaky" blood vessels such as liver and spleen, choroid plexus and uveal tract, and highly restrictive in the CNS. Here the NVU provides a complex physical, molecular, cellular and immunological barrier, in which pericytes, glia,

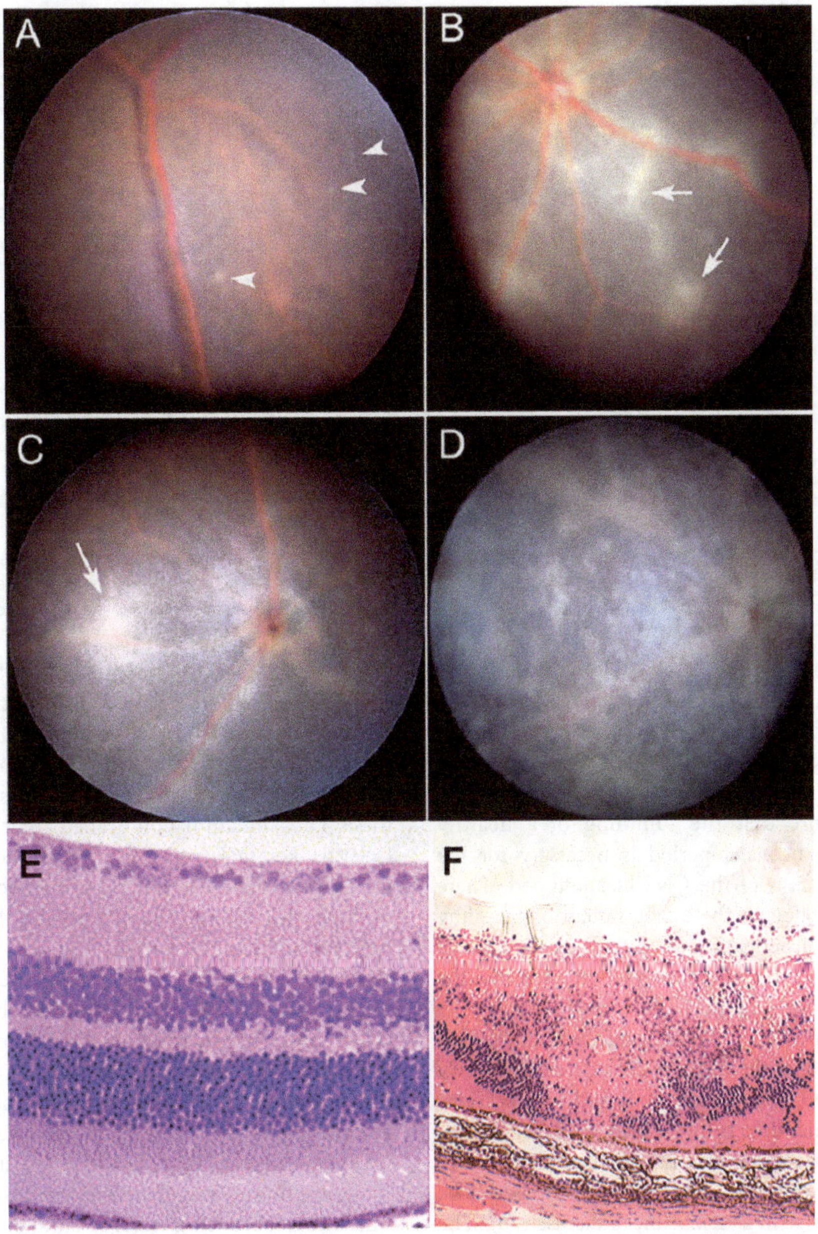

FIGURE 3 | Experimental Autoimmune Uveoretinitis (EAU): a model for sight-threatening posterior uveitis. Clinical and histological signs of EAU in mice. EAU may be induced by subcutaneous injection of interphotoreceptor retinol binding protein (IRBP) peptide 161–180 in B10.RIII mice or peptide 1–20 in C57BL/6 mice with Complete Freund's Adjuvant (CFA) and pertussis toxin (Ptx). Disease is mediated by a Th1/IL12 and/or a Th17/IL23 mechanism with dominant effect being Th17 mediated disease. The images are from the C57/BL6 mouse model. Clinical images are shown: **(A)** early focal chorioretinal infiltrate (arrowhead); **(B)** developing retinal vasculitis shown as focal perivascular "sheathing" (arrows); **(C)** extensive retinal vasculitis and large granulomatous infiltrate; **(D)** severe retinal inflammation, damage and atrophy; **(E)** Section of normal mouse retina; **(F)** EAU showing severe inflammation with large central area of retinal necrosis and loss of photoreceptors.

perivascular macrophages and microglia collaborate (**Figure 2**). The microbiome has a significant role to play in the development of the BBB and perhaps also in the BRB [discussed in (68)]. Mice reared in germ-free conditions have increased permeability of the BBB, continuing on into adult life and appear to have reductions in tight junction proteins including occludin and claudin 5 (13), indicating a role for the microbiome in maturation of the endothelial tight junctions. Similar control may also be exerted by the microbiome over the development of the blood-testis barrier (69). We have mentioned that maturation of CNS barriers occurs during the first months/year of life under the control of the developing microbiome and disruption of this critical process in the neonatal period renders infants susceptible to infections, particularly common viral infections such as herpes

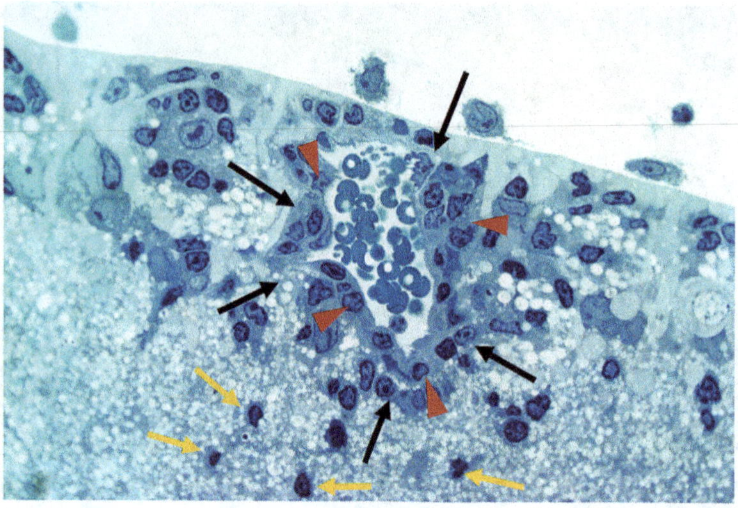

FIGURE 4 | Experimental Autoimmune Uveoretinitis (EAU) in the rat model. EAU was induced in Lewis rats using retinal S antigen as described in (49). The image is a toluidine blue-stained thin section of the inner retina showing perivascular inflammatory cells (large arrows, black) retained within the glia limitans (arrow heads, red). Cells which have entered the retinal parenchyma have pyknotic nuclei and appear to be undergoing apoptosis (small arrows, yellow). Image provided by permission of the authors.

simplex (HSV) and cytomegalovirus (CMV). It is at this time that lifelong viral latency is frequently established [for review see (11)]. Remarkably, these effects can be modified *in utero* since stabilizing the maternal microbiome can have beneficial effects on weanling BBB tight junction formation promoting reduced permeability (70). It is clear therefore that the founding of a healthy microbiome in the early neonatal period is necessary for the establishment of the IP status of the CNS in adulthood. There are many factors which influence the establishment of a healthy microbiome in this critical perinatal period such as the type of delivery, the use of antibiotics, and breast- vs. bottle feeding, the significance of which is now being fully appreciated (71).

Interestingly, at the opposite end of the aging spectrum, defects in the integrity of the NVU of the BBB are considered to underly neurodegenerative disease (72) and may be linked to conditions such as diabetes (73). Similar defects in the BRB are linked to age-related disease in the eye which have an underlying inflammatory pathogenesis (74, 75). Some of these conditions are proposed to be driven *via* a gut-CNS axis such as Alzheimer's disease (76). The nature of the CNS immune response ("privilege") may make it more susceptible to latent infections (see **Figure 1**) with pathogens such as CMV acquired in childhood and prions acquired in adulthood liable to reactivation as immune defenses weaken in old age [reviewed in (11)].

UVEITIS, IMMUNE PRIVILEGE, AND THE BLOOD RETINAL BARRIER

The above considerations allow an interpretation of ocular inflammation, in particular uveitis, in the context of IP. Uveitis has been classified anatomically (anterior vs. posterior), etiologically (infectious vs. non-infections) and pathogenetically (autoimmune vs. autoinflammatory), most recently as part of the standardization of uveitis nomenclature (SUN) project (77) and has been reviewed elsewhere (68, 77, 78). Since the eye is composed of a range of discrete tissue types, inflammation may involve one or more of these tissues individually or together and "uveitis" (i.e. swelling and leakage of uveal blood vessels) is necessarily part of these. Thus, inflammation of the parenchyma of the ocular coats (scleritis, keratitis, iritis, cyclitis, and choroiditis) always involves inflammation of the uveal tract and its blood vessels. Inflammation at these sites does not usually involve the retinal vasculature. In contrast, inflammation of the retina (retinitis, retinal vasculitis) almost always involves uveal vessels. Acute AU is a self-limiting disease in which the retina is not usually involved. Anterior and intermediate uveitis may be complicated by cytokine-mediated secondary macular edema (swelling of the retina at its thinnest central region) in a bystander fashion if these conditions persist and become chronic but the retina is not usually directly under attack.

Thus, one can view AU, and associated conditions such as keratouveitis and sclerouveitis as ocular inflammatory conditions which do not break high level-IP since they do not breach the BRB. In this sense, the level of IP (see above comments on relative IP) expressed by tissues such as the cornea and sclera is not significantly different from other tissues which sit behind the external barriers of the skin and mucosa but outside the highly developed CNS barriers. Similar considerations apply to the coverings/surrounding tissues of the brain, i.e. the meninges. A possible "protective" role for IP can thus be considered specifically for CNS neural tissue (retina and brain parenchyma) but much less so for ocular and brain tissues outside the CNS barrier such as the uvea and meninges, and this is reflected in the much greater frequency of AU over PU (posterior uveitis) and meningitis over encephalomyelitis (11).

When IP is lost and the BRB and the BBB are breached, the outcome is sight-threatening and life-threatening, respectively. The most dangerous time is during development of the BBB and BRB in the prenatal and neonatal periods and in early infancy/childhood (see above section). Many infections acquired at this time are cleared only partially by the developing immune system; where tissues have lower levels of IP, infections are cleared quite efficiently and completely e.g. from the gut and its secondary lymphoid organs. However, from areas with higher levels of IP such as the CNS, the testes/ovaries and stem cell niches in the bone marrow, organisms which have made it through both the external and internal barriers, may further respond to the unfavorable CNS environment by becoming latent [reviewed in (11)]. Here, the immunological component of the IP-dependent CNS barrier comes into play in which Treg sustain latency by suppressing potential Teff and TRM cells, thereby preventing damaging immune responses in essential tissues and organs. The strongest evidence that this mechanism is functioning in immune defense is the "experiment of nature" brought on by the AIDS epidemic. Only when the global circulating T cell numbers, which includes Teff, TRM and Treg cells decline below 200 cells/ml and especially when they are less than 50 cells/ml, do latent infections, including those acquired in early life, become active infections and spread through the tissues (79, 80). This is particularly so for viral infections, such as CMV, HSV and varicella zoster virus (VZV) but also for infections acquired in adulthood which were held in check by the immune system such as *Mycobacterium tuberculosis* (Mtb) and *Toxoplasma gondii* (81–83). Even more convincing is that opportunistic infections by pathogens which would normally present no threat to the host, and in many cases would be regarded as "commensals," come to the fore, particularly as brain and retinal infections, when T cell immunity in particular is compromised (e.g. pneumocystis) (84).

IP, therefore, as it affects the eye, is retina-centric and is primarily an immunological device whereby Treg and other immune regulatory cells, as major components of the BRB, control the activity of Teff cells. If engaged in clearing infection, Teff would generate excessive tissue damage. The gut microbiome not only plays a major role in development and maintenance of the physical BRB and its tight junctions but is central to the generation of the all-important Treg which underpin IP. When retina-centric IP breaks down retina-damaging sight-threatening uveoretinitis takes place.

In contrast, IP is relatively less important in non-retinal forms of ocular inflammation including autoimmune anterior uveitis (AAU) and corneal inflammation. Inflammation of the anterior segment is managed by the host in much the same way as inflammation at other sites including joints, muscle, and connective tissues generally. Indeed, the most common form of AAU is that associated with SpA and its etiology is similar (16, 56). Many cases of presumed non-infectious uveitis have recently been shown to be linked to infection and may in fact be due to persistent/latent infections delivered to the eye and other tissues *via* latently infected bone marrow precursors (85–88).

PATHOGENESIS OF UVEITIS

The pathogenesis of uveitis can be considered by defining the conditions in which the disease occurs. Firstly, uveitis is a blanket term which applies to all forms of ocular inflammation involving any of the coats of the eye (**Table 1**). In infectious uveitis, where a replicating pathogen has been identified, the etiology is quite clear. In this context, endophthalmitis, including post-surgical endophthalmitis caused by bacterial or fungal infection is a particular form of uveitis. HSV stromal keratitis (HSK) is another characteristic and relatively common form of inflammation in which significant cell infiltration in the anterior chamber of the eye can be observed and indeed the entire uveal tract may be involved as has been observed in mouse models (46, 89). Scleritis caused by infection, such as Mtb produces a sclero-choroiditis which similarly involves the uveal tract, preferentially locating in the choroid (90, 91). As indicated in the section above, infectious retinitis in immunocompromised individuals invariably involves the uveal tract but the reverse is much less common, i.e. most forms of uveitis do not involve the retina. Infectious AU and PU can thus be defined quite clearly by the BRB.

Terminology of Ocular inflammation (Uveitis)

In the absence of infection, the etiology of ocular inflammation is less clear. Autoimmunity as a mechanism has been championed for many decades of the 20th century, initially focusing on the uveal tract as a source of antigen [reviewed in (92, 93)]. The discovery of retinal antigens as potent inducers of PU (uveoretintitis, EAU) (94, 95) in animal models, similar in pathogenesis to other models of autoimmunity (experimental autoimmune encephalomyelitis, EAE; experimental autoimmune thyroiditis, EAT) (96–98) opened the door to a rich field of discovery relating to the pathogenic antigen-specific T cells (Th1, Th17), antigen presenting DC, effector macrophages and other myeloid cells as well as pro-inflammatory cytokines (TNFα, IL1, IL12, IL23) all participating one way or another with the mechanism of uveitis [reviewed in (99)]. Autoantigens in AU have been much more difficult to identify: perhaps the best model is the proteoglycan transgenic mouse in which there is a predominance of T cells expressing a T cell receptor (TCR) specific for the arthritogenic epitope of the G1 domain of the proteoglycan aggrecan (100). These mice develop a joint disease resembling spondylo-arthritis. A proportion of the mice also develop AU but, importantly, the uveitis does not involve the retina, once more emphasizing the divide between AU and PU, buttressed by the BRB.

However, evidence for autoimmunity in human uveitis, either anterior or posterior, is thin. While adaptive immune B and T cell reactivity to ocular antigens has been amply documented in patients with uveitis, similar activity has been reported in healthy

TABLE 1 | Terminology of ocular inflammation in uveitis.

Terminology of ocular inflammation (uveitis)		
Type of uveitis	**Etiology**	**Tissues affected**
Anterior	Infectious Non-infectious	Iris, ciliary body, sclera, cornea
Intermediate	Infectious Non-infectious	Ciliary body, vitreous, peripheral retina
Posterior	Infectious Non-infectious	Retina, retinal vessels, optic nerve

Disease classification is based on type, etiology and affected tissues in uveitis.

individuals without disease [reviewed in (68)], and pathogenicity has been impossible to prove so far. Probably the best evidence might come from interventions such as cellular therapies (antigen-primed DC or Treg cell therapy) to demonstrate antigen specificity conclusively [reviewed in (101)].

Dysregulated innate immunity, or autoinflammatory disease, has more recently been proposed as a mechanism for many forms of uveitis. Endotoxic uveitis is a standard model in which local or systemic inoculation of endotoxin induces a short-lived ocular inflammation [reviewed in (102)]. Peptidoglycan and other pathogen-associated molecular patterns (PAMPs) such as CpG induce a similar type of inflammation, acting through pathogen recognition receptors including toll-like receptors (TLR) and C-type lectins and are mediated by downstream signaling pathways such as PI3 Kinase/Akt/NFκB, Syk-CARD9, and the Asc/NLRP3/inflammasome pathways (103–106). Most of these models resemble AU and do not involve the retina except in a bystander fashion. Similarly, uveitis associated with many of the human autoinflammatory syndromes and proposed autoinflammatory diseases such as SpA, is almost exclusively restricted to AU [reviewed in (68)]. The main exception to this is Behçet's disease (BD), which can include AU, PU or panuveitis in its manifestations, as well as neuro-Behçet's symptoms (cerebral vasculitis) (107–110).

Interestingly, recent studies have linked EAU, a recognized experimental autoimmune disease induced by specific antigen (50, 95), with gut microbiota. IRBP-TCR transgenic B10.RIII mice with a high precursor frequency (~25%) of T cells specific for peptide $IRBP_{161-180}$ of the retinal antigen interphotoreceptor retinol binding protein (IRBP) develop spontaneous uveoretinitis gradually from p20 (post-natal day 20) and reaching an incidence of 100% by 2 months of age (111). However, disease severity is reduced if the mice are reared in a germ free environment (112). Similarly, C57BL/6 mice immunized with IRBP peptide $IRBP_{1-20}$ emulsified in Complete Freund's adjuvant (CFA) develop EAU but not in a germ free environment (113). Furthermore, treatment of mice with antibiotics prior to induction of EAU prevents disease but cannot stop disease once it has been induced (113). These data indicate that the microbiome strongly influences the risk of BRB breakdown and the immunological component of so-called IP depends on the condition of the microbiome. The question which remains is whether particular microbiota/commensals which constitute the microbiome specifically annul the protection of CNS IP. Studies in humans indicate that certain diseases such as BD and ankylosing spondylitis (AS) are associated with specific microbiome composition (16, 109, 110), although, if the above dependence of IP on the BRB is to hold true, retinal vasculitis in BD but not AU in AS might expect to be covered by IP.

A case has been made that retinal antigens are sequestered behind the BRB (114) and are not recognized by the peripheral immune system (immunological ignorance). In this scenario, a healthy BRB prevents access by autoreactive T cells to the retina and so, retinal inflammation is prevented. However, in the presence of dysbiosis commensal antigen-specific T cells are activated and circulate systemically. It is suggested that such T cells are cross-reactive with retinal antigens and have the potential to cross the BRB and initiate inflammation. How activated T cells cross the BRB is not clear, but it is well established that non-activated, naïve T cells do not enter the tissues. The question is whether all activated T cells can enter the tissue. Prevailing dogmata support a pathogenesis which depends on precursor frequency and antigen dosage/availability, both of which determine whether, stochastically, such cells will become pathogenic (115–118). Most recently, in a neoantigen transgenic model of spontaneous uveo-retinitis, an absolute requirement for antigen-specific T cell activation has been demonstrated while non-specifically TCR-activated T cells fail to induce disease (119). These questions have exercised researchers over many years and the concept that cross-reactive T cells, activated by a dysbiotic microbiome, might be the guilty party adds significantly to pathogenetic possibilities. Candidate mechanisms include bystander damage, molecular mimicry, dual TCR expression and TCR promiscuity due to variable TCR-peptide MHC affinity. In addition, a possible innate immune, microbiome-based adjuvant effect has been proposed. In the case of the retina and EAU some of these questions have been addressed. In a transgenic model in which the foreign antigen Hen Egg Lysozyme (HEL) has been expressed in the retina under control of the promoter for IRBP (single transgenic IRBP-HEL, sTg : IRBP-HEL mice), adoptive transfer of HEL-TCR specific (3A9) T cells failed to induce EAU, even when the mice were co-infected with cytomegalovirus (MCMV) to induce a proinflammatory background microenvironment. However, when the mice were co-infected with MCMV which had been genetically modified to express the pathogenic HEL_{41-60} peptide, EAU developed within 7 days of adoptive transfer of 3A9 cells and the severity of uveitis depended on the level of HEL expression in the retina (41). T cell cross reactivity/molecular mimicry between retinal and viral antigen therefore appeared to be the dominant mechanism generating pathogenicity, while bystander activation was essentially discounted. These data indicate that T cell activation by specific antigen underpins their pathogenicity in this model of autoimmune disease. Interestingly, a recent study has shown that chimeric human-viral proteins can be generated during viral infection in humans which may offer a further novel explanation for how infection and autoimmunity may overlap (120).

The other side of the microbiome coin is the abundant evidence that a healthy microbiome maintains a proportionate peripheral Treg population through mediators such as SCFA and folate (see below), and Treg are known to be central to the maintenance of immune tolerance and the prevention of autoimmunity (121) (see below). In addition, there is accruing data from human studies that autoimmune/autoinflammatory uveitis syndromes such as Vogt-Koyanagi-Harada disease (VKH) and BD are associated with unsuspected dysbiosis (109, 122) and the failure/lack of Treg cells.

The concept that the gut might drive autoimmune disease in the eye, as has been shown for gut-associated segmented filamentous bacteria in the joint (123), deserves careful examination in relation to IP. Disturbed microbiota has been linked to numerous non ocular as well as ocular inflammatory conditions [reviewed in (54)] and a direct relationship to gut-derived T cells, cross reactive with tissue antigens has not been reported in other models. In addition, a link between a dysregulated microbiome and systemic autoimmune/autoinflammatory disease is not restricted to conditions associated with disrupted IP. Thus, if the microbiome is implicated in the pathogenesis of uveitis, this would appear to be irrespective of IP status, thus relegating IP to a lesser, if any, role. While microbiome-based antigens are currently being evaluated for a role in ocular inflammatory disease, the precise relationship is likely to be complex.

ROLE OF TREG AND THE MICROBIOME IN IMMUNE REGULATION/PREVENTION OF UVEITIS

The gastrointestinal tract is now recognized as a major immune organ, containing an abundance of innate and adaptive immune cells which influence immune responses locally and at distant sites (124). The microbiome with its superabundance of micro-organisms directs the development of T cell populations particularly Th17 cells and Treg, responsive in an antigen-specific manner to microbial antigens. The innate immune system responds in an antigen non-specific manner to produce anti-microbial peptides such as α- and β-defensins in response to cytokines such as IL22, IL18, and INFγ (125). From the moment of birth and even prenatally, microbial colonization shapes the developing immune system and reciprocal interactions benefit (or otherwise) the development of a healthy immune system. The influence of the microbiome on IP therefore relates to several of the components of the blood-CNS barrier: in addition to guiding maturation of tight junctions between BBB endothelial cells (13), the microbiome induces the generation of commensal antigen-specific Treg (126–128), which not only act locally but have a specific gut phenotype combining RORγt and FoxP3 transcription factors (129, 130), and are central to the prevention of intestinal inflammation and IBD (131, 132). In addition, they may have an extra-intestinal effect in the regulation of systemic autoimmune disease such as collagen-induced arthritis (133).

Treg are antigen-specific in their generation but not so in their effector function where they have broader regulatory properties (134). Importantly, the plasticity of Treg both in their generation and their activity is relevant to the above concepts of how commensal antigens might cross-react with tissue-specific antigens through molecular mimicry and induce uveitis (114). Peripheral Treg (pTreg) develop in the secondary lymphoid tissues, including the gut, from naïve T cells under the influence of their cytokine environment which includes both proinflammatory cytokines such as IL6 and regulatory cytokines such as TGFβ and IL22. Generation of Treg in the gut has been linked to the process of T cell education in the thymus although clearly there are differences (135). In the presence of antigen (here we are considering commensal antigen rather than self-antigen as in thymus) T cells may develop along a Teff pathway to generate Th17 cells and then undergo antigen-induced cell death (AICD). Alternatively, in the presence of folate such Teff either convert to homeostatic Th17 cells which generate IL22 (135), or they may become anergic (Tan) and continue on to convert to $FoxP3^+$ Treg (136–138). Both thymus-like $Helios^+$, $neuropilin^+$ (natural, n) Treg and "peripheral," induced (i) $Helios^-$ Treg occur in the gut but iTreg are induced by the microbiome while nTreg are present from a pre-weaning stage (139–141). In addition, there are intraepithelial $FoxP3^-$ Treg and $CD4^+$ $CD8\alpha\alpha^+$ Treg which have an important regulatory role to play (142, 143). However, if the milieu is not conducive, commensal antigen-generated Teff (Th17) cells may clonally expand and enter the circulation as activated cells, with the risk of causing disease if they meet cognate antigen (similar to thymic autoreactive T cells which have escaped deletion). Disease may then ensue where access to tissue antigen is possible and co-stimulation is available. However, for tissues behind "heavy duty" barriers such as the BRB and the BBB, where access may be dependent on a sufficient precursor frequency of activated Teff, released from the constraints of Treg, additional factors to antigen specificity are required. These may be delivered through upregulated innate immune responses (41) and in the case of dysbiotic commensal antigens, through an "adjuvant" effect (114).

In homeostasis, Treg induced by the microbiome promote tolerance rather than immunity. The beneficial/tolerance-inducing role of the microbiome and secreted bacterial products in this scenario is becoming better understood. Mention has already been made of the range of SCFA (propionate, acetate, and butyrate) and other bacterial products which apart from promoting epithelial integrity, promote Treg homeostasis [reviewed in (135)]. In addition, the labile, plastic Th17 cell which can develop into a Treg in the colon is induced by resident DC and other myeloid cells in the small intestine (144, 145). This, however, is a double-edged sword since some intestinal T cells possess dual TCR reactivity and under certain circumstances, can induce autoimmune disease in distant organs such as the lung (146). Dual TCR-expressing T cells are a recognized hazard for the development of autoimmunity by limiting the generation of self-reactive Treg, as has been shown in the non-obese diabetes-prone mouse (NOD) (147). This possible mechanism may also apply to autoimmune uveitis induced by commensal antigen-activated retina-specific T cells although the evidence currenlty appears to be against this notion (114).

GENETIC SUSCEPTIBILITY TO UVEITIS IN THE CONTEXT OF THE MICROBIOME AND TREG: ASSOCIATION BETWEEN DYSBIOSIS AND UVEITIS

The genetics of uveitis also raises questions about the role of IP in conditions in which uveitis features. IP as a phenomenon was hypothesized during the time when MHC antigens were being discovered and was based on failure of the host to react to alloantigens transplanted to the anterior chamber of the eye. Since then the importance of MHC antigen has been revealed particularly in corneal graft rejection (148–150) suggesting that MHC antigens themselves were not the IP-responsive antigens but that the host responded to some tissue allografts through alternative limited polymorphisms. This undermines the original notion of IP as it was conceived but supports the concept of tissues modulating the host response to foreign antigens including alloantigens. To extend

Matzinger and Kamala's concept of tissues in control of the immune response (2), not only do different tissues such as the skin, gut, adrenal gland and retina modify the immune response in different ways, but each individual minor polymorphism in each tissue's proteins will have an influence on the host response. This is borne out by the variable pattern of disease found in different individuals and contributes to the overall variability, exemplified by the current Corona virus (Sars-CoV-2) pandemic in which the upper respiratory tract and the lungs are the main target of attack but the individual outcome varies from fatal Covid-19 disease to severe cases with long-lasting effects [individuals referred to as "long-haulers" (151)] to no symptoms depending on the severity of the associated host immune response (152, 153). Large scale "big data studies" performed through consortia such as *The Infection and Immunity Immunophenotyping* (3i) consortium have revealed the influence of a large number of immunoregulatory genes (>140) on the properties of different tissues underpinning immune variation which resonate with a much broader interpretation of how different cells and tissues influence the outcomes of immune challenge (154), and the future invites further similar study to reveal how CNS tissues including the eye fit with these paradigms.

Both human uveitis and experimental models of uveitis have quite specific and wide-ranging genetic susceptibilities. Caspi's initial studies in mice confirmed the importance of minor antigens in murine susceptibility to induction of EAU (51). Further studies defined the roles of a range of innate immune genes such as TLR, C-type lectins, and genes regulating the inflammasome and IL1 production (103, 155–158). Indeed, an essential role for IL1 in EAU induction has been shown (159).

In human uveitis, strong genetic links have been established with certain types of uveitis. The long known association of the MHC antigen HLA-B27 with AU has been extended with more recent information on susceptibility links to antigen processing genes such as endoplasmic reticulum peptidase 1 (ERAP1) but also to genes more closely associated with innate immunity such as nitric oxide synthase 2 (NOS2) as well as less strong links to a number of other proteins such as Mer Proto-oncogene tyrosine kinase (MERTK), kinesin-associated protein 3 (KAP3) and acetyl-Coenzyme A acyltransferase 2 (ACAA2) (160) The strongest association of MHC antigens and any human disease is that between HLA-A29 and the rare uveitis condition birdshot chorioretinopathy (BCR) (161). Further linkages with BCR have been found with functionally distinct ERAP-1 and -2 genes in a large population of BCR patients (162). BD has linkage with HLA-B51 while sympathetic ophthalmia and VKH disease have common associations with HLA-DR0405 and, interestingly, T cells from patients with VKH show cross-reactivity with peptides from CMV and the melanocyte protein tyrosinase (163), once more implicating infection in a well-defined autoimmune disease.

In many of these conditions, shared linkages with innate immune response (IR) genes, such as the IL23 receptor (164) and cytokine genes of myeloid cells (52, 165–167) have been observed. However, most of the associations are particular to specific disease entities and no clear pattern emerges for adaptive or IR genes for ocular inflammation as a whole, whether it be retina-centric, i.e. behind the BRB or not. No MHC or non-MHC association has been described for IP *per se*. IP was originally attributed to a lack of MHC expression in the relevant tissues (cornea, brain parenchyma, retina, hair follicle, testis etc.) which, in terms of MHC Class I and II still has some relevance due to the paucity of overall expression in these tissues. However, an analysis of CD11c expression on myeloid cells in brain vs. other tissues revealed a significant down regulation in CNS myeloid cells, indicating that while such cells were present in the tissues, the microenvironment of the tissue had the greater influence on whether IR genes were likely to be activated (168).

In contrast to genetic associations with IP, clear connections with some types of uveitis and a disturbed microbiome have been described. For instance, VKH (122), HLA-B27-associated AU [reviewed in (169)], and uveitis in BD (110) have all been linked to dysregulated microbiota with *Prevotella* sp. being identified as a consensus bacterial community in which further stratification linked *Clostridiales* sp. to neuro-BD and *Bacteroides* with multiple sclerosis (170). Importantly, Treg which are considered to play a role in maintaining IP in the retina (43, 44, 171, 172) and brain (173–175) have demonstrated clear tissue adaptation at the barrier sites of the skin and the intestine (176) and it is likely that they do so at sites of the BRB and BBB. Thus, in terms of uveitis there is no clear pattern of disease susceptibility. Indeed, the range of genetic susceptibilities based on MHC Class I and II, and minor/tissue antigen polymorphisms do not support the concept of a unique property of IP for any particular tissue. Tissues' abilities to deal with pathogen invasion and foreign antigens depend on the tissue as well as the genetic make-up of the individual, but probably more importantly it depends on the tissue/cell tropism and virulence of the pathogen.

RESTORING MICROBIOME-ASSOCIATED GUT IMMUNE PRIVILEGE TO PREVENT AND TREAT UVEITIS

As indicated above, IP, when considered as a process whereby tissues modulate immune responses, is by definition a property of most if not all tissues and the gut is no exception (60, 177). Commensal microbial and dietary antigens are "tolerated" in a privileged manner in the gut, mediated by a unique set of Treg (130, 139) which exert control over potential Teff cells. In this, they are assisted by a range of innate immune lymphocytes (124), "tolerant" DC and specialized T cells such as $\gamma\delta$T cells and $CD8\alpha\alpha^+$ mucosal epithelial T cells [reviewed in (178)]. As discussed above, disturbance of the gut microbiota (i.e. dysbiosis) is linked to disease, particularly IBD but is also implicated in various autoimmune diseases such as rheumatoid arthritis, type 1 diabetes mellitus, multiple sclerosis and autoimmune liver disease [reviewed in (179)]. Caspi's group has shown that spontaneous EAU in IRBP-TCR transgenic mice can be prevented and/or suppressed in microbiota-deficient mice, as well as in mice treated with an antibiotic cocktail and has proposed that retina-specific T cells are activated by microbiome-derived antigens which escape through a "leaky gut" epithelium and are presented to T cells by gut or mesenteric lymph node DC (112). The activated T cells then enter the circulation and cross the BRB where they connect with cognate antigen (IRBP) and become pathogenic. Precisely why retina-specific T cells should become activated by microbiota-associated antigen is not clear, but several mechanisms have been proposed. Bystander activation is unlikely but molecular mimicry/antigen cross-reactivity are genuine possibilities (41), while dual TCR expression discussed above is also an interesting option (147) although unlikely as argued by Horai and Caspi (114). Hybrid self-foreign antigen is a novel paradigm (120). Similar studies in the IRBP-inducible model of uveitis have also been reported, showing that EAU can be suppressed in antibiotic-treated mice (180) while IRBP-induced EAU is completely suppressed in germ-free mice (113). In this model, the effect of antibiotic administration is essentially preventive and not therapeutic, i.e. once the disease is active, antibiotic treatment is ineffective (113). These studies, in both the spontaneous and inducible models of EAU, implicate an underlying dysbiosis which permits translocation of bacterial antigen across the lining epithelium, and indeed this is the case. In CFA/IRBP-induced EAU where an antigenic peptide (IRBP) and CFA-mixed emulsion is inoculated subcutaneously, defects in the gut epithelium have been demonstrated with inflammatory cell infiltration in the gut wall (181). Interestingly, these effects on the bowel did not seem to be IRBP-specific since similar findings were observed with CFA-mycobacterial antigen alone. In addition, the numbers of circulating IRBP-specific T cells (Teff or Treg) when CFA/IRBP was inoculated were vanishingly low while the numbers of microbial antigen-specific cells were significantly higher, as might be expected. However, an associated dysbiosis may not be required for microbiota-antigen reactive/activated cells to be present in the circulation. Hegazy et al (182). have shown that in healthy humans, microbiota-specific activated CD4 T cells are present in the blood, and are responsive to a range of commensal bacteria. In patients with IBD, the frequency and specificity of these T cells is increased (182).

WHAT DOES THE GUT–CENTRAL NERVOUS SYSTEM AXIS IMPLY FOR THERAPEUTIC INTERVENTION?

Several groups suggest that there are significant opportunities to intervene, particularly by promoting Treg induction in the gut to eliminate dysbiosis and restore a healthy microbiome. Commensal bacteria provide many mediators of immune and metabolic homeostasis including SCFA. Attempts to ameliorate autoimmune disease by administration of SCFA have been quite successful experimentally in models of multiple sclerosis, hepatitis and diabetes (109, 183–187) as well as uveitis (188). The mechanism of action appears to be through induction of Treg which act locally in the gut as well as at a distance on barrier structures such as the BRB (189–191).

Bacteria produce other metabolites and nutrients. These include bacterial metabolites derived from bile acids, tryptophan, indole and activators of the aryl hydrocarbon receptor (AhR) and folic acid (FA). The latter is of particular interest since it has a direct impact on the survival of intestinal Treg (65) predominantly mediated *via* one of the folate receptors (FR4). FA deficiency is intrinsically damaging to the eye and has been linked to amblyopia (192), optic neuropathy (193), senile cataracts (194), and retinal hyper-homocysteinemia (195) along with its secondary complications (196–198). Hyper-homocysteinemia is connected to specific polymorphisms in FA metabolism-associated genes (199) and has been reported to occur in autoinflammatory BD patients (200). A role for FA in autoimmune uveitis is therefore recognized [for review see (201)].

The direct effects of FA on the eye are delivered *via* several routes including folate receptors (FR; folate-binding proteins) (202), the reduced folate carrier, and the proton-coupled folate transporter (203). FA transport proteins are ubiquitously expressed, and are abundant in retinal pigment epithelium (RPE) and retina (204), suggesting a potential direct immune-modulating role for folate at these sites, particularly as the immunoregulatory BRB cell (the RPE) has the potential to convert naïve T cells to Treg. In humans, there are four known FR isoforms (α, β, γ, and δ) with tissue-specific expression patterns (202, 205). Most recently the human receptor homolog for murine FRδ (also known as FR4 or folate binding protein 3) has been found most abundantly expressed on Treg cells (206). In mice (and possibly in humans), FR4 is expressed under the control of the transcription factor FoxP3 (206), whose sustained expression is a key factor in Treg functional stability (206–210). FoxP3$^+$ Treg populations in the colon are sustained by oral FA supplementation; in contrast, a diet deficient in folate leads to a marked reduction of FoxP3$^+$ Treg selectively in the colon and increased autoimmune bowel inflammation.

The induction of Treg in the periphery, including the gut, is a major control mechanism in the resolving stages of inflammation. Peripheral Treg are generated from naïve T cells but may also be derived from anergic T effector cells (Tan) through a reciprocal induction process (211). T cell anergy is a major contributor to peripheral tolerance mechanisms, wherein CD4$^+$ T cells lose the capacity to produce autocrine growth factor and proliferate in response to antigen (212, 213). A subset of FoxP3$^-$ CD44^{hi} CD73^{hi} FR4^{hi} anergic CD4$^+$ T cells has been identified (214) which upon adoptive transfer, gave rise to Treg cells in an autoimmune arthritis model (211), thereby functioning as progenitors for Treg cell differentiation following TCR-mediated anergy reversal. It has been hypothesized that upon recurrent antigen encounter, anergic CD4$^+$ FoxP3$^-$ FR4$^+$ CD73$^+$ Nrp1$^+$ T cells are prone to partial de-methylation in a specific signature gene, generating ideal progenitors for the peripheral differentiation of stable FoxP3$^+$ Treg (211, 215). These anergy-derived Treg suppress immunopathology and reinforce anergy induction (215). In this context, we have recently shown, in a transgenic model of spontaneous uveitis due to failure of Treg induction, that Tan convert to Treg cells as the inflammation resolves (119). Furthermore, adoptive transfer of antigen-experienced Treg completely prevented development of this spontaneous disease, showing the importance of Treg in the control of uveoretinitis. In the development of cell therapies, such as Treg, for autoimmune disease it would seem there should be a role for FA.

Alternatively, FA may be included in the proposed use of probiotics for control of autoimmune disease (216). Probiotics are preparations which deliver bacteria beneficial to the host through mechanisms such as improving gut epithelial integrity and promoting a balanced immune system. In contrast, prebiotics such as dietary fiber feed the gut microbiome. Probiotics act by becoming part of the commensal community of the microbiome and thus may promote intestinal Treg generation. Some probiotics such as those containing *Lactobacillus (L.) reuteri* WH1689 (217) and *Streptococcus gallolyticus subsp. macedonicus (S. macedonicus)* CRL415 (218), have genes conferring specific beneficial properties affecting metabolism and FA biosynthesis. Recently, probiotic *L. reuteri* has been shown to convert CD4 T cells into $CD4^+$ $CD8\alpha\alpha^+$ double positive intraepithelial cells, which as indicated above are immunoregulatory cells, by decreasing the transcription factor THPOK through activation of the AhR (219). Probiotics have been shown to be effective in certain autoimmune conditions [reviewed in (220)] and are part of what has been termed "the global preclinical pipeline" which includes small molecules such as SCFA as well as engineered probiotics and phages (221). Both probiotics and prebiotics (such as glucans and fructans) are under intense investigation as regulators of general health and homeostasis (222).

Despite the avalanche of studies and projects evaluating probiotics, there is still continuing uncertainty about their overall effectiveness in the context of active autoimmune disease. For this reason, preclinical studies are important. Heat-killed *L. reuteri GMNL*-263 was found to be effective in preventing cardiac damage in a model of systemic lupus erythematosus (223); in a second study, a commercially prepared probiotic, *Lactibiane Iki*, controlled active EAE by promoting tolerogenic DC (224); and the combined administration of two *Bifidobacteria* and *Lactobacilli* probiotic strains prevented experimental myasthenia gravis (225). Preclinical studies of probiotics are in progress but to date no randomized controlled trials of probiotics in patients with uveitis have been reported. However, the opportunities for such studies are becoming clearer (226).

CONCLUSION

The concept of IP in the context of uveitis is difficult to sustain. The pathogenesis of uveitis (whether it be infectious or "non-infectious") (68, 78, 114, 227) is different depending on whether the inflammation occurs in front of or behind the BRB. Even if the site of inflammation is in a tissue which presents a greater immunomodulatory microenvironment, as in the retina compared to the iris, the classical IP properties of the tissue (such as immunosuppressive mediators and lack of resident MHC Class II^+ DC) are not overly effective in preventing inflammatory disease (uveoretinitis). Perhaps a fresh look at what IP as an immunological concept entails is required, specifically asking the question: is IP intrinsically different from mainstream mechanisms which deliver immunological tolerance? Relative degrees of IP can be applied essentially to all tissues and are very highly developed in healthy tissues such as the skin and the gut where a multitude of immunoregulatory mechanisms and cell types are positioned to control the immunostimulatory potential of vast colonies of commensal bacteria. Breakdown of these protective shields is the initial stage of development of systemic and organ-specific inflammatory diseases. This is dependent on the cross reactivity (or other mechanisms as discussed above) of microbiome/ commensal pathogenic antigens to activate and sufficiently expand tissue-specific T cells which can cross internal barriers and cause disease on encountering cognate antigen. Therapies directed toward generation of regulatory cells (Treg or other) which will restore immune homeostasis, particularly in the bowel, may be the way forward to restoring the IP status of all tissues, including those of the CNS.

AUTHOR CONTRIBUTIONS

CM researched, collated, and summarized available literature, drafted the article, and wrote parts of it. JVF conceptualized and wrote the main body of the manuscript. CM edited and formatted the manuscript and figures. JH, HMW, and LK provided expert opinion, edited and critically revised the article. All authors contributed to the article and approved the submitted version.

REFERENCES

1. Forrester JV, Xu H. Good news-bad news: the Yin and Yang of immune privilege in the eye. *Front Immunol* (2012) 3:338. doi: 10.3389/fimmu.2012.00338
2. Matzinger P, Kamala T. Tissue-based class control: the other side of tolerance. *Nat Rev Immunol* (2011) 11(3):221–30. doi: 10.1038/nri2940
3. Forrester JV. Ebola virus and persistent chronic infection: when does replication cease? *Ann Trans Med* (2018) 6(Suppl 1):S39. doi: 10.21037/atm.2018.09.60
4. Streilein JW. Ocular immune privilege: the eye takes a dim but practical view of immunity and inflammation. *J Leukocyte Biol* (2003) 74(2):179–85. doi: 10.1189/jlb.1102574
5. Caspi RR. Ocular autoimmunity: the price of privilege? *Immunol Rev* (2006) 213:23–35. doi: 10.1111/j.1600-065X.2006.00439.x
6. Hazlett LD, Hendricks RL. Reviews for Immune Privilege in the Year 2010: Immune Privilege and Infection. *Ocular Immunol Inflammation* (2010) 18 (4):237–43. doi: 10.3109/09273948.2010.501946
7. Stein-Streilein J. Mechanisms of immune privilege in the posterior eye. *Int Rev Immunol* (2013) 32(1):42–56. doi: 10.3109/08830185.2012.740535
8. Dick AD. Doyne lecture 2016: intraocular health and the many faces of inflammation. *Eye* (2017) 31(1):87–96. doi: 10.1038/eye.2016.177
9. Gery I, Caspi RR. Tolerance Induction in Relation to the Eye. *Front Immunol* (2018) 9:2304. doi: 10.3389/fimmu.2018.02304
10. Williams KA, Esterman AJ, Bartlett C, Holland H, Hornsby NB, Coster DJ. How effective is penetrating corneal transplantation? Factors influencing long-term outcome in multivariate analysis. *Transplantation* (2006) 81 (6):896–901. doi: 10.1097/01.tp.0000185197.37824.35
11. Forrester JV, McMenamin PG, Dando SJ. CNS infection and immune privilege. *Nat Rev Neurosci* (2018) 19(11):655–71. doi: 10.1038/s41583-018-0070-8
12. Jabs DA. Epidemiology of uveitis. *Ophthalmic Epidemiol* (2008) 15(5):283–4. doi: 10.1080/09286580802478724
13. Braniste V, Al-Asmakh M, Kowal C, Anuar F, Abbaspour A, Tóth M, et al. The gut microbiota influences blood-brain barrier permeability in mice. *Sci*

Trans Med (2014) 6(263):263ra158–263ra158. doi: 10.1126/scitranslmed.3009759

14. Bhattarai Y. Microbiota-gut-brain axis: Interaction of gut microbes and their metabolites with host epithelial barriers. *Neurogastroenterol Motil* (2018) 30 (6):e13366. doi: 10.1111/nmo.13366
15. Michel L, Prat A. One more role for the gut: microbiota and blood brain barrier. *Ann Trans Med* (2016) 4(1):15–5. doi: 10.3978/j.issn.2305-5839.2015.10.16
16. Rosenbaum JT, Asquith M. The microbiome and HLA-B27-associated acute anterior uveitis. *Nat Rev Rheumatol* (2018) 14(12):704–13. doi: 10.1038/s41584-018-0097-2
17. Niederkorn JY. Immune privilege of corneal allografts, in *Cornea and External Eye Disease*. Berlin, Heidelberg: Springer (2010) p.1–12. doi: 10.1097/00007890-199906270-00001
18. Medawar PB. The immunology of transplantation. *Harvey Lectures* (1956) (Series 52):144–76.
19. Medawar PB. Immunological tolerance. *Science* (1961) 133(3449):303–6. doi: 10.1126/science.133.3449.303
20. Medawar PB. Immunity to homologous grafted skin; the fate of skin homografts transplanted to the brain, to subcutaneous tissue, and to the anterior chamber of the eye. *Br J Exp Pathol* (1948) 29(1):58–69.
21. Gregerson DS, Torseth JW, McPherson SW, Roberts JP, Shinohara T, Zack DJ. Retinal expression of a neo-self antigen, beta-galactosidase, is not tolerogenic and creates a target for autoimmune uveoretinitis. *J Immunol* (1999) 163(2):1073–80.
22. Carson MJ, Doose JM, Melchior B, Schmid CD, Ploix CC. CNS immune privilege: hiding in plain sight. *Immunol Rev* (2006) 213(1):48–65. doi: 10.1111/j.1600-065X.2006.00441.x
23. Cobbold SP. Regulatory T cells and transplantation tolerance. *J Nephrol* (2008) 21(4):485–96.
24. Niederkorn JY. Corneal transplantation and immune privilege. *Int Rev Immunol* (2013) 32(1):57–67. doi: 10.3109/08830185.2012.737877
25. Louveau A, Harris TH, Kipnis J. Revisiting the mechanisms of CNS immune privilege. *Trends Immunol* (2015) 36(10):569–77. doi: 10.1016/j.it.2015.08.006
26. Engelhardt B, Vajkoczy P, Weller RO. The movers and shapers in immune privilege of the CNS. *Nat Immunol* (2017) 18(2):123. doi: 10.1038/ni.3666
27. Wildner G, Diedrichs-Möhring M. Resolution of uveitis. *Semin Immunopathol* (2019) 41(6):727–36. doi: 10.1007/s00281-019-00758-z
28. Ferguson TA, Herndon JM. The immune response and the eye: the ACAID inducing signal is dependent on the nature of the antigen. *Invest Ophthalmol Visual Sci* (1994) 35(7):3085–93.
29. Stein-Streilein J, Streilein JW. Anterior chamber associated immune deviation (ACAID): regulation, biological relevance, and implications for therapy. *Int Rev Immunol* (2002) 21(2-3):123–52. doi: 10.1080/08830180212066
30. Wenkel H, Streilein JW, Young MJ. Systemic Immune Deviation in the Brain That Does Not Depend on the Integrity of the Blood-Brain Barrier. *J Immunol* (2000) 164(10):5125. doi: 10.4049/jimmunol.164.10.5125
31. Li XY, D'orazio T, Niederkorn J. Role of Th1 and Th2 cells in anterior chamber-associated immune deviation. *Immunology* (1996) 89(1):34–40. doi: 10.1046/j.1365-2567.1996.d01-714.x
32. Zhang-Hoover J, Stein-Streilein J. Therapies based on principles of ocular immune privilege. *Immune Response Eye* (2007) 92:317–27. doi: 10.1159/000099281
33. Streilein JW, Niederkorn JY. Induction of anterior chamber-associated immune deviation requires an intact, functional spleen. *J Exp Med* (1981) 153(5):1058–67. doi: 10.1084/jem.153.5.1058
34. Niederkorn JY, Streilein JW, Kripke ML. Promotion of Syngeneic Intraocular Tumor Growth in Mice by Anterior Chamber-Associated Immune Deviation. *JNCI: J Natl Cancer Institute* (1983) 71(1):193–9. doi: 10.1093/jnci/71.1.193
35. Dang Z, Kuffova L, Liu L, Forrester JV. Soluble antigen traffics rapidly and selectively from the corneal surface to the eye draining lymph node and activates T cells when codelivered with CpG oligonucleotides. *J Leukocyte Biol* (2014) 95(3):431–40. doi: 10.1189/jlb.0612294
36. Kuffová L, Lumsden L, Veselá V, Taylor JA, Filipec M, Holán V, et al. Kinetics of leukocyte and myeloid cell traffic in the murine corneal allograft response. *Transplantation* (2001) 72(7):1292–8. doi: 10.1097/00007890-200110150-00019
37. Kuffová L, Netuková M, Duncan L, Porter A, Stockinger B, Forrester JV. Cross Presentation of Antigen on MHC Class II via the Draining Lymph Node after Corneal Transplantation in Mice. *J Immunol* (2008) 180(3):1353. doi: 10.4049/jimmunol.180.3.1353
38. Plsková J, Duncan L, Holán V, Filipec M, Kraal G, Forrester JV. The immune response to corneal allograft requires a site-specific draining lymph node. *Transplantation* (2002) 73(2):210–5. doi: 10.1097/00007890-200201270-00010
39. Gregerson DS. Immune privilege in the retina. *Ocular Immunol Inflammation* (1998) 6(4):257–67. doi: 10.1076/ocii.6.4.257.4029
40. Harris MG, Hulseberg P, Ling C, Karman J, Clarkson BD, Harding JS, et al. Immune privilege of the CNS is not the consequence of limited antigen sampling. *Sci Rep* (2014) 4:4422. doi: 10.1038/srep04422
41. Voigt V, Wikstrom ME, Kezic JM, Schuster IS, Fleming P, Makinen K, et al. Ocular antigen does not cause disease unless presented in the context of inflammation. *Sci Rep* (2017) 7(1):14226. doi: 10.1038/s41598-017-14618-z
42. Keino H, Sugita S. Immune Privilege and Eye-Derived T-Regulatory Cells. *J Immunol Res* (2018) 2018:1679197. doi: 10.1155/2018/1679197
43. McPherson SW, Heuss ND, Gregerson DS. Local "on-demand" generation and function of antigen-specific Foxp3+ regulatory T cells. *J Immunol* (2013) 190(10):4971–81. doi: 10.4049/jimmunol.1202625
44. McPherson SW, Heuss ND, Pierson MJ, Gregerson DS. Retinal antigen-specific regulatory T cells protect against spontaneous and induced autoimmunity and require local dendritic cells. *J Neuroinflamm* (2014) 11:205. doi: 10.1186/s12974-014-0205-4
45. Engelhardt B, Carare RO, Bechmann I, Flügel A, Laman JD, Weller RO. Vascular, glial, and lymphatic immune gateways of the central nervous system. *Acta Neuropathol* (2016) 132(3):317–38. doi: 10.1007/s00401-016-1606-5
46. Forrester JV, Xu H, Kuffova L, Dick AD, McMenamin PG. Dendritic cell physiology and function in the eye. *Immunol Rev* (2010) 234(1):282–304. doi: 10.1111/j.0105-2896.2009.00873.x
47. Dua H, McKinnon A, McMenamin P, Forrester J. Ultrastructural pathology of the'barrier sites' in experimental autoimmune uveitis and experimental autoimmune pinealitis. *Br J Ophthalmol* (1991) 75(7):391–7. doi: 10.1136/bjo.75.7.391
48. Xu H, Koch P, Chen M, Lau A, Reid DM, Forrester JV. A clinical grading system for retinal inflammation in the chronic model of experimental autoimmune uveoretinitis using digital fundus images. *Exp Eye Res* (2008) 87(4):319–26. doi: 10.1016/j.exer.2008.06.012
49. McMenamin P, Forrester J, Steptoe R, Dua H. Ultrastructural pathology of experimental autoimmune uveitis. Quantitative evidence of activation and possible high endothelial venule-like changes in retinal vascular endothelium. *Lab Invest J Tech Methods Pathol* (1992) 67(1):42–55.
50. Mattapallil MJ, Silver PB, Mattapallil JJ, Horai R, Karabekian Z, McDowell JH, et al. Uveitis-associated epitopes of retinal antigens are pathogenic in the humanized mouse model of uveitis and identify autoaggressive T cells. *J Immunol (Baltimore Md: 1950)* (2011) 187(4):1977–85. doi: 10.4049/jimmunol.1101247
51. Caspi RR. Immunogenetic aspects of clinical and experimental uveitis. *Regional Immunol* (1992) 4(5):321–30.
52. Atan D, Heissigerova J, Kuffová L, Hogan A, Kilmartin DJ, Forrester JV, et al. Tumor necrosis factor polymorphisms associated with tumor necrosis factor production influence the risk of idiopathic intermediate uveitis. *Mol Vision* (2013) 19:184.
53. Kilmartin DJ, Wilson D, Liversidge J, Dick AD, Bruce J, Acheson RW, et al. Immunogenetics and clinical phenotype of sympathetic ophthalmia in British and Irish patients. *Br J Ophthalmol* (2001) 85(3):281–6. doi: 10.1136/bjo.85.3.281
54. Belkaid Y, Harrison OJ. Homeostatic immunity and the microbiota. *Immunity* (2017) 46(4):562–76. doi: 10.1016/j.immuni.2017.04.008
55. Belkaid Y, Tamoutounour S. The influence of skin microorganisms on cutaneous immunity. *Nat Rev Immunol* (2016) 16(6):353–66. doi: 10.1038/nri.2016.48
56. Berlinberg A, Kuhn KA. Barrier lymphocytes in spondyloarthritis. *Curr Opin Rheumatol* (2020) 32(4):343–48. doi: 10.1097/BOR.0000000000000716
57. Taylor AW, Ng TF. Negative regulators that mediate ocular immune privilege. *J Leukocyte Biol* (2018) 103(6):1179–87. doi: 10.1002/JLB.3MIR0817-337R

58. van den Berg TK. On the origin and function of immune 'self recognition. *Immunol Lett* (2010) 1(128):24–5. doi: 10.1016/j.imlet.2009.09.013
59. Lucca LE, Dominguez-Villar M. Modulation of regulatory T cell function and stability by co-inhibitory receptors. *Nat Rev Immunol* (2020) p:1–14. doi: 10.1038/s41577-020-0296-3
60. Spadoni I, Fornasa G, Rescigno M. Organ-specific protection mediated by cooperation between vascular and epithelial barriers. *Nat Rev Immunol* (2017) 17(12):761. doi: 10.1038/nri.2017.100
61. Priyadarshini M, Kotlo KU, Dudeja PK, Layden BT. Role of short chain fatty acid receptors in intestinal physiology and pathophysiology. *Compr Physiol* (2011) 8(3):1091–115. doi: 10.1002/cphy.c170050
62. Amabebe E, Robert FO, Agbalalah T, Orubu ESF. Microbial dysbiosis-induced obesity: role of gut microbiota in homoeostasis of energy metabolism. *Br J Nutr* (2020) 123(10):1127–37. doi: 10.1017/S0007114520000380
63. Engevik MA, Morra CN, Röth D, Engevik K, Spinler JK, Devaraj S, et al. Microbial Metabolic Capacity for Intestinal Folate Production and Modulation of Host Folate Receptors. *Front Microbiol* (2019) 10:2305–5. doi: 10.3389/fmicb.2019.02305
64. Fukuda S, Toh H, Hase K, Oshima K, Nakanishi Y, Yoshimura K, et al. Bifidobacteria can protect from enteropathogenic infection through production of acetate. *Nature* (2011) 469(7331):543–7. doi: 10.1038/nature09646
65. Kinoshita M, Kayama H, Kusu T, Yamaguchi T, Kunisawa J, Kiyono H, et al. Dietary Folic Acid Promotes Survival of Foxp3+ Regulatory T Cells in the Colon. *J Immunol* (2012) 189(6):2869. doi: 10.4049/jimmunol.1200420
66. Trujillo-Vargas CM, Schaefer L, Alam J, Pflugfelder SC, Britton RA, de Paiva CS. The gut-eye-lacrimal gland-microbiome axis in Sjögren Syndrome. *Ocular Surface* (2020) 18(2):335–44. doi: 10.1016/j.jtos.2019.10.006
67. Chun E, Lavoie S, Fonseca-Pereira D, Bae S, Michaud M, Hoveyda HR, et al. Metabolite-sensing receptor Ffar2 regulates colonic group 3 innate lymphoid cells and gut immunity. *Immunity* (2019) 51(5):871–884. e6. doi: 10.1016/j.immuni.2019.09.014
68. Forrester JV, Kuffova L, Dick AD. Autoimmunity, Autoinflammation and Infection in Uveitis. *Am J Ophthalmol* (2018) 189:77–85. doi: 10.1016/j.ajo.2018.02.019
69. Al-Asmakh M, Hedin L. Microbiota and the control of blood-tissue barriers. *Tissue Barriers* (2015) 3(3):e1039691. doi: 10.1080/21688370.2015.1039691
70. Lu J, Lu L, Yu Y, Baranowski J, Claud EC. Maternal administration of probiotics promotes brain development and protects offspring's brain from postnatal inflammatory insults in C57/BL6J mice. *Sci Rep* (2020) 10(1):1–16. doi: 10.1038/s41598-020-65180-0
71. Weström B, Arévalo Sureda E, Pierzynowska K, Pierzynowski SG, Pérez-Cano F-J. The Immature Gut Barrier and Its Importance in Establishing Immunity in Newborn Mammals. *Front Immunol* (2020) 11:1153. doi: 10.3389/fimmu.2020.01153
72. Michalicova A, Majerova P, Kovac A. Tau Protein and Its Role in Blood–Brain Barrier Dysfunction. *Front Mol Neurosci* (2020) 13:178. doi: 10.3389/fnmol.2020.570045
73. Yan C, Zhou Y, Chen Q, Luo Y, Zhang JH, Huang H, et al. Dysfunction of the neurovascular unit in diabetes-related neurodegeneration. *Biomed Pharmacother* (2020) 131:110656. doi: 10.1016/j.biopha.2020.110656
74. Chen M, Luo C, Zhao J, Devarajan G, Xu H. Immune regulation in the aging retina. *Prog Retinal Eye Res* (2019) 69:159–72. doi: 10.1016/j.preteyeres.2018.10.003
75. Xu H, Chen M, Forrester JV. Para-inflammation in the aging retina. *Prog Retinal Eye Res* (2009) 28(5):348–68. doi: 10.1016/j.preteyeres.2009.06.001
76. Jiang C, Li G, Huang P, Liu Z, Zhao B. The gut microbiota and Alzheimer's disease. *J Alzheimer's Dis* (2017) 58(1):1–15. doi: 10.3233/JAD-161141
77. Jabs DA, Nussenblatt RB. J T Rosenbaum, and G Standardization of Uveitis Nomenclature Working, Standardization of uveitis nomenclature for reporting clinical data. Results of the First International Workshop. *Am J Ophthalmol* (2005) 140(3):509–16. doi: 10.1016/j.ajo.2005.03.057
78. Cunningham ET Jr., Forrester JV, Rao NA, Zierhut M. Post-infectious uveitis. *Ocular Immunol Inflammation* (2016) 24:603–6. doi: 10.1080/09273948.2016.1253983
79. Song A, Liu X, Huang X, Meyers K, Oh D-Y, Hou J, et al. From CD4-based initiation to treating all HIV-infected adults immediately: an evidence-based meta-analysis. *Front Immunol* (2018) 9:212. doi: 10.3389/fimmu.2018.00212
80. Aldrete S, Jang JH, Easley KA, Okulicz J, Dai T, Chen YN, et al. CD4 rate of increase is preferred to CD4 threshold for predicting outcomes among virologically suppressed HIV-infected adults on antiretroviral therapy. *PloS One* (2020) 15(1):e0227124. doi: 10.1371/journal.pone.0227124
81. Sudharshan S, Nair N, Curi A, Banker A, Kempen JH. Human immunodeficiency virus and intraocular inflammation in the era of highly active anti retroviral therapy-An update. *Indian J Ophthalmol* (2020) 68 (9):1787–98. doi: 10.4103/ijo.IJO_1248_20
82. Joao I, Bujdáková H, Jordao L. Opportunist Coinfections by Nontuberculous Mycobacteria and Fungi in Immunocompromised Patients. *Antibiotics* (2020) 9(11):771. doi: 10.3390/antibiotics9110771
83. Nizami S, Morales C, Hu K, Holzman R, Rapkiewicz A. Trends in Mortality From Human Immunodeficiency Virus Infection, 1984–2016: An Autopsy-Based Study. *Arch Pathol Lab Med* (2020) 144(5):572–9. doi: 10.5858/arpa.2019-0144-OA
84. Bowen LN, Smith B, Reich D, Quezado M, Nath A. HIV-associated opportunistic CNS infections: pathophysiology, diagnosis and treatment. *Nat Rev Neurol* (2016) 12(11):662. doi: 10.1038/nrneurol.2016.149
85. Yasunaga J, Matsuoka M. Molecular mechanisms of HTLV-1 infection and pathogenesis. *Int J Hematol* (2011) 94(5):435–42. doi: 10.1007/s12185-011-0937-1
86. Carmichael A. Cytomegalovirus and the eye. *Eye* (2012) 26(2):237–40. doi: 10.1038/eye.2011.327
87. Lee JH, Agarwal A, Mahendradas P, Lee CS, Gupta V, Pavesio CE, et al. Viral posterior uveitis. *Survey Ophthalmol* (2017) 62(4):404–45. doi: 10.1016/j.survophthal.2016.12.008
88. Chan NS-W, Chee S-P, Caspers L, Bodaghi B. Clinical features of CMV-associated anterior uveitis. *Ocular Immunol Inflammation* (2018) 26(1):107–15. doi: 10.1080/09273948.2017.1394471
89. Wang H-M, Sheu M-M, Stulting RD, Kaplan HJ. Immunohistochemical evaluation of murine HSV-1 keratouveitis. *Curr Eye Res* (1989) 8(1):37–46. doi: 10.3109/02713688909013892
90. Gineys R, Bodaghi B, Carcelain G, Cassoux N, Amoura Z, Lehoang P, et al. QuantiFERON-TB gold cut-off value: implications for the management of tuberculosis-related ocular inflammation. *Am J Ophthalmol* (2011) 152 (3):433–440. e1. doi: 10.1016/j.ajo.2011.02.006
91. Nora RLD, Van Velthoven ME, Ninette H, Misotten T, Bakker M, Van Hagen MP, et al. Clinical manifestations of patients with intraocular inflammation and positive QuantiFERON–TB Gold In-Tube Test in a country nonendemic for tuberculosis. *Am J Ophthalmol* (2014) 157 (4):754–61. doi: 10.1016/j.ajo.2013.11.013
92. Lee RW, Nicholson LB, Sen HN, Chan CC, Wei L, Nussenblatt RB, et al. Autoimmune and autoinflammatory mechanisms in uveitis. *Semin Immunopathol* (2014) 36(5):581–94. doi: 10.1007/s00281-014-0433-9
93. Nussenblatt R. Proctor Lecture. Experimental autoimmune uveitis: mechanisms of disease and clinical therapeutic indications. *Invest Ophthalmol Visual Sci* (1991) 32(13):3131–41.
94. Wacker WB, Donoso LA, Kalsow CM, Yankeelov JA, Organisciak DT. Experimental allergic uveitis. Isolation, characterization, and localization of a soluble uveitopathogenic antigen from bovine retina. *J Immunol* (1977) 119(6):1949–58.
95. Caspi RR, Chan C-C, Wiggert B, Chader GJ. The mouse as a model of experimental autoimmune uveoretinitis (EAU). *Curr Eye Res* (1990) 9 (supl):169–74. doi: 10.3109/02713689008999438
96. Wan Q, McCormick D, Shah R, Giraldo A, David C, Kong Y. Induction of autoimmune thyroiditis by unique human thyroglobulin epitopes in H2E transgenic mice. *FASEB J* (1998) 12(5):A1051.
97. Baxter AG. The origin and application of experimental autoimmune encephalomyelitis. *Nat Rev Immunol* (2007) 7(11):904–12. doi: 10.1038/nri2190
98. Schlüter A, Flögel U, Diaz-Cano S, Görtz G-E, Stähr K, Oeverhaus M, et al. Graves' orbitopathy occurs sex-independently in an autoimmune hyperthyroid mouse model. *Sci Rep* (2018) 8(1):1–13. doi: 10.1038/s41598-018-31253-4
99. Caspi RR. A look at autoimmunity and inflammation in the eye. *J Clin Invest* (2010) 120(9):3073–83. doi: 10.1172/JCI42440
100. Kezic JM, Glant TT, Rosenbaum JT, Rosenzweig HL. Neutralization of IL-17 ameliorates uveitis but damages photoreceptors in a murine model of spondyloarthritis. *Arthritis Res Ther* (2012) 14(1):R18. doi: 10.1186/ar3697

101. Forrester JV, Steptoe RJ, Klaska IP, Martin-Granados C, Dua HS, Degli-Esposti MA, et al. Cell-based therapies for ocular inflammation. *Prog Retinal Eye Res* (2013) 35:82–101. doi: 10.1016/j.preteyeres.2013.02.002
102. Klaska IP, Forrester JV. Mouse models of autoimmune uveitis. *Curr Pharm Design* (2015) 21(18):2453–67. doi: 10.2174/1381612821666150316122928
103. Fang J, Fang D, Silver PB, Wen F, Li B, Ren X, et al. The role of TLR2, TRL3, TRL4, and TRL9 signaling in the pathogenesis of autoimmune disease in a retinal autoimmunity model. *Invest Ophthalmol Visual Sci* (2010) 51 (6):3092–9. doi: 10.1167/iovs.09-4754
104. Chinnery HR, Leong CM, Chen W, Forrester JV, McMenamin PG. TLR9 and TLR7/8 activation induces formation of keratic precipitates and giant macrophages in the mouse cornea. *J Leukocyte Biol* (2015) 97(1):103–10. doi: 10.1189/jlb.3AB0414-216R
105. Basu S, Rao N, Elkington P. Animal Models of Ocular Tuberculosis: Implications for Diagnosis and Treatment. *Ocular Immunol Inflammation* (2020) p:1–7. doi: 10.1080/09273948.2020.1746358
106. Bridgewood C, Sharif K, Sherlock J, Watad A, McGonagle D. Interleukin-23 pathway at the enthesis: The emerging story of enthesitis in spondyloarthropathy. *Immunol Rev* (2020) 294(1):27–47. doi: 10.1111/imr.12840
107. Ghasemi Y, Dabbagh F, Rasoul-Amini S, Haghighi AB, Morowvat MHmedicine. The possible role of HSPs on Behçet's disease: a bioinformatic approach. *Comput Biol* (2012) 42(11):1079–85. doi: 10.1016/j.compbiomed.2012.08.009
108. Consolandi C, Turroni S, Emmi G, Severgnini M, Fiori J, Peano C, et al. Behçet's syndrome patients exhibit specific microbiome signature. *Autoimmun Rev* (2015) 14(4):269–76. doi: 10.1016/j.autrev.2014.11.009
109. Shimizu J, Kubota T, Takada E, Takai K, Fujiwara N, Arimitsu N, et al. Bifidobacteria abundance-featured gut microbiota compositional change in patients with Behcet's disease. *PloS One* (2016) 11(4):e0153746. doi: 10.1371/journal.pone.0153746
110. Ye Z, Zhang N, Wu C, Zhang X, Wang Q, Huang X, et al. A metagenomic study of the gut microbiome in Behcet's disease. *Microbiome* (2018) 6(1):135. doi: 10.1186/s40168-018-0520-6
111. Horai R, Silver PB, Chen J, Agarwal RK, Chong WP, Jittayasothorn Y, et al. Breakdown of immune privilege and spontaneous autoimmunity in mice expressing a transgenic T cell receptor specific for a retinal autoantigen. *J Autoimmun* (2013) 44:21–33. doi: 10.1016/j.jaut.2013.06.003
112. Horai R, Zarate-Blades CR, Dillenburg-Pilla P, Chen J, Kielczewski JL, Silver PB, et al. Microbiota-Dependent Activation of an Autoreactive T Cell Receptor Provokes Autoimmunity in an Immunologically Privileged Site. *Immunity* (2015) 43(2):343–53. doi: 10.1016/j.immuni.2015.07.014
113. Heissigerova J, Seidler Stangova P, Klimova A, Svozilkova P, Hrncir T, Stepankova R, et al. The Microbiota Determines Susceptibility to Experimental Autoimmune Uveoretinitis. *J Immunol Res* (2016) 2016:5065703. doi: 10.1155/2016/5065703
114. Horai R, Caspi RR. Microbiome and autoimmune uveitis. *Front Immunol* (2019) 10:232. doi: 10.3389/fimmu.2019.00232
115. Prendergast RA, Iliff CE, Coskuncan NM, Caspi RR, Sartani G, Tarrant TK, et al. T cell traffic and the inflammatory response in experimental autoimmune uveoretinitis. *Invest Ophthalmol Visual Sci* (1998) 39(5):754–62.
116. Xu H, Manivannan A, Goatman KA, Jiang HR, Liversidge J, Sharp PF, et al. Reduction in shear stress, activation of the endothelium, and leukocyte priming are all required for leukocyte passage across the blood—retina barrier. *J Leukocyte Biol* (2004) 75(2):224–32. doi: 10.1189/jlb.1002479
117. Xu H, Manivannan A, Liversidge J, Sharp PF, Forrester JV, Crane IJ. Requirements for passage of T lymphocytes across non-inflamed retinal microvessels. *J Neuroimmunol* (2003) 142(1-2):47–57. doi: 10.1016/S0165-5728(03)00258-3
118. Crane IJ, Xu H, Wallace C, Manivannan A, Mack M, Liversidge J, et al. Involvement of CCR5 in the passage of Th1-type cells across the blood-retina barrier in experimental autoimmune uveitis. *J Leukocyte Biol* (2006) 79 (3):435–43. doi: 10.1189/jlb.0305130
119. Liu Y-H, Mölzer C, Makinen K, Kamoi K, Corbett CLC, Klaska IP, et al. Treatment With FoxP3+ Antigen-Experienced T Regulatory Cells Arrests Progressive Retinal Damage in a Spontaneous Model of Uveitis. *Front Immunol* (2020) 11(2071). doi: 10.3389/fimmu.2020.02071
120. Ho JSY, Angel M, Ma Y, Sloan E, Wang G, Martinez-Romero C, et al. Hybrid gene origination creates human-virus chimeric proteins during infection. *Cell* (2020) 181(7):1502 17.e23. doi: 10.1016/j.cell.2020.05.035
121. Klein L, Robey EA, Hsieh C-S. Central CD4+ T cell tolerance: deletion versus regulatory T cell differentiation. *Nat Rev Immunol* (2019) 19(1):7–18. doi: 10.1038/s41577-018-0083-6
122. Ye Z, Wu C, Zhang N, Du L, Cao Q, Huang X, et al. Altered gut microbiome composition in patients with Vogt-Koyanagi-Harada disease. *Gut Microbes* (2020) p:1–17. doi: 10.1080/19490976.2019.1700754
123. Wu H-J, Ivanov III, Darce J, Hattori K, Shima T, Umesaki Y, et al. Gut-residing segmented filamentous bacteria drive autoimmune arthritis via T helper 17 cells. *Immunity* (2010) 32(6):815–27. doi: 10.1016/j.immuni.2010.06.001
124. Vivier E, Artis D, Colonna M, Diefenbach A, Di Santo JP, Eberl G, et al. Innate Lymphoid Cells: 10 Years On. *Cell* (2018) 174(5):1054–66. doi: 10.1016/j.cell.2018.07.017
125. Thaiss CA, Zmora N, Levy M, Elinav E. The microbiome and innate immunity. *Nature* (2016) 535(7610):65–74. doi: 10.1038/nature18847
126. Atarashi K, Tanoue T, Shima T, Imaoka A, Kuwahara T, Momose Y, et al. Induction of Colonic Regulatory T Cells by Indigenous Clostridium Species. *Science* (2011) 331(6015):337. doi: 10.1126/science.1198469
127. Geuking MB, Cahenzli J, Lawson MAE, Ng DCK, Slack E, Hapfelmeier S, et al. Intestinal Bacterial Colonization Induces Mutualistic Regulatory T Cell Responses. *Immunity* (2011) 34(5):794–806. doi: 10.1016/j.immuni.2011.03.021
128. Mosconi I, Geuking M, Zaiss M, Massacand J, Aschwanden C, Chung CK, et al. Intestinal bacteria induce TSLP to promote mutualistic T-cell responses. *Mucosal Immunol* (2013) 6(6):1157–67. doi: 10.1038/mi.2013.12
129. Ohnmacht C, Park J-H, Cording S, Wing JB, Atarashi K, Obata Y, et al. The microbiota regulates type 2 immunity through RORγt+ T cells. *Science* (2015) 349(6251):989–93. doi: 10.1126/science.aac4263
130. Sefik E, Geva-Zatorsky N, Oh S, Konnikova L, Zemmour D, McGuire AM, et al. Individual intestinal symbionts induce a distinct population of RORγ+ regulatory T cells. *Science* (2015) 349(6251):993–7. doi: 10.1126/science.aaa9420
131. Zhong Y, Cantwell A, Dube PHJ. Transforming Growth Factor β and CD25 Are Important for Controlling Systemic Dissemination following Yersinia enterocolitica Infection of the Gut. *Infect Immun* (2010) 78(9):3716–25. doi: 10.1128/IAI.00203-10
132. Sujino T, London M, Hoytema van Konijnenburg DP, Rendon T, Buch T, Silva HM, et al. Tissue adaptation of regulatory and intraepithelial CD4(+) T cells controls gut inflammation. *Science* (2016) 352(6293):1581–6. doi: 10.1126/science.aaf3092
133. Tong B, Yu J, Wang T, Dou Y, Wu X, Kong L, et al. Sinomenine suppresses collagen-induced arthritis by reciprocal modulation of regulatory T cells and Th17 cells in gut-associated lymphoid tissues. *Mol Immunol* (2015) 65 (1):94–103. doi: 10.1016/j.molimm.2015.01.014
134. Zeng H, Chi H. Metabolic control of regulatory T cell development and function. *Trends Immunol* (2015) 36(1):3–12. doi: 10.1016/j.it.2014.08.003
135. Zhao Q, Elson CO. Adaptive immune education by gut microbiota antigens. *Immunology* (2018) 154(1):28–37. doi: 10.1111/imm.12896
136. Gagliani N, Huber S. Basic aspects of T helper cell differentiation. *T-Cell Differ* (2017) 1514:19–30. doi: 10.1007/978-1-4939-6548-9_2
137. Gagliani N, Vesely MCA, Iseppon A, Brockmann L, Xu H, Palm NW, et al. T H 17 cells transdifferentiate into regulatory T cells during resolution of inflammation. *Nature* (2015) 523(7559):221–5. doi: 10.1038/nature14452
138. Josefowicz SZ, Niec RE, Kim HY, Treuting P, Chinen T, Zheng Y, et al. Extrathymically generated regulatory T cells control mucosal TH2 inflammation. *Nature* (2012) 482(7385):395–9. doi: 10.1038/nature10772
139. Panduro M, Benoist C, Mathis D. Tissue Tregs. *Annu Rev Immunol* (2016) 34:609–33. doi: 10.1146/annurev-immunol-032712-095948
140. Torres J, Hu J, Seki A, Eisele C, Nair N, Huang R, et al. Infants born to mothers with IBD present with altered gut microbiome that transfers abnormalities of the adaptive immune system to germ-free mice. *Gut* (2020) 69(1):42–51. doi: 10.1136/gutjnl-2018-317855
141. Al Nabhani Z, Dulauroy S, Marques R, Cousu C, Al Bounny S, Déjardin F, et al. A weaning reaction to microbiota is required for resistance to immunopathologies in the adult. *Immunity* (2019) 50(5):1276–1288. e5. doi: 10.1016/j.immuni.2019.02.014
142. Das G, Augustine MM, Das J, Bottomly K, Ray P, Ray A. An important regulatory role for CD4+ CD8αα T cells in the intestinal epithelial layer in the prevention of inflammatory bowel disease. *Proc Natl Acad Sci* (2003) 100 (9):5324–9. doi: 10.1073/pnas.0831037100

143. Qiu Y, Peng K, Liu M, Xiao W, Yang H. CD8αα TCRαβ intraepithelial lymphocytes in the mouse gut. *Digest Dis* (2016) 61(6):1451–60. doi: 10.1007/s10620-015-4016-y
144. Goto Y, Panea C, Nakato G, Cebula A, Lee C, Diez MG, et al. Segmented filamentous bacteria antigens presented by intestinal dendritic cells drive mucosal Th17 cell differentiation. *Immunity* (2014) 40(4):594–607. doi: 10.1016/j.immuni.2014.03.005
145. Atarashi K, Tanoue T, Ando M, Kamada N, Nagano Y, Narushima S, et al. Th17 cell induction by adhesion of microbes to intestinal epithelial cells. *Cell* (2015) 163(2):367–80. doi: 10.1016/j.cell.2015.08.058
146. Bradley CP, Teng F, Felix KM, Sano T, Naskar D, Block KE, et al. Segmented filamentous bacteria provoke lung autoimmunity by inducing gut-lung axis Th17 cells expressing dual TCRs. *Cell Host Microbe* (2017) 22(5):697–704. e4. doi: 10.1016/j.chom.2017.10.007
147. Schuldt NJ, Auger JL, Spanier JA, Martinov T, Breed ER, Fife BT, et al. Cutting edge: Dual TCRα expression poses an autoimmune hazard by limiting regulatory T cell generation. *J Immunol* (2017) 199(1):33–8. doi: 10.4049/jimmunol.1700406
148. Sano Y, Ksander BR, Wayne SJ. Minor H, rather than MHC, alloantigens offer the greater barrier to successful orthotopic corneal transplantation in mice. *Transplant Immunol* (1996) 4(1):53–6. doi: 10.1016/S0966-3274(96)80035-9
149. Haskova Z, Sproule TJ, Roopenian DC, Ksander BR. An immunodominant minor histocompatibility alloantigen that initiates corneal allograft rejection1. *Transplantation* (2003) 75(8):1368–74. doi: 10.1097/01.TP.0000063708. 26443.3B
150. Vitova A, Kuffová L, Klaska IP, Holan V, Cornall RJ, Forrester JV. The high-risk corneal regraft model: a justification for tissue matching in humans. *Transplant Int* (2013) 26(4):453–61. doi: 10.1111/tri.12055
151. Godlee F. Living with covid-19. *BMJ* (2020) 370:m3392. doi: 10.1136/ bmj.m3392
152. İnandıklıoğlu N, Akkoc T. Immune Responses to SARS-CoV, MERS-CoV and SARS-CoV-2. *Cell Biol Trans Med* (2020) 9:5–12. doi: 10.1007/ 5584_2020_549
153. Sangith N. Unique fibrinogen-binding motifs in the nucleocapsid phosphoprotein of SARS CoV-2: Potential implications in host-pathogen interactions. *Med Hypotheses* (2020) 144:110030. doi: 10.1016/j.mehy.2020.110030
154. Abeler-Dorner L, Laing AG, Lorenc A, Ushakov DS, Clare S, Speak AO, et al. High-throughput phenotyping reveals expansive genetic and structural underpinnings of immune variation. *Nat Immunol* (2020) 21(1):86–100. doi: 10.1038/s41590-019-0549-0
155. Stoppelkamp S, Reid DM, Yeoh J, Taylor J, McKenzie EJ, Brown GD, et al. Murine pattern recognition receptor dectin-1 is essential in the development of experimental autoimmune uveoretinitis. *Mol Immunol* (2015) 67(2):398–406. doi: 10.1016/j.molimm.2015.07.002
156. Brown B, Lee E, Snow P, Vance E, Iwakura Y, Ohno N, et al. Fungal-derived cues promote ocular autoimmunity through a Dectin-2/Card9-mediated mechanism. *Clin Exp Immunol* (2017) 190(3):293–303. doi: 10.1111/ cei.13021
157. Lee EJ, Brown BR, Vance EE, Snow PE, Silver PB, Heinrichs D, et al. Mincle activation and the Syk/Card9 signaling axis are central to the development of autoimmune disease of the eye. *J Immunol* (2016) 196(7):3148–58. doi: 10.4049/jimmunol.1502355
158. Bing SJ, Shemesh I, Chong WP, Horai R, Jittayasothorn Y, Silver PB, et al. AS101 ameliorates experimental autoimmune uveitis by regulating Th1 and Th17 responses and inducing Treg cells. *J Autoimmun* (2019) 100:52–61. doi: 10.1016/j.jaut.2019.02.006
159. Wan C-K, He C, Sun L, Egwuagu CE, Leonard WJ. Cutting edge: IL-1 receptor signaling is critical for the development of autoimmune uveitis. *J Immunol* (2016) 196(2):543–6. doi: 10.4049/jimmunol.1502080
160. Huang X-F, Li Z, De Guzman E, Robinson P, Gensler L, Ward MM, et al. Genomewide Association Study of Acute Anterior Uveitis Identifies New Susceptibility Loci. *Invest Ophthalmol Visual Sci* (2020) 61(6):3–3. doi: 10.1167/iovs.61.6.3
161. Nussenblatt RB, Mittal KK, Ryan S, Green WR, Maumenee AE. Birdshot retinochoroidopathy associated with HLA-A29 antigen and immune responsiveness to retinal S-antigen. *Am J Ophthalmol* (1982) 94(2):147–58. doi: 10.1016/0002-9394(82)90069-1
162. Kuiper JJ, v Setten J, Devall M, Cretu-Stancu M, Hiddingh S, Ophoff RA, et al. Functionally distinct ERAP1 and ERAP2 are a hallmark of HLA-A29-(Birdshot) Uveitis. *Hum Mol Genet* (2018) 27(24):4333–43. doi: 10.1101/ 338228
163. Sugita S, Takase H, Kawaguchi T, Taguchi C, Mochizuki M. Cross-reaction between tyrosinase peptides and cytomegalovirus antigen by T cells from patients with Vogt-Koyanagi-Harada disease. *Int Ophthalmol* (2007) 27(2-3):87–95. doi: 10.1007/s10792-006-9020-y
164. Hou S, Kijlstra A, Yang P. Molecular genetic advances in uveitis. *Prog Mol Biol Trans Sci* (2015) 134:283–98. doi: 10.1016/bs.pmbts.2015.04.009
165. Atan D, Turner SJ, Kilmartin DJ, Forrester JV, Bidwell J, Dick AD, et al. Cytokine gene polymorphism in sympathetic ophthalmia. *Invest Ophthalmol Visual Sci* (2005) 46(11):4245–50. doi: 10.1167/iovs.05-0126
166. Atan D, Fraser-Bell S, Plskova J, Kuffova L, Hogan A, Tufail A, et al. Cytokine polymorphism in noninfectious uveitis. *Invest Ophthalmol Visual Sci* (2010) 51(8):4133–42. doi: 10.1167/iovs.09-4583
167. Atan D, Fraser-Bell S, Plskova J, Kuffová L, Hogan A, Tufail A, et al. Punctate inner choroidopathy and multifocal choroiditis with panuveitis share haplotypic associations with IL10 and TNF loci. *Invest Ophthalmol Visual Sci* (2011) 52(6):3573–81. doi: 10.1167/iovs.10-6743
168. Immig K, Gericke M, Menzel F, Merz F, Krueger M, Schiefenhövel F, et al. CD11c-positive cells from brain, spleen, lung, and liver exhibit site-specific immune phenotypes and plastically adapt to new environments. *Glia* (2015) 63(4):611–25. doi: 10.1002/glia.22771
169. Rosenbaum JT, Lin P, Asquith M, The microbiome HLA. and the pathogenesis of uveitis. *Japanese J Ophthalmol* (2016) 60(1):1–6. doi: 10.1007/s10384-015-0416-y
170. Oezguen N, Yalcinkaya N, Kücükali C, Dahdouli M, Hollister E, Luna R, et al. Microbiota stratification identifies disease-specific alterations in neuro-Behçet's disease and multiple sclerosis. *Clin Exp Rheumatol* (2019) 37(121): S58–66.
171. Silver PB, Horai R, Chen J, Jittayasothorn Y, Chan CC, Villasmil R, et al. Retina-specific T regulatory cells bring about resolution and maintain remission of autoimmune uveitis. *J Immunol* (2015) 194(7):3011–9. doi: 10.4049/jimmunol.1402650
172. Zhou R, Horai R, Silver PB, Mattapallil MJ, Zárate-Bladés CR, Chong WP, et al. The Living Eye "Disarms" Uncommitted Autoreactive T Cells by Converting Them to Foxp3<sup<+</sup< Regulatory Cells following Local Antigen Recognition. *J Immunol* (2012) 188(4):1742. doi: 10.4049/ jimmunol.1102415
173. Ito M, Komai K, Nakamura T, Srirat T, Yoshimura A. Tissue regulatory T cells and neural repair. *Int Immunol* (2019) 31(6):361–9. doi: 10.1093/ intimm/dxz031
174. Malviya M, Saoudi A, Bauer J, Fillatreau S, Liblau R. Treatment of experimental autoimmune encephalomyelitis with engineered bi-specific Foxp3+ regulatory CD4+ T cells. *J Autoimmun* (2020) 108:102401. doi: 10.1016/j.jaut.2020.102401
175. O'Brien CA, Harris TH. ICOS-deficient and ICOS YF mutant mice fail to control Toxoplasma gondii infection of the brain. *PloS One* (2020) 15(1): e0228251. doi: 10.1371/journal.pone.0228251
176. Whibley N, Tucci A, Powrie F. Regulatory T cell adaptation in the intestine and skin. *Nat Immunol* (2019) 20(4):386–96. doi: 10.1038/s41590-019-0351-z
177. Iweala OII, Nagler CR. Immune privilege in the gut: the establishment and maintenance of non-responsiveness to dietary antigens and commensal flora. *Immunol Rev* (2006) 213(1):82–100. doi: 10.1111/j.1600-065X.2006.00431.x
178. Kurashima Y, Kiyono H. Mucosal ecological network of epithelium and immune cells for gut homeostasis and tissue healing. *Annu Rev Immunol* (2017) 35:119–47. doi: 10.1146/annurev-immunol-051116-052424
179. Li B, Selmi C, Tang R, Gershwin ME, Ma X. The microbiome and autoimmunity: a paradigm from the gut–liver axis. *Cell Mol Immunol* (2018) 15(6):595–609. doi: 10.1038/cmi.2018.7
180. Nakamura YK, Metea C, Karstens L, Asquith M, Gruner H, Moscibrocki C, et al. Gut Microbial Alterations Associated With Protection From Autoimmune Uveitis. *Invest Ophthalmol Visusal Sci* (2016) 57(8):3747–58. doi: 10.1167/iovs.16-19733
181. Janowitz C, Nakamura YK, Metea C, Gligor A, Yu W, Karstens L, et al. Disruption of Intestinal Homeostasis and Intestinal Microbiota During Experimental Autoimmune Uveitis. *Invest Ophthalmol Visual Sci* (2019) 60(1):420–9. doi: 10.1167/iovs.18-24813
182. Hegazy AN, West NR, Stubbington MJ, Wendt E, Suijker KII, Datsi A, et al. Circulating and tissue-resident CD4+ T cells with reactivity to intestinal

microbiota are abundant in healthy individuals and function is altered during inflammation. *Gastroenterology* (2017) 153(5):1320–37.e16. doi: 10.1053/j.gastro.2017.07.047
183. Mariño E, Richards JL, McLeod KH, Stanley D, Yap YA, Knight J, et al. Gut microbial metabolites limit the frequency of autoimmune T cells and protect against type 1 diabetes. *Nat Immunol* (2017) 18(5):552–62. doi: 10.1038/ni.3713
184. Wu J-L, Zou J-Y, Hu E-D, Chen D-Z, Chen L, Lu F-B, et al. Sodium butyrate ameliorates S100/FCA-induced autoimmune hepatitis through regulation of intestinal tight junction and toll-like receptor 4 signaling pathway. *Immunol Lett* (2017) 190:169–76. doi: 10.1016/j.imlet.2017.08.005
185. Gill P, Van Zelm M, Muir J, Gibson P. Short chain fatty acids as potential therapeutic agents in human gastrointestinal and inflammatory disorders. *Aliment Pharmacol Ther* (2018) 48(1):15–34. doi: 10.1111/apt.14689
186. Hu E-D, Chen D-Z, Wu J-L, Lu F-B, Chen L, Zheng M-H, et al. High fiber dietary and sodium butyrate attenuate experimental autoimmune hepatitis through regulation of immune regulatory cells and intestinal barrier. *Cell Immunol* (2018) 328:24–32. doi: 10.1016/j.cellimm.2018.03.003
187. Melbye P, Olsson A, Hansen TH, Søndergaard HB, Bang Oturai A. Short-chain fatty acids and gut microbiota in multiple sclerosis. *Acta Neurologica Scand* (2019) 139(3):208–19. doi: 10.1111/ane.13045
188. Nakamura YK, Janowitz C, Metea C, Asquith M, Karstens L, Rosenbaum JT, et al. Short chain fatty acids ameliorate immune-mediated uveitis partially by altering migration of lymphocytes from the intestine. *Sci Rep* (2017) 7 (1):11745. doi: 10.1038/s41598-017-12163-3
189. Erny D, Hrabě de Angelis AL, Jaitin D, Wieghofer P, Staszewski O, David E, et al. Host microbiota constantly control maturation and function of microglia in the CNS. *Nat Neurosci* (2015) 18(7):965–77. doi: 10.1038/nn.4030
190. Haghikia A, Jörg S, Duscha A, Berg J, Manzel A, Waschbisch A, et al. Dietary fatty acids directly impact central nervous system autoimmunity via the small intestine. *Immunity* (2015) 43(4):817–29. doi: 10.1016/j.immuni.2015.09.007
191. Marungruang N, Arévalo Sureda E, Lefrançoise A, Weström B, Nyman M, Prykhodko O, et al. Impact of dietary induced precocious gut maturation on cecal microbiota and its relation to the blood-brain barrier during the postnatal period in rats. *Neurogastroenterology* (2018) 30(6):e13285. doi: 10.1111/nmo.13285
192. Knox DL, Chen MF, Guilarte TR, Dang CV, Burnette J. Nutritional amblyopia. Folic acid, vitamin B-12, and other vitamins. *Retina* (1982) 2 (4):288–93. doi: 10.1097/00006982-198202040-00014
193. de Silva P, Jayamanne G, Bolton R. Folic acid deficiency optic neuropathy: A case report. *J Med Case Rep* (2008) 2(1):299. doi: 10.1186/1752-1947-2-299
194. Sen SK, Pukazhvanthen P, Abraham R. Plasma Homocysteine, Folate and Vitamin B(12) levels in senile cataract. *Indian J Clin Biochem* (2008) 23 (3):255–7. doi: 10.1007/s12291-008-0057-8
195. Selhub J, Bagley LC, Miller J, Rosenberg IH, vitamins B. homocysteine, and neurocognitive function in the elderly. *Am J Clin Nutr* (2000) 71(2):614S–20S. doi: 10.1093/ajcn/71.2.614s
196. Bleich S, Kornhuber J, Junemann AG. Homocysteine in primary and secondary open-angle glaucoma. *J Glaucoma* (2003) 12(6):498–9; author reply 499. doi: 10.1097/00061198-200312000-00013
197. Xu C, Wu Y, Liu G, Liu X, Wang F, Yu J. Relationship between homocysteine level and diabetic retinopathy: a systematic review and meta-analysis. *Diagn Pathol* (2014) 9:167. doi: 10.1186/s13000-014-0167-y
198. Huang P, Wang F, Sah BK, Jiang J, Ni Z, Wang J, et al. Homocysteine and the risk of age-related macular degeneration: a systematic review and meta-analysis. *Sci Rep* (2015) 5:10585. doi: 10.1038/srep10585
199. Messedi M, Frigui M, Chaabouni K, Turki M, Neifer M, Lahiyani A, et al. Methylenetetrahydrofolate reductase C677T and A1298C polymorphisms and variations of homocysteine concentrations in patients with Behcet's disease. *Gene* (2013) 527(1):306–10. doi: 10.1016/j.gene.2013.06.041
200. Elbay AE, Topalkara A, Elbay A, Erdoğan H, Vural A, Bahadır Çetin A. Evaluation of Serum Homocysteine and Leptin Levels in Patients with Uveitis. *Turkish J Ophthalmol* (2015) 45(4):146–51. doi: 10.4274/tjo.26539
201. Sijilmassi O. Folic acid deficiency and vision: a review. *Graefe's Arch Clin Exp Ophthalmol* (2019) 257(8):1573–80. doi: 10.1007/s00417-019-04304-3
202. Elnakat H, Ratnam M. Distribution, functionality and gene regulation of folate receptor isoforms: implications in targeted therapy. *Adv Drug Delivery Rev* (2004) 56(8):1067–84. doi: 10.1016/j.addr.2004.01.001
203. Zhao R, Qiu A, Tsai E, Jansen M, Akabas MH, Goldman ID. The Proton-Coupled Folate Transporter: Impact on Pemetrexed Transport and on Antifolates Activities Compared with the Reduced Folate Carrier. *Mol Pharmacol* (2008) 74(3):854. doi: 10.1124/mol.108.045443
204. Smith SB, Kekuda R, Gu X, Chancy C, Conway SJ, Ganapathy V. Expression of folate receptor alpha in the mammalian retinol pigmented epithelium and retina. *Invest Ophthalmol Visual Sci* (1999) 40(5):840–8.
205. Weitman SD, Weinberg AG, Coney LR, Zurawski VR, Jennings DS, Kamen BA. Cellular Localization of the Folate Receptor: Potential Role in Drug Toxicity and Folate Homeostasis. *Cancer Res* (1992) 52(23):6708.
206. Yamaguchi T, Hirota K, Nagahama K, Ohkawa K, Takahashi T, Nomura T, et al. Control of immune responses by antigen-specific regulatory T cells expressing the folate receptor. *Immunity* (2007) 27(1):145–59. doi: 10.1016/j.immuni.2007.04.017
207. Kim JM, Rasmussen JP, Rudensky AY. Regulatory T cells prevent catastrophic autoimmunity throughout the lifespan of mice. *Nat Immunol* (2007) 8(2):191–7. doi: 10.1038/ni1428
208. Sakaguchi S, Yamaguchi T, Nomura T, Ono M. Regulatory T Cells and Immune Tolerance. *Cell* (2008) 133(5):775–87. doi: 10.1016/j.cell.2008.05.009
209. Simpson TR, Li F, Montalvo-Ortiz W, Sepulveda MA, Bergerhoff K, Arce F, et al. Fc-dependent depletion of tumor-infiltrating regulatory T cells co-defines the efficacy of anti–CTLA-4 therapy against melanoma. *J Exp Med* (2013) 210(9):1695–710. doi: 10.1084/jem.20130579
210. Zamiri P, Sugita S, Streilein JW. Immunosuppressive properties of the pigmented epithelial cells and the subretinal space. *Chem Immunol Allergy* (2007) 92:86–93. doi: 10.1159/000099259
211. Kalekar LA, Schmiel SE, Nandiwada SL, Lam WY, Barsness LO, Zhang N, et al. CD4(+) T cell anergy prevents autoimmunity and generates regulatory T cell precursors. *Nat Immunol* (2016) 17(3):304–14. doi: 10.1038/ni.3331
212. Chappert P, Schwartz RH. Induction of T cell anergy: integration of environmental cues and infectious tolerance. *Curr Opin Immunol* (2010) 22(5):552–9. doi: 10.1016/j.coi.2010.08.005
213. Mueller DL. Mechanisms maintaining peripheral tolerance. *Nat Immunol* (2010) 11(1):21–7. doi: 10.1038/ni.1817
214. Martinez RJ, Zhang N, Thomas SR, Nandiwada SL, Jenkins MK, Binstadt BA, et al. Arthritogenic Self-Reactive CD4+ T Cells Acquire an FR4+CD73+ Anergic State in the Presence of Foxp3+ Regulatory T Cells. *J Immunol* (2012) 188(1):170. doi: 10.4049/jimmunol.1101311
215. Kalekar LA, Mueller DL. Relationship between CD4 Regulatory T Cells and Anergy In Vivo. *J Immunol* (2017) 198(7):2527–33. doi: 10.4049/jimmunol.1602031
216. Rossi M, Amaretti A, Raimondi S. Folate Production by Probiotic Bacteria. *Nutrients* (2011) 3(1):118–34. doi: 10.3390/nu3010118
217. Chen L, Gu Q, Li P, Chen S, Li Y. Genomic analysis of Lactobacillus reuteri WHH 1689 reveals its probiotic properties and stress resistance. *Food Sci Nutr* (2019) 7(2):844–57. doi: 10.1002/fsn3.934
218. Laiño JE, Levit R, d M de LeBlanc A, de Giori GS, LeBlanc JG. Characterization of folate production and probiotic potential of Streptococcus gallolyticus subsp. macedonicus CRL415. *Food Microbiol* (2019) 79:20–6. doi: 10.1016/j.fm.2018.10.015
219. Cervantes-Barragan L, Chai JN, Tianero MD, Di Luccia B, Ahern PP, Merriman J, et al. Lactobacillus reuteri induces gut intraepithelial CD4+ CD8αα+ T cells. *Science* (2017) 357(6353):806–10. doi: 10.1126/science.aah5825
220. Lavelle A, Sokol H. Gut microbiota-derived metabolites as key actors in inflammatory bowel disease. *Nat Rev Gastroentero* (2020) p:1–15. doi: 10.1038/s41575-019-0258-z
221. Theuretzbacher U, Outterson K, Engel A, Karlén A. The global preclinical antibacterial pipeline. *Nat Rev Microbiol* (2019) 18(5):275–85. doi: 10.1038/s41579-019-0288-0
222. Sanders ME, Merenstein DJ, Reid G, Gibson GR, Rastall RA. Probiotics and prebiotics in intestinal health and disease: from biology to the clinic. *Nat Rev Gastroentero* (2019) 16(10):605–16. doi: 10.1038/s41575-019-0173-3
223. Yeh Y-L, Lu M-C, Tsai B, Tzang B-S, Cheng S-M, Zhang X, et al. Heat-Killed Lactobacillus reuteri GMNL-263 Inhibits Systemic Lupus Erythematosus–Induced Cardiomyopathy in NZB/W F1 Mice. *Probiotics Antimicrob Proteins* (2020). doi: 10.1007/s12602-020-09668-1

224. Calvo-Barreiro L, Eixarch H, Ponce-Alonso M, Castillo M, Lebrón-Galán R, Mestre L, et al. A Commercial Probiotic Induces Tolerogenic and Reduces Pathogenic Responses in Experimental Autoimmune Encephalomyelitis. *Cells* (2020) 9(4):906. doi: 10.3390/cells9040906
225. Rinaldi E, Consonni A, Cordiglieri C, Sacco G, Crasà C, Fontana A, et al. Therapeutic Effect of Bifidobacterium Administration on Experimental Autoimmune Myasthenia Gravis in Lewis Rats. *Front Immunol* (2019) 10:2949. doi: 10.3389/fimmu.2019.02949
226. Fitzgibbon G, Mills KH. The microbiota and immune-mediated diseases: Opportunities for therapeutic intervention. *Eur J Immunol* (2020) 50(3):326–37. doi: 10.1002/eji.201948322
227. Lin P. Importance of the intestinal microbiota in ocular inflammatory diseases: A review. *Clin Exp Ophthalmol* (2019) 47(3):418–22. doi: 10.1111/ceo.13493

16

Polymorphisms and Circulating Plasma Protein Levels of Immune Checkpoints (CTLA-4 and PD-1) are Associated with Posner-Schlossman Syndrome in Southern Chinese

Xiaosheng Huang[1,2†], Xinhua Liu[1,2†], Ye Ye[2], Tong Zhang[1], Shaoyi Mei[1,2], Tianhui Zhu[1,2], Shiming Peng[1,2], Jiamin Cai[2], Zonghui Yan[1,2], Kun Zeng[1,2], Danyao Nie[1,2], Liangnan Sun[1,2], Xiaofeng Hou[1] and Jun Zhao[3]*

[1] Shenzhen Eye Institute, Shenzhen Eye Hospital, Jinan University, Shenzhen, China, [2] School of Ophthalmology, Optometry, Shenzhen Eye Hospital, Shenzhen University, Shenzhen, China, [3] Department of Ophthalmology, Shenzhen People's Hospital (The Second Clinical Medical College, Jinan University; The First Affiliated Hospital, Southern University of Science and Technology), Shenzhen, China

***Correspondence:** Jun Zhao doctorzhaojun@163.com

†These authors have contributed equally to this work

Cytotoxic T-lymphocyte associated protein 4 (CTLA-4) and programmed cell death 1 (PD-1) are well-known key immune checkpoints that play a crucial dampening effect on regulating T-cell homeostasis and self-tolerance. In this study, we aimed to evaluate the association between immune checkpoints (CTLA-4 and PD-1) and Posner-Schlossman syndrome (PSS) in a southern Chinese population. A total of 137 patients with PSS and 139 healthy controls from a southern Chinese population were recruited. Five single nucleotide polymorphisms (SNPs) of *CTLA-4* (rs733618, rs4553808, rs5742909, rs231775, and rs3087243) and five SNPs of *PD-1* (rs10204525, rs2227981, rs2227982, rs41386349, and rs36084323) were genotyped by SNaPshot technique. Soluble CTLA-4 (sCTLA-4) and soluble PD-1 (sPD-1) were determined by ELISA and antibody array assay, respectively. The frequencies of T allele at rs733618 and A allele at rs231775 of *CTLA-4* were significantly higher in PSS patients than in healthy controls (corrected p (P_c) = 0.037; P_c = 0.044, respectively). The haplotype frequencies of CACGG haplotype (rs733618-rs4553808-rs5742909-rs231775-rs3087243) of *CTLA-4* and TGAGC haplotype (rs10204525-rs2227981-rs2227982-rs41386349-rs36084323) of *PD-1* in the PSS group was significantly lower than those in the control group (P_c = 0.015, p = 0.034, respectively). Circulating plasma levels of sCTLA-4 and sPD-1 in PSS patients were significantly higher than those in controls (all $p < 0.001$). The present study suggests that *CTLA-4* and *PD-1* genetic polymorphisms are associated with the susceptibility to PSS in a southern Chinese population. The upregulated circulating plasma protein levels of sCTLA-4 and sPD-1 might provide some hints regarding the dysfunction of immune checkpoints in PSS during the active status.

Keywords: Posner-Schlossman syndrome, CTLA-4, PD-1, genetic variants, soluble molecular

INTRODUCTION

Posner-Schlossman syndrome (PSS) is eponymously named after Posner and Schlossman who first described this condition in 1948 (1). PSS is characterized by recurrent unilateral non-granulomas anterior uveitis with elevated intraocular pressure (IOP) (1). The endothelial cell density and progression of retinal nerve fiber layer loss of young adult patients with PSS is caused by frequent attacks of high IOP (2, 3). The mechanism of PSS is still unclear. Many previous studies have reported evidence of cytomegalovirus (CMV) in the aqueous humor and serum (3, 4). Ganciclovir eyedrop (2%) is a novel and effective treatment for PSS patients with high frequent attacks (3). Some previous studies have found that the adaptive immune system was dysfunctional in patients with PSS. Pohlmann et al. found that the expression level of Th1 immune mediator significantly increased in the aqueous humor of patients with PSS (5). Our previous research showed that the Th1- and Th17-related cytokines in the serum might not contribute to PSS (4). Human leukocyte antigen (HLA) allelic heterogenicity might contribute to some differences in PSS prevalence among ethnic populations. Hirose et al. reported that the HLA-Bw54 and HLA-Bw54-Cw1 haplotype were overrepresented in patients with PSS in a Japanese population (6). In previous studies, we found that the *HLA-C*14:02* and *HLA-E*01:03* alleles, and the *HLA-A*11:01-C*14:02*, *HLA-B*51:01-C*14:02*, and *HLA-E*01:03-G*01:04* haplotypes confer susceptibility to PSS in a southern Chinese population (7, 8). However, the role of non-HLA genetic variants in PSS still needs to be investigated.

The adaptive immune system maintaining normal function needs appropriate balance between the stimulatory and inhibitory signals (9). The positive costimulatory signal involves the peptide-HLA engagement of the T cell receptor, which is associated with PSS (6–9). The inhibitory signal is caused by the negative immune checkpoints (e.g., CTLA-4 and PD-1) to spare healthy cells and maintain self-tolerance (9). CTLA-4, a close homolog to CD28 and located on chromosome 2q33, competes with CD28 to bind B7.1/7.2 to provide an inhibitory counterbalance at the initial stage of naive T-cell activation (10). PD-1, located on chromosome 2q37, interacts with its ligands to suppress activated T-cell at the later stage of the immune response (9). CTLA-4 and PD-1 contribute to maintaining ocular homeostasis of the immune microenvironment, including ocular immune privilege and anterior chamber-associated immune deviation (11, 12). CTLA-4 and PD-1 are associated with several autoimmune eye diseases. The G allele of rs231775 in *CTLA-4* is associated with Vogt-Koyanagi-Harada (VKH) syndrome and thyroid-associated ophthalmopathy, and the G allele of rs3087243 in *CTLA-4* is associated with scleritis (13–15). The G/G genotype of rs10204525 in *PD-1* is associated with acute anterior uveitis, and the G/G genotype of rs2227981 in *PD-1* is associated with sympathetic ophthalmia and the occurrence of extraocular manifestations of VKH syndrome (16, 17). Splenic $CD4^+$ T cells expressing CTLA-4 and PD-1 contributed to the induction of anterior chamber-associated immune deviation (11, 12). High expression of PD-1 mitigated inflammation during the active phase of experimental autoimmune uveitis mouse model (18). PD-1 is highly expressed in the inflammation sites of herpes simplex, keratitis, autoimmune uveitis, diabetic retinopathy, and thyroid-associated ophthalmopathy (19). Thus, CTLA-4 and PD-1 might contribute to the progression of some eye diseases.

However, the association between the immune checkpoints (CTLA-4 and PD-1) and PSS is unclear. In the present study, we investigated 10 SNPs of CTLA-4 and PD-1 and quantitatively assessed soluble CTLA-4 (sCTLA-4) and soluble PD-1 (sPD-1) from circulating plasma in a southern Chinese population with PSS. We aimed to evaluate whether genetic heterogeneity of immune checkpoints (CTLA-4 and PD-1) and their protein expression levels contribute to PSS during the active status.

MATERIALS AND METHODS

Study Participants

A total of 137 patients with PSS attending the Clinic of Shenzhen Eye Hospital were included in the study between January 2018 and March 2020. Patients were diagnosed with PSS according to the following classical criteria and amendments (1, 3, 4): i) recurrent attacks of mild discomfort in one eye; ii) elevated IOP > 21 mmHg with duration of attack. The IOP may reach 50 mmHg without peripheral anterior synechia; iii) a few white mutton-fat keratic precipitates; iv) no significant decrease or slight decrease in visual acuity, no visual field loss, and optic nerve damage in patients with shorter course of disease; and v) no history of other eye diseases except for refractive error. All patients were in the active disease phase with either a first attack or in the early stage of a recurrent one. One hundred and thirty-nine unrelated subjects were recruited at the Shenzhen Blood Center from healthy volunteer blood donors without eye disease. Patients and controls were all southern Han Chinese and matched for age, sex, and ethnicity. Written informed consent was obtained from all study participants.

Specimen Collection

The peripheral blood of all participants was collected in EDTA vial. Plasma was separated by centrifugation (3,000×g, 20 min, 4°C) within 2 h after blood collection. The peripheral venous blood and plasma were stored at −80°C until further analysis.

DNA Extraction, Polymerase Chain Reaction Amplification, and Genotyping

The SNPs, that we selected for genotyping in this study could potentially regulate the function and expression of these genes based on previous studies in **Supplementary Table 1** (13, 15–17). Genomic DNA was extracted from peripheral blood samples of all participants using the TIANamp Blood DNA Kit (TIANGEN Biotech, Beijing, China). PCR amplification was performed in a 20 μl reaction system, including 1 μl genomic DNA, 0.5 μl of each PCR primer in a total volume of 20 μl containing 1× HotStarTaq buffer, 2.0 mM Mg^{2+}, 0.3 mM dNTP, and 1 U HotStarTaq polymerase (Qiagen, Hilden, Germany).

The cycling conditions for *CTLA-4* and *PD-1* were 95°C for 2 min; followed by 35 cycles at 96°C for 20 s, 62°C; for 2 min, and 72°C for 3 min; and a final extension at 72°C for 10 min. The amplified samples were maintained at 4°C. SNaPshot multiplex single-base extension reaction primer sequences of each SNP are listed in **Supplementary Table 2**. The extension reaction was performed in a 10 µl reaction system, including 2 µl purified PCR product, 1 µl primer (final concentration: 0.8 mM), 5 µl SNaPshot Multiplex Kit (Applied Biosystems, Foster City, CA, USA), and 2 µl ultrapure water. The cycling conditions for extension for *CTLA-4* and *PD-1* were 96°C for 1 min; followed by 28 cycles at 96°C for 10 s, 52°C for 5 s, and 60°C for 30 s; with a final hold at 4°C. Finally, 10 µl of the extension product was purified with 1 U SAP for 1 h at 37°C and inactivated for 15 min at 75°C. The resulting data were analyzed with an ABI3130XL sequencer and GeneMapper version 4.0 Software (Applied Biosystems, Co. Ltd., USA).

Determination of Plasma Protein Levels of sCTLA-4 and sPD-1 by Double Antibody Sandwich ELISA and Confirmed by Antibody Array Assay

Commercially available ELISA kits were used to measure the concentrations of sCTLA-4 and sPD-1 (Jianglai Bio, Shanghai, China) according to the manufacturer's instructions. The assay sensitivities for sCTLA-4 and sPD-1 were 0.1 and 1.0 pg/ml, respectively. The range of detection was 0.25–8 ng/ml and 7.5–240 pg/ml for sCTLA-4 and sPD-1, respectively. Plasma samples were added into the microplate wells and incubated at 37°C for 30 min according to the manufacturer's instructions (Jianglai Bio, Shanghai, China). The horseradish peroxidase-labeled antibody was then added and incubated at 37°C for 30 min. TMB (3,3',5,5'-tetramethylbenzidine) solution was added to each well and incubated for 15 min for the color reaction. The reaction was terminated by adding stop solution. The absorbance (A) at 450 nm was measured using a microplate reader (Model 680, Bio-Rad Laboratories Inc., Japan). The plasma levels of sCTLA-4 and sPD-1 were calculated based on the A values of the samples.

The plasma protein levels of sCTLA-4 and sPD-1 were contained using the human immune checkpoint molecule array (RayBiotech, USA, QAH-ICM-1-1) according to the manufacturer's instructions, as described by Chang et al. (20).

Detection of CMV-IgG and CMV-IgM Antibodies by Indirect ELISA and Chemiluminescent Immunoassay

The CMV-IgG and -IgM antibodies were determined in the plasma of a subset of samples including 50 patients with PSS and 54 heathy controls by indirect ELISA (Virion/Serion, Germany) and chemiluminescent immunoassay (LIASON®, DiaSorin, Italy) according to the manufacturer's recommendations.

Statistical Analysis

Statistical analysis was performed using SPSS (version 22.0, SPSS Inc., Chicago, IL, USA). Age and IOP were compared between patients with PSS and controls, using independent-samples *t*-test. Hardy-Weinberg equilibrium (HWE) was evaluated using the chi-squared test. The frequencies of alleles and genotypes were obtained through direct counting. We used using PLINK (ver 1.07, http://pngu.mgh.harvard.edu/purcell/plink/) to construct haplotypes and estimate haplotype frequencies for both cases and controls (21). Linkage disequilibrium (LD) and haplotype blocks were estimated using the Haploview 4.2 program (22). Since sCTLA-4 and sPD-1 were not consistent with normal distribution as suggested by the Shapiro-Wilk test, the data were presented as median and interquartile range (Q1, Q3), and Mann-Whitney U test was used to compare the differences between the two groups. The differences in sex, allele frequency, genotype frequency, and haplotype frequency between cases and controls were evaluated using the chi-squared test or Fisher's exact test. We used Benjamin & Hochberg step-up false discovery rate (FDR) to correct multiple testing. The value of $p < 0.05$ was considered to indicate statistical significance. Odds ratio (OR) and 95% confidence interval (CI) were calculated whenever applicable.

RESULTS

Demographic and Clinical Features of Study Participants

The mean age of the PSS group [72 males (52.5%) and 65 females (47.5%)] was 39.6±12.5 years. The mean age of the control group [74 males (53.2%) and 65 females (46.8%)] was 41.3±10.4 years. No significant intergroup differences were found with respect to age and sex (p = 0.89 and 0.32, respectively, **Table 1**). The mean IOP of the PSS group was 40.9±5.7 mmHg, which was significantly higher than that of the controls (15.3±3.2 mmHg) ($p < 0.001$, **Table 1**).

CTLA-4 Genotype and Allele Frequencies

Genotype and allele frequencies of *CTLA-4* rs733618, rs4553808, rs5742909, rs231775, and rs3087243 are depicted in **Table 2**. The genotype distributions of *CTLA-4* SNPs in control groups did not violate the HWE (all $p > 0.05$). The frequencies of T/T genotype at rs733618 and the A/A genotype at rs231775 and rs3087243 of *CTLA-4* were significantly higher in PSS patients than in healthy controls, but did not survive the FDR correction (51.82 *vs.* 35.52%, p = 0.005, corrected p (P_c) = 0.082, OR = 1.81; 21.90 *vs.* 9.35%, p = 0.004, P_c = 0.122, OR = 2.72; 8.76 *vs.* 2.88%,

TABLE 1 | The demographic and clinical features of the patients with PSS and controls.

Feature	PSS (n = 137)	Control (n = 139)	p
Sex (M/F)	72/65	74/65	0.89[a]
Age (year, mean ± SD)	39.6±12.5	41.3±10.4	0.32[b]
IOP (mmHg, mean ± SD)	40.9±5.7	15.3±3.2	<0.001[b]
KPs (Y/N)	Y	N	

[a]*Chi-squared test;* [b]*independent-samples t-test; PSS, Posner-Schlossman syndrome; M, male, F, female; IOP, intraocular pressure; KPs, keratic precipitates; Y, yes; N, no.*

TABLE 2 | Genotype and allele frequencies of *CTLA-4* SNPs in the PSS patients and healthy controls.

	PSS *n* = 137 (%)	Control *n* = 139 (%)	*p*	P_c	OR	95% CI
rs733618						
Genotype						
TT	**71 (51.82)**	**49 (35.25)**	**0.005**	0.082	**1.81**	**1.12–2.92**
CT	52 (37.96)	66 (47.48)	0.110	0.550	0.68	0.42–1.10
CC	14 (10.22)	24 (17.27)				
Allele						
T	**194 (70.80)**	**164 (58.99)**	**0.004**	**0.037**	**1.56**	**1.11–2.21**
C	80 (29.20)	114 (41.01)				
rs4553808						
Genotype						
AA	103 (75.18)	112 (80.58)	0.280	0.560	0.73	0.41–1.29
AG	28 (20.44)	25 (17.99)	0.605	0.726	1.17	0.67–2.13
GG	6 (4.38)	2 (1.44)				
Allele						
A	234 (85.40)	249 (89.57)	0.139	0.278	0.68	0.41–1.12
G	40 (14.60)	29 (10.43)				
rs5742909						
Genotype						
CC	104 (75.91)	113 (81.29)	0.275	0.635	0.71	0.40–1.26
CT	27 (19.71)	24 (17.27)	0.605	0.698	1.22	0.67–2.22
TT	6 (4.38)	2 (1.44)				
Allele						
C	235 (85.44)	250 (89.93)	0.134	0.336	0.67	0.40–1.12
T	39 (14.23)	28 (10.07)				
rs231775						
Genotype						
AA	**30 (21.90)**	**13 (9.35)**	**0.004**	0.122	**2.72**	**1.35–5.47**
AG	52 (37.96)	58 (41.73)	0.522	0.746	0.87	0.53–1.38
GG	55 (40.15)	68 (48.92)				
Allele						
A	**112 (40.88)**	**84 (30.22)**	**0.009**	**0.044**	**1.553**	**1.10–2.20**
G	162 (59.12)	194 (69.78)				
rs3087243						
Genotype						
AA	**12 (8.76)**	**4 (2.88)**	**0.037**	0.370	**3.24**	**1.028–10.31**
AG	48 (35.04)	48 (34.53)	0.930	0.930	1.02	0.62–1.68
GG	77 (56.20)	87 (62.59)				
Allele						
A	72 (26.28)	56 (20.14)	0.088	0.293	1.36	0.92–2.02
G	202 (73.72)	222 (79.86)				

Values in bold indicate significant differences. p value was calculated using $\chi 2$ test or Fisher's exact test and corrected for multiple testing using the FDR method. PSS, Posner-Schlossman syndrome; P_c, corrected p value; OR, odds ratio; CI, confidence interval.

$p = 0.037$, $P_c = 0.37$, OR = 3.24, respectively). The frequencies of T allele at rs733618 and A allele at rs231775 of *CTLA-4* were significantly higher in PSS patients than in healthy controls, and these associations survived the FDR correction (70.80 *vs.* 58.99%, $P_c = 0.037$, OR = 1.56; 40.88 *vs.* 30.22%, $P_c = 0.044$, OR = 1.55, respectively). Our results showed that there were no significant differences in the genotype and allele frequencies of rs4553808 and rs5742909 in *CTLA-4* between PSS patients and controls (all $p > 0.05$). The raw genotype data of the samples was shown in the **Supplementary Table 3**.

PD-1 Genotype and Allele Frequencies

Genotype and allele frequencies of *PD-1* rs10204525, rs2227981, rs2227982, rs41386349, and rs36084323 are depicted in **Table 3**. The genotype distributions of *PD-1* SNPs in control groups did not violate HWE (all $p > 0.05$). Our results showed that there were no significant differences in the genotype and allele frequencies of rs10204525, rs2227981, rs2227982, rs41386349, and rs36084323 in *PD-1* between PSS patients and controls (all $p > 0.05$). The raw genotype data of the samples was shown in the **Supplementary Table 3**.

CTLA-4 and *PD-1* Haplotype Frequencies and Linkage Disequilibrium

Four haplotypes of *CTLA-4* and six haplotypes of *PD-1* were detected (**Table 4**). The haplotype frequency of CACGG haplotype (rs733618-rs4553808-rs5742909-rs231775-rs3087243) of *CTLA-4* in the PSS group was significantly lower than that in the control group (29.30 *vs.* 41.16%, $P_c = 0.015$, OR = 0.60). The haplotype frequency of TGAGC haplotype

TABLE 3 | Genotype and allele frequencies of *PD-1* SNPs in the PSS patients and healthy controls.

	PSS *n* = 137 (%)	Control *n* = 139 (%)	*p*	P_c	OR	95% CI
rs10204525						
Genotype						
TT	70 (52.45)	83 (59.71)	0.150	0.500	0.71	0.44–1.14
CT	59 (41.96)	50 (35.97)	0.228	0.570	1.35	0.83–2.19
CC	8 (5.59)	6 (4.32)				
Allele						
T	199 (72.63)	216 (77.70)	0.168	0.240	0.76	0.52–1.12
C	75 (27.37)	62 (22.30)				
rs2227981						
Genotype						
AA	17 (12.41)	9 (6.47)	0.092	0.552	2.05	0.88–4.77
AG	45 (32.85)	52 (37.41)	0.427	0.641	0.82	0.50–1.34
GG	75 (54.74)	78 (56.21)				
Allele						
A	79 (28.83)	70 (25.18)	0.334	0.417	1.20	0.83–1.75
G	195 (71.17)	208 (74.82)				
rs2227982						
Genotype						
AA	40 (29.20)	47 (33.81)	0.409	0.646	0.81	0.49–1.34
AG	60 (43.80)	65 (46.76)	0.621	0.690	0.89	0.55–1.43
GG	37 (27.01)	27 (19.42)				
Allele						
A	140 (51.09)	159 (57.19)	0.150	0.251	0.78	0.56–1.09
G	134 (48.91)	119 (42.81)				
rs41386349						
Genotype						
AA	10 (7.30)	6 (4.32)	0.289	0.510	1.75	6.62–4.94
AG	39 (28.47)	48 (34.78)	0.278	0.596	0.75	0.45–1.26
GG	88 (64.23)	85 (61.15)				
Allele						
A	59 (21.53)	58 (21.01)	0.882	0.882	1.03	0.69–1.55
G	215 (78.47)	218 (78.99)				
rs36084323						
Genotype						
CC	36 (26.28)	30 (21.58)	0.361	0.602	1.30	0.74–2.26
CT	62 (45.26)	65 (46.76)	0.802	0.859	0.94	0.59–1.51
TT	39 (28.47)	44 (31.65)				
Allele						
C	134 (48.91)	125 (44.96)	0.354	0.553	1.17	0.84–1.64
T	140 (51.09)	153 (55.04)				

The p value was calculated using $\chi 2$ test or Fisher's exact test and corrected for multiple testing using the FDR method. PSS, Posner-Schlossman syndrome; P_c, corrected p value; OR, odds ratio; CI, confidence interval.

(rs10204525-rs2227981-rs2227982-rs41386349-rs36084323) of *PD-1* in the PSS group was significantly lower than that in the control group (0.73 *vs.* 3.27%, p = 0.034, OR = 0.22), although this association did not survive the FDR correction (P_c = 0.204). No significant difference in the other haplotypes was found between the two groups (all $p > 0.05$).

LD analysis among five SNPs of *CTLA-4* and five SNPs of *PD-1* showed that all pair-wise LD between *CTLA-4* SNPs and *PD-1* SNPs had strong LD (D' > 0.9), expect for the weak LD between rs10204525 and rs2227981 (D' = 0; **Figure 1**).

Circulating Plasma Protein Levels of sCTLA-4 and sPD-1

The circulating plasma protein levels of sCTLA-4 and sPD-1 in PSS patients (n = 81) were significantly higher than those in controls (n = 83) by ELISA (2.76±0.43 *vs.* 1.78±0.63 ng/ml, $p < 0.0001$; 110.31±30.60 *vs.* 47.98±27.72 pg/ml, $p < 0.0001$, respectively; **Figure 2**). Our study did not find any significant difference in plasma protein levels of sCTLA-4 and sPD-1 according to the genotypes of *CTLA-4* and *PD-1* (all $p > 0.05$; data not shown).

The circulating plasma protein levels of sCTLA-4 and sPD-1 were confirmed by the human immune checkpoint molecular array. The circulating plasma protein levels of sCTLA-4 in PSS patients (n = 52) were significantly higher than those in controls (n = 55) (16.37±22.73 *vs.* 4.99±23.53 pg/ml, $p < 0.0001$; **Figure 3A**). The circulating plasma protein levels of sPD-1 in PSS patients (n = 56) were significantly higher than those in controls (n = 55) (373.35±314.27 *vs.* 112.40±176.20 pg/ml, $p < 0.0001$; **Figure 3B**).

TABLE 4 | *CTLA-4* and *PD-1* haplotype frequencies of the PSS patients and healthy controls.

	Frequency (%)		p	P_c	OR	95% CI
	PSS $2n = 274$	Control $2n = 278$				
CTLA-4 rs733618-rs4553808-rs5742909-rs231775-rs3087243						
TACAA	26.37	19.86	0.070	0.139	1.45	0.97–2.15
TGTAG	14.29	10.11	0.134	0.179	1.48	0.88–2.49
CACGG	**29.30**	**41.16**	**0.004**	**0.015**	**0.60**	**0.42–0.85**
TACGG	30.04	28.88	0.767	0.766	1.06	0.73–1.53
PD-1 rs10204525-rs2227981-rs2227982-rs41386349-rs36084323						
TAGAC	20.80	19.11	0.639	0.639	1.11	0.73–1.68
CAGGC	7.30	4.52	0.203	0.609	1.61	0.77–3.35
CGGGC	20.07	17.46	0.420	0.630	1.19	0.78–1.83
TGAGC	**0.73**	**3.27**	**0.034**	0.204	**0.22**	**0.05–1.02**
TAGAT	0.73	1.82	0.450	0.540	0.40	0.08–2.07
TGAGT	50.36	53.82	0.395	0.790	0.87	0.62–1.21

Values in bold indicate significant differences. The p value was calculated using $\chi 2$ test or Fisher's exact test and corrected for multiple testing using the FDR method. PSS, Posner-Schlossman syndrome; P_C: corrected p value; OR, odds ratio; CI, confidence interval.

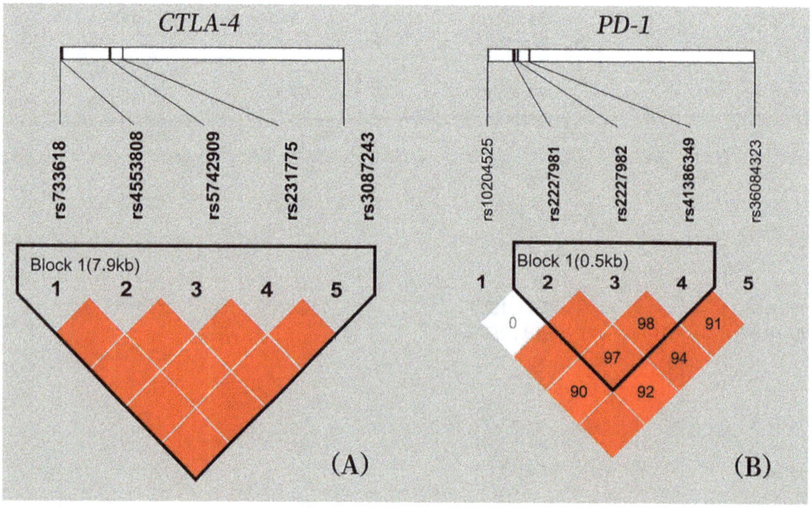

FIGURE 1 | Location and pair-wise linkage disequilibrium values of CTLA-4 and PD-1 SNPs in all study participants. **(A)** These five SNPs span 7 kb of *CTLA-4* gene region. **(B)** These five SNPs of *PD-1* gene region. Values of the pair-wise D' (x100) are shown in blocks (D' values of 1.0 are not presented). Haplotype blocks were estimated with the Haploview program.

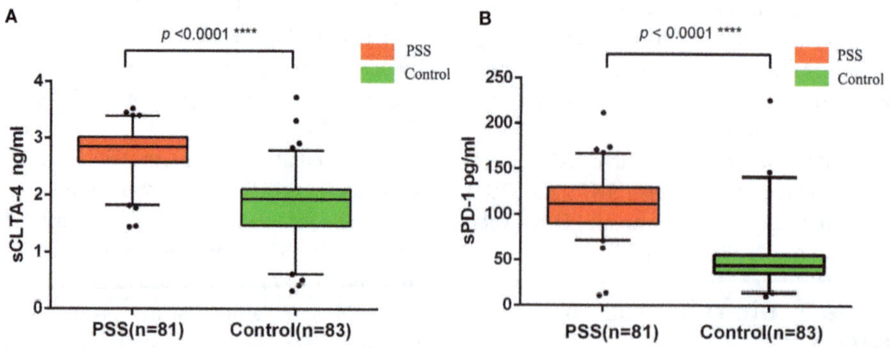

FIGURE 2 | Expression anaysis of sCTLA-4 and sPD-1 by ELISA. **(A)** Comparison of circulating plasma protein levels of sCTLA-4 between PSS patients and controls. **(B)** Comparison of circulating plasma protein levels of sPD-1 between PSS patients and controls. PSS: Posner-Schlossman syndrome; sCTLA-4: soluble Cytotoxic T-lymphocyte associated protein 4; sPD-1: soluble programmed cell death 1.

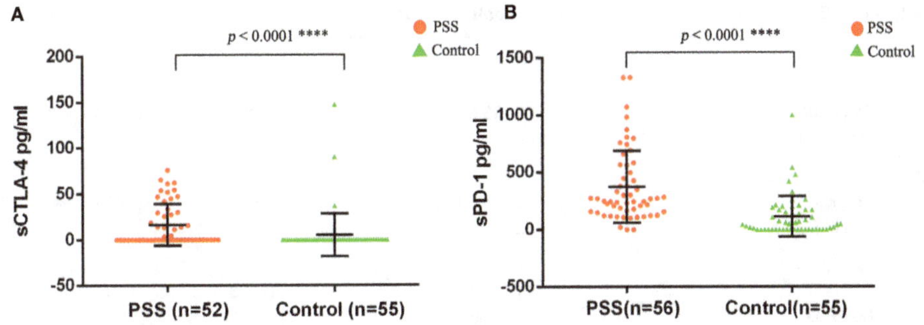

FIGURE 3 | Expression anaysis of sCTLA-4 and sPD-1 by antibody array assay. **(A)** Comparison of circulating plasma protein levels of sCTLA-4 between PSS patients and controls. **(B)** Comparison of circulating plasma protein levels of sPD-1 between PSS patients and controls. PSS: Posner-Schlossman syndrome; sCTLA-4: soluble Cytotoxic T-lymphocyte associated protein 4; sPD-1: soluble programmed cell death 1.

Comparison of *CTLA-4* and *PD-1* Allele Frequencies and Levels of sCTLA-4 and sPD-1 Between CMV-IgG (+) PSS Patients and CMV-IgG (+) Controls

A subset of samples including 50 patients with PSS and 54 heathy controls were available for detection of the CMV antibodies. None of these samples was positive for CMV-IgM, and all these samples were positive for CMV-IgG. The frequencies of T allele of rs733618, A allele of rs231775, and A allele of rs3087243 in *CTLA-4* were significantly higher in CMV-IgG (+) PSS patients than in CMV-IgG (+) controls, although these associations did not survive the correction for multiple testings (71.0 *vs.* 55.6%, $p = 0.021$, $P_c = 0.21$, OR=1.96; 46.0 *vs.* 29.6%, $p = 0.015$, $P_c = 0.075$, OR=2.02; 32.0 *vs.* 19.4%, $p = 0.038$, $P_c = 0.13$, OR=1.95, respectively; **Table 5**). No significant difference was found in allele frequencies of rs10204525, rs2227981, rs2227982, rs41386349, and rs36084323 in *PD-1* between CMV-IgG (+) PSS patients and CMV-IgG (+) controls (all $p > 0.05$). Circulating plasma levels of sCTLA-4 and sPD-1 in CMV-IgG (+) PSS patients were significantly higher than those in controls ($p < 0.0001$; **Table 6**).

DISCUSSION

Immune checkpoints prevent the excessive immune response by transferring the inhibitory signals to spare healthy cells and maintain self-tolerance (9). CTLA-4 and PD-1, the most widely investigated checkpoints, are reportedly upregulated by the tumor to escape from immune system monitoring (10). The HLA polymorphism confers susceptibility to PSS. However, little is known about the non-HLA genetic background of PSS (3).

In the present study, we genotyped five *CTLA-4* SNPs and five *PD-1* SNPs in 137 patients with PSS and 139 healthy controls from a southern Chinese population. The frequencies of T allele of rs733618 and A allele of rs231775 in *CTLA-4* were significantly higher in PSS patients than in controls, and these associations survived multiple testings correction. The frequencies of T/T genotype of rs733618 and A/A genotype of rs231775 and rs3087243 in *CTLA-4* were significantly higher in PSS patients than in controls, but did not survive the FDR correction. The CACGG haplotype (rs733618-rs4553808-rs5742909-rs231775-rs3087243) in *CTLA-4* might be the protective haplotype for PSS. Du et al. reported that the G allele at rs231775 and ACGG at *CTLA-4* rs4553808-rs5742909-rs231775-rs3087243 might be risk factors for VKH syndrome (13). Since the risk genotype of rs733618 and rs231775, and the haplotype of rs4553808-rs5742909-rs231775-rs3087243 of *CTLA-4* in PSS were completely different from those in VKH syndrome, we considered that *CTLA-4* genetic background might be different between PSS and VKH syndrome (13). SNP rs231775 of the *CTLA-4* gene causes adenine-guanine dimorphism at codon 17 in the peptide leader sequence (23). The A and G alleles of rs231775 encodes the CTLA-4 ^{17}Thr and CTLA-4 ^{17}Ala, respectively. Sun et al. reported that the CTLA-4 ^{17}Thr enhances the interaction between CTLA-4 and B7.1 molecule, and carries greater inhibitory effects on the proliferation and activation process of $CD25^+/CD4^+$ T cell in PBMCs treated with or without phytohemagglutinin, than the CTLA-4^{17} Ala (23, 24). SNP rs733618 is located upstream of the *CTLA-4* gene and is a part of the gene's activator sequence. The substitution of C allele to T allele of rs733618 could affect the gene expression by changing the sequence of transcription factor regulated NF-1 and c/EBPβ binding sites (25). We hypothesized that the A allele of rs231775 and T allele of rs733618 could confer susceptibility to PSS in the southern Chinese population by impacting the expression and function of *CTLA-4*. The circulating plasma protein levels of sCTLA-4 were increased during the onset of disease in PSS patients compared with healthy controls, which also occurs in other autoimmune diseases (e.g., autoimmune thyroid disease, Graves' ophthalmopathy, myasthenia gravis, and spondyloarthropathies) (26–28). The relevance of sCTLA-4, primarily secreted by Treg cell, to immune regulation remains controversial. The sCTLA-4 maintains the ability to bind to the B7 ligand *via* the MYPPPY motif on antigen presenting cells, and prevents the B7 ligand from combining with CD28 to inhibit T cell responses (29). Furthermore, the selective blockade of sCTLA-4

TABLE 5 | Allele frequencies of *CTLA-4* and *PD-1* SNPs in the CMV IgG (+) PSS patients and healthy controls.

	CMV IgG (+) PSS *n* = 50 (%)	CMV IgG (+) control *n* = 54 (%)	*p*	P_c	OR	95% CI
CTLA-4						
rs733618						
T	**71 (71.00)**	**60 (55.56)**	**0.021**	0.210	**1.959**	**1.11–2.21**
C	29 (29.00)	48 (44.44)				
rs4553808						
A	86 (86.00)	96 (88.89)	0.529	0.756	0.768	0.34–1.75
G	14 (14.00)	12 (11.11)				
rs5742909						
T	14 (14.00)	11 (10.19)	0.398	0.796	1.436	0.62–3.33
C	86 (86.00)	97 (89.81)				
rs231775						
A	**46 (46.00)**	**32 (29.63)**	**0.015**	0.075	**2.023**	**1.14–3.58**
G	54 (54.00)	76 (70.37)				
rs3087243						
A	**32 (32.00)**	**21 (19.44)**	**0.038**	0.127	**1.95**	**1.03–3.68**
G	68 (68.00)	87 (80.56)				
PD-1						
rs10204525						
T	73 (73.00)	83 (76.85)	0.522	0.870	0.814	0.43–1.53
C	27 (27.00)	25 (23.15)				
rs2227981						
A	27 (27.00)	32 (29.63)	0.674	0.843	0.878	0.48–1.61
G	73 (73.00)	76 (70.37)				
rs2227982						
A	53 (53.00)	56 (51.85)	0.868	0.868	1.047	0.61–1.81
G	47 (47.00)	52 (48.15)				
rs41386349						
A	20 (20.00)	27 (25.00)	0.389	0.973	0.750	0.39–1.45
G	80 (80.00)	81 (75.00)				
rs36084323						
T	53 (53.00)	55 (50.93)	0.765	0.850	1.087	0.63–1.87
C	47 (47.00)	53 (49.07)				

Values in bold indicate significant differences. The p value was calculated using $\chi 2$ test or Fisher's exact test and corrected for multiple testing using the FDR method. PSS, Posner-Schlossman syndrome; CMV, cytomegalovirus; P_c, corrected p value; OR, odds ratio; CI, confidence interval.

TABLE 6 | Comparison of plasma levels of sCTLA-4 and sPD-1 between CMV IgG (+) PSS patients and healthy controls.

	n	sCTLA-4 (ng/ml)	sPD-1 (pg/ml)
CMV IgG (+) PSS	50	2.75±0.46	108.85±29.57
CMV IgG (+) Control	54	1.77±0.63	49.01±32.54
Z		6.848	7.664
p		**<0.0001**	**<0.0001**

Values in bold indicate significant differences. The p value was calculated using Mann-Whitney U test. PSS, Posner-Schlossman syndrome; CMV, cytomegalovirus.

activates the proliferation of T cells and upregulated the expression of Th1/Th17-related cytokines (30). The significant antigen-specific immune responses were increased by using the anti-sCTLA-4-mAb *in vitro* and *in vivo* (30). However, we did not find significant association between the genotype and expression of sCTLA-4 (data not shown), probably because we only investigated a limited number of SNPs in this study. More related SNPs, the transcriptional regulation and protein modification of CTLA-4 in the onset of PSS are needed to be investigated in the future. We concluded that the A allele of rs231775 and T allele of rs733618 were risk factors for PSS, and the expression of sCTLA-4 increased the participation of T-cell regulation in the B7/CTLA-4/CD28 signaling pathway during the onset of PSS.

With regard to another important immune checkpoint, PD-1, we found that the polymorphisms of *PD-1* were not associated with PSS, except that the TGAGC haplotype (rs10204525-rs2227981-rs2227982-rs41386349-rs36084323) of *PD-1* was lower in patients with PSS than in the controls. Interestingly, the expression of sPD-1 increased during the onset of PSS compared to controls. High expression of sPD-1 might contribute to the process of PSS through transforming the PD-1/PD-L1 signaling pathway or regulating the immune response of the T cell. In some chronic viral infections, higher PD-1 likely converts effector cytotoxic T lymphocytes into exhausted cytotoxic T lymphocytes (e.g., human immunodeficiency virus, hepatitis B virus, hepatitis C virus) (31). High PD-1 expression is associated with emerging and evident CMV disease and with viremia in liver transplant recipients (32). PD-1 was also associated with the viremia caused by chronic CMV infection, and blocking PD-1 signaling might help recover the function of exhausted T cells in chronic CMV infection (33).

High expression of PD-1 is related to CMV infection, which might be the potential crucial factor for PSS (3). The sPD-1 enhanced the immune response by enhancing co-delivered antigen-specific $CD8^+$ T-cell responses and *in vivo* maturation of DCs during activation of naive $CD8^+$ T cells, and inhibited the PD-1/PD-L1 interaction (34, 35). However, the mechanisms of upregulated expression of sPD-1 in the onset of PSS require future investigation.

Since the CMV infection might be an important risk factor for PSS, we analyzed the associations of the *CTLA-4* and *PD-1* SNPs and the expression levels of sCTLA-4 and sPD-1 with PSS in the CMV-IgG (+) samples. Our results showed that rs733618, rs231775, and rs3087243 in *CTLA-4* were significantly associated with PSS in the CMV-IgG (+) individuals, although these associations did not survive the FDR correction, probably due to the limited sample sizes available for detection of the CMV antibodies (**Table 5**). The circulating plasma protein levels of sCTLA-4 and sPD-1 were increased during the onset of disease in CMV-IgG (+) PSS patients compared with CMV-IgG (+) healthy controls (**Table 6**). Our study did not find any significant difference when plasma protein levels of sCTLA-4 and sPD-1 were analyzed according to the genotypes of CTLA-4 and PD-1 (all $p > 0.05$). We hypothesize that the mechanisms of increased expression of sCTLA-4 and sPD-1 might be complex in the onset of PSS. Moreover, the transcriptional regulation and protein modification of sCTLA-4 and sPD-1 worth to be investigated in the onset of PSS.

In summary, the results of the present study suggest that the T allele of rs733618 and the A allele of rs231775 in *CTLA-4* might contribute to the process of PSS in a southern Chinese population. The CACGG haplotype (rs733618-rs4553808-rs5742909-rs231775-rs3087243) of *CTLA-4* and TGAGC haplotype (rs10204525-rs2227981-rs2227982-rs41386349-rs36084323) of *PD-1* might be protective factors against PSS in southern Chinese patients. Moreover, sCTLA-4 and sPD-1 were increased in the onset of PSS. These findings suggest that the polymorphism and soluble levels of *CTLA-4* and *PD-1* might shed further light on the dysfunction of immune checkpoints in PSS.

ETHICS STATEMENT

The studies involving human participants were reviewed and approved by the local Ethics Committee of Shenzhen Eye Hospital. The patients/participants provided their written informed consent to participate in this study.

AUTHOR CONTRIBUTIONS

XHu, XL, and JZ conceived and designed the experiments. XHu, YY, TZ, XHo, and JZ performed the experiments and analyzed the data. XHu, XL, YY, SM, SP, JC, ZY, KZ, DN, LS, and JZ contributed to patients and control recruitments. XHu and JZ wrote the paper. All authors contributed to the article and approved the submitted version.

ACKNOWLEDGMENTS

We would like to thank all patients who participated in this study. We want to thank the volunteer blood donors for generously supplying blood samples for this study. We also thank Baojian Fan for his insightful comments on this manuscript. Finally, we thank the Center for Human Genetics Research, Shanghai Genesky Bio-Tech Co., Ltd for their genotyping work.

REFERENCES

1. Posner A, Schlossman A. Syndrome of unilateral recurrent attacks of glaucoma with cyclitic symptoms. *Arch Ophthalmol* (1948) 39(4):517–35. doi: 10.1001/archopht.1948.00900020525007
2. Maruyama K, Maruyama Y, Sugita S, Mori K, Yokoyama Y, Sanuki-Kunimatsu S, et al. Characteristics of cases needing advanced treatment for intractable Posner-Schlossman syndrome. *BMC Ophthalmol* (2017) 17(1):45. doi: 10.1186/s12886-017-0438-y
3. Megaw R, Agarwal PK. Posner-Schlossman syndrome. *Surv Ophthalmol* (2017) 62(3):277–85. doi: 10.1016/j.survophthal.2016.12.005
4. Zhao J, Chen W, Huang X, Peng S, Zhu T, Deng Z, et al. Serum Th1 and Th17 related cytokines and autoantibodies in patients with Posner-Schlossman syndrome. *PloS One* (2017) 12(4):e0175519. doi: 10.1371/journal.pone.0175519
5. Pohlmann D, Schlickeiser S, Metzner S, Lenglinger M, Winterhalter S, Pleyer U. Different composition of intraocular immune mediators in Posner-Schlossman-Syndrome and Fuchs' Uveitis. *PloS One* (2018) 13(6):e0199301. doi: 10.1371/journal.pone.0199301
6. Hirose S, Ohno S, Matsuda H. HLA-Bw54 and glaucomatocyclitic crisis. *Arch Ophthalmol* (1985) 103(12):1837–9. doi: 10.1001/archopht.1985.01050120071023
7. Zhao J, Zhu T, Chen W, Fan BJ, He L, Yang B, et al. Human leukocyte antigens-B and -C loci associated with Posner-Schlossman syndrome in a southern Chinese population. *PloS One* (2015) 10(7):e0132179. doi: 10.1371/journal.pone.0132179
8. Huang X, Xu Y, Chen W, Zhu T, He L, Wang S, et al. The genetic contribution of HLA-E*01:03 and HLA-E*01:03-G*01:01 to Posner-Schlossman syndrome in southern Chinese. *Ann Trans Med* (2019) 7(23):749. doi: 10.21037/atm.2019.11.70
9. Sharpe AH, Pauken KE. The diverse functions of the PD1 inhibitory pathway. *Nat Rev Immunol* (2018) 18(3):153–67. doi: 10.1038/nri.2017.108
10. Gu D, Ao X, Yang Y, Chen Z, Xu X. Soluble immune checkpoints in cancer: production, function and biological significance. *J Immunother Cancer* (2018) 6(1):132. doi: 10.1186/s40425-018-0449-0
11. Zhu X, Yang P, Zhou H, Li B, Huang X, Meng Q, et al. CD4+CD25+Tregs express an increased LAG-3 and CTLA-4 in anterior chamber-associated immune deviation. *Graefe's Arch Clin Exp Ophthalmol* (2007) 245(10):1549–57. doi: 10.1007/s00417-007-0591-8
12. Meng Q, Yang P, Li B, Zhou H, Huang X, Zhu L, et al. CD4+PD-1+ T cells acting as regulatory cells during the induction of anterior chamber-associated immune deviation. *Invest Ophthalmol Visual Sci* (2006) 47(10):4444–52. doi: 10.1167/iovs.06-0201
13. Du L, Yang P, Hou S, Lin X, Zhou H, Huang X, et al. Association of the CTLA-4 gene with Vogt-Koyanagi-Harada syndrome. *Clin Immunol* (2008) 127 (1):43–8. doi: 10.1016/j.clim.2008.01.004
14. Wang H, Zhu LS, Cheng JW, Cai JP, Li Y, Ma XY, et al. Meta-analysis of association between the +49A/G polymorphism of cytotoxic T-lymphocyte antigen-4 and thyroid associated ophthalmopathy. *Curr eye Res* (2015) 40 (12):1195–203. doi: 10.3109/02713683.2014.993767

15. Li F, Ma X, Du L, Shi L, Cao Q, Li N, et al. Identification of susceptibility SNPs in CTLA-4 and PTPN22 for scleritis in Han Chinese. *Clin Exp Immunol* (2019) 197(2):230–6. doi: 10.1111/cei.13298
16. Li Y, Hong M, Huang X, Zhong L, Gu Y, Wang D, et al. PD-1 Polymorphisms are associated with susceptibility of acute anterior uveitis in Chinese population. *DNA Cell Biol* (2019) 38(2):121–8. doi: 10.1089/dna.2018.4417
17. Meng Q, Liu X, Yang P, Hou S, Du L, Zhou H, et al. PDCD1 genes may protect against extraocular manifestations in Chinese Han patients with Vogt-Koyanagi-Harada syndrome. *Mol Vision* (2009) 15:386–92.
18. Chen L, Pai V, Levinson R, Sharpe AH, Freeman GJ, Braun J, et al. Constitutive neuronal expression of the immune regulator, programmed death 1 (PD-1), identified during experimental autoimmune uveitis. *Ocular Immunol Inflammation* (2009) 17(1):47–55. doi: 10.1080/09273940802491884
19. Wang X, Wu M, Cao Y, Zhang Z, Guo F, Li X, et al. Exploring the role of programmed cell death protein 1 and its ligand 1 in eye diseases. *Crit Rev Clin Lab Sci* (2019) 56(1):18–32. doi: 10.1080/10408363.2018.1522292
20. Chang B, Huang T, Wei H, Shen L, Zhu D, He W, et al. The correlation and prognostic value of serum levels of soluble programmed death protein 1 (sPD-1) and soluble programmed death-ligand 1 (sPD-L1) in patients with hepatocellular carcinoma. *Cancer Immunol Immunother CII* (2019) 68 (3):353–63. doi: 10.1007/s00262-018-2271-4
21. Purcell S, Neale B, Todd-Brown K, Thomas L, Ferreira MA, Bender D, et al. PLINK: a tool set for whole-genome association and population-based linkage analyses. *Am J Hum Genet* (2007) 81(3):559–75. doi: 10.1086/519795
22. Barrett JC, Fry B, Maller J, Daly MJ. Haploview: analysis and visualization of LD and haplotype maps. *Bioinf (Oxford England)* (2005) 21(2):263–5. doi: 10.1093/bioinformatics/bth457
23. Sun T, Zhou Y, Yang M, Hu Z, Tan W, Han X, et al. Functional genetic variations in cytotoxic T-lymphocyte antigen 4 and susceptibility to multiple types of cancer. *Cancer Res* (2008) 68(17):7025–34. doi: 10.1158/0008-5472.Can-08-0806
24. Mäurer M, Loserth S, Kolb-Mäurer A, Ponath A, Wiese S, Kruse N, et al. A polymorphism in the human cytotoxic T-lymphocyte antigen 4 (CTLA4) gene (exon 1 +49) alters T-cell activation. *Immunogenetics* (2002) 54(1):1–8. doi: 10.1007/s00251-002-0429-9
25. Wang XB, Pirskanen R, Giscombe R, Lefvert AK. Two SNPs in the promoter region of the CTLA-4 gene affect binding of transcription factors and are associated with human myasthenia gravis. *J Internal Med* (2008) 263(1):61–9. doi: 10.1111/j.1365-2796.2007.01879.x
26. Daroszewski J, Pawlak E, Karabon L, Frydecka I, Jonkisz A, Slowik M, et al. Soluble CTLA-4 receptor an immunological marker of Graves' disease and severity of ophthalmopathy is associated with CTLA-4 Jo31 and CT60 gene polymorphisms. *Eur J Endocrinol* (2009) 161(5):787–93. doi: 10.1530/eje-09-0600
27. Wang XB, Kakoulidou M, Giscombe R, Qiu Q, Huang D, Pirskanen R, et al. Abnormal expression of CTLA-4 by T cells from patients with myasthenia gravis: effect of an AT-rich gene sequence. *J Neuroimmunol* (2002) 130(1-2):224–32. doi: 10.1016/s0165-5728(02)00228-x
28. Toussirot E, Saas P, Deschamps M, Pouthier F, Perrot L, Perruche S, et al. Increased production of soluble CTLA-4 in patients with spondylarthropathies correlates with disease activity. *Arthritis Res Ther* (2009) 11(4):R101. doi: 10.1186/ar2747
29. Linsley PS, Greene JL, Brady W, Bajorath J, Ledbetter JA, Peach R. Human B7-1 (CD80) and B7-2 (CD86) bind with similar avidities but distinct kinetics to CD28 and CTLA-4 receptors. *Immunity* (1994) 1(9):793–801. doi: 10.1016/s1074-7613(94)80021-9
30. Ward FJ, Dahal LN, Wijesekera SK, Abdul-Jawad SK, Kaewarpai T, Xu H, et al. The soluble isoform of CTLA-4 as a regulator of T-cell responses. *Eur J Immunol* (2013) 43(5):1274–85. doi: 10.1002/eji.201242529
31. Hofmeyer KA, Jeon H, Zang X. The PD-1/PD-L1 (B7-H1) pathway in chronic infection-induced cytotoxic T lymphocyte exhaustion. *J Biomed Biotechnol* (2011) 2011:451694. doi: 10.1155/2011/451694
32. La Rosa C, Krishnan A, Longmate J, Martinez J, Manchanda P, Lacey SF, et al. Programmed death-1 expression in liver transplant recipients as a prognostic indicator of cytomegalovirus disease. *J Infect Dis* (2008) 197(1):25–33. doi: 10.1086/523652
33. Sester U, Presser D, Dirks J, Gärtner BC, Köhler H, Sester M. PD-1 expression and IL-2 loss of cytomegalovirus- specific T cells correlates with viremia and reversible functional anergy. *Am J Transplant* (2008) 8(7):1486–97. doi: 10.1111/j.1600-6143.2008.02279.x
34. Song MY, Park SH, Nam HJ, Choi DH, Sung YC. Enhancement of vaccine-induced primary and memory CD8(+) T-cell responses by soluble PD-1. *J Immunother* (2011) 34(3):297–306. doi: 10.1097/CJI.0b013e318210ed0e
35. Shin SP, Seo HH, Shin JH, Park HB, Lim DP, Eom HS, et al. Adenovirus expressing both thymidine kinase and soluble PD1 enhances antitumor immunity by strengthening CD8 T-cell response. *Mol Ther* (2013) 21 (3):688–95. doi: 10.1038/mt.2012.252

17

Behçet's Disease—Do Microbiomes and Genetics Collaborate in Pathogenesis?

*Nafeesa Mehmood, Liying Low and Graham R. Wallace**

Institute of Inflammation and Ageing, College of Medical and Dental Sciences, University of Birmingham, Birmingham, United Kingdom

***Correspondence:**
Graham R. Wallace
g.r.wallace@bham.ac.uk

Behçet's disease (BD) is a multisystem autoinflammatory condition characterized by mucosal ulceration, breakdown of immune privilege sites and vasculitis. A genetic basis for BD has been described in genome-wide and validation studies. Similarly, dysbiosis of oral and gut microbiomes have been associated with BD. This review will describe links between genetic polymorphisms in genes encoding molecules involved in gut biology and changes seen in microbiome studies. A potential decrease in bacterial species producing short chain fatty acids linked to mutations in genes involved in their production suggests a potential therapy for BD.

Keywords: Behçet's disease, microbiome, genetic polymorphism, gut, butyrate

INTRODUCTION

Behçet's Disease (BD) is a multisystem autoinflammatory disorder characterized by inflammation at mucosal surfaces and break down of barriers at privileged sites including the eye, brain and joint (1). Many of the mucosal surfaces involved in BD host a community of microorganisms, and collectively their genetic content is known as the microbiome. The largest and most diverse of these microbial communities reside in the gut and have been shown to be important in the development and regulation of the immune system (2). Changes in the gut microbiome, also known as dysbiosis, have been associated with many human diseases including chronic kidney disease, diabetes, multiple sclerosis (3–5). The gut microbiome has also been shown to modulate the efficacy of immunotherapies in cancer patients (6, 7).

Since the first description of the disease triad in the 1930s, infectious microbial agents have always been speculated to be involved in the pathogenesis of BD, however, so far, no single pathogenic etiology has been found. Recent studies have investigated the association between the composition of the microbiomes and BD, which may provide a useful insight to the role of the microbiome in the disease process.

Gut Microbiome in Behçet's Disease

The gut microbiome profile in BD was first reported by Consolandi and associates, whereby they compared the fecal microbiota of 22 patients with 16 age-matched cohabitating individuals. Recruiting healthy controls who lived in the same house as the BD patients is of particular importance as it is known that several factors contribute to variations in gut microbiota composition, including environmental factors, geographical location, diet, age and host genetics (6). There was significant reduction in the alpha diversity and depletion of butyrate-producing bacteria, such as *Roseburia* and *Subdoligranulum* genera, in the gut microbiome of BD patients compared to healthy controls (**Table 1**). The short chain fatty acid (SCFA) profile, by chromatography-mass spectrometry (GC-MS), revealed a significant reduction of butyrate levels in fecal samples of BD patients. Butyrate is important in regulating the host immune system and is responsible for inhibiting intestinal pro-inflammatory cytokines and promoting T cell differentiation into a T regulatory cell (Treg) lineage. Thus, it can be hypothesized that the dysbiotic microbiota seen in BD patients could have an important role in the pathogenesis of BD, whereby a reduction in butyrate causes downstream effects of promoting immune-pathological T-effector responses, leading to gut inflammation (18). Interestingly, a similar pattern is seen in patients with inflammatory bowel disease (IBD) and oral administration of butyrate in experimental IBD mice, has shown to enhance Treg differentiation and reduce colitis (8, 19).

In a pilot 16S gut microbiome study of 12 Japanese patients with BD and 12 healthy controls (HC), Shimizu and colleagues reported a significant increase in the relative abundance of *Bifidobacterium* and *Eggerthella*, and decrease in the relative abundance of *Megamonas* and *Prevotella* in BD patients compared with controls, however there was correlation between the bacterial taxa and clinical manifestation of BD (9).

TABLE 1 | Summary of microbiome dysbiosis in Behçet's Disease patients compared to healthy controls or disease controls.

Author	MicrobiomeBody Site (Country)	Increased bacterial abundance in BD patients	Reduced bacterial abundance in BD patients
Consolandi, C., et al. (7)	**Gut** (Italy) P=22 HC=16		***Roseburia (Clostridium* genus)** ***Subdoligranulum (Clostridium* genus)**
Shimizu, J., et al. (8)	**Gut** (Japan) P=12 HC=12	*Bifidobacterium* *Eggerthella*	*Megamonas* *Prevotella*
Shimizu, J., et al. (9)	**Gut** (Japan) P=13 HC=27	*Eggerthella lenta* *Acidaminococcus* spp. *Lactobacillus* spp. *Bifidobacterium bifidum* *Streptococus* spp.	*Megamonas hypermegale* ***Butyrivibrio* spp.** *Filifactor* spp.
Ye, Z., et al. (10)	**Gut** (active ocular BD patients from China) P=24 HC=52	*Bilophila* spp. *(Sulfate-reducing)* *Parabacteroides* spp. *Paraprevotella* spp.	***Clostridium* spp. *(Butyrate-producing bacteria)*** *Methanoculleus* spp. *Methanomethylophilus* spp.
Oezguen N., et al. (11)	**Gut** (neuro-BD patients Turkey)	*Parabacteroides* *Clostridiales* *Gemminger* *Butyricimonas* *Actinobacteria*	*Vampirovibrio* *Unclassified Lachnospiraceae*
Tecer D, et al. (12)	**Gut** (BD-uveitis, FMF, CD patients Turkey) BD=7 FMF=12 CD=9 HC=16	*Veionellaceae* *Succinivibrionaceae* *Succinivibrio* *Mitsuokella*	
Yaser Bilge et al. (13)	**Gut** (Turkey) P=27 HC=10	*Actinomyces* *Libanicoccus* *Collinsella* *Eggerthella* *Enetrohabdus* *Catenibacterium* *Enterobacter*	*Bacteroides* *Cricetibacter* *Alistipes* *Lachnospira* *Dielma* ***Akkermansia*** *Sutterella* *Anaerofilum* *Ruminococcease Acetanaerobacterium* *Copropaacter*
Van der Houwen J. et al. (14)	**Gut** (Italy and Netherlands; IgA coated bacteria- Netherlands only) BD Dutch=19 HC Dutch=17 BD Italy=13 HC Italy=15	*Bifidobacterium* spp., *Dorea* spp., *Ruminoccoccus bromei* spp. (all IgA coating in Netherlands cohort)	*Barnesiellaceae* *Lachnospira* *(Italy only)* *Erysipelotrichaceae* spp. (IgA coating in Netherlands cohort)
Coit, P., et al. (15)	**Oral** (Turkey) P=31 HC=15	*Haemophilus parainfluenza*	*Alloprevotella rava* *Leptotrichia*
Seoudi, N., et al. (16)	**Oral** (UK) BD=54 RAS=8 HC=25	*Rothia denticariosa* *Streptococcus salivarius* *Streptococcus sanguinis*	*Neisseria* *Veillonella*
Balt J. et al. (17)	**Oral** (Mongolia) P=47 HC=48		***Akkermansia***

The table shows the relative abundance of microbial species in the microbiota (gut and oral microbiota) of BD patients when compared to HCs. ***Bold*** *= species or genera linked to T regulatory cells. Abbreviations: BD, Behçet's Disease; HC, healthy control; FMF, Familial Mediterranean Fever; CD, Chron's Disease CD; MS, Multiple Sclerosis, RAS, Recurrent aphthous ulcer.*

(**Table 1**) Fecal soluble immunoglobulin A (sIgA) concentrations were also significantly increased in BD patients but did not correlate with any specific bacterial species (9). In a follow up study analysis of the taxonomic and predicted metagenome functional composition in the fecal sample of 13 Japanese patients with BD and 27 HC, the relative abundance of *Lactobacillus, Bifidobacterium* and *Streptococcus* spp. was significantly increased in patients with BD compared to HC, whilst *Megamonas hypermegale* and *Butyrivibrio* species were less abundant, which correlated with the previous study (**Table 1**). The latter species were suggested to produce SCFA, particularly butyrate and propionate, in the human intestine. Such a reduction in butyrate-producing-SCFA may be responsible for the skewed T cell differentiation, ie. an increase in Th17 with a concomitant reduction in Treg cells. Functional annotation analysis found links to the pentose phosphate pathway and inosine monophosphate biosynthesis, suggesting that changes in the microbiome could affect metabolic processes in patients with BD. Nevertheless, intestinal microbiome interactions with the immune response are complex and SCFA depletion may only be one of many contributing factors to BD pathogenesis (10).

Ye et al. compared the DNA extracted from fecal samples of 24 patients with active BD, who had only received topical steroids, and 52 gender, body mass index (BMI) and aged-matched healthy controls (HC) (11). Metagenomic analysis revealed significant differences in gut microbial composition between the two cohorts with sulfate-reducing bacteria (SRB) and opportunistic pathogens significantly enriched, and methanogens, *Methanoculleus* spp. and *methanomethylophilus* ssp. and butyrate-producing bacteria, *Clostridium* spp. were reduced in BD patients compared to controls. SRB are pro-inflammatory bacteria that can inhibit butyrate. The shortage of butyrate and methane, combined with an abundance of hydrogen sulphide, creates an atypical environment that may contribute to intestinal epithelial barrier damage. This may allow for subsequent invasion by Th1 and Th17 cells, reduction in Tregs, thus triggering downstream inflammatory processes within the gut in patients with BD. To address this Ye *et al.* used the animal model of experimental autoimmune uveitis in B10RIII mice. Mice were treated with antibiotics (ampicillin, neomycin, metronidazole and vancomycin) for 3 weeks, prior to daily transplantation of pooled fecal suspension either from patients with active BD or from healthy controls. After one week of daily fecal transplants, mice were immunized with an interphotoreceptor retinoid binding protein peptide (161-180) to induce EAU and the severity of uveitis was reported on day 14 following immunization. The results showed that severe uveitis (corneal oedema, posterior synechiae and infiltrates of inflammatory cells in retina, choroid and vitreous humor) was observed in the active BD-recipient group, whilst the HC-recipient group displayed a slight intraocular inflammatory reaction with very few inflammatory cells in the vitreous cavity, indicating that the components within the fecal samples from BD patients exacerbated the development of intraocular inflammation in these mice (11). This supports the hypothesis that gut microbiome composition may contribute to BD pathogenesis and severity.

In a novel study the gut microbiome composition of Turkish patients with neuro-BD was compared to patients with multiple sclerosis, an autoimmune condition, and to healthy controls. 16S rRNA gene sequencing revealed that neuro-BD patients had an increased relative abundance of *Parabacteroides, Geminger* and *Prevotella*, whilst *Vampirovibrio* and *Lachnospiraceae* were decreased (**Table 1**), although the differences did not reach statistical significance, probably due to the small cohort sizes. However, it is of interest that two neurological conditions were linked to different changes in the intestinal microbiota. Whether this is due to the different disease processes or treatment regimens for participants, as those with neuro-BD had commenced azathioprine (with or without colchicine treatment), whilst MS patients had commenced immunomodulatory drug treatment (drug treatment not specified), will have to be investigated further (12).

The gut microbiome was compared in patients with BD uveitis to patients with Familial Mediterranean Fever (FMF) and Crohn's Disease (CD), both which have autoinflammatory processes, as well as healthy controls. In total seven patients with BD, 12 patients with FMF, 9 patients with CD and 16 healthy controls (HC) were analyzed by 16S rRNA gene sequencing. The results showed that *Veionellaceae, Succinivibrionaceae* families and *Succinivibrio* and *Mitsuokella* genera were enriched in patients with BD compared to the other groups. The relevance to uveitis is not yet elucidated (15).

Oral Microbiome in Behçets Disease

Oral ulceration is an important manifestation of BD and maintains a specific microbiome. To investigate the involvement of the oral microbiome in BD pathogenesis, Coit et al. collected stimulated saliva samples from 31 BD patients and 15 HCs, after 5 minutes of paraffin chewing, between 9-11am to address circadian rhythm of saliva secretion. Microbial DNA was isolated and sequencing revealed a significant difference in bacterial communities between the two cohorts. *Haemophilus parainfluenzae* and *Alloprevotella* were increased in BD patients, whilst *Leptotrichia* and *Clostridiales* were decreased compared to control samples. *H. parainfluenzae*, a gram-negative bacterium, is commonly linked to endocarditis, meningitis, septicaemia and gingival inflammation. While use of immunosuppressants (cyclosporin, azathioprine and prednisolone) had an impact on abundances of bacteria, there was no differences in bacterial communities between drug treatments (16).

In a second study, the oral microbiome profiles of BD patients (active vs. inactive disease) were compared to patients with recurrent aphthous ulcers (RAS), used as disease control, and healthy individuals. In total, unstimulated saliva samples were collected from 54 patients with BD, 8 patients with RAS and 25 HC together with mucosal samples from some patients. The results showed differences between the cohorts, with *Neisseria* more commonly isolated from HC compared to BD patients, whereas *Staphylococcus salivarius* and *Streptococcus sanguinis* were more abundant in BD patients with active oral disease when compared to those with inactive disease, patients with RAS and HC. *Candida albicans* was more frequently isolated from salivary samples taken from orally inactive BD patients when compared to HCs and RAS, however this could be attributed to steroid treatment. Samples taken from ulcerated and non-ulcerated mucosa of active BD patients was compared to those from HCs and RAS and revealed *Rothia dentocariosa* as the abundant organism in non-ulcerated mucosa of active BD patients, with a trend toward *Rothia mucilaginosa* from the ulcer sites of active BD patients (17).

In a recent study the oral microbiome in Mongolian patients with BD was compared to healthy controls. Saliva samples were obtained from 47 patients and 48 healthy individuals and the V3-V4 region of 16S RNA was amplified. Specifically, Prevotella, Veillonella, Streptococcus, and Haemophilus were the most abundant species in all samples However, three genera including, Akkermansia were significantly lower in patients compared to controls (20).

Gut and Oral Microbiomes in BD—Summary

These studies support a possible role for gut or oral dysbiosis in BD. Common features such as the reduction in butyrate producing species can be found in most studies, although different bacterial species are reported in different studies. Despite the evidence of microbial dysbiosis in BD patients, it is difficult to ascertain whether such differences are causative or reactive in BD. This is due to many confounding factors that could affect the microbiome including the type and duration of drug treatment, sampling and sequencing methodology, or host genetics. This could also be linked to the different manifestations of BD, which could only be addressed through large longitudinal studies.

To distinguish disease-associated determinants from country and methodology, the gut microbiomes of patients with BD from the Netherlands and Italy were analyzed by the same method and compared to each other and healthy controls. In both cohorts, alpha diversity were similar to controls. Beta-diversity analysis did not show clustering based on disease, however, there was segregation by country of origin. The Italian cohort showed a significant decrease in *Barnesiellaceae* and *Lachnospira* genera, which in the Netherlands cohort was only a trend. IgA coated of intestinal bacteria analyzed by RNA sequencing can identify distinct disease-associated species in fecal samples. Increased IgA coating of *Bifidobacterium* spp., *Dorea* spp., and *Ruminoccoccus bromei* spp. and reduced presence of IgA-coated *Erysipelotrichaceae* spp. in the Dutch BD cohort compared to healthy controls, although this was not analyzed in the Italian cohort (14). These data support the requirement for more, larger studies to determine the geographical and environmental changes compared to disease-induced changes in the BD gut microbiome.

Behçet's Disease often involves variable disease manifestations at different body sites, such as the oral, skin, eyes, gastrointestinal, or nervous system, over time. To identify the clinical clusters of BD, Soejima and associates investigated the clinical phenotype of 657 patients with BD from the Yokohama City Hospital database and 6754 patients with BD from the Japanese Ministry of Health, Labour and Welfare database. They identified that gastrointestinal BD was associated with vascular but not eye involvement, while a second cluster had high incidence of eye involvement but no vascular or neurological involvement (13). Chronological analyses showed expansion of the gastrointestinal cluster in BD patients over 27 years in a relatively stable genetic cohort in Japan, indicating that environmental factors might be involved in the disease manifestation of BD.

Changes in the gut microbiome could drive the clinical phenotype in BD. To answer this, Yasar Bilge and associates compared the gut microbiome of 27 patients with BD (ocular, mucocutaneous, and vascular involvement), and 10 age- and sex-matched healthy controls. Linear discriminant analysis of this small patient cohort revealed a difference in the bacterial genera according to the manifestations of BD: *Lachnospiraceae NK4A136* enriched in BD patients with eye involvement, *Dialister*, *Intestinomonas*, and *Marvinbryantia* enriched in BD patients with predominant mucocutaneous disease, *Gemella* in vascular BD. However, larger studies and functional relevance of such associations should be investigated (21).

This data, if validated in other patient cohorts, supports the stratification of individuals in relation to their gut microbiome profile (i.e. to determine if specific bacterial species are associated with specific manifestations or whether general alterations to the microbiome influences all manifestations). In either process, factors that may potentially influence the gut microbiome, such as diet, can be addressed by the potential of re-establishing a more balanced, symbiotic relationship might prove to be important in reducing the severity of active BD phases. To test this concept a randomized controlled trial the Modulation of Gut Microbiota through Nutritional Invention in Behçet's Syndrome Patients (MAMBA) study, will recruit 90 patients with BD, to investigate the impact of three dietary interventions, a lacto-ovo-vegetarian diet, a Mediterranean diet, or a Mediterranean diet supplemented with butyrate on the severity of clinical manifestations of BD (22).

There is increasing evidence that the host genetic background shapes the gut microbiome profile (23, 24).

Link Between Gut Microbiome and Genetics in BD

There are more than 20 genetic susceptibility loci that meet the threshold for genome-wide level of significance in patients with Behçet's disease and several other loci that have been associated with BD (25). To address the potential role of genetics in BD gut dysbiosis we have selected a potential pathway associated with production of SCFA in the gut and mutations in the genes involved. Activation of Toll-like receptors on systemic dendritic cells induces the release of IL-23, which activates innate lymphoid cells to release IL-22 which leads to a rapid α (1,2)-fucosylation of small intestine epithelial cells *via* the release of fucosyltransferase 2 (FUT2). Fucosylated proteins enter into the lumen of the gut where they release fucose molecules which are metabolized by bacteria present. As stated, products from these bacteria include short chain fatty acids, including butyrate which supports T regulatory cells (26). This complex series of interactions involve several of the gene mutations in which have been associated with BD.

Toll-Like Receptors

Toll-like receptors (TLR) are a family of transmembrane sensors for bacteria, fungi and viruses that are a vital component of innate immunity. The strongest associations between TLR and BD is in with TLR4 which recognizes bacterial lipopolysaccharide. Nine single nucleotide polymorphisms previously detected in TLR4 by direct sequencing were analyzed for an association with BD in Korean patients. The most frequent haplotype, TAGCGGTAA, was significantly increased in HLA-B*51-positive patients compared with healthy control participants and potential linked to joint disease (27). This was supported by targeted exonic resequencing of specific genes identified in the original GWAS, from 2,461 BD cases compared with 2,458 controls where a SNP in TLR4 was significantly associated with BD (28). In buccal lesions from patients with BD, TLR expression was increased compared with healthy controls, however, a similar increase was seen in lesion tissue from patients with lichen planus or gingivitis, suggesting that this was a generalized inflammatory response as opposed to a BD-specific response. In these patients no significant associations were seen with TLR4, but a gain of function mutation in the TLR adaptor molecule, TIR-adaptor protein (TIRAP) was significantly associated with BD in UK, but not Middle Eastern, patients (29). This mutation is associated with an more potent cytokine response to TLR stimulation.

In a study of 400 patients with ocular BD compared to 600 healthy Han Chinese controls frequencies of genotypes of TLR2 rs2289318 and rs3804099 were significantly higher in ocular BD patients compared with controls. A validation cohort of 438 patients with BD uveitis and 1000 healthy controls confirmed the associations. TLR2 mRNA expression in PBMC was increased in healthy carriers of the certain genotypes, although this did not affect the release of TNF-α, IL-6, IL-10, and IL-1β could be detected (30).

In Tunisians patients with Behcet's Disease expression of SNP in TLR9 (1486 T/C) was different between BD patients and healthy controls but did not reach statistical significance (31). In Chinese patients with BD TLR7 had an increased copy number and increased expression in PBMC compared to healthy controls (32).

These data support a role for bacterial sensing in BD.

Interleukin-23

Two major GWAS studies in Turkish and Japanese patients with BD identified SNP at the IL23R-IL12RB2 locus (rs924080 and rs12119179) respectively. Meta-analysis of both data sets further identified rs1495965 as associated with BD (33, 34). These associations have been supported in several other studies in different patient cohorts (35–39). These mutations have been linked to enhanced expression of IL-23R and potential upregulation of the IL-17 pathway.

Lymphocytes isolated from the intestinal mucosa of 8 patients with intestinal symptoms, that had started within 6 months of collection, were cloned and analyzed for surface phenotype and cytokine production. Results showed more $CD4^+$ clones compared to $CD8^+$ with the majority of both showing Th1 profile secreting IFN-γ and TNF-α, with a substantial population produced both IFN-γ and IL-17 (Th1/Th17 profile). Most of the T-cell clones showed perforin-mediated cytotoxicity and Fas–Fas Ligand-mediated pro-apoptotic activity. Therefore, in the early stages of intestinal BD both Th1 cytokines, IL-17 and cytotoxicity are involved in inflammation of the mucosal tissue. This data would support the use of anti-TNF treatment and potentially anti-IL-17 in controlling intestinal BD (40).

In support of treatment altering the Th17 pathway, twenty-seven patients who received interferon alfa-2a for active BD uveitis and Treg and Th17 cells were assessed. Treg, Th17 cell frequencies and Th17 RORγt expression were significantly elevated, although IL-10 concentration in Treg culture supernatants was significantly lower with cells from BD patients compared to controls. IFN alfa-2a treatment led to clinical remission in 70% of patients which correlated with a significant reversal in Treg and Th17 cell frequencies, Treg IL-10 and Th17 cytokine production (41).

Interleukin-22

IL-22 is a member of the IL-10 cytokine family that is involved in inflammatory processes. Th22-type T cell clones from ocular samples taken from Behçet's disease patients with active uveitis, produced IL-22 and TNF-a but not IFN-γ or IL-17. IL-22 can affect epithelial and stromal cells and has been involved the pathogenesis of inflammatory skin disorders, such as psoriasis, atopic eczema, and allergic contact dermatitis (42). Healthy IL-22-deficient mice had altered microbiome, with decreased abundance of *Lactobacillus*, and increased levels of others. Induction of experimental colitis caused more sever disease in deficient mice compared to controls. When the microbiome from IL-22 deficient mice was transmitted to wild-type animals along this led to an increased susceptibility to colitis, suggesting an important role for IL-22 the balance between immunity and colonic microbiota (43). Therefore, although no polymorphisms in *IL22* have been reported in BD, a potential role in pathogenesis is likely.

Fucosyltransferase-2

Genome-wide array analysis of Iranian patients with BD and controls identified an association with five coding polymorphisms of the gene encoding fucosyltransferase -2 (FUT2), including the rs601338 nonsense variant which, in Caucasians, determines the secretion of the H antigen (precursor of the ABO blood group antigens) in body fluids and on the intestinal mucosa. These results were validated by comparison with GWAS analysis of Turkish patients with BD. A non-secretor phenotype is suggested to link with intestinal glycosylation (44). The association with FUT2 polymorphisms and BD was supported in an larger study of three populations. The rs601338 A allele, in Turkish and Iranian patients and the rs1047781 T allele in Japanese patients for which homozygosity leads to an ABO non-secretor phenotype were confirmed in this study. These non-secretor genotypes are also associated with Crohn's disease risk (45).

The process by which FUT2 polymorphisms influence the gut microbiome is not yet clear. Secretor mothers produce milk containing α1-2 fucosylated human milk oligosaccharides and several strains of bacteria in the infant gut have the capacity to utilize these oligosaccharides (46). In vaginally born infants, the mother's secretor status had no effect on the infants' microbiome. By comparison, in children delivered by caesarean section several differences were seen in infants from secretor mothers compared to non-secretor mothers. In particular, *Bifidobacteria* were depleted and Enterococci increased among the caesarean-born infants of non-secretor mothers. *Akkermansia* was increased in infants of secretor mothers. In a study of 14 non-secretor (FUT2 rs601338 genotype AA) and 57 secretor (genotypes GG and AG) adult individuals of western European descent, the gut microbiota was analyzed. Results showed a several differences between the two groups with nonsecretors presenting lower species richness than secretors and different enterotypes in the two groups (46). This data supports the concept that FUT2 polymorphism can influence the composition of the gut microbiota and variation between individuals (47). By comparison, the association of rs601338 and intestinal microbiota composition was analyzed in 1,190 healthy individuals, and the results showed no association of the FUT2 genotype, secretor status and microbial alpha diversity, microbial composition or inferred microbial function after correction for multiple testing (48).

Non-secretors, who are homozygous for the loss-of-function alleles of FUT2 gene, have increased susceptibility to Crohn's disease (CD). From 39 healthy individuals, 75 endoscopic lavage samples were profiled for microbiome, proteome and metabolome composition based on FUT2 genotype. Metagenomic analysis revealed differences in energy metabolism in the microbiome of non-secretor and heterozygote individuals, in particular enrichment of carbohydrate, vitamin and lipid metabolism, and depletion of amino-acid biosynthesis and metabolism. Metabolomic analysis of human specimens showed changes of many metabolites related to the different genotype groups. These results support compositional and functional differences in the microbiota of non-secretors that may be relevant for CD susceptibility (49).

Taken together polymorphisms in all genes encoding proteins in the pathway TLR-IL-23-IL-22- FUT2 have all been reported in patients with BD. Systemic activation of this pathway could lead to a reduction in beneficial SCFA either by increased targeting of SCFA-producing species or *via* reduced fucosylation and SCFA generation. This is one potential pathway initiated by systemic activation of tissue dendritic cells. The best direct evidence of cause and effect remains the induction of uveitis in B10RIII mice following transplantation of fecal material from patients with active BD (11). However, it is not known what induced the changes in the microbiome of these patients nor what processes drove ocular inflammation even in this genetically susceptible mouse model.

Summary

A possible link between gut and oral microbiome dysbiosis is supported by several studies and the involvement of the FUT2 pathway and gene polymorphisms in molecules involved may be relevant. However, there are several aspects that must be addressed. First, that different bacterial species and genera have been identified in the different studies. While there may be a commonality in decreased abundance of species linked to short chain fatty acid regulation that could link the studies more work needs to be done in larger cohorts with the same collection and preparation procedures. Second, certain demographic analysis does not support a link between manifestations of BD form

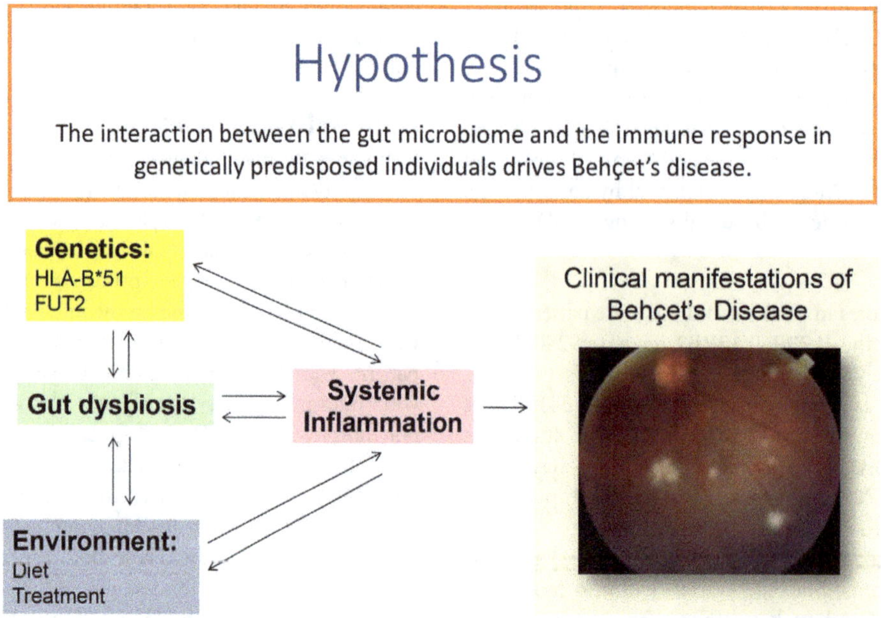

FIGURE 1 | Systemic inflammation leading to clinical features in Behçet's disease may either be initiated by of causing changes in the gut microbiome in patients who are genetically predisposed to the condition.

example ocular involvement not associated with intestinal BD (13). Thirdly, many patients with BD do not have intestinal-BD, therefore there is no direct association between gut inflammation, the microbiome and other manifestations of BD. Fourth, several other sites affected by BD including oral and genital mucosa and skin harbor their own microbiome, which will need to be analyzed for association with manifestations of BD. Fifth, there is a significant non-genetic component in Behçet's Disease. As stated, the MAMBA study (22) will address dietary influences on the gut microbiome. Recently the numbers of new patients being diagnosed with BD in Japan and Korea have been steadily decreasing (50, 51). Whether such changes involve factors such as a move to a more westernized diet would be interesting to address. Effects of different treatment regimes on the gut microbiome should be investigated. Finally, there are other gene loci that have been associated with BD that could impact on the composition of or the response to the gut microbiome, including HLA-B*51 and *IL-10* and cells such as natural killer cells which can produce IL-10 when stimulated. Moreover, IL-10 production by Treg has been linked to *Akkermansia* which is altered in several studies.

In conclusion, while it is clear that dysbiosis of the gut microbiome is associated with Behçet's disease and a role for known genetic mutations can be linked to these changes (**Figure 1**), further research is required to understand the combinations involved in the manifestations of this complex disease.

AUTHOR CONTRIBUTIONS

All authors contributed equally to this manuscript. All authors contributed to the article and approved the submitted version.

REFERENCES

1. Leccese P, Alpsoy E. Behçet's Disease: An Overview of Etiopathogenesis. *Front Immunol* (2019) 10:1067. doi: 10.3389/fimmu.2019.01067
2. Belkaid Y, Harrison OJ. Homeostatic Immunity and the Microbiota. *Immunity* (2017) 46:562–76. doi: 10.1016/j.immuni.2017.04.008
3. Massey W, Brown JM. The Gut Microbial Endocrine Organ in Type 2 Diabetes. *Endocrinol (United States)* (2021) 162:bqaa235. doi: 10.1210/endocr/bqaa235
4. Kishikawa T, Ogawa K, Motooka D, Hosokawa A, Kinoshita M, Suzuki K, et al. A Metagenome-Wide Association Study of Gut Microbiome in Patients With Multiple Sclerosis Revealed Novel Disease Pathology. *Front Cell Infect Microbiol* (2020) 10:585973. doi: 10.3389/fcimb.2020.585973
5. Horai R, Caspi RR. Microbiome and Autoimmune Uveitis. *Front Immunol* (2019) 10:232. doi: 10.3389/fimmu.2019.00232
6. Gupta VK, Paul S, Dutta C. Geography, Ethnicity or Subsistence-Specific Variations in Human Microbiome Composition and Diversity. *Front Microbiol* (2017) 8:1162. doi: 10.3389/fmicb.2017.01162
7. Gopalakrishnan V, Spencer CN, Nezi L, Reuben A, Andrews MC, Karpinets TV, et al. Gut Microbiome Modulates Response to Anti-PD-1 Immunotherapy in Melanoma Patients. *Science* (2018) 359:97–103. doi: 10.1126/science.aan4236
8. Atarashi K, Tanoue T, Oshima K, Suda W, Nagano Y, Nishikawa H, et al. Treg Induction by a Rationally Selected Mixture of Clostridia Strains From the Human Microbiota. *Nature* (2013) 500:232–6. doi: 10.1038/nature12331
9. Shimizu J, Kubota T, Takada E, Takai K, Fujiwara N, Arimitsu N, et al. Bifidobacteria Abundance-Featured Gut Microbiota Compositional Change in Patients With Behcet's Disease. *PloS One* (2016) 11:e0153746. doi: 10.1371/journal.pone.0153746
10. Shimizu J, Kubota T, Takada E, Takai K, Fujiwara N, Arimitsu N, et al. Relative Abundance of Megamonas Hypermegale and Butyrivibrio Species Decreased in the Intestine and Its Possible Association With the T Cell Aberration by Metabolite Alteration in Patients With Behcet's Disease. *Clin Rheumatol* (2019) 38:1437–45. doi: 10.1007/s10067-018-04419-8
11. Ye Z, Zhang N, Wu C, Zhang X, Wang Q, Huang X, et al. A Metagenomic Study of the Gut Microbiome in Behcet's Disease. *Microbiome* (2018) 6:135. doi: 10.1186/s40168-018-0520-6
12. Oezguen N, Yalcinkaya N, Kücükali CI, Dahdouli M, Hollister EB, Luna RA, et al. Microbiota Stratification Identifies Disease-Specific Alterations in Neuro-Behçet's Disease and Multiple Sclerosis. *Clin Exp Rheumatol* (2019) 37 Suppl 121:58–66.
13. Soejima Y, Kirino Y, Takeno M, Kurosawa M, Takeuchi M, Yoshimi R, et al. Changes in the Proportion of Clinical Clusters Contribute to the Phenotypic Evolution of Behçet's Disease in Japan. *Arthritis Res Ther* (2021) 23:49. doi: 10.1186/s13075-020-02406-6
14. van der Houwen TB, van Laar JAM, Kappen JH, van Hagen PM, de Zoete MR, van Muijlwijk GH, et al. Behçet's Disease Under Microbiotic Surveillance? a Combined Analysis of Two Cohorts of Behçet's Disease Patients. *Front Immunol* (2020) 11:1192. doi: 10.3389/fimmu.2020.01192
15. Tecer D, Gogus F, Kalkanci A, Erdogan M, Hasanreisoglu M, Ergin Ç, et al. Succinivibrionaceae is Dominant Family in Fecal Microbiota of Behçet's Syndrome Patients With Uveitis. *PloS One* (2020) 15(10):e0241691. doi: 10.1371/journal.pone.0241691
16. Coit P, Mumcu G, Ture-Ozdemir F, Unal AU, Alpar U, Bostanci N, et al. Sequencing of 16S Rrna Reveals a Distinct Salivary Microbiome Signature in Behçet's Disease. *Clin Immunol* (2016) 169:28–35. doi: 10.1016/j.clim.2016.06.002
17. Seoudi N, Bergmeier LA, Drobniewski F, Paster B, Fortune F. The Oral Mucosal and Salivary Microbial Community of Behçet's Syndrome and Recurrent Aphthous Stomatitis. *J Oral Microbiol* (2015) 7:27150. doi: 10.3402/jom.v7.27150
18. Consolandi C, Turroni S, Emmi G, Severgnini M, Fiori J, Peano C, et al. Behçet's Syndrome Patients Exhibit Specific Microbiome Signature. *Autoimmun Rev* (2015) 14:269–76. doi: 10.1016/j.autrev.2014.11.009
19. Moco S, Candela M, Chuang E, Draper C, Cominetti O, Montoliu I, et al. Systems Biology Approaches for Inflammatory Bowel Disease: Emphasis on Gut Microbial Metabolism. *Inflammation Bowel Dis* (2014) 20:2104–14. doi: 10.1097/MIB.0000000000000116
20. Balt J, Uehara O, Abiko Y, Jamyanjav B, Jav S, Nagasawa T, et al. Alteration of Oral Flora in Mongolian Patients With Behçet's Disease: A Multicentre Study. *Clin Exp Rheumatol* (2020) 38(Suppl 127(5):80–5.
21. Yasar Bilge NS, Pérez Brocal V, Kasifoglu T, Bilge U, Kasifoglu N, Moya A, et al. Intestinal Microbiota Composition of Patients With Behçet's Disease: Differences Between Eye, Mucocutaneous and Vascular Involvement. the Rheuma-BIOTA Study. *Clin Exp Rheumatol* (2020) 38 Suppl 127:60–8. doi: 10.1136/annrheumdis-2020-eular.3626
22. Pagliai G, Dinu M, Fiorillo C, Becatti M, Turroni S, Emmi G, et al. Modulation of Gut Microbiota Through Nutritional Interventions in Behçet's Syndrome Patients (the MAMBA Study): Study Protocol for a Randomized Controlled Trial. *Trialss* (2020) 21:511. doi: 10.1186/s13063-020-04444-6
23. Olivares M, Neef A, Castillejo G, De Palma G, Varea V, Capilla A, et al. The HLA-DQ2 Genotype Selects for Early Intestinal Microbiota Composition in Infants At High Risk of Developing Coeliac Disease. *Gut* (2015) 64:406–17. doi: 10.1136/gutjnl-2014-306931
24. Zhernakova A, Kurilshikov A, Bonder MJ, Tigchelaar EF, Schirmer M, Vatanen T, et al. Population-Based Metagenomics Analysis Reveals Markers for Gut Microbiome Composition and Diversity. *Science* (2016) 352:565–56. doi: 10.1126/science.aad3369

25. Ortiz-Fernández L, Sawalha AH. Genetics of Behçet's Disease: Functional Genetic Analysis and Estimating Disease Heritability. *Front Med* (2021) 8:625710. doi: 10.3389/fmed.2021.625710
26. Pickard JM, Maurice CF, Kinnebrew MA, Abt MC, Schenten D, Golovkina TV, et al. Rapid Fucosylation of Intestinal Epithelium Sustains Host-Commensal Symbiosis in Sickness. *Nature* (2014) 514:638641. doi: 10.1038/nature13823
27. Horie Y, Meguro A, Ota M, Kitaichi N, Katsuyama Y, Takemoto Y, et al. Association of TLR4 Polymorphisms With Behçet's Disease in a Korean Population. *Rheumatology* (2009) 48:638–42. doi: 10.1093/rheumatology/kep077
28. Kirino Y, Zhou Q, Ishigatsubo Y, Mizuki N, Tugal-Tutkun I, Seyahie E, et al. Targeted Resequencing Implicates the Familial Mediterranean Fever Gene MEFV and the Toll-Like Receptor 4 Gene TLR4 in Behçet Disease. *Proc Natl Acad Sci USA* (2013) 110:8134–9. doi: 10.1073/pnas.1306352110
29. Durrani O, Banahan K, Sheedy FJ, McBride L, Ben-Chetrit E, Greiner K, et al. Tirap Ser180Leu Polymorphism is Associated With Behçet's Disease. *Rheumatology* (2011) 50:1760–5. doi: 10.1093/rheumatology/ker200
30. Fang J, Hu R, Hou S, Ye Z, Xiang Q, Qi J, et al. Association of TLR2 Gene Polymorphisms With Ocular Behcet's Disease in a Chinese Han Population. *Invest Ophthalmol Vis Sci* (2013) 54:8384–92. doi: 10.1167/iovs.13-12878
31. Dhifallah IB, Lachheb J, Houman H, Hamzaoui K. Toll-Like-Receptor Gene Polymorphisms in a Tunisian Population With Behçet's Disease. *Clin Exp Rheumatol* (2009) 27(Suppl 53):S58–62.
32. Fang J, Chen L, Tang J, Hou S, Liao D, Ye Z, et al. Association Between Copy Number Variations of TLR7 and Ocular Behçet's Disease in a Chinese Han Population. *Investig Ophthalmol Vis Sci* (2015) 56:1517–23. doi: 10.1167/iovs.14-15030
33. Remmers EF, Cosan F, Kirino Y, Ombrello MJ, Abaci N, Satorius C, et al. Genome-Wide Association Study Identifies Variants in the MHC Class I, IL10, and IL23R-IL12RB2 Regions Associated With Behçet's Disease. *Nat Genet* (2010) 42:698–702. doi: 10.1038/ng.625
34. Mizuki N, Meguro A, Ota M, Ohno S, Shiota T, Kawagoe T, et al. Genome-Wide Association Studies Identify Il23r-IL12RB2 and IL10 as Behçet's Disease Susceptibility Loci. *Nat Genet* (2010) 42:703–6. doi: 10.1038/ng.624
35. Xavier JM, Shahram F, Davatchi F, Rosa A, Crespo J, Abdollahi BS, et al. Association Study of IL10 and IL23r-IL12RB2 in Iranian Patients With Behçet's Disease. *Arthritis Rheum* (2012) 64:2761–72. doi: 10.1002/art.34437
36. Çavuş F, Ulusoy C, Örçen A, Gül A, Tüzün E, Vural B. Increased IL-23 Receptor, Tnf-Alpha and IL-6 Expression in Individuals With the IL23R-IL12RB2 Locus Polymorphism. *Immunol Lett* (2014) 160:96–8. doi: 10.1016/j.imlet.2014.01.001
37. Kang EH, Kim S, Park MY, Choi JY, Choi IA, Kim MJ, et al. Behçet's Disease Risk Association Fine-Mapped on the IL23R-IL12RB2 Intergenic Region in Koreans. *Arthritis Res Ther* (2017) 19(1):227–36. doi: 10.1186/s13075-017-1435-5
38. Kramer M, Hasanreisoglu M, Weiss S, Kumova D, Schaap-Fogler M, Guntekin-Ergun S, et al. Single-Nucleotide Polymorphisms in IL23R-IL12RB2 (Rs1495965) are Highly Prevalent in Patients With Behcet's Uveitis and Vary Between Populations. *Ocul Immunol Inflamm* (2019) 27:766–73. doi: 10.1080/09273948.2018.1467463
39. Yu H, Zheng M, Zhang L, Li H, Zhu Y, Cheng L, et al. Identification of Susceptibility Snps in IL10 and IL23R-IL12RB2 for Behçet's Disease in Han Chinese. *J Allergy Clin Immunol* (2017) 139(2):621–7. doi: 10.1016/j.jaci.2016.05.024
40. Emmi G, Silvestri E, Della BC, Grassi A, Benagiano M, Cianchi F, et al. Cytotoxic Th1 and Th17 Cells Infiltrate the Intestinal Mucosa of Behcet Patients and Exhibit High Levels of TNF-Alpha in Early Phases of the Disease. *Med (United States)* (2016) 95:e5516. doi: 10.1097/MD.0000000000005516
41. Albayrak O, Oray M, Can F, Kirimli GU, Gul A, Tugal-Tutkun I, et al. Effect of Interferon Alfa-2a Treatment on Adaptive and Innate Immune Systems in Patients With Behçet Disease Uveitis. *Investig Ophthalmol Vis Sci* (2019) 60:52–63. doi: 10.1167/iovs.18-25548
42. Sugita S, Kawazoe Y, Imai A, Kawaguchi T, Horie S, Keino H, et al. Role of IL-22- and TNF-Alpha–Producing Th22 Cells in Uveitis Patients With Behçet's Disease. *J Immunol* (2013) 190:5799–808. doi: 10.4049/jimmunol.1202677
43. Zenewicz LA, Yin X, Wang G, Elinav E, Hao L, Zhao L, et al. Il-22 Deficiency Alters Colonic Microbiota to Be Transmissible and Colitogenic. *J Immunol* (2013) 190:5306–12. doi: 10.4049/jimmunol.1300016
44. Xavier JM, Shahram F, Sousa I, Davatchi F, Matos M, Abdollahi BS, et al. Fut2: Filling the Gap Between Genes and Environment in Behçet's Disease? *Ann Rheum Dis* (2015) 74:618–24. doi: 10.1136/annrheumdis-2013-204475
45. Takeuchi M, Mizuki N, Meguro A, Ombrello MJ, Kirino Y, Satorius C, et al. Dense Genotyping of Immune-Related Loci Implicates Host Responses to Microbial Exposure in Behçet's Disease Susceptibility. *Nat Genet* (2017) 49:438–43. doi: 10.1038/ng.3786
46. Korpela K, Salonen A, Hickman B, Kunz C, Sprenger N, Kukkonen K, et al. Fucosylated Oligosaccharides in Mother's Milk Alleviate the Effects of Caesarean Birth on Infant Gut Microbiota. *Sci Rep* (2018) 8:13757. doi: 10.1038/s41598-018-32037-6
47. Wacklin P, Tuimala J, Nikkilä J, Tims S, Mäkivuokko H, Alakulppi N, et al. Faecal Microbiota Composition in Adults is Associated With the FUT2 Gene Determining the Secretor Status. *PloS One* (2014) 9:e94863. doi: 10.1371/journal.pone.0094863
48. Turpin W, Bedrani L, Espin-Garcia O, Xu W, Silverberg MS, Smith MI, et al. Fut2 Genotype and Secretory Status are Not Associated With Fecal Microbial Composition and Inferred Function in Healthy Subjects. *Gut Microbes* (2018) 9:357–68. doi: 10.1080/19490976.2018.1445956
49. Tong M, McHardy I, Ruegger P, Goudarzi M, Kashyap PC, Haritunians T, et al. Reprograming of Gut Microbiome Energy Metabolism by the FUT2 Crohn's Disease Risk Polymorphism. *ISME J* (2014) 8:2193–206. doi: 10.1038/ismej.2014.64
50. Goto H, Mochizuki M, Yamaki K, Kotake S, Usui M, Ohno S. Epidemiological Survey of Intraocular Inflammation in Japan. *Jpn J Ophthalmol* (2007) 51:41–4. doi: 10.1007/s10384-006-0383-4
51. Jun J, Kim HJ, Kazmi SZ, Kang T, Kim K, Kang MJ, et al. Significant Decline in the Incidence of Behcet's Disease in South Korea: A Nationwide Population-Based Study (2004-2017). *Arthritis Care Res (Hoboken)* (2020). doi: 10.1002/acr.24408

18

Pathogenesis of Non-Infectious Uveitis Elucidated by Recent Genetic Findings

Masaki Takeuchi[1], *Nobuhisa Mizuki*[1] *and Shigeaki Ohno*[2*]

[1] *Department of Ophthalmology and Visual Science, Yokohama City University Graduate School of Medicine, Yokohama, Japan,* [2] *Department of Ophthalmology, Faculty of Medicine and Graduate School of Medicine, Hokkaido University, Sapporo, Japan*

Correspondence:
Shigeaki Ohno
sohno@med.hokudai.ac.jp

Uveitis is a generic term for inflammation of the uvea, which includes the iris, ciliary body, and choroid. Prevalence of underlying non-infectious uveitis varies by race and region and is a major cause of legal blindness in developed countries. Although the etiology remains unclear, the involvement of both genetic and environmental factors is considered important for the onset of many forms of non-infectious uveitis. Major histocompatibility complex (MHC) genes, which play a major role in human immune response, have been reported to be strongly associated as genetic risk factors in several forms of non-infectious uveitis. Behçet's disease, acute anterior uveitis (AAU), and chorioretinopathy are strongly correlated with MHC class I-specific alleles. Moreover, sarcoidosis and Vogt-Koyanagi-Harada (VKH) disease are associated with MHC class II-specific alleles. These correlations can help immunogenetically classify the immune pathway involved in each form of non-infectious uveitis. Genetic studies, including recent genome-wide association studies, have identified several susceptibility genes apart from those in the MHC region. These genetic findings help define the common or specific pathogenesis of ocular inflammatory diseases by comparing the susceptibility genes of each form of non-infectious uveitis. Interestingly, genome-wide association of the interleukin (IL)23R region has been identified in many of the major forms of non-infectious uveitis, such as Behçet's disease, ocular sarcoidosis, VKH disease, and AAU. The interleukin-23 (IL-23) receptor, encoded by *IL23R*, is expressed on the cell surface of Th17 cells. IL-23 is involved in the homeostasis of Th17 cells and the production of IL-17, which is an inflammatory cytokine, indicating that a Th17 immune response is a common key in the pathogenesis of non-infectious uveitis. Based on the findings from the immunogenetics of non-infectious uveitis, a personalized treatment approach based on the patient's genetic make-up is expected.

Keywords: acute anterior uveitis, Behcet's disease, birdshot chorioretinopathy, GWAS - genome-wide association study, immunogenetics, ocular sarcoidosis, uveitis, Vogt-Koyanagi-Harada disease

INTRODUCTION

Uvea is the middle layer of three concentric layers of the eye, including the iris, ciliary body, and choroid. Uvea plays an important role in providing diffusible nutrients in the outer layer of the retina and homeostasis of the temperature of the eye. Conversely, because of the abundant blood flow, it tends to be the primary site of inflammatory reaction in the eye, leading to uveitis. Uveitis can be clinically divided into infectious uveitis and non-infectious uveitis. Non-infectious uveitis often develops as an ocular symptom of systemic disease.

Uveitis is one of the major causes of visual impairment in developed countries. Severe eye inflammation irreversibly damages the retina and optic nerve. Uveitis accounts for 5%–20% of legal blindness in the United States and Europe and leads to irreversible blindness in approximately 35% of patients in developed countries (1, 2).

Although the pathophysiology of non-infectious uveitis has not yet been clarified, the involvement of genetic predisposition and environmental factors has been suggested. With the recent development of genome analysis research, several susceptibility genes involved in the pathophysiology of each non-infectious uveitis have been identified, contributing to the understanding of the pathophysiology of non-infectious uveitis. Here we describe immunogenetics of non-infectious uveitis elucidated by genetic analysis focusing on genome-wide association studies (GWASs).

GENETIC EVIDENCE OF NON-INFECTIOUS UVEITIS

Behçet's Disease

Behçet's disease (BD) is a systemic inflammatory disease with repeated attacks and remissions that causes inflammation of various organs of the body, including oral aphtous ulcers, uveitis, skin lesions, and genital ulcers (3). BD is relatively common in countries that fall on the ancient silk route, including the Mediterranean basin, Middle East, Central Asia, and East Asia. BD is genetically one of the most studied causes of non-infectious uveitis. The geoepidemiological features of BD suggest that both environmental and genetic factors are likely involved in the development of BD. Familial aggregation and high sibling recurrence observed in multiple populations also support the involvement of genetic factors in its pathogenesis (4, 5).

In 1973, Ohno et al. reported a strong association of HL-A5 (later termed HLA-B5) in the Japanese population. HLA-B5 is a broad antigen subsuming *HLA-B*51* and *HLA-B*52* (6). After finding this initial genetic evidence, the association between BD and *HLA-B*51* has been confirmed in multiple populations (7–18). A systematic review and meta-analysis including 4,800 patients and 16,289 controls from 78 independent studies reported the pooled odds ratio for the susceptibility of HLA-B5/HLA-B51 and *HLA-B*51*, 5.78 (95% confidence interval [CI], 5.00–6.67) and 5.90 (95% CI, 4.87–7.16), respectively. Other than *HLA-B*51*, other MHC class I alleles also show some disease susceptibility (19). A GWAS targeting microsatellites by Meguro et al. identified *HLA-A*26* susceptibility in the Japanese population (20). Due to the strong linkage disequilibrium, it is difficult to reveal the true association of HLA alleles. Stepwise conditional analysis of Turkish GWAS-predicted HLA alleles revealed associations of *HLA-B*15*, *HLA-B*27* as risk alleles and *HLA-A*03* as protective alleles, which were independent from *HLA-B*51* susceptibility (20, 21).

The summary of susceptible single nucleotide polymorphisms (SNPs) outside of the MHC region for diseases with non-infectious uveitis with $P<5 \times 10^{-8}$, thus exceeding the threshold for genome-wide significance, is shown in **Table 1**. In 2010, Mizuki et al. and Remmers et al. conducted GWASs for BD in the Japanese and Turkish populations, respectively. The GWASs initially reported genome-wide associations in loci of *IL23R-IL12RB2* and *IL10* by GWASs in the Japanese and Turkish populations, respectively (22, 23). Genetic association of *UBAC2* was reported in a candidate gene approach based on results of the previous GWAS by a meta-analysis of Turkish and Italian populations, although the p-value did not achieve a general threshold of genome-wide association ($P=1.69 \times 10^{-7}$) (48). The susceptibility of *UBAC2* were confirmed in Han Chinese and Japanese populations (49, 50).

A GWAS in the Han Chinese population reported a susceptibility locus of *STAT4* and *TNFAIP3* (29, 32). Imputation of Turkish GWAS data additionally identified *CCR1*, *KLRC4*, and *ERAP1* (27). Meta-analysis of the *IL12A* susceptibility in a mixed population with Turkish GWAS data reached a genome-wide significant association level (31). In 2017, Takeuchi et al., conducted a large-scale genetic analysis, including 3,477 patients and 3,342 controls from Turkish, Japanese, and Iranian populations using the Immunochip (Illumina), which has 200,000 markers designed from previous GWASs of other immune-related diseases. This dense genotyping of immune-related loci identified six novel loci, *IL1A-IL1B*, *RIPK2*, *ADO-EGR2*, *LACC1*, *IRF8*, and *CEBPB-PTPN1* (26). Another Immunochip study in the European Spanish population identified a novel association in the locus of *JRKL-CNTN5* (24). The disease susceptibility of ancestry specific FUT2 non-secretor alleles, which influence gut microbiome composition and susceptibility to viral and bacterial infections, was reported in Turks, Japanese and Iranian (26, 34, 51–53). A targeted sequencing approach revealed genome-wide association of a missense variant of *MEFV* M694V, which is one of the causative mutations for familial Mediterranean fever (35).

Sarcoidosis

Sarcoidosis is a systemic inflammatory disease characterized by non-caseating granuloma formation affecting multiple organs, such as lungs, eyes, skin, and heart (54). In a Danish and Finnish twin cohort study, when one proband of monozygotic twins has sarcoidosis, the risk of the second twin developing sarcoidosis is 80 times higher than in the general population. This observation indicates that genetic factors are involved in the development of sarcoidosis (55).

The MHC region also confers the strongest susceptibility to sarcoidosis. Among the HLA genes, multiple allele forms of

TABLE 1 | Summary of susceptibility SNPs with genome-wide significance for non-infectious uveitis.

Traits	Variant	Gene	OR	Population		Function of the risk allele	Ref
				Discovery	Replication		
BD	rs1495965	*IL23R-IL12RB2*	1.35	Japanese	Turkish		(22, 23)
BD	rs924080	*IL23R-IL12RB2*	1.28	Turkish, Japanese			(22, 23)
BD	rs10889664	*IL23R*	2.00	Spanish			(24)
BD	rs1518111	*IL10*	1.45	Turkish	Greek, UK, Iranian, Middle Eastern Arab, Japanese, Han Chinese	Reduces expression in monocytes	(23)
BD	rs1800871	*IL10*	1.45	Japanese	Turkish, Korean, Han Chinese		(22, 25)
BD	rs3783550	*IL1A-IL1B*	1.33	Turkish		rs4420765 (r2 = 0.97) increases IL-1β and decreases IL-1α in PBMCs	(26)
BD	rs7574070	*STAT4*	1.27	Turkish	Japanese, Iranian	Increases expression	(27, 28)
BD	rs897200	*STAT4*	1.45	Han Chinese		Increases expression of *STAT4* and *IL17*	(29)
BD	rs17006292	*TFCP2L1*	4.17	Han Chinese			(29)
BD	rs7616215	*CCR1*	1.39	Turkish	Japanese, Iranian	Decreases expression in monocytes Reduces monocyte chemotaxis	(27, 28)
BD	rs13092160	*CCR1-CCR3*	3.13	Han Chinese		Decreases expression in PBMCs	(30)
BD	rs17810546	*IL12A*	1.66	Turkish, Mixed populations			(31)
BD	rs1874886	*IL12A*	1.61	Spanish			(24)
BD	rs17482078	*ERAP1*[1]	4.56	Turkish	Iranian	Reduces enzymatic activity	(27, 28)
BD	rs9494885	*TNFAIP3*	1.81	Han Chinese		No difference in expression in PBMCs	(32)
BD	rs2230801	*RIPK2*	1.53	Turkish, Iranian, Japanese		Possibly damaging (I259T)	(26)
BD	rs10094579	*RIPK2*	1.32	Turkish, Han Chinese			(26, 33)
BD	rs224127	*ADO-ZNF365-EGR2*	1.27	Turkish, Japanese	Han Chinese		(26, 33)
BD	rs1509966	*ADO-ZNF365-EGR2*	1.13	Turkish, Iranian			(26)
BD	rs2848479	*JRKL-CNTN5*	1.66	Spanish			(24)
BD	rs2617170	*KLRC4*	1.28	Turkish	Japanese, Iranian		(27, 34)
BD	rs2121033	*LACC1*	1.32	Turkish, Iranian, Japanese		r2 = 0.93 with a missense variant (I254V)	(26)
BD	rs9316059	*LACC1*	1.37	Japanese, Han Chinese		r2 = 0.93 with a missense variant (I254V)	(26, 33)
BD	rs61752717	*MEFV*	2.65	Turkish, Japanese		Missense variant (M694V), which increases response to LPS	(35)
BD	rs7203487	*IRF8*	1.39	Turkish, Iranian			(26)
BD	rs142105922	*IRF8*	1.61	Turkish, Japanese			(26)
BD	rs11117433	*IRF8*	1.59	Turkish			(26)
BD	rs681343	*FUT2*	1.30	Iranian, Turkish	Turkish	r^2 = 1 with a nonsecretor allele (rs601338)	(34)
BD	rs913678	*CEBPB-PTPN1*	1.32	Turkish, Iranian	Han Chinese		(26, 33)
Sarcoidosis	rs3762318	*IL23R-C1orf141*	1.65	Japanese	Czech	Decreases expression	(36)
Sarcoidosis	rs12069782	*IL23R-C1orf141*	1.24	German			(37)
Sarcoidosis	rs6748088	*FAM117B*	1.18	German			(37)
Sarcoidosis	rs1499506	*MAGI1*	1.98	African American		Associated with ocular sarcoidosis	(38)
Sarcoidosis	rs223498	*NFKB1-MANBA*	1.19	German			(37)
Sarcoidosis	rs4921492	*IL12B*	1.20	German			(37)
Sarcoidosis	rs715299	*NOTCH4*	1.14	African American			(39)
Sarcoidosis	rs2302006	*CCL24*	1.31	Japanese	Czech	Decreases expression	(36)
Sarcoidosis	rs3779419	*STYXL1-SRRM3*	1.37	Japanese	Czech	Increases *POR* expression	(36)
Sarcoidosis	rs2789679	*ANXA11*	1.67	German	African American, European American, Han Chinese	High LD with a missense variant R230C	(39, 40)
Sarcoidosis	rs479777	*CCDC88B*	1.18	German			(37)
Sarcoidosis	rs653178	*SH2B3-ATXN2*	1.19	German			(37)
VKH disease	rs117633859	*IL23R*	1.82	Han Chinese	Singaporean, Japanese	Decreases expression in PBMCs	(41–43)
VKH disease	rs442309	*ADO-ZNF365-EGR2*	1.37	Han Chinese	Thai, Japanese		(41–43)
AAU	rs79755370	*IL23R*	1.80	European			(44)
AAU	rs2032890	*ERAP1*	1.51	European			(44)
BCR	rs7705093	*ERAP2*	2.20	Dutch, Spanish	British	rs10044354 T (r^2 = 0.98) increases ERAP2 in B-cell lines	(45)

(Continued)

TABLE 1 | Continued

Traits	Variant	Gene	OR	Population		Function of the risk allele	Ref
				Discovery	Replication		
BCR	rs2287987-rs10044354	*ERAP1, ERAP2*[2]	2.75	Dutch, Spanish		Decreases *ERAP1* expression Increases *ERAP2* expression	(46) (45)
BCR	rs150571175	*TECPR2*	6.10	Dutch, Spanish			(45)
Crohn's disease uveitis	rs4766697	*RBM19*	3.31	United States[3]			(47)

[1]*Risk allele homozygotes of rs17482078 showed genome wide significance in BD patients with uveitis.*
[2]*Haplotype analysis of rs2287987 in the ERAP1 locus and rs10044354 in the ERAP2 locus showed disease susceptibility for BCR.*
[3]*Patients with IBD who were enrolled in the cedars-Sinai IBD Research Repository (MIRAD) were evaluated.*
OR, odds ratio; Ref, reference,; BD, Behçet's disease; VKH disease,: Vogt-Koyanagi-Harada disease; AAU, acute anterior uveitis; BCR, birdshot chorioretinopathy.

HLA-DRB1 (*HLA-DRB1*03, 11, 12, 14,* and *15*), which is an MHC class II molecule, and *BTNL2* have been associated with sarcoidosis (56–61). A GWAS in the German population identified genome-wide association in *ANXA11*, which has since been confirmed in Han Chinese, European American, and Portuguese populations (40, 59, 62–64). Meta-analysis of SNPs in the *ANXA11* locus, rs2573346 T and rs2789679 T showed protective association (OR;0.66 and 0.70, respectively) (65).

An African ancestry GWAS additionally identified susceptibilities in the loci of *CCDC88B*, and *NOTCH4*, and suggestive associations ($1 \times 10^{-5} > P > 5 \times 10^{-8}$) in the loci of *RAB23*, *OS9*, and *XAF1* (66). In 2015, an Immunochip genetic study was performed in the European population, and four loci of *SH2B3-ATXN2*, *IL12B*, *NFKB1-MANBA*, and *FAM117B* were identified (37). Recently, a GWAS in a Japanese cohort with replication in independent samples from Japan and the Czech Republic newly identified *CCL24* and *STYXL1-SRRM3* and confirmed disease susceptibility of *IL23R* (36). GWAS of ocular sarcoidosis was reported by Garman et al., and the association of the locus of *MAGI1* in African Americans was identified, which also showed suggestive association when comparing ocular-sarcoidosis to non-ocular sarcoidosis (38).

Vogt-Koyanagi-Harada Disease

Vogt-Koyanagi-Harada (VKH) disease is a systemic immune-mediated disorder that affects melanocytes contained in pigmented tissues, such as the uvea, inner ear, meninges, skin, and hair (67). Although the etiology of VKH disease is still unknown, it is thought that certain environmental factors, for instance, viral infection, provoke aberrant activation of the immune response through Th1 and Th17 pathways in individuals with a predisposing genetic background.

As in other non-infectious uveitis cases, the involvement of the MHC region has been reported. Disease susceptibility has been reported for MHC class II genes, such as *HLA-DR4/DRw53*, and *HLA-DQ4* In VKH disease (68). A systematic review of the association of *HLA-DR4/HLA-DRB1*04* from 21 studies including 1853 patients with VKH disease and 4164 controls showed an odds ratio (OR) of 8.42 (95% CI, 5.69–12.45) with interethnic heterogeneity (69). The suballele analysis showed increased risk in *HLA-DRB1*04:04* (OR=2.57), *HLA-DRB1*04:05* (OR=10.31), and *HLA-DRB1*04:10* (OR=6.52), but a protective effect in *HLA-DRB1*04:01* (OR=0.21) (69).

A GWAS of a Chinese cohort including 1,538 cases and 5,603 controls reported disease susceptibility loci of *IL23R* and *ADO-EGR2* (41). Disease susceptibility of *IL23R* was confirmed in the Han Chinese Singaporean and Japanese populations, and *ADO-EGR2* was confirmed in the Japanese and Thai populations (42, 43).

Acute Anterior Uveitis

Acute anterior uveitis (AAU) is a uniocular fibrinous iridocyclitis that develops acutely with fibrin precipitation and anterior chamber hypopyon. AAU is the most common cause of non-infectious uveitis in European countries, affecting 0.2% of the general population (70–73). Spondyloarthropathies (SpAs) comprising ankylosing spondylitis (AS), psoriatic arthritis, reactive arthritis, and inflammatory bowel disease are frequently found in AAU patients (74). Especially, AS is the most common condition with 30%–50% prevalence in patients with AAU (75).

AAU has been known to be associated with *HLA-B*27* (76). *HLA-B*27* is positive in > 50% of AAU cases in the Caucasian population compared to 8%–10% of the general population. Another study reported the frequency of *HLA-B*27* positive was 81.8% and 92.0% in patients with ophthalmologist-diagnosed AAU and self-reported AAU, respectively (44). In contrast, the prevalence of AAU is lower in the Asian population, which has a commensurately low frequency of *HLA-B*27*.

A genetic analysis by Immunochip in the European population showed an OR of 66.8 for heterozygosity of *HLA-B*27* and 130.6 for homozygosity, indicating that the *HLA-B*27* molecule plays a key role in the pathogenesis of AAU (44). This study also identified susceptibility outside the MHC region, *IL23R*, *ERAP1*, 2p15 (44). A recent GWAS of AAU in the European population found genome-wide association at rs9378248 in *HLA-B*. The GWAS also found suggestive association in the previously reported locus of *ERAP1* and novel loci of *NOS2, MERTK, KIFAP3, CLCN7, ACAA2*, and 5 intergenic loci (77).

Birdshot Chorioretinopathy

Birdshot chorioretinopathy (BCR) is a bilateral chronic posterior uveitis with creamy ovoid choroidal spots called "birdshot" on the fundus (78). It is predominant in middle age and slightly more common in women by sex, and most patients are

Caucasian, especially of northern European ancestry. Conversely, there are few studies from other races.

A strong association between BCR and *HLA-A*29* has been reported. Of the *HLA-A*29* subtypes, *HLA-A*29:01* and *HLA-A*29:02* are common in the general population (0.2% and 4.3% in the Caucasian population, respectively). *HLA-A*29:02* is positive in > 95% of BCRs, indicating that this HLA allele is strongly involved in the development of BCRs. However, patients with *HLA-A*29:01*-positive BCR are rarely observed. Unlike other non-infectious uveitis involving HLA genetic predisposition, BCR does not show predominant extraocular manifestations (79).

In GWASs conducted in Dutch and Spanish populations, HLA imputation analysis identified the strongest susceptibility of *HLA-A*29:02* with OR of 157.5 among all markers including HLA alleles, amino acid changes, and SNPs (45). From outside the MHC region, a genome-wide association was observed in *TECPR2* (45). In addition, a meta-analysis in the British population revealed susceptibility of *ERAP2* to BCR (45). A haplotype analysis revealed genome-wide significance of an *ERAP1-ERAP2* haplotype (45).

Tubulointerstitial Nephritis and Uveitis Syndrome

Tubulointerstitial nephritis and uveitis syndrome (TINU) is a bilateral sudden-onset anterior uveitis accompanied by tubulointerstitial nephritis (80). An HLA analysis of acute tubulointerstitial nephritis (ATIN) including patients with TINU and drug hypersensitivity-related ATIN (D-ATIN) in the Chinese population identified genome-wide significant association of *HLA-DQA1*01:04*, and *HLA-DRB1*14:05* in both TINU and D-ATIN and *HLA-DQB1*05:03* in D-ATIN (81).

Other Systemic Immune-Related Diseases

Uveitis is also observed in systemic immune-related diseases such as juvenile idiopathic arthritis (JIA) and inflammatory bowel disease (IBD). Several susceptibility genes have been identified in these diseases. However, the frequency of uveitis in these diseases is not high, i.e., 10–30% in JIA (82) and 2–4% in IBD (47). Therefore, whether the reported susceptibility genes are really involved in the pathogenesis of uveitis remains unclear.

Haasnoot et al. compared patients with JIA with and without uveitis and reported that amino acid serine at position 11 (serine 11) of HLA-DRβ1 was strongly correlated with uveitis in JIA (OR=2.60, P=5.43×10^{-10}) (82). In addition, the susceptibility of serine 11 was found only in girls and not in boys (P_{girls}=7.61×10-10, P_{boys}=0.18). Epidemiologically, uveitis is more prevalent in girls with JIA (83), and this genotype-sex interaction may be a factor to elucidate this sexual dimorphism.

Taleban et al. identified the susceptibility of a region of *RBM19* according to GWAS of uveitis in IBD (47). While the novel susceptibility locus was detected, none were identified from the several known regions of IBD in the study, due in part to the small sample size and low statistical power. Although little is known on the function of RBM19, it is probably involved in the regulation of ribosomal biogenesis. Replication studies are warranted to confirm the susceptibility of *RBM19* to IBD uveitis.

IMMUNOGENETICS OF NON-INFECTIOUS UVEITIS

MHC

The genetic findings from several GWASs provide evidence to elucidate pathogenesis of non-infectious uveitis (**Figure 1**). To date, studies have consistently found that all major non-infectious uveitis diseases were genetically most strongly associated with HLA alleles, classified into the MHC class I and MHC class II. MHC molecules play an essential role in the adaptive immune system by presenting peptide antigens derived from pathogens and self-proteins on the surface of cells, specialized antigen-presenting cells for MHC class II and nearly all cells for MHC class I.

From the point of view of MHC susceptibility, non-infectious uveitis can be divided into two groups. BD, AAU and BCR are associated with MHC I molecules and sarcoidosis, VKH and TINU are associated with MHC II molecules.

The MHC class I molecule is involved in cell-mediated immunity by presenting antigens to CD8-positive cytotoxic T cells. In contrast, MHC class II molecules influence humoral immunity by presenting antigens to CD4-positive helper T cells. However, there is not a one-to-one correspondence between each non-infectious uveitis and abnormality in one immune pathway. For instance, for BD, although the strong MHC class I association suggests a role of CD8-positve T cell-mediated immunity, the associations of *IL23R-IL12RB2* and *IL10*, identified by the initial GWAS for BD, are genes involved in the immune pathway of CD4-positive T cells (22, 23). In addition, several genes identified thereafter were genes involved in innate immunity (26, 27). These findings indicate that abnormalities in multiple immune pathways intricately contribute to each disease pathogenesis.

In BD, independent risk or protective variants of HLA-B amino acids identified by the stepwise conditional analysis were mainly located within the antigen-binding grove of the HLA molecule (21, 84).. The strongest association was observed for threonine at position 97, including HLA-B*51, followed by leucine at 116, glutamic acid at 152, and phenylalanine at 67, with independent associations (21). Amino acid position 97 also showed the most significant association in patients with AS and AAU compared with patients with AS without AAU (77). After the conditioning on amino acid position 97, independent associations of positions 67 and 70 in HLA-B were revealed (77). Amino acid positions 116, 67, and 97 located in the HLA-B antigen-binding groove are known to be key determinants that remotely influence the HLA-B alleles binding affinity of KIR3DL1 and KIR3DS1 receptors (85). These findings further implicate peptide binding on MHC molecules in the pathogenesis of non-infectious uveitis.

While MHC class I molecules are present in all nucleated cells and present with intracellular antigens, MHC class II molecules are expressed on dendritic cells, macrophages, and B cells and present extracellular antigens such as bacteria, viruses, and soluble proteins to CD4-positive T cells. Considering that flu-like symptoms are often observed in the prodromal phase of

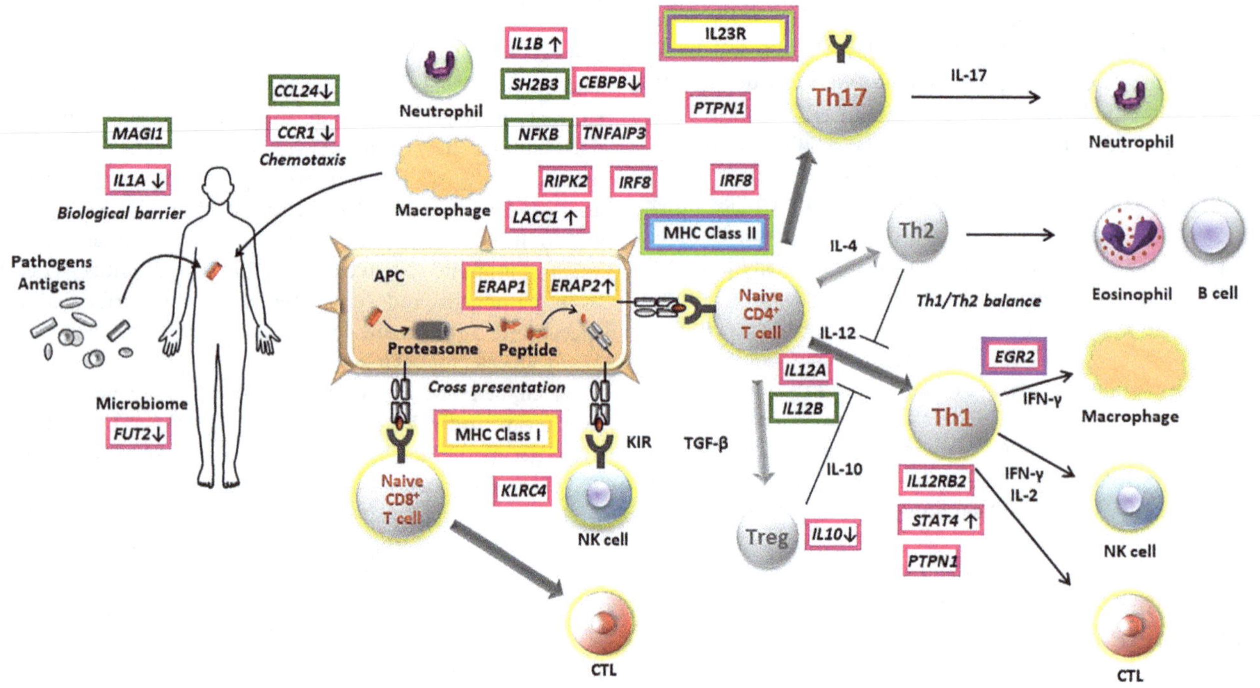

FIGURE 1 | Pathogenesis of non-infectious non-infectious uveitis elucidated by immunogenetic findings. Susceptibility genes of Behçet's disease (red boxes), sarcoidosis (green boxes), Vogt-Koyanagi-Harada disease (purple boxes), acute anterior uveitis (yellow boxes), birdshot chorioretinopathy (orange boxes), and tubulointerstitial nephritis and uveitis syndrome (light blue boxes) are indicated in the figure. The direction on gene expression or function of risk alleles are described with arrows, where identified. APC, antigen presenting cell; CTL, cytotoxic T cell; NK, natural killer cell; Treg, regulatory T cell.

patients with VKH, a viral infection is considered to be a trigger for disease development. In this hypothesis, MHC class II molecules that recognize specific viral antigens that may elicit an immune response by cross-reaction with self-proteins associated with melanocytes (67). Patients with VKH are sensitized to melanocyte antigens, and the melanocyte peptide binding capacity of the *HLA-DRB1* allele is thought to influence disease susceptibility. Susceptible *HLA-DRB1* alleles such as *HLA-DRB1*0405* may broadly recognize melanocyte associated antigens (86), whereas protective alleles such as *HLA-DRB1*0401* showed a vulnerable binding capacity (87).

Genetic Interaction With MHC Class I

ERAP1/ERAP2

ERAP1, which is a common susceptibility gene to AAU and BD, and *ERAP2*, identified in the GWAS of birdshot retinopathy, encode endoplasmic reticulum aminopeptidase 1 and 2 proteins (ERAP1 and 2), respectively. ERAP1 and ERAP2 are enzymes that trim proteasome-processed precursor peptides in the ER for loading onto the MHC I molecule. The rs1044354 C allele in high linkage disequilibrium (LD) with the rs7705093 T allele, which is associated with susceptibility to BCR, is associated with high mRNA expression of *ERAP2* in LCL cells and homozygotes of the non-risk allele showed little or no protein expression in B cells from controls (45).

A missense mutation in *ERAP1* p.Asp725Gln showed susceptibility in patients with BD uveitis only under *HLA-B*51* positivity, and *ERAP1* susceptibility was abolished in *HLA-B*51*-negative patients (27). Analysis of *ERAP1* haplotypes in BD showed strong susceptibility to Hap10 in *HLA-B*51*-positive patients with OR of 10.96 compared with those with neither *HLA-B*51* nor *ERAP1* Hap10 (88). It is suggested that polymorphisms in *ERAP1* Hap10 affect trimming efficiency and peptide length (89).

Epistasis between *ERAP1* and MHC class I was also observed in other MHC-I-opathies, such as AS and psoriasis (74, 90, 91). In contrast to BD, *ERAP1* p.Asp725Gln acts protectively for AS under *HLA-B*27* positivity and also for psoriasis under HLA-Cw6 positivity (27). The differential effects of *ERAP1* variants in conjunction with disease-specific MHC class I alleles among these diseases may be explained by differential availability of disease-specific peptides.

In BD, an inefficient ERAP1 enzyme could fail to degrade a disease-promoting peptide. Majority of the position 2 of the peptidome bound to HLA-B51:01 is Ala with lower affinity or Pro with higher affinity for HLA-B*51:01 (92). Guasp et al. compared the peptidome of HLA-B*51 trimmed by homozygotes of ERAP1 Hap10 and ERAP1 Hap1/Hap8 and found that Hap10 increased the Ala/Pro ratio at position 2 in addition to affecting the amino acid length distribution (92). In HLA-B51/ERAP1 Hap10 individuals, the low affinity of the HLA-B51-peptide complex is assumed to enhance the activation of NK cells.

On the other hand, in AS and psoriasis, an inefficient ERAP1 enzyme could fail to produce a disease-promoting peptide.

Agene interaction was analyzed between a nonsynonymous SNP located in *ERAP1* rs30187, which showed suggestive association with AAU, and *HLA-B*27*. Genome-wide association was revealed when comparing patients with *HLA-B*27*-positive AS with AAU and without AAU. In contrast, *ERAP1* susceptibility disappeared when comparing patients with *HLA-B*27*-negative AS with AAU and without AAU (77).

Both a tag SNP of *ERAP1* Hap10 haplotype, which is associated with decreased ERAP1 protein expression and enzymatic activity, and rs10044354, which is associated with increased ERAP2 expression, showed strong association in patients with HLA-A*29-associated BCR. The combined haplotype of *ERAP1-ERAP2* resulted in a genome-wide association with BCR by meta-analysis (OR 2.75, $P=2.6 \times 10^{-8}$) (46).

Killer Immunoglobulin-Like Receptors

Killer cell immunoglobulin-like receptors (KIR) are receptors on natural killer cells, which ligate to the MHC class I molecules (93). The KIR family clustered on chromosome 19q13.4 is divided into activating KIRs (aKIRs) and inhibitory KIRs (iKIRs) according to the length of the cytoplasmic tail, short (S) and long (L), respectively.

Although the role of KIRs may be critical in the pathogenesis of BD, an MHC-I-opathy, GWASs of non-infectious uveitis have not revealed genome-wide association with KIRs, and many candidate gene approach studies did not find a statistical association with KIRs (94–96). A recent study showed the frequency of *KIR3DL1*004*, which encodes a misfolded protein of this iKIR, was decreased in patients with BD with or without *HLA-B*51* (97). Evaluating functional *KIRD3L1/S1* alleles, increasing risk of BD was observed in individuals with *KIR3DL1*^{LOW}*/KIR3DS1*genotypes (OR = 2.47), and individuals with *KIR3DL1*^{HIGH}*/KIR3DL1*^{NULL} genotypes showed a protective effect to the disease (OR=0.53) (98).

Evaluated by absence or presence of 16 KIR genes, KIR3DL1$^-$/2DS3$^-$ was significantly associated with increased risk of uveitis in patients with AS (96).

The association between KIR and VKH disease has also been evaluated despite the lack of evidence of association with MHC class I. No statistical difference of KIRs was identified in Mestizo individuals living in Southern California by Levinson et al. (99). They also conducted KIR analysis in the Japanese population, a more genetically homogeneous population. A high frequency of aKIRs, KIR3DS1, 2DS1, and 2DS5 and a low frequency of an iKIR of KIR3DL1 were observed in Japanese patients with VKH disease compared with healthy controls (42.2% vs 21.4% and 76.9% vs 98.8%, respectively) (100). Sheereen et al. reported a high frequency of KIR2DS3 and KIR Bx genotypes, which includes 2DS2, 2DS3, and 2DS4, in Saudi Arabian patients with VKH disease (101). They also found weak associations of MHHHC class I genes, HLA-Cw*14 and -Cw*17, and protective association in the combination of KIR2DL2/2DL3 and HLA-C1 (101).

Immunogenetics of the MHC genes, ERAP1/ERAP2, and KIRs strongly suggest that pathways influencing peptide-MHC class I binding affinity and regulation of CTL and NK cell activation play crucial roles in the pathogenesis of several causes of non-infectious uveitis.

IL-23/Th17 Pathway

The most common susceptibility gene outside the MHC region is IL23R, encoding interleukin 23 receptor (IL-23R), identified from GWASs of several major non-infectious uveitis causes, such as BD, sarcoidosis, VKH, and AAU. Although disease risk alleles of BD and sarcoidosis were located in the IL23R locus, those are not in the same LD block, and the BD-associated SNP was not associated with susceptibility to sarcoidosis (36).

The IL-23 receptor is expressed on the surface of Th17 cells and involved in the maintenance of Th17 homeostasis and IL-17 production with recognition of IL-23 as a ligand (102). IL-23 is a key checkpoint for naïve T cell to differentiate into pathogenic Th17 cells and also contribute to homeostasis of Th17 cells and Th17 cell cytokine production, such as IL-17, IL-6, interferon γ, and granulocyte macrophage colony-stimulating factor (103).

In vivo studies on each non-infectious uveitis have supported these genetic findings. The serum IL-17 level was increased in patients with BD uveitis, and the IL-23 level was also elevated in peripheral blood mononuclear cells (PBMCs) from patients with active BD and VKH disease compared with inactive patients and healthy controls (104). The proportions of IL-17A+ cells contained in circulating memory CD4+ T cell populations were increased in patients with sarcoidosis (105). Increased IL-17A+ cells were also observed in the lamina propria from biopsies containing granulomas compared with those from biopsies from healthy controls or non-granulomas biopsies (105). Elevated IL-23p19 mRNA and IL-23 protein production levels in PBMCs, increased serum IL-23 level, and increased IL-17 level in polyclonally stimulated PBMCs and CD4+ T cells were reported in patients with VKH disease (106). Serum IL-23 level was elevated in patients with BCR with active disease naïve to systemic treatment compared with that in controls (107). These data suggest that IL-23/Th17 pathway cells, in which the IL-23 receptor is involved, are the basis of a common pathophysiology of non-infectious uveitis, regardless of inflammatory properties, such as serous and granulomatous properties, or the class of MHC association with the disease.

Biological Defense

Functional studies have revealed how susceptible polymorphisms affect the expression or function of genes in the locus. The risk allele of rs1518111 for BD, the lead SNP in the IL10 locus, is associated with decreased IL10 expression in monocytes (23). This polymorphism may decrease IL-10 production, which is an anti-inflammatory cytokine, leading to Th1 polarization. The risk allele of rs7574070 is associated with increased gene expression of *STAT4*, which plays a role in the differentiation of naïve T cells into Th1 and Th17 cells (108). These functional findings of risk alleles may lead to hyperinflammation of immune pathways, contributing to the development of non-infectious uveitis.

Interestingly, it is reported that some risk alleles for BD in gene loci involved in innate immunity act in the opposite direction, which could suppress inflammation and impair the biological defenses against pathogens. For example, risk alleles of SNPs in the *CCR1* locus reduce CCR1 expression levels and monocyte migration in PBMC from healthy controls (48). The risk allele of the lead SNP, rs4402765 in the locus of *IL1A-IL1B*, is associated with reduced production of IL-1α, which is an important contributor to biological defense in the skin, but interestingly, it is also associated with increased production of IL-1β (26), an important antimicrobial inflammatory molecule. The evidence that a BD-associated genetic locus downregulates IL-1α production in conjunction with upregulation of IL-1β raises the intriguing possibility that the combination of impaired barrier function and excessive inflammatory response to invading microorganisms contribute to BD risk.

The risk allele of rs117633859, a disease-associated SNP for sarcoidosis in both the Chinese and Japanese populations, and VKH disease in the Han Chinese population reduced IL23R transcription activity in HEK-293A cells and *IL23* expression (36, 41). This suggests that impairing host defense against pathogens by downregulating the IL-23R/Th17 axis plays an important role in the development of VKH disease and sarcoidosis.

Although consensus has yet to be reached, it has been thought that transient or occult microbial infection may play a role as a trigger in disease onset of non-infectious uveitis (67, 109). These immunogenetic findings may help clarify the involvement of pathogens in the development of non-infectious uveitis.

BENCH TO BEDSIDE

Genetics and Clinical Manifestation

Disease susceptibility genes identified by genetic approaches, such as GWAS, help clarify pathways leading to the onset of non-infectious uveitis. Moreover, the identified genes and pathways have the potential to be applied to drug discovery as targets for new treatments and for prediction of prognosis and drug efficacy based on the genetic attributes of individual patients. Because subgrouping by clinical manifestations results in analyses with smaller sample size that may limit the detection of statistical associations, the evidence connecting genetics to clinical manifestations has been seldom reported.

Although the evidence connecting genetics to clinical manifestations has not been sufficiently reported yet, some studies showed that HLA alleles may affect disease clinical features and prognosis. Uveitis is more common in patients with *HLA-B*51*-positive BD compared with those with *HLA-B*51*-negative BD (110). In addition, HLA-A*26-positive patients have a poor visual prognosis (111).

In patients with sarcoidosis, *HLA-DRB1*04* is associated with eye involvement (112). The association between HLA alleles and extraocular manifestations of non-infectious uveitis has been reported. *HLA-DQB1*06:01* was more common in Japanese patients with cardiac sarcoidosis (113). *HLA DRB1*04/*15* increased the risk of extrapulmonary involvement (including uveitis) in the European population (114). *HLA-DRB1*03:01* showed association with Löfgren syndrome, a subtype of sarcoidosis with acute onset of systemic inflammation disorder (58). Mackensen et al. performed HLA analysis on European patients with TINU and TIN and reported that the incidence of *HLA-DRB1*01:02* was increased only in patients with TINU compared with those with TIN and healthy controls (115).

Meguro reported that, in Japanese and Czech populations, the OR of the rs4728493 risk allele at the *CCL24* locus decreases with the progression of the sarcoidosis chest X-ray (CXR) when compared in the CXR stage 0 + I, stage II, and stage III + IV subgroups (36). The highest OR was observed for susceptible SNPs in both *CCL24* and *STYXL1-SRRM3* in the acute systemic Lofgren's syndrome compared with sarcoidosis with any chest X-ray stage in the Czech population (36). The risk allele of rs4728493 was associated with decreased *CCL24* expression in fibroblasts and skin. CCL24 is an eotaxin, which is upregulated by Th2-biased immune responses; thus, these findings indicate that Th1 polarization associated with decreased expression of CCL24 might be important in onset and maintenance of the early stage and acute subtype of sarcoidosis (36, 116).

Treatment Based on Immunogenetics

Anti-inflammatory treatment by topical or systemic administration of corticosteroids and immunosuppressants have been the basic treatment for non-infectious uveitis (117). In recent years, the development of biologics targeting specific molecules involved in pathological conditions has progressed, and multiple biologics have been used in the treatment of non-infectious uveitis (118). In particular, anti-TNF reagents have significantly improved the visual acuity prognosis of patients with intractable uveitis due to their strong anti-inflammatory effect. Multicenter double-masked randomized clinical trials of adalimumab for non-infectious uveitis with insufficient control by corticosteroids (VISUAL I, VISUAL II, and VISUAL III) reported efficacy of adalimumab with a lower risk of ocular flare and visual impairment (119–121).

However, while the efficacy of TNF inhibitors is noteworthy, there are still cases of refractory non-infectious uveitis who do not respond to TNF inhibitors. Therefore, it is desirable to establish treatment based on the pathogenesis of each disease and the genetic factors of the individual as precision medicine.

IL-1β encoded from IL1B, identified in the BD Immunochip study, is an inflammatory cytokine and plays an important role in biological defense through activating NF-κB. In healthy donor PBMCs homozygous for rs4402765, the lead SNP for BD in the IL1B region, IL-1β was expressed higher than in cells homozygous for the non-risk allele (26). IL-1 inhibitors, anakinra and canakinumab, showed a significant reduction of ocular attacks, resolution of active retinal vasculitis, and a decrease in steroid dosages in patients with BD uveitis (122). Other studies with a small sample size also reported the effectiveness of IL-1 inhibitors in BD uveitis (123–125).

Other candidate treatment targets for non-infectious uveitis may be molecules involved in the IL-23R/Th17 pathway according to the susceptibility of IL-23R in BD, sarcoidosis, VKH disease, and AAU as previously described. Ustekinumab, an inhibitor of the p40 subunit of IL-23, effectively suppressed eye inflammation in patients with BD in concurrence with its efficacy in psoriasis (126–128). Ustekinumab also showed effectiveness for oral ulcers in patients with BD, which were resistant to colchicine (129, 130). IL-6 is a pleiotropic cytokine involved in the differentiation of TH17 cells and activation of STAT3 in the JAK-STAT pathway (131). A multicenter study including 11 patients with BD treated by tocilizumab, an IL-6 inhibitor, reported 8 of 11 achieved a complete remission at 9.5 months with two withdrawn due to severe infusion reaction (132). Secukinumab is a fully human monoclonal antibody that binds to IL-17A, leading to neutralization. Hueber et al. reported that secukinumab suppressed ocular inflammation in 11 of 16 patients with active non-infectious uveitis (133). Letko et al. reported efficacy and safety for the treatment of intravenous secukinumab in remission rates of non-infectious uveitis compared with subcutaneous administration (134, 135). However, three multicenter RCTs, including 118 patients with BD uveitis, 31 patients with active non-BD uveitis, and 125 inactive non-BD uveitis reported that no statistical effectiveness in recurrence of non-infectious uveitis was observed in all three studies compared with placebo groups (136). The authors noted that patients in both groups were treated with high doses of concomitant immunosuppressive drugs with and without secukinumab in the study and that these may have contributed to the lack of significant differences between secukinumab and placebo groups (136). In addition, for non-infectious uveitis with variable clinical manifestation, a larger sample size and longer observation period may be necessary to accurately evaluate the anti-inflammatory effect of secukinumab.

CONCLUSIONS

We have described the immunogenetics of major non-infectious uveitis, focusing on the genetic findings by GWASs. Similar to other immune-related disorders, HLA genes are the strongest genetic factors in major non-infectious uveitis, and evidence from studies on ERAP1/ERAP2 and KIR suggests that the binding of peptides to MHC molecules and immune response through MHC antigen presentation are considered central to these pathological conditions. Outside of the MHC, the fact that disease susceptibility of IL23R has been reported for several non-infectious uveitis conditions at a genome-wide significant level, suggests that the IL-23/TH17 pathway may be a common basis for the pathogenesis of non-infectious uveitis. Based on the immunogenetics of non-infectious uveitis, it is expected that the development of molecular-targeted drugs based on the pathophysiology of non-infectious uveitis and selection of treatment options based on the genetic attributes of individual patients are required to increase efficacy and reduce side effects.

AUTHOR CONTRIBUTIONS

MT wrote this manuscript. NM and SO revised manuscript. All authors contributed to the article and approved the submitted version.

ACKNOWLEDGMENTS

The authors deeply appreciate Dr. Elaine F. Remmers and Dr. Akira Meguro for insightful discussion in writing this review. The authors deeply appreciate that our studies were supported by the Grants from Japanese Behcet's Disease Research Committee of the Ministry of Health, Labor and Welfare.

REFERENCES

1. de Smet MD, Taylor SR, Bodaghi B, Miserocchi E, Murray PI, Pleyer U, et al. Understanding uveitis: the impact of research on visual outcomes. *Prog Retin Eye Res* (2011) 30(6):452–70. doi: 10.1016/j.preteyeres.2011.06.005
2. Bodaghi B, Cassoux N, Wechsler B, Hannouche D, Fardeau C, Papo T, et al. Chronic severe uveitis: etiology and visual outcome in 927 patients from a single center. *Med (Baltimore)* (2001) 80(4):263–70. doi: 10.1097/00005792-200107000-00005
3. Sakane T, Takeno M, Suzuki N, Inaba G. Behcet's disease. *New Engl J Med* (1999) 341(17):1284–91. doi: 10.1056/NEJM199910213411707
4. Dundar SV, Gencalp U, Simsek H. Familial cases of Behcet's disease. *Br J Dermatol* (1985) 113(3):319–21. doi: 10.1111/j.1365-2133.1985.tb02084.x
5. Gul A, Inanc M, Ocal L, Aral O, Konice M. Familial aggregation of Behcet's disease in Turkey. *Ann Rheumatic Dis* (2000) 59(8):622–5. doi: 10.1136/ard.59.8.622
6. Ohno S, Aoki K, Sugiura S, Nakayama E, Itakura K. Letter: HL-A5 and Behcet's disease. *Lancet* (1973) 2(7842):1383–4. doi: 10.1016/S0140-6736(73)93343-6
7. Ersoy F, Berkel I, Firat T, Kazokoglu H. HLA antigens associated with Behcet's disease. *Arch Dermatol* (1977) 113(12):1720–1. doi: 10.1001/archderm.113.12.1720
8. Haim S, Gideoni O, Barzilai A. The histocompatibility antigens in patients with Behcet's disease. *Acta Derm Venereol* (1977) 57(3):243–5.
9. Djawari D, Lang B, Hornstein OP. [HLA typing in patients of German origin with recurrent benign aphthosis and Behcet's disease]. *Z Hautkr* (1984) 59(15):1005–9.
10. Al-Rawi ZS, Sharquie KE, Khalifa SJ, Al-Hadithi FM, Munir JJ. Behcet's disease in Iraqi patients. *Ann Rheumatic Dis* (1986) 45(12):987–90. doi: 10.1136/ard.45.12.987
11. Lee S, Koh YJ, Kim DH, Bang D, Nam IW, Lee KH, et al. A study of HLA antigens in Behcet's syndrome. *Yonsei Med J* (1988) 29(3):259–62. doi: 10.3349/ymj.1988.29.3.259
12. Balboni A, Pivetti-Pezzi P, Orlando P, Rubini M, Selvatici R, Accorinti M, et al. Serological and molecular HLA typing in Italian Behcet's patients: significant association to B51-DR5-DQw3 haplotype. *Tissue Antigens* (1992) 39(3):141–3. doi: 10.1111/j.1399-0039.1992.tb01925.x
13. Mineshita S, Tian D, Wang LM, Jian XY, Li SY, Fang GZ, et al. Histocompatibility antigens associated with Behcet's disease in northern Han Chinese. *Internal Med (Tokyo Japan)* (1992) 31(9):1073–5. doi: 10.2169/internalmedicine.31.1073
14. Yabuki K, Ohno S, Mizuki N, Ando H, Tabbara KF, Goto K, et al. HLA class I and II typing of the patients with Behçet's disease in Saudi Arabia. *Tissue Antigens* (1999) 54(3):273–7. doi: 10.1034/j.1399-0039.1999.540308.x
15. Verity DH, Wallace GR, Vaughan RW, Kondeatis E, Madanat W, Zureikat H, et al. HLA and tumour necrosis factor (TNF) polymorphisms in ocular Behcet's disease. *Tissue Antigens* (1999) 54(3):264–72. doi: 10.1034/j.1399-0039.1999.540307.x
16. Yabuki K, Mizuki N, Ota M, Katsuyama Y, Palimeris G, Stavropoulos C, et al. Association of MICA gene and HLA-B*5101 with Behcet's disease in Greece. *Invest Ophthalmol Visual Sci* (1999) 40(9):1921–6.
17. Mizuki N, Ota M, Katsuyama Y, Yabuki K, Ando H, Yoshida M, et al. HLA class I genotyping including HLA-B*51 allele typing in the Iranian patients with Behcet's disease. *Tissue Antigens* (2001) 57(5):457–62. doi: 10.1034/j.1399-0039.2001.057005457.x
18. Munoz-Saa I, Cambra A, Pallares L, Espinosa G, Juan A, Pujalte F, et al. Allelic diversity and affinity variants of MICA are imbalanced in Spanish patients with Behcet's disease. *Scand J Immunol* (2006) 64(1):77–82. doi: 10.1111/j.1365-3083.2006.01780.x

19. de Menthon M, Lavalley MP, Maldini C, Guillevin L, Mahr A. HLA-B51/B5 and the risk of Behcet's disease: a systematic review and meta-analysis of case-control genetic association studies. *Arthritis Rheum* (2009) 61 (10):1287–96. doi: 10.1002/art.24642
20. Meguro A, Inoko H, Ota M, Katsuyama Y, Oka A, Okada E, et al. Genetics of Behcet disease inside and outside the MHC. *Ann Rheumatic Dis* (2010) 69 (4):747–54. doi: 10.1136/ard.2009.108571
21. Ombrello MJ, Kirino Y, de Bakker PI, Gul A, Kastner DL, Remmers EF. Behcet disease-associated MHC class I residues implicate antigen binding and regulation of cell-mediated cytotoxicity. *Proc Natl Acad Sci USA* (2014) 111(24):8867–72. doi: 10.1073/pnas.1406575111
22. Mizuki N, Meguro A, Ota M, Ohno S, Shiota T, Kawagoe T, et al. Genome-wide association studies identify IL23R-IL12RB2 and IL10 as Behcet's disease susceptibility loci. *Nat Genet* (2010) 42(8):703–6. doi: 10.1038/ng.624
23. Remmers EF, Cosan F, Kirino Y, Ombrello MJ, Abaci N, Satorius C, et al. Genome-wide association study identifies variants in the MHC class I, IL10, and IL23R-IL12RB2 regions associated with Behcet's disease. *Nat Genet* (2010) 42(8):698–702. doi: 10.1038/ng.625
24. Ortiz-Fernandez L, Carmona FD, Montes-Cano MA, Garcia-Lozano JR, Conde-Jaldon M, Ortego-Centeno N, et al. Genetic Analysis with the Immunochip Platform in Behcet Disease. Identification of Residues Associated in the HLA Class I Region and New Susceptibility Loci. *PloS One* (2016) 11(8):e0161305. doi: 10.1371/journal.pone.0161305
25. Wu Z, Zheng W, Xu J, Sun F, Chen H, Li P, et al. IL10 polymorphisms associated with Behcet's disease in Chinese Han. *Hum Immunol* (2014) 75 (3):271–6. doi: 10.1016/j.humimm.2013.11.009
26. Takeuchi M, Mizuki N, Meguro A, Ombrello MJ, Kirino Y, Satorius C, et al. Dense genotyping of immune-related loci implicates host responses to microbial exposure in Behcet's disease susceptibility. *Nat Genet* (2017) 49 (3):438–43. doi: 10.1038/ng.3786
27. Kirino Y, Bertsias G, Ishigatsubo Y, Mizuki N, Tugal-Tutkun I, Seyahi E, et al. Genome-wide association analysis identifies new susceptibility loci for Behcet's disease and epistasis between HLA-B*51 and ERAP1. *Nat Genet* (2013) 45(2):202–7. doi: 10.1038/ng.2520
28. Sousa I, Shahram F, Francisco D, Davatchi F, Abdollahi BS, Ghaderibarmi F, et al. CCR1, KLRC4, IL12A-ASN1, STAT4, and ERAP1 are associated with Behcet's disease in Iranian. *Arthritis Rheumatol (Hoboken NJ)* (2015) 67:2742–8. doi: 10.1002/art.39240
29. Hou S, Yang Z, Du L, Jiang Z, Shu Q, Chen Y, et al. Identification of a susceptibility locus in STAT4 for Behcet's disease in Han Chinese in a genome-wide association study. *Arthritis Rheum* (2012) 64(12):4104–13. doi: 10.1002/art.37708
30. Hou S, Xiao X, Li F, Jiang Z, Kijlstra A, Yang P. Two-stage association study in Chinese Han identifies two independent associations in CCR1/CCR3 locus as candidate for Behcet's disease susceptibility. *Hum Genet* (2012) 131 (12):1841–50. doi: 10.1007/s00439-012-1200-4
31. Kappen JH, Medina-Gomez C, van Hagen PM, Stolk L, Estrada K, Rivadeneira F, et al. Genome-wide association study in an admixed case series reveals IL12A as a new candidate in Behcet disease. *PloS One* (2015) 10 (3):e0119085. doi: 10.1371/journal.pone.0119085
32. Li H, Liu Q, Hou S, Du L, Zhou Q, Zhou Y, et al. TNFAIP3 gene polymorphisms confer risk for Behcet's disease in a Chinese Han population. *Hum Genet* (2013) 132(3):293–300. doi: 10.1007/s00439-012-1250-7
33. Wu P, Du L, Hou S, Su G, Yang L, Hu J, et al. Association of LACC1, CEBPB-PTPN1, RIPK2 and ADO-EGR2 with ocular Behcet's disease in a Chinese Han population. *Br J Ophthalmol* (2018) 102(9):1308–14. doi: 10.1136/bjophthalmol-2017-311753
34. Xavier JM, Shahram F, Sousa I, Davatchi F, Matos M, Abdollahi BS, et al. FUT2: filling the gap between genes and environment in Behcet's disease? *Ann Rheumatic Dis* (2015) 74(3):618–24. doi: 10.1136/annrheumdis-2013-204475
35. Kirino Y, Zhou Q, Ishigatsubo Y, Mizuki N, Tugal-Tutkun I, Seyahi E, et al. Targeted resequencing implicates the familial Mediterranean fever gene MEFV and the toll-like receptor 4 gene TLR4 in Behcet disease. *Proc Natl Acad Sci USA* (2013) 110(20):8134–9. doi: 10.1073/pnas.1306352110
36. Meguro A, Ishihara M, Petrek M, Yamamoto K, Takeuchi M, Mrazek F, et al. Genetic control of CCL24, POR, and IL23R contributes to the pathogenesis of sarcoidosis. *Commun Biol* (2020) 3(1):465. doi: 10.1038/s42003-020-01185-9
37. Fischer A, Ellinghaus D, Nutsua M, Hofmann S, Montgomery CG, Iannuzzi MC, et al. Identification of Immune-Relevant Factors Conferring Sarcoidosis Genetic Risk. *Am J Respir Crit Care Med* (2015) 192(6):727–36. doi: 10.1164/rccm.201503-0418OC
38. Garman L, Pezant N, Pastori A, Savoy KA, Li C, Levin AM, et al. Genome-Wide Association Study of Ocular Sarcoidosis Confirms HLA Associations and Implicates Barrier Function and Autoimmunity in African Americans. *Ocular Immunol Inflamm* (2020), 1–6. doi: 10.1080/09273948.2019.1705985
39. Adrianto I, Lin CP, Hale JJ, Levin AM, Datta I, Parker R, et al. Genome-wide association study of African and European Americans implicates multiple shared and ethnic specific loci in sarcoidosis susceptibility. *PloS One* (2012) 7 (8):e43907. doi: 10.1371/journal.pone.0043907
40. Hofmann S, Franke A, Fischer A, Jacobs G, Nothnagel M, Gaede KI, et al. Genome-wide association study identifies ANXA11 as a new susceptibility locus for sarcoidosis. *Nat Genet* (2008) 40(9):1103–6. doi: 10.1038/ng.198
41. Hou S, Du L, Lei B, Pang CP, Zhang M, Zhuang W, et al. Genome-wide association analysis of Vogt-Koyanagi-Harada syndrome identifies two new susceptibility loci at 1p31.2 and 10q21.3. *Nat Genet* (2014) 46(9):1007–11. doi: 10.1038/ng.3061
42. Cao S, Chee SP, Yu HG, Sukavatcharin S, Wu L, Kijlstra A, et al. Investigation of the association of Vogt-Koyanagi-Harada syndrome with IL23R-C1orf141 in Han Chinese Singaporean and ADO-ZNF365-EGR2 in Thai. *Br J Ophthalmol* (2016) 100(3):436–42. doi: 10.1136/bjophthalmol-2015-307366
43. Sakono T, Meguro A, Takeuchi M, Yamane T, Teshigawara T, Kitaichi N, et al. Variants in IL23R-C1orf141 and ADO-ZNF365-EGR2 are associated with susceptibility to Vogt-Koyanagi-Harada disease in Japanese population. *PloS One* (2020) 15(5):e0233464. doi: 10.1371/journal.pone.0233464
44. Robinson PC, Claushuis TA, Cortes A, Martin TM, Evans DM, Leo P, et al. Genetic dissection of acute anterior uveitis reveals similarities and differences in associations observed with ankylosing spondylitis. *Arthritis Rheumatol (Hoboken NJ)* (2015) 67(1):140–51. doi: 10.1002/art.38873
45. Kuiper JJ, Van Setten J, Ripke S, Van TSR, Mulder F, Missotten T, et al. A genome-wide association study identifies a functional ERAP2 haplotype associated with birdshot chorioretinopathy. *Hum Mol Genet* (2014) 23 (22):6081–7. doi: 10.1093/hmg/ddu307
46. Kuiper JJW, Setten JV, Devall M, Cretu-Stancu M, Hiddingh S, Ophoff RA, et al. Functionally distinct ERAP1 and ERAP2 are a hallmark of HLA-A29-(Birdshot) Uveitis. *Hum Mol Genet* (2018) 27(24):4333–43. doi: 10.1101/338228
47. Taleban S, Li D, Targan SR, Ippoliti A, Brant SR, Cho JH, et al. Ocular Manifestations in Inflammatory Bowel Disease Are Associated with Other Extra-intestinal Manifestations, Gender, and Genes Implicated in Other Immune-related Traits. *J Crohns Colitis* (2016) 10(1):43–9. doi: 10.1093/ecco-jcc/jjv178
48. Sawalha AH, Hughes T, Nadig A, Yilmaz V, Aksu K, Keser G, et al. A putative functional variant within the UBAC2 gene is associated with increased risk of Behcet's disease. *Arthritis Rheum* (2011) 63(11):3607–12. doi: 10.1002/art.30604
49. Hou S, Shu Q, Jiang Z, Chen Y, Li F, Chen F, et al. Replication study confirms the association between UBAC2 and Behçet's disease in two independent Chinese sets of patients and controls. *Arthritis Res Ther* (2012) 14(2):R70. doi: 10.1186/ar3789
50. Yamazoe K, Meguro A, Takeuchi M, Shibuya E, Ohno S, Mizuki N. Comprehensive analysis of the association between UBAC2 polymorphisms and Behcet's disease in a Japanese population. *Sci Rep* (2017) 7(1):742. doi: 10.1038/s41598-017-00877-3
51. Payne DC, Currier RL, Staat MA, Sahni LC, Selvarangan R, Halasa NB, et al. Epidemiologic Association Between FUT2 Secretor Status and Severe Rotavirus Gastroenteritis in Children in the United States. *JAMA Pediatr* (2015) 169(11):1040–5. doi: 10.1001/jamapediatrics.2015.2002
52. Wacklin P, Makivuokko H, Alakulppi N, Nikkila J, Tenkanen H, Rabina J, et al. Secretor genotype (FUT2 gene) is strongly associated with the composition of Bifidobacteria in the human intestine. *PloS One* (2011) 6 (5):e20113. doi: 10.1371/journal.pone.0020113
53. Marionneau S, Airaud F, Bovin NV, Le Pendu J, Ruvoen-Clouet N. Influence of the combined ABO, FUT2, and FUT3 polymorphism on susceptibility to Norwalk virus attachment. *J Infect Dis* (2005) 192(6):1071–7. doi: 10.1086/432546

54. Arkema EV, Cozier YC. Epidemiology of sarcoidosis: current findings and future directions. *Ther Adv Chron Dis* (2018) 9(11):227–40. doi: 10.1177/2040622318790197
55. Sverrild A, Backer V, Kyvik KO, Kaprio J, Milman N, Svendsen CB, et al. Heredity in sarcoidosis: a registry-based twin study. *Thorax* (2008) 63 (10):894–6. doi: 10.1136/thx.2007.094060
56. Ishihara M, Ohno S, Ishida T, Ando H, Naruse T, Nose Y, et al. Molecular genetic studies of HLA class II alleles in sarcoidosis. *Tissue Antigens* (1994) 43(4):238–41. doi: 10.1111/j.1399-0039.1994.tb02331.x
57. Rossman MD, Thompson B, Frederick M, Maliarik M, Iannuzzi MC, Rybicki BA, et al. HLA-DRB1*1101: a significant risk factor for sarcoidosis in blacks and whites. *Am J Hum Genet* (2003) 73(4):720–35. doi: 10.1086/378097
58. Grunewald J, Eklund A. Lofgren's syndrome: human leukocyte antigen strongly influences the disease course. *Am J Respir Crit Care Med* (2009) 179 (4):307–12. doi: 10.1164/rccm.200807-1082OC
59. Levin AM, Iannuzzi MC, Montgomery CG, Trudeau S, Datta I, McKeigue P, et al. Association of ANXA11 genetic variation with sarcoidosis in African Americans and European Americans. *Genes Immun* (2013) 14(1):13–8. doi: 10.1038/gene.2012.48
60. Valentonyte R, Hampe J, Huse K, Rosenstiel P, Albrecht M, Stenzel A, et al. Sarcoidosis is associated with a truncating splice site mutation in BTNL2. *Nat Genet* (2005) 37(4):357–64. doi: 10.1038/ng1519
61. Rybicki BA, Walewski JL, Maliarik MJ, Kian H, Iannuzzi MC, Group AR. The BTNL2 gene and sarcoidosis susceptibility in African Americans and Whites. *Am J Hum Genet* (2005) 77(3):491–9. doi: 10.1086/444435
62. Morais A, Lima B, Peixoto M, Melo N, Alves H, Marques JA, et al. Annexin A11 gene polymorphism (R230C variant) and sarcoidosis in a Portuguese population. *Tissue Antigens* (2013) 82(3):186–91. doi: 10.1111/tan.12188
63. Feng X, Zang S, Yang Y, Zhao S, Li Y, Gao X, et al. Annexin A11 (ANXA11) gene polymorphisms are associated with sarcoidosis in a Han Chinese population: a case-control study. *BMJ Open* (2014) 4(7):e004466. doi: 10.1136/bmjopen-2013-004466
64. Mrazek F, Stahelova A, Kriegova E, Fillerova R, Zurkova M, Kolek V, et al. Functional variant ANXA11 R230C: true marker of protection and candidate disease modifier in sarcoidosis. *Genes Immun* (2011) 12(6):490–4. doi: 10.1038/gene.2011.27
65. Zhou H, Diao M, Zhang M. The Association between ANXA11 Gene Polymorphisms and Sarcoidosis: a Meta-Analysis and systematic review. *Sarcoidosis Vasc Diffuse Lung Dis* (2016) 33(2):102–11.
66. Fischer A, Grunewald J, Spagnolo P, Nebel A, Schreiber S, Muller-Quernheim J. Genetics of sarcoidosis. *Semin Respir Crit Care Med* (2014) 35(3):296–306. doi: 10.1055/s-0034-1376860
67. Du L, Kijlstra A, Yang P. Vogt-Koyanagi-Harada disease: Novel insights into pathophysiology, diagnosis and treatment. *Prog Retin Eye Res* (2016) 52:84–111. doi: 10.1016/j.preteyeres.2016.02.002
68. Silpa-Archa S, Silpa-Archa N, Preble JM, Foster CS. Vogt-Koyanagi-Harada syndrome: Perspectives for immunogenetics, multimodal imaging, and therapeutic options. *Autoimmun Rev* (2016) 15(8):809–19. doi: 10.1016/j.autrev.2016.04.001
69. Shi T, Lv W, Zhang L, Chen J, Chen H. Association of HLA-DR4/HLA-DRB1*04 with Vogt-Koyanagi-Harada disease: a systematic review and meta-analysis. *Sci Rep* (2014) 4:6887. doi: 10.1038/srep06887
70. Jakob E, Reuland MS, Mackensen F, Harsch N, Fleckenstein M, Lorenz HM, et al. Uveitis subtypes in a german interdisciplinary uveitis center–analysis of 1916 patients. *J Rheumatol* (2009) 36(1):127–36. doi: 10.3899/jrheum.080102
71. Palmares J, Coutinho MF, Castro-Correia J. Uveitis in northern Portugal. *Curr Eye Res* (1990) 9 Suppl:31–4. doi: 10.3109/02713689008999416
72. Smit RL, Baarsma GS, de Vries J. Classification of 750 consecutive uveitis patients in the Rotterdam Eye Hospital. *Int Ophthalmol* (1993) 17(2):71–6. doi: 10.1007/BF00942778
73. Tran VT, Auer C, Guex-Crosier Y, Pittet N, Herbort CP. Epidemiology of uveitis in Switzerland. *Ocular Immunol Inflamm* (1994) 2(3):169–76. doi: 10.3109/09273949409057073
74. McGonagle D, Aydin SZ, Gul A, Mahr A, Direskeneli H. 'MHC-I-opathy'-unified concept for spondyloarthritis and Behcet disease. *Nat Rev Rheumatol* (2015) 11(12):731–40. doi: 10.1038/nrrheum.2015.147
75. Monnet D, Breban M, Hudry C, Dougados M, Brezin AP. Ophthalmic findings and frequency of extraocular manifestations in patients with HLA-B27 uveitis: a study of 175 cases. *Ophthalmology* (2004) 111(4):802–9. doi: 10.1016/j.ophtha.2003.07.011
76. Brewerton DA, Caffrey M, Nicholls A, Walters D, James DC. Acute anterior uveitis and HL-A 27. *Lancet* (1973) 302(7836):994–6. doi: 10.1016/S0140-6736(73)91090-8
77. Huang XF, Li Z, De Guzman E, Robinson P, Gensler L, Ward MM, et al. Genomewide Association Study of Acute Anterior Uveitis Identifies New Susceptibility Loci. *Invest Ophthalmol Visual Sci* (2020) 61(6):3. doi: 10.1167/iovs.61.6.3
78. Minos E, Barry RJ, Southworth S, Folkard A, Murray PI, Duker JS, et al. Birdshot chorioretinopathy: current knowledge and new concepts in pathophysiology, diagnosis, monitoring and treatment. *Orphanet J Rare Dis* (2016) 11(1):61. doi: 10.1186/s13023-016-0429-8
79. Pagnoux C, Mahr A, Aouba A, Berezne A, Monnet D, Cohen P, et al. Extraocular manifestations of birdshot chorioretinopathy in 118 French patients. *Presse Med* (2010) 39(5):e97–e102. doi: 10.1016/j.lpm.2009.12.005
80. Amaro D, Carreño E, Steeples LR, Oliveira-Ramos F, Marques-Neves C, Leal I. Tubulointerstitial nephritis and uveitis (TINU) syndrome: a review. *Br J Ophthalmol* (2020) 104(6):742–7. doi: 10.1136/bjophthalmol-2019-314926
81. Jia Y, Su T, Gu Y, Li C, Zhou X, Su J, et al. HLA-DQA1, -DQB1, and -DRB1 Alleles Associated with Acute Tubulointerstitial Nephritis in a Chinese Population: A Single-Center Cohort Study. *J Immunol (Baltimore Md 1950)* (2018) 201(2):423–31. doi: 10.4049/jimmunol.1800237
82. Haasnoot AJW, Schilham MW, Kamphuis S, Hissink Muller PCE, Heiligenhaus A, Foell D, et al. Identification of an Amino Acid Motif in HLA-DRbeta1 That Distinguishes Uveitis in Patients With Juvenile Idiopathic Arthritis. *Arthritis Rheumatol (Hoboken NJ)* (2018) 70(7):1155–65. doi: 10.1101/140954
83. Moradi A, Amin RM, Thorne JE. The role of gender in juvenile idiopathic arthritis-associated uveitis. *J Ophthalmol* (2014) 2014:461078. doi: 10.1155/2014/461078
84. Takeuchi M, Kastner DL, Remmers EF. The immunogenetics of Behcet's disease: A comprehensive review. *J Autoimmunity* (2015) 64:137–48. doi: 10.1016/j.jaut.2015.08.013
85. Sanjanwala B, Draghi M, Norman PJ, Guethlein LA, Parham P. Polymorphic sites away from the Bw4 epitope that affect interaction of Bw4+ HLA-B with KIR3DL1. *J Immunol (Baltimore Md 1950)* (2008) 181(9):6293–300. doi: 10.4049/jimmunol.181.9.6293
86. Damico FM, Cunha-Neto E, Goldberg AC, Iwai LK, Marin ML, Hammer J, et al. T-cell recognition and cytokine profile induced by melanocyte epitopes in patients with HLA-DRB1*0405-positive and -negative Vogt-Koyanagi-Harada uveitis. *Invest Ophthalmol Visual Sci* (2005) 46(7):2465–71. doi: 10.1167/iovs.04-1273
87. Shah J, Shah A, Hassman L, Gutierrez A. Ocular Manifestations of Inflammatory Bowel Disease. *Inflamm bowel Dis* (2021). doi: 10.1093/ibd/izaa359
88. Takeuchi M, Ombrello MJ, Kirino Y, Erer B, Tugal-Tutkun I, Seyahi E, et al. A single endoplasmic reticulum aminopeptidase-1 protein allotype is a strong risk factor for Behcet's disease in HLA-B*51 carriers. *Ann Rheumatic Dis* (2016) 75(12):2208–11. doi: 10.1136/annrheumdis-2015-209059
89. York IA, Brehm MA, Zendzian S, Towne CF, Rock KL. Endoplasmic reticulum aminopeptidase 1 (ERAP1) trims MHC class I-presented peptides in vivo and plays an important role in immunodominance. *Proc Natl Acad Sci USA* (2006) 103(24):9202–7. doi: 10.1073/pnas.0603095103
90. Evans DM, Spencer CC, Pointon JJ, Su Z, Harvey D, Kochan G, et al. Interaction between ERAP1 and HLA-B27 in ankylosing spondylitis implicates peptide handling in the mechanism for HLA-B27 in disease susceptibility. *Nat Genet* (2011) 43(8):761–7. doi: 10.1038/ng0911-919a
91. Strange A, Capon F, Spencer CC, Knight J, Weale ME, Allen MH, et al. A genome-wide association study identifies new psoriasis susceptibility loci and an interaction between HLA-C and ERAP1. *Nat Genet* (2010) 42 (11):985–90. doi: 10.1038/ng.694
92. Guasp P, Barnea E, González-Escribano MF, Jiménez-Reinoso A, Regueiro JR, Admon A, et al. The Behçet's disease-associated variant of the aminopeptidase ERAP1 shapes a low affinity HLA-B*51 peptidome by differential subpeptidome processing. *J Biol Chem* (2017) 292:9680–9. doi: 10.1074/jbc.M117.789180

93. Trowsdale J. Genetic and functional relationships between MHC and NK receptor genes. *Immunity* (2001) 15(3):363–74. doi: 10.1016/S1074-7613(01)00197-2
94. Erer B, Takeuchi M, Ustek D, Tugal-Tutkun I, Seyahi E, Ozyazgan Y, et al. Evaluation of KIR3DL1/KIR3DS1 polymorphism in Behcet's disease. *Genes Immun* (2016) 17(7):396–9. doi: 10.1038/gene.2016.36
95. Middleton D, Meenagh A, Sleator C, Gourraud PA, Ayna T, Tozkir H, et al. No association of KIR genes with Behcet's disease. *Tissue Antigens* (2007) 70(5):435–8. doi: 10.1111/j.1399-0039.2007.00929.x
96. Moon SJ, Oh EJ, Kim Y, Kim KS, Kwok SK, Ju JH, et al. Diversity of killer cell immunoglobulin-like receptor genes in uveitis associated with autoimmune diseases: ankylosing spondylitis and Behcet disease. *Ocular Immunol Inflammation* (2013) 21(2):135–43. doi: 10.3109/09273948.2012.754905
97. Castaño-Núñez Á, Montes-Cano MA, García-Lozano JR, Ortego-Centeno N, García-Hernández FJ, Espinosa G, et al. Association of Functional Polymorphisms of KIR3DL1/DS1 With Behçet's Disease. *Front Immunol* (2019) 10:2755. doi: 10.3389/fimmu.2019.02755
98. Petrushkin H, Norman PJ, Lougee E, Parham P, Wallace GR, Stanford MR, et al. KIR3DL1/S1 Allotypes Contribute Differentially to the Development of Behcet Disease. *J Immunol (Baltimore Md 1950)* (2019) 203(6):1629–35. doi: 10.4049/jimmunol.1801178
99. Levinson RD, Du Z, Luo L, Holland GN, Rao NA, Reed EF, et al. KIR and HLA gene combinations in Vogt-Koyanagi-Harada disease. *Hum Immunol* (2008) 69(6):349–53. doi: 10.1016/j.humimm.2008.04.005
100. Levinson RD, Okada AA, Ashouri E, Keino H, Rajalingam R. Killer cell immunoglobulin-like receptor gene-cluster 3DS1-2DL5-2DS1-2DS5 predisposes susceptibility to Vogt-Koyanagi-Harada syndrome in Japanese individuals. *Hum Immunol* (2010) 71(2):192–4. doi: 10.1016/j.humimm.2009.11.001
101. Sheereen A, Gaafar A, Iqneibi A, Eldali A, Tabbara KF, Adra C, et al. A study of KIR genes and HLA-C in Vogt-Koyanagi-Harada disease in Saudi Arabia. *Mol Vision* (2011) 17:3523–8.
102. Murphy CA, Langrish CL, Chen Y, Blumenschein W, McClanahan T, Kastelein RA, et al. Divergent pro- and antiinflammatory roles for IL-23 and IL-12 in joint autoimmune inflammation. *J Exp Med* (2003) 198(12):1951–7. doi: 10.1084/jem.20030896
103. Gaffen SL, Jain R, Garg AV, Cua DJ. The IL-23-IL-17 immune axis: from mechanisms to therapeutic testing. *Nat Rev Immunol* (2014) 14(9):585–600. doi: 10.1038/nri3707
104. Zhong Z, Su G, Kijlstra A, Yang P. Activation of the interleukin-23/interleukin-17 signalling pathway in autoinflammatory and autoimmune uveitis. *Prog Retin Eye Res* (2020) 100866:1–24. doi: 10.1016/j.preteyeres.2020.100866
105. Ten Berge B, Paats MS, Bergen IM, van den Blink B, Hoogsteden HC, Lambrecht BN, et al. Increased IL-17A expression in granulomas and in circulating memory T cells in sarcoidosis. *Rheumatol (Oxford England)* (2012) 51(1):37–46. doi: 10.1093/rheumatology/ker316
106. Chi W, Yang P, Li B, Wu C, Jin H, Zhu X, et al. IL-23 promotes CD4+ T cells to produce IL-17 in Vogt-Koyanagi-Harada disease. *J Allergy Clin Immunol* (2007) 119(5):1218–24. doi: 10.1016/j.jaci.2007.01.010
107. Yang P, Foster CS. Interleukin 21, interleukin 23, and transforming growth factor beta1 in HLA-A29-associated birdshot retinochoroidopathy. *Am J Ophthalmol* (2013) 156(2):400–6:e2. doi: 10.1016/j.ajo.2013.03.004
108. Nishikomori R, Usui T, Wu CY, Morinobu A, O'Shea JJ, Strober W. Activated STAT4 has an essential role in Th1 differentiation and proliferation that is independent of its role in the maintenance of IL-12R beta 2 chain expression and signaling. *J Immunol (Baltimore Md 1950)* (2002) 169(8):4388–98. doi: 10.4049/jimmunol.169.8.4388
109. Zierhut M, Mizuki N, Ohno S, Inoko H, Gul A, Onoe K, et al. Immunology and functional genomics of Behcet's disease. *Cell Mol Life Sci CMLS* (2003) 60(9):1903–22. doi: 10.1007/s00018-003-2333-3
110. Horie Y, Meguro A, Ohta T, Lee EB, Namba K, Mizuuchi K, et al. HLA-B51 Carriers are Susceptible to Ocular Symptoms of Behçet Disease and the Association between the Two Becomes Stronger towards the East along the Silk Road: A Literature Survey. *Ocular Immunol Inflammation* (2017) 25(1):37–40. doi: 10.3109/09273948.2015.1136422
111. Kaburaki T, Takamoto M, Numaga J, Kawashima H, Araie M, Ohnogi Y, et al. Genetic association of HLA-A*2601 with ocular Behcet's disease in Japanese patients. *Clin Exp Rheumatol* (2010) 28(4 Suppl 60):S39–44.
112. Darlington P, Tallstedt L, Padyukov L, Kockum I, Cederlund K, Eklund A, et al. HLA-DRB1* alleles and symptoms associated with Heerfordt's syndrome in sarcoidosis. *Eur Respir J* (2011) 38(5):1151–7. doi: 10.1183/09031936.00025011
113. Naruse TK, Matsuzawa Y, Ota M, Katsuyama Y, Matsumori A, Hara M, et al. HLA-DQB1*0601 is primarily associated with the susceptibility to cardiac sarcoidosis. *Tissue Antigens* (2000) 56(1):52–7. doi: 10.1034/j.1399-0039.2000.560107.x
114. Darlington P, Gabrielsen A, Sorensson P, Tallstedt L, Padyukov L, Eklund A, et al. HLA-alleles associated with increased risk for extra-pulmonary involvement in sarcoidosis. *Tissue Antigens* (2014) 83(4):267–72. doi: 10.1111/tan.12326
115. Mackensen F, David F, Schwenger V, Smith LK, Rajalingam R, Levinson RD, et al. HLA-DRB1*0102 is associated with TINU syndrome and bilateral, sudden-onset anterior uveitis but not with interstitial nephritis alone. *Br J Ophthalmol* (2011) 95(7):971–5. doi: 10.1136/bjo.2010.187955
116. Lezcano-Meza D, Dávila-Dávila B, Vega-Miranda A, Negrete-García MC, Teran LM. Interleukin (IL)-4 and to a lesser extent either IL-13 or interferon-gamma regulate the production of eotaxin-2/CCL24 in nasal polyps. *Allergy* (2003) 58(10):1011–7. doi: 10.1034/j.1398-9995.2003.00174.x
117. Gamalero L, Simonini G, Ferrara G, Polizzi S, Giani T, Cimaz R. Evidence-Based Treatment for Uveitis. *Isr Med Assoc J* (2019) 21(7):475–9.
118. Duica I, Voinea LM, Mitulescu C, Istrate S, Coman IC, Ciuluvica R. The use of biologic therapies in uveitis. *Rom J Ophthalmol* (2018) 62(2):105–13. doi: 10.22336/rjo.2018.16
119. Jaffe GJ, Dick AD, Brezin AP, Nguyen QD, Thorne JE, Kestelyn P, et al. Adalimumab in Patients with Active Noninfectious Uveitis. *New Engl J Med* (2016) 375(10):932–43. doi: 10.1056/NEJMoa1509852
120. Nguyen QD, Merrill PT, Jaffe GJ, Dick AD, Kurup SK, Sheppard J, et al. Adalimumab for prevention of uveitic flare in patients with inactive non-infectious uveitis controlled by corticosteroids (VISUAL II): a multicentre, double-masked, randomised, placebo-controlled phase 3 trial. *Lancet* (2016) 388(10050):1183–92. doi: 10.1016/S0140-6736(16)31339-3
121. Suhler EB, Adan A, Brezin AP, Fortin E, Goto H, Jaffe GJ, et al. Safety and Efficacy of Adalimumab in Patients with Noninfectious Uveitis in an Ongoing Open-Label Study: VISUAL III. *Ophthalmology* (2018) 125(7):1075–87. doi: 10.1016/j.ophtha.2017.12.039
122. Fabiani C, Vitale A, Emmi G, Lopalco G, Vannozzi L, Guerriero S, et al. Interleukin (IL)-1 inhibition with anakinra and canakinumab in Behcet's disease-related uveitis: a multicenter retrospective observational study. *Clin Rheumatol* (2017) 36(1):191–7. doi: 10.1007/s10067-016-3506-4
123. Cantarini L, Vitale A, Scalini P, Dinarello CA, Rigante D, Franceschini R, et al. Anakinra treatment in drug-resistant Behcet's disease: a case series. *Clin Rheumatol* (2015) 34(7):1293–301. doi: 10.1007/s10067-013-2443-8
124. Caso F, Costa L, Rigante D, Lucherini OM, Caso P, Bascherini V, et al. Biological treatments in Behcet's disease: beyond anti-TNF therapy. *Mediators Inflammation* (2014) 2014:107421. doi: 10.1155/2014/107421
125. Vitale A, Rigante D, Caso F, Brizi MG, Galeazzi M, Costa L, et al. Inhibition of interleukin-1 by canakinumab as a successful mono-drug strategy for the treatment of refractory Behcet's disease: a case series. *Dermatology* (2014) 228(3):211–4. doi: 10.1159/000358125
126. Baerveldt EM, Kappen JH, Thio HB, van Laar JA, van Hagen PM, Prens EP. Successful long-term triple disease control by ustekinumab in a patient with Behcet's disease, psoriasis and hidradenitis suppurativa. *Ann Rheumatic Dis* (2013) 72(4):626–7. doi: 10.1136/annrheumdis-2012-202392
127. Langley RG, Armstrong AW, Lebwohl MG, Blauvelt A, Hsu S, Tyring S, et al. Efficacy and safety of brodalumab in patients with psoriasis who had inadequate responses to ustekinumab: subgroup analysis of two randomized phase III trials. *Br J Dermatol* (2019) 180(2):306–14. doi: 10.1111/bjd.17318
128. Langley RG, Tsai TF, Flavin S, Song M, Randazzo B, Wasfi Y, et al. Efficacy and safety of guselkumab in patients with psoriasis who have an inadequate response to ustekinumab: results of the randomized, double-blind, phase III NAVIGATE trial. *Br J Dermatol* (2018) 178(1):114–23. doi: 10.1111/bjd.15750

129. Mirouse A, Barete S, Desbois AC, Comarmond C, Sene D, Domont F, et al. Long-Term Outcome of Ustekinumab Therapy for Behcet's Disease. *Arthritis Rheumatol (Hoboken NJ)* (2019) 71(10):1727–32. doi: 10.1002/art.40912
130. Mirouse A, Barete S, Monfort JB, Resche-Rigon M, Bouyer AS, Comarmond C, et al. Ustekinumab for Behçet's disease. *J Autoimmun* (2017) 82:41–6. doi: 10.1016/j.jaut.2017.05.002
131. Weinstein JE, Pepple KL. Cytokines in uveitis. *Curr Opin Ophthalmol* (2018) 29(3):267–74. doi: 10.1097/ICU.0000000000000466
132. Atienza-Mateo B, Calvo-Rio V, Beltran E, Martinez-Costa L, Valls-Pascual E, Hernandez-Garfella M, et al. Anti-interleukin 6 receptor tocilizumab in refractory uveitis associated with Behcet's disease: multicentre retrospective study. *Rheumatol (Oxford England)* (2018) 57(5):856–64. doi: 10.1093/rheumatology/kex480
133. Hueber W, Patel DD, Dryja T, Wright AM, Koroleva I, Bruin G, et al. Effects of AIN457, a fully human antibody to interleukin-17A, on psoriasis, rheumatoid arthritis, and uveitis. *Sci Transl Med* (2010) 2(52):52ra72. doi: 10.1126/scitranslmed.3001107
134. Di Scala G, Bettiol A, Cojan RD, Finocchi M, Silvestri E, Emmi G. Efficacy of the anti-IL 17 secukinumab in refractory Behçet's syndrome: A preliminary study. *J Autoimmunity* (2019) 97:108–13. doi: 10.1016/j.jaut.2018.09.002
135. Letko E, Yeh S, Foster CS, Pleyer U, Brigell M, Grosskreutz CL. Efficacy and safety of intravenous secukinumab in noninfectious uveitis requiring steroid-sparing immunosuppressive therapy. *Ophthalmology* (2015) 122(5):939–48. doi: 10.1016/j.ophtha.2014.12.033
136. Dick AD, Tugal-Tutkun I, Foster S, Zierhut M, Melissa Liew SH, Bezlyak V, et al. Secukinumab in the treatment of noninfectious uveitis: results of three randomized, controlled clinical trials. *Ophthalmology* (2013) 120(4):777–87. doi: 10.1016/j.ophtha.2012.09.040

19

Ocular Microbiota and Intraocular Inflammation

Jing Jing Li, Sanjun Yi and Lai Wei**

State Key Laboratory of Ophthalmology, Zhongshan Ophthalmic Center, Sun Yat-sen University, Guangzhou, China

Correspondence:
Jing Jing Li
lijingjing@gzzoc.com
Lai Wei
weil9@mail.sysu.edu.cn

The term ocular microbiota refers to all types of commensal and pathogenic microorganisms present on or in the eye. The ocular surface is continuously exposed to the environment and harbors various commensals. Commensal microbes have been demonstrated to regulate host metabolism, development of immune system, and host defense against pathogen invasion. An unbalanced microbiota could lead to pathogenic microbial overgrowth and cause local or systemic inflammation. The specific antigens that irritate the deleterious immune responses in various inflammatory eye diseases remain obscure, while recent evidence implies a microbial etiology of these illnesses. The purpose of this review is to provide an overview of the literature on ocular microbiota and the role of commensal microbes in several eye diseases. In addition, this review will also discuss the interaction between microbial pathogens and host factors involved in intraocular inflammation, and evaluate therapeutic potential of targeting ocular microbiota to treat intraocular inflammation.

Keywords: ocular microbiota, ocular surface microbiome, intraocular inflammation, eye, ocular inflammatory disease

INTRODUCTION

As the term microbiota refers to all types of microorganisms present in or on human body, the term ocular microbiota refers to all types of microorganisms present in or on the eyes. Ever since the launch of the Human Microbiome Project, our understanding toward the diversity and composition of commensal microbiota has been expanding. It has been evidenced that commensal microbiota plays fundamental roles in regulating host physiology, induction and development of immune

Abbreviations: AMD, age-related macular degeneration; DR, diabetic retinopathy; CNS, central nervous system; RGC, retinal ganglion cell; BD, Behcet's disease; rRNA, ribosomal RNA; ITS, internal transcribed spacer; PMNs, polymorphonuclear leukocytes; ACAID, anterior chamber-associated immune deviation; cfu, colony-forming unit; HLA-B27, human leukocyte antigen-B27; MHC, major histocompatability complex; EAU, experimental autoimmune uveitis; IRBP, interphotoreceptor retinoid binding protein; TCR, T cell receptor; CF, complement factor H; ARMS2, age-related maculopathy susceptibility 2; TIMP3, tissue inhibitor of metalloproteinases-3; MMP9, matrix metallopeptidase 9; APOE, apolipoprotein E; LIPC, lipase C; CETP, cholesteryl ester transfer protein; ABCA1, ATP-binding cassette transporter; RPE, retinal pigment epithelium; LPS, lipopolysaccharide; TLR, Toll-like receptor; PAMP, pathogen-associated molecular pattern; DAMP, damage-associated molecular pattern; APC, antigen presenting cells; PRR, pattern recognition receptors; TIR, Toll/IL-1 receptor; MyD88, Myeloid differentiating factor 88; TRIF, TIR domain containing adaptor inducing interferon β; TIRAP, TIR domain-containing adaptor protein; TRAM, TRIF-related adaptor molecule; IRF, interferon regulatory factor; MAPK, mitogen-activate protein kinase; AAU, acute anterior uveitis; DC, dendritic cells; VCAM-1, vascular cell adhesion molecule-1; ICAM-1, intercellular cell adhesion molecule-1; MIP, macrophage inflammatory protein; MCP-1, monocyte chemotactic protein-1.

system, as well as host defense against pathogen invasion, albeit dysbiosis (unbalanced microbiota) could lead to pathogenic microbial overgrowth and cause local or systemic inflammation (1). The ocular surface is directly exposed to the external environment and endangered by various pathogenic microorganisms. These facts combined with our recent findings of intraocular microbes raise intense research interest in clarifying the role of ocular microbiota in ocular health and diseases.

The ocular immune system is composed of a complex network of innate and adaptive components. Infection or autoimmunity could lead to intraocular inflammation which is associated with a multitude of sight-threatening diseases, which include but may not be limited to endophthalmitis, uveitis, age-related macular degeneration (AMD), glaucoma, and diabetic retinopathy (DR). Intraocular inflammation exerts deleterious effects on vision integrity since the delicate ocular components, such as the retina and the cornea, are unable to regenerate. The eye is an immunologically privileged organ. Up to date, the specific antigens that irritate the deleterious immune responses in the immune privileged site in those diseases remain obscure. A growing body of research has shown that commensal microbes might be the trigger of intraocular inflammation. Here, we discuss evidence for the relationship between microbes and ocular diseases, discuss microbial pathogen and host factors, including the molecular and cellular interactions, involved in non-infectious intraocular inflammation, and evaluate therapeutic potential of targeting ocular microbiota to treat intraocular inflammation.

THE OCULAR MICROBIOTA

The ocular surface is the interface between the eye and the environment which comprises the cornea, the conjunctiva, the tear film, and the eyelids. It has been much debated whether the microorganisms in our environment are able to adhere to and colonize the ocular surface, because during eye blinking, tears secreted from the lacrimal gland of the eyes contain lysozyme that could kill bacteria and wash the ocular surface (1). Supporting evidence for the existence of ocular surface microorganisms arises from microbial cultivation studies documented first in 1930 (2). Many subsequent results from similar studies are in line with the first discovery. Swabs from different parts of the ocular surface were incubated in bacteria growth media (mostly blood and chocolate agar). The incubations occur in aerobic, anaerobic, or 5% CO_2 for up to 14 days at body temperature (3). These culture-based methods are invaluable in a historical perspective in confirming the existence of a microbiota and identifying microorganisms. The common bacteria isolated from these sites of the eye are Gram-positive genera, including coagulase-negative *Staphylococcus*, *Streptococcus*, *Propionibacterium*, *Diphtheroid bacteria* and *Micrococcus* (4). Some genera that are abundant in the gut flora, such as *Escherichia*, *Enterococcus*, *Lactobacillus*, and *Bacillus* are less common on the normal ocular surface (4). Gram-negative genera, such as *Haemophilus*, *Neisseria*, *Pseudomonas*, and fungal isolates are even rarer but can also be isolated and cultured from the surface of eyes without obvious signs of inflammation or infection (4, 5). The most common ocular surface bacteria are coagulase-negative *Staphylococci* which present in 20–80% of the swabs from the conjunctiva and 30–100% of the swabs from the lids (4). The density of microbes recovered are usually lowest from tears while higher from conjunctiva and eye lid (3). Types of the ocular surface microbes identified are consistent with results from studies of cultivable microbiota from contact lenses, which also suggest that coagulase-negative *Staphylococcus* is the most common genera, and less commonly *Bacillus*, *Micrococcus*, and fungi (3).

The ocular surface and the sclera enwrap the interior ocular cavity. The cavity enclosed by the ocular outer compartments mainly consists of the anterior chamber, the posterior chamber, the ciliary body, and the vitreous body (**Figure 1**). Historically, the intraocular environment has been deemed sterile on account of its closed anatomical structure as well as protection provided

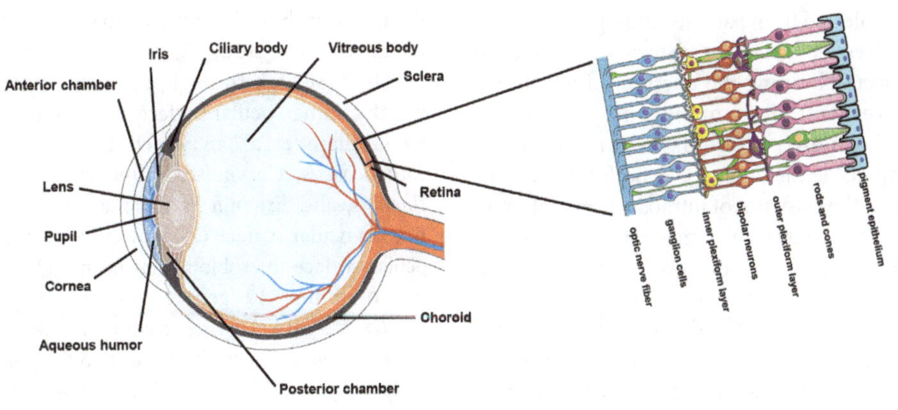

FIGURE 1 | Anatomy of the eye.

by the tight and restrictive blood-retina barrier unless it is invaded by pathogens due to unnatural circumstances. Contamination could occur when the outer ocular compartments are damaged during an intraocular surgical procedure or following an injury caused by a penetrating foreign object (6, 7). For example, post-operative infectious endophthalmitis is a rare but serious vision-threatening complication of ocular surgery (e.g., cataract extraction) which involves inflammation of both the anterior and posterior segments of the eye. Post-operative endophthalmitis is presumably attributed to the diffusion of microorganisms from the patient's conjunctival or skin flora into the sterile intraocular compartments of the eye during surgery and cause overwhelming inflammation (8). Besides, diseased conditions that are associated with retinal vascular lesions could introduce microbial invasions from the circulating blood as normal human blood contains appreciable numbers of microorganisms (9–12). For example, one of the early pathological features of DR, a common diabetes complication in the eye, is retinal vascular leakage (13). Coincidently, DR has been demonstrated to be affected by microbiome (14, 15). Furthermore, some microbes (mainly viruses) could spread along the nerves. Cases of infections occurred in the central nervous system (CNS) by neurological spread are not sparse. Ocular infection could be secondary to a CNS infection. For instance, it has been reported that rabies virus infected in the hind limbs of mice could travel along the peripheral nerve and the axon to the brain and then spread to the eye through the optic nerve where it infects the retinal ganglion cell (RGC) but not the photoreceptors (16).

The vitreous humor and aqueous humor contain a variety of organic and anorganic components that form an excellent cultivating medium for microorganisms (17, 18). In the late 19th century, researchers found that microorganisms, such as *Bacillus Subtilis* and *Bacillus Megaterium* grew extremely well in the aqueous humor withdrawn from living body (18). In some studies by others, *Propionibacterium acnes* (*P. acnes*) was detected in the granuloma of the retina in patients with ocular sarcoidosis where accumulated $CD4^+$ cells and $CD68^+$ cells were also nearby, suggesting that *P. acnes* could be associated with sarcoid uveitis (19, 20). In line with their findings, we were able to detect the expression of *P. acnes* mRNA in most aqueous humor specimens we collected from patients undergoing cataract surgeries who were free of active or history of intraocular inflammation and infection, raising the question of whether *P. acnes* is a benign resident or a pathogenic intraocular microorganism and whether there is a community of microorganisms living inside the human eye. So far, there is no direct documentation of the existence of intraocular microbiome. This is possibly because the intraocular materials from healthy human eye are difficult to acquire. In our preliminary study, the intraocular microbial communities were significantly different among patients with distinct ocular diseases. Whether the intraocular microbiome lives in symbiosis with the host just as the intestinal microbiome and whether alteration of intraocular microbiome contributes to the ocular health and the etiology of ocular diseases in general remain to be examined.

DEFINING THE OCULAR MICROBIOTA

Methods to define a microbiota can be generally divided into culture-based techniques and non-culture-based techniques. The culture-based techniques depend on phenotypic characteristics of microbes to estimate the microbial load, for example, the ability of microbes in a sample to proliferate in or on a specified growth medium under a specified growth condition (21, 22). Although it provides a rough evaluation of microbial density and diversity in specimens, these measures are often inaccurate and biased. The cultivable species may only represent a small proportion of the real microbial populations in the samples which are prone to grow under the applied cultivation conditions (23, 24). In addition, the estimation of microbial density in a certain sample also varies according to a wide range of factors that may affect the proliferation ability of microbes. Some microbes are even uncultivable on traditional laboratory medium. Currently, only half of the bacterial phyla have cultivated representatives (25). Indeed, variations in types and density of microorganisms that can be cultured from the ocular surface exist in many published studies (23, 26).

The more advanced non-culture diagnostic methods are immunoassays, which target microbe-secreted peptides or microbial antigen, and metagenomic sequencing, which target microbial RNA or DNA. Both methods allow study of the community of the microbes present without obtaining pure cultures. Methods targeting microbial nucleic acids do not require specific antibodies making them more readily available for laboratory study. 16S ribosomal RNA (rRNA) is commonly used for taxonomic purposes for bacteria, while 18S rRNA and internal transcribed spacer (ITS) are used for fungi. To define microbial species, the 16S/18S/ITS gene amplicons are usually sequenced and the sequence will be matched with the repository of existing sequence to yield taxonomic information. Nowadays, more than 9,000 16S rRNA gene sequences have been deposited in GenBank, rendering 16S rRNA gene sequence analysis a better tool to identify those rarely isolated, poorly described, and uncultivable bacteria (27). Another sequencing method called shotgun metagenomics can achieve species- and strain-level resolution. It examines the entire genome as opposed to only the 16S/18S/ITS amplicons, but its high costs and heavy demands on bioinformatic analyses precluded its extensive use for microbiome study (28).

The first high-throughput study to explore the diversity of healthy human ocular surface microbiome was published in 2007 by Graham et al. in which they identified *Staphylococcus*, *Rhodococcus*, *Corynebacterium*, *Propionibacterium*, *Klebsiella*, *Bacillus*, and *Erwinia* as the main bacterial genera on healthy human ocular surface (2). However, the composition of the "core ocular surface microbiota" has been highly contested. Dong et al. proposed that 12 genera—*Pseudomonas*, *Propionibacterium*, *Bradyrhizobium*, *Corynebacterium*, *Acinetobacter*, *Brevundimonas*, *Staphylococcus*, *Aquabacterium*, *Sphingomonas*, *Streptococcus*, *Streptophyta*, and *Methylobacterium*—represented the putative "core" of conjunctival microbiota (29). Another study claimed that *Corynebacterium*, *Streptococcus*, *Propionibacterium*, *Bacillus*,

Staphylococcus, and *Ralsontia* were detected in 80% of the 105 samples tested and together accounted for more than a third of the entire bacterial community characterized (30). The core conjunctival microbial communities were later shown to be composed of *Corynebacterium*, *Pseudomonas*, *Staphylococcus*, *Acinetobacter*, *Streptococcus*, *Millisia*, *Anaerococcus*, *Finegoldia*, *Simonsiella*, and *Veillonella* (31). Doan et al. applied three different techniques to explore the healthy human conjunctiva microbiome: bacterial culture, 16S rDNA gene deep sequencing, and biome representational in silico karyotyping. They found that *Corynebacteria*, *Propionibacterium*, and coagulase-negative *Staphylococcus* were the predominant organisms (32). A study by Ozkan et al. reported that *Corynebacterium*, *Acinetobacteria*, *Pseudomonas*, *Sphingomonas*, *Streptococcus*, *Massilia*, and *Rothia* accounted for 80% of the operational taxanomic units (OTUs) and microbial genera on the ocular surface (24). The metagenomic data collected from our laboratory revealed that *Propionibacterium*, *Staphylococcus*, *Escherichia*, and *Micrococcus* were the most abundant ocular surface microbial genera in healthy humans (33). Li et al. found the predominant genera to be *Pseudomonas*, *Acinetobacter*, *Bacillus*, *Chryseobacterium*, and *Corynebacterium* (34). The more recent study carried out by Suzuki et al. demonstrated that the ocular surface was typically dominated by *Propionibacterium* in the young subjects and by *Corynebacterium* or *Neisseriaceae* in the elderly subjects (35).

Although metagenomic sequencing offers substantial information about the diversity of the ocular microbiome and reveal previously unidentified microbial species by the traditional culture-based methods, inconsistency remains between several studies using similar sequencing techniques (**Table 1**). Therefore, culture-based methods are sometimes combined with non-culture-based methods to prove the existence of a microbe. Most of the metagenomic sequencing results support *Corynebacterium*, *Propionibacterium*, and *Staphylococcus* as the dominant taxons of healthy ocular surface. This expands the list of the most common genera recovered by culture-based methods, *i.e.* the coagulase-negative *Staphylococcus*. Noteworthy, metagenomic sequencing results could also be complicated by several factors, such as small sample size (36), depth of swabs (37, 38), and contaminations from DNA extraction kit and PCR reagents (39, 40) and so forth. Nonetheless, it remains the best state-of-the-art tool for *in situ* profiling of a microbiota. Utilizing this powerful metagenomic sequencing tool, we have also characterized the intraocular microbiota of the aqueous humor from patients with ocular diseases that required surgical intervention. We found that each disease has a unique intraocular microbial signature, suggesting a potential link between intraocular microbiota and ocular health and diseases.

FACTORS CHANGING THE OCULAR MICROBIOTA

The ocular surface microbiota can be influenced by environmental conditions, age, gender, personal habits, contact lens wear, disease states, antibiotics, and infection etc (41). Understanding toward the factors that alter the intraocular microbiota is still in its infancy. As the intraocular space is relatively separated from the outer environment, it is reasonable to speculate that the intraocular microbiota is more imaginably associated with host factors.

Age and sex hormone have significant impacts on immune regulation and ocular health (33). Our study showed that age groups differs significantly in bacterial composition and metabolic functions, and that gender factor only affects β but not α diversity of bacterial composition. Our data suggest that age and gender can collectively shape the ocular surface microbiome, while age appears to be a stronger factor in reshaping the ocular surface microbiome (33). However, some earlier studies showed contradictory findings: Ozkan et al (24). found no effect of age on the microbial a diversity and a higher Shannon diversity index in males; Zhou et al. found no effect of sex on the microbial diversity and a higher richness and Shannon diversity index in children less than 10 years old (30). This inconsistency may be explained by the fact that the techniques used were different in these studies. We used metagenomic sequencing approach which may detect a much broader range of microbes (33).

Dry eye syndrome is a multi-pathogenic factorial disease of the ocular surface characterized by loss of homeostasis of the tear film which results in excessive evaporation of tears in most of the

TABLE 1 | Core ocular surface microbiome in healthy adults.

Genera of bacteria	Number of samples	Reference
Staphylococcus, Bacillus, Rhodococcus, Corynebacterium, Propionibacterium, Klebsiella, and *Erwinia*	57	(2)
Pseudomonas, Propionibacterium, Bradyrhizobium, Corynebacterium, Acinetobacter, Brevundimonas, Staphylococcus, Aquabacterium, Sphingomonas, Streptococcus, Streptophyta, and *Methylobacterium*	4	(29)
Corynebacterium, Streptococcus, Propionibacterium, Bacillus, Staphylococcus, and *Ralsontia*	105	(30)
Corynebacterium, Pseudomonas, Staphylococcus, Acinetobacter, Streptococcus, Millisia, Anaerococcus, Finegoldia, Simonsiella, and *Veillonella*	31	(31)
Corynebacteria, Propionibacteria, and *Staphylococcus*	107	(32)
Corynebacterium, Acinetobacteria, Pseudomonas, Sphingomonas, Streptococcus, Massilia, and *Rothia*	45	(24)
Propionibacterium, Staphylococcus, Escherichia, and *Micrococcus*	90	(33)
Pseudomonas, Acinetobacter, Bacillus, Chryseobacterium, and Corynebacterium	54	(34)
Propionibacterium, Corynebacterium, and *Neisseriaceae*	36	(35)

cases. Meibomian glands located in the eyelids are responsible for the secretion of oily components for the tear film to protect the ocular surface from overt dryness, discomfort, or damage. Meibomian gland dysfunction often leads to evaporative dry eye syndrome. Inconsistencies in the microbial species that changed by dry eye syndrome and meibomian gland dysfunction remain in several studies (34, 42, 43). This may again be explained by sample size, sequencing approach, and different diagnostic criteria. For example, it has been reported that some cases of meibomian gland dysfunction overlap with not only dry eye syndrome but also blepharitis (44). No conclusive results have been achieved by these analyses, yet the results hinted that the ocular surface "resident microbiota", *Corynebacterium*, is likely associated with these diseases. However, it is still unclear that whether the change of the ocular surface microbiota is a cause or a consequence of the ocular surface disorders.

Patients with other diseases such as diabetes, high cholesterol and triglycerides, conjunctivitis, autoimmune diseases like Behcet's disease (BD), rheumatoid arthritis, and Sjögren's syndrome, which are linked with meibomian gland dysfunction and dry eye syndrome have also been reported with altered ocular surface microbiota (45–53). These suggest that endogenous host factors other than age and gender may be equally important in shaping the ocular surface microbiome, or the change of ocular surface microbiome may be secondary to meibomian gland dysfunction or dry eye syndrome. Further investigations are needed to dissociate data of patients with meibomian gland dysfunction or dry eye syndrome from those without in order to provide insights into finding the endogenous host factors that alter ocular surface microbiome.

INTRAOCULAR INFLAMMATION

Intraocular inflammation has two types: acute and chronic. The acute intraocular inflammation as observed in post-operative or post-traumatic endophthalmitis is normally caused by pathogenic microbes and is capable of inducing robust changes in blood-retina barrier permeability and subsequent infiltration of non-resident immune cells, such as polymorphonuclear leukocytes (PMNs) and macrophages (**Figure 2**) (54). The chronic form accounting for most intraocular inflammation appears to arise from a combination of predisposing genetic and environmental factors. A break of immune tolerance against endogenous antigens, followed by autoantibody production, dysregulation of effector and regulatory T cells, and infiltration of T lymphocytes and macrophages, is usually the mechanistic basis for chronic intraocular inflammation associated with inflammatory ocular diseases, particularly uveitis.

The eye is an immunologically privileged organ. The anterior chamber, the vitreous cavity, and the subretinal space of the eyes, are immune privileged sites where multiple mechanisms work together to inhibit overt immune responses (55). The conjunctiva and the interior of the eye are highly vascularized and home to many immune cells, suggesting that the eyes are under sophisticated regulation by immune system. Presumably due to an evolutionary adaption, our immune system uses several strategies to avoid intraocular inflammation, for example, immunological ignorance of eye-derived antigens, immune tolerance, and a local immunosuppressive or anti-inflammatory microenvironment created by blood-retina barriers and immunosuppressive/anti-inflammatory molecules

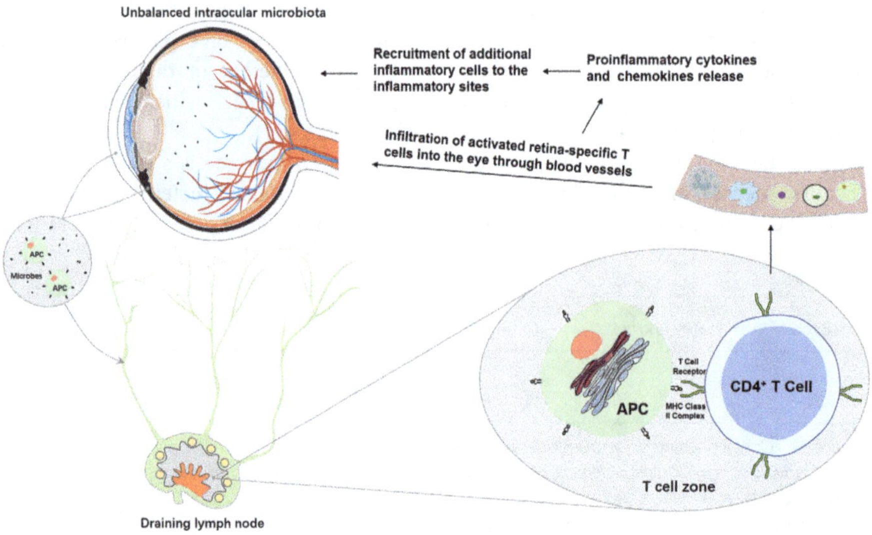

FIGURE 2 | Potential mechanisms of intraocular microbiome-mediated intraocular inflammation. Unbalanced intraocular microbiota can lead to overgrowth of pathogenic microbes which are surveyed by resident ocular APCs, such as ocular DCs. Immature APCs take up either the microbe as a whole or the microbial antigens in the eye to become mature. Through afferent lymphatic vessels, mature APCs migrate to the closest draining lymph nodes where they are recognized by $CD4^+$ T cells. Activated retina-specific T cells migrate into the eyes to secret proinflammatory cytokines and chemokines which may disrupt the blood-retina barrier and recruit additional inflammatory cells and mediators to the eyes to cause intraocular inflammation.

in ocular fluids or constitutively expressed by ocular parenchymal cells (55). These strategies are collectively known as ocular immune privilege. By virtue of ocular immune privilege, transplants into the eyes are not subjected to sight-destroying immune responses and inflammation. Antigen injected into these places induces peripheral tolerance to that antigen (56). A classic phenomenon is the anterior chamber-associated immune deviation (ACAID) in which injection of an antigen to the anterior chamber of the eye induces systemic immunoregulatory responses that are believed to protect the eye from future immune-mediated damage (57). Similarly, adeno-associated virus delivery to the subretinal space elicits only limited immune response (58, 59). However, in the face of antigen overload, the mechanisms of immune privilege cannot always effectively restrain the immune cells from infiltrating and responding. The C56BL/6 mice eyes intravitreally injected with 500 colony-forming unit (cfu) of *Staphylococcus aureus* were observed to reach 10^7 cfu 24 hours post injection and eventually reduced the number to 5×10^3 cfu by 72 hours. During the 3 day course, mice had few infiltrating inflammatory cells and no microscopic retinal damage. By contrast, eyes intravitreally injected with 5,000 cfu of the same microbes resulted in massive infiltration and severe damage to ocular structures (60).

OCULAR INFLAMMATORY DISEASES ARE ASSOCIATED WITH NON-OCULAR MICROBIOTA

The microbiota was once considered to be inert in immune homeostasis. However, over the past decades, pivotal roles of dysbiosis (changes in the gut commensal microbiota) in human health have been established. Dysbiosis has been implicated in various diseases associated with systemic inflammation, including rheumatoid arthritis, multiple sclerosis, inflammatory bowel disease, and type 1 diabetes (61–67). In recent years, gut commensals have also been involved in the pathogenesis of several non-infectious eye diseases like autoimmune uveitis, AMD, and glaucoma.

The eye is protected by a prompt immune response to clear pathogens or antigens. However, inappropriate intraocular inflammation, such as those occurs in various forms of uveitis could be fatal to the eye and its visual function. Uveitis is a group of eye diseases characterized by acute or chronic intraocular inflammation of infectious or non-infectious origin. Autoimmune uveitis arises without known infectious stimuli. In humans, uveitis has been associated with human leukocyte antigen-B27 (HLA-B27), a prominent major histocompatibility complex (MHC) class I-allele expressed on the white blood cell surface, suggesting innate etiology (68). Patients with acute anterior uveitis have distinct intestinal microbial signature (69). Animal models have provided tremendous insights into its mechanistic basis. HLA-B27 transgenic rats exhibited altered cecal microbiota compared to healthy controls (70). Other mouse models of induced or spontaneous uveitis also showed ameliorated inflammation when commensals were removed or reduced. A classic mouse model of autoimmune uveitis is the experimental autoimmune uveitis (EAU) in which interphotoreceptor retinoid binding protein (IRBP) and heat-killed *Mycobacterium tuberculosis* are co-administered in complete Freund's adjuvant and ocular inflammation begins around day 10. Fecal microbiota transplantation with feces from BD patients significantly exacerbated EAU and increased the production of inflammatory cytokines (71). In EAU, an intestinal dysbiosis accompanies a disruption in intestinal homeostasis was demonstrated (72). Microbial ablation by raising mice in germ-free environment or microbial reduction by the treatment of a combination of broad-spectrum antibiotics in EAU reduce the severity of ocular inflammation (73). The direct connection between intestinal microbiota and the eye was confirmed in a spontaneous uveitis mouse model in R161H mice which are engineered to express a transgene for T cell receptor (TCR) specific for IRBP. In these mice, retina-specific T cells are first activated by intestinal commensals in the gut through the autoreactive TCR and then trigger inflammation in the retina, implying that a commensal microbial antigen may mimic a retinal antigen to trigger autoimmune uveitis (**Figure 2**) (74). In line with this evidence, another study demonstrated that broad-spectrum oral antibiotics could attenuate EAU by increasing Tregs and decreasing effector T cells in the gut and extraintestinal tissues (75).

AMD is a progressive retinal degeneration and often associated with chronic low-grade intraocular inflammation. A substantial genome-wide association studies revealed that genetic variants in complement and various inflammatory pathway such as *complement factor* (*CF*) *H*, *CFI*, *age-related maculopathy susceptibility 2* (*ARMS2*), *tissue inhibitor of metalloproteinases-3* (*TIMP3*), and *matrix metallopeptidase 9* (*MMP9*), as well as in lipid pathway such as *apolipoprotein E* (*APOE*), *lipase C* (*LIPC*), *cholesteryl ester transfer protein* (*CETP*), and *ATP-binding cassette transporter* (*ABCA1*) were associated with the disease (76, 77). The identified variants, however, explain only 46–71% of the genomic heritability of AMD (78). This may be attributed to additional variation not identified, or to genetic interaction with environmental factors such as smoking, diet or sunlight exposure (76). Commensal bacteria as one potential environmental influence could play a role in AMD development. There are several reasons for such presumption: (i) Microbes are involved in the regulation of host immunity and lipid metabolism both of which have profound effects on chronic low-grade inflammation and are important in the pathogenesis of AMD. (ii) Drusen in AMD eyes contain anti-infectious components such as complement components, apolipoprotein E, amyloid β, vitronectin, immunoglobulins and C1Q (79). (iii) As discussed earlier, gut microorganisms could send signals that exert distal effects on a remote organ like the eye. Indeed, several studies have linked commensal microbiota to AMD pathogenesis. Patients with AMD have shown distinct intestinal, oral, nasal, and pharyngeal microbial communities, highlighting potential role of mucosal surface microbes in the pathogenesis of AMD (80–82). Mice fed a high-glycemic diet developed hallmarks of AMD, such as retinal pigment epithelium (RPE) hypopigmentation and atrophy, lipofuscin accumulation, and photoreceptor degeneration, whereas mice fed the lower-glycemia diet did no (83, 84). High-fat diet feeding in mice significantly influenced gut microbiota composition and exacerbated laser-induced model of neovascular AMD, also known as choroidal neovascularization (85). In our preliminary study, we observed that several intraocular bacteria were associated specifically with AMD and significantly enriched in soft drusen from AMD patients implying that bacterial infection may be a previously unappreciated etiology of early AMD.

Gut and oral commensals have been implicated in glaucoma which involves local inflammatory response. Astafurov et al. demonstrated that patients with glaucoma had higher oral bacterial load than patients without glaucoma, and that low-dose subcutaneous lipopolysaccharide (LPS) in two separate animal models of glaucoma resulted in enhanced glaucomatous neural degeneration (86). DBA/2J mice, which spontaneously develop high intraocular pressure, mild intraocular inflammation and glaucoma by 6–8 months of age, have been frequently used as a murine model for glaucoma (87). Interestingly, DBA/2J mice raised in germ-free environment do not display typical axonal degeneration and neuronal loss at 12 months of age (88). The study demonstrated that T cells at least partially mediated the glaucomatous pathology in DBA/2J mice raised under specific-pathogen-free conditions (88). A more recent study found that compared to healthy subjects, the gut microbiota of patients with primary open-angle glaucoma had a different gut microbiota profile (89).

The molecular mechanisms underlying the altered gut microbiota and the progression of these ocular inflammatory diseases remain obscure. Further investigations are required to elucidate whether translocation of microbes and/or microbial products (e.g., LPS, peptidoglycan, short-chain fatty acids, and microbial DNA) from the gastrointestinal tract or other mucosal surfaces to the eye through blood circulation or ocular lymphatics occurs during the progression of diseases.

MICROBIAL PATHOGENS AND HOST FACTORS IN INTRAOCULAR INFLAMMATION

During an event of intraocular inflammation, the immunosuppressive environment of the eye is compromised when pathogens or antigens are detected by local immune surveillance. An immune response is usually initiated by innate receptors, such as Toll-like receptors (TLRs), located in the retina. TLRs generally recognize pathogen-associated molecular patterns (PAMPs) and damage-associated molecular patterns (DAMPs). The former comprise microbial structures/nucleic acid sequences, while the latter are usually molecules released from host cells following tissue injury or damage. The complex interactions between PAMPs/DAMPs and host immune system are mediated through multiple host factors including antigen presenting cells (APCs), MHCs, and inflammatory mediators (**Figure 2**).

Toll-Like Receptors

The activation of an innate immune response is followed by the recognition of PAMPs on the surface of microbes by a group of receptors called pattern recognition receptors (PRRs). Of the several different families of PRRs which includes TLRs, NOD-like receptors, and mannose receptors, TLRs are the most important members and have been extensively researched in the field of intraocular inflammation. The TLRs are type 1 integral membrane receptors with an N-terminal extracellular domain for ligand binding composed of leucine rich repeats and a C-terminal cytoplasmic Toll/IL-1 receptor (TIR) domain for intracellular signaling (90). Bacterial structural components such as LPS, peptidoglycan, lipids, and lipoproteins can be detected by TLRs on RPE cells, retinal microglia, astrocytes, and Müller cells. As of today, 10 functional TLRs have been identified in humans, while 12 TLRs have been identified in mice (91). TLR1, 2, 4, 5 and 6 are expressed on the cell surface and mainly recognize PAMPs derived from bacteria, fungi and protozoa. In contrast, TLR3, 7, 8 and 9 are expressed in the cytoplasmic compartment and primarily recognize nucleic acids derived from virus and bacteria (91). Upon ligand-receptor interactions, TLRs recruit adaptor molecules including Myeloid differentiating factor 88 (MyD88) and TIR domain containing adaptor inducing interferon β (TRIF), TIR domain-containing adaptor protein (TIRAP) and TRIF-related adaptor molecule (TRAM). Stimulation of TLR signaling further induces nuclear factor kappa-B (NF-κB) nuclear translocation, or activation of interferon regulatory factors (IRFs), or mitogen-activate protein kinases (MAPKs) pathways to promote the expression of inflammatory mediators (92).

Previous studies have linked TLR signaling to inflammatory eye diseases (93–96). Significantly higher expression of TLR 2, 3, 4, and 8 has been observed in BD patients as compared with healthy controls (93). A selective perturbation in the expression and function of TLR2 and 4 was observed on the neutrophils and monocytes of patients with acute anterior uveitis (AAU) (96), suggestive of microbial triggers and TLRs in the pathogenesis of AAU, as TLR2 or TLR4 stimulation by their ligands results in internalization of the cell surface receptors (97, 98). The activation of TLR4 by endotoxin induces a standard model of uveitis in rats, referred to as endotoxin-induced uveitis (99), although the molecular mechanisms by which endotoxin induces uveitis remain unknown. Injection of different TLR agonists into iris/ciliary body explants increased production of inflammatory cytokines TNF-α, IL-6, IP-10/CXCL10, MCP-1. Intraocular injection of TLR agonist increased leukocyte interactions with the endothelium of the iris vasculature and chemotaxis into the iris tissue (100). Contradictorily, studies utilizing genetic mouse models demonstrated that TLR2, 3, 4, and 9 are highly redundant in the adjuvant effect needed to induce EAU and that diverse microbial infections may contribute to the pathogenesis of uveitis (101). TLRs may partially explain the experimental and clinical manifestations of immune-mediated uveitis implicating microbial triggers (102, 103).

Antigen-Presenting Cells

Professional APCs include dendritic cells (DCs), macrophages and B cells. APCs express and use antigen-specific surface receptors, such as PRRs, to recognize and bind their targets, such as PAMPs or DAMPs. Binding of surface PRRs to microbial PAMPs or whole bacteria induces phagocytosis of microbial pathogens by DCs or macrophages. A previous study demonstrated that the protein expression of functional endotoxin receptor TLR4 and its associated LPS receptor complex (CD14 and MD-2) was restricted to resident APCs in the normal human uvea, consisting mainly of HLA-DR$^+$ DCs. These APCs appeared to be strategically located in perivascular and subepithelial sites to detect and respond to blood-borne or intraocular LPS of Gram-negative bacteria (104). These observations were confirmed by another study showing the expression of the functional TLR4 and CD14 in human ciliary body and TLR4 in human iris endothelial cells (105), supporting the notion that microbial triggers, in particular LPS of Gram-negative bacteria may trigger AAU by activating TLR4-expressing resident uveal APCs. RPE cells *in vitro* display many characteristics typical of APC yet are poor inducers of lymphocyte proliferation (106). RPE cells express proteins for TLR1-6 and 9, and are capable of secreting IL-8 after stimulation by PAMPs (107). APCs themselves may release cytokines to directly influence the development of uveitis (108) or may pathogenically link to uveitis through regulating the function of T cells (109, 110).

Major Histocompatibility Complexes

After binding to respective PRR ligands, APCs internalize and degrade their targets by initiating phagocytosis or clathrin-mediated endocytosis, and then display the epitope by MHCs for recognition by immunologic structures like TCRs on appropriate T cells. MHCs are cell surface proteins essential for adaptive immune response. Two types of MHCs display antigens: class I MHCs and class II MHCs. Class I MHC receptors are produced by all nucleated cells and display endogenous antigens to activate CD8$^+$ cytotoxic T cells. Class II MHC receptors normally express only on professional APCs (111). HLA-B27 is present in about 50% of all patients with AAU and is the strongest genetic factor for AAU. Both HLA-B27 transgenic Lewis rats and HLA-B27 transgenic Fischer rats developed gut inflammation (112). The rats develop diarrhea, peripheral arthritis, and spondylitis, while removal of microbiota significantly reduces the symptoms, however, these rats do not develop uveitis (68, 113). Similarly, in humans, the majority of individuals who are HLA-B27-positive do not develop AAU or other autoimmune diseases, implying the involvement of other genes or environmental factors in the development of uveitis. Some literature suggests the involvement of microbial triggers in disease development, in particular Gram-negative bacteria (114, 115).

Inflammatory Mediators

Proinflammatory mediators released by retinal microglia, endothelial, or Müller cells are critical for recruiting PMNs and macrophages to sites of inflammation or infection. In addition to pathogen clearance, PMNs and macrophages produce cytokines and chemokines to increase blood-retinal barrier permeability, facilitate migration of cells, and recruit additional inflammatory cells and mediators to the inflammatory sites. Many of the proinflammatory mediators increased in experimental animal models of intraocular inflammation are also diagnosed with increased levels in the aqueous and vitreous humor of humans with inflammatory eye diseases (116). Several inflammatory mediators play essential roles in mounting an inflammatory response. TNFα is a pleiotropic cytokine that rapidly upregulates following tissue injury and can be produced by activated macrophages, T cells, and natural killer cells (117). In the eye, TNFα appears to mediate the pathogenesis of intraocular inflammation, neovascular and retinal degeneration by stimulating other retinal cells to produce cytokines, such as interferon γ, IL-1β, IL-2, IL-4, IL-6, IL-8, and IL-10, and other proinflammatory molecules, such as vascular cell adhesion molecule-1 (VCAM-1), intercellular cell adhesion molecule-1 (ICAM-1), and macrophage inflammatory protein (MIP)-1α, MIP-2, monocyte chemotactic protein-1 (MCP-1), and CXCL1 (117–120). During an intraocular inflammation, elevated levels of TNFα correlated with worsen visual acuity (120). TNFα$^{-/-}$ mice were subjected to greater bacterial growth, intraocular inflammation, and ocular structural damage after an infection (121). While bacterial growth was similar between wild-type controls and IL-6$^{-/-}$ and CXCL1$^{-/-}$ mice, the intraocular inflammation was attenuated in mice lacking CXCL-1, but not IL-6 (122).

TARGETING OCULAR MICROBIOTA AS NOVEL THERAPIES FOR INTRAOCULAR INFLAMMATION

Current treatment for intraocular inflammation includes steroids, anti-cytokine biologics, and non-biologic immunosuppressive agents therapies. While corticosteroids remain the most potent and efficacious drug for treating intraocular inflammation, results from the corticosteroids use are not optimal and poor control in some cases (123). Patients diagnosed with uveitis require prolonged repeated intravitreal injections which usually leads to many side effects, such as hyperglycemia and dysregulated bone metabolic homeostasis (124). The drugs most commonly used in replacement of corticosteroids are non-biologic immunosuppressive agents including azathioprine, methotrexate, mycophenolate and cyclosporine, all of which have been reported with potentials for significant side effects (123). The more recent anti-cytokine biologics have greatly changed the therapeutic options for non-infectious uveitis. In 2016, adalimumab as the first anti-TNFα biologic, was approved by the FDA in the treatment of non-infectious intermedia uveitis, posterior uveitis, and panuveitis. Similar anti-TNFα biologics, such as infliximab and golimumab, could also exert significant anti-inflammatory effects. In TNFα$^{-/-}$ mice, the intraocular inflammation and cytokine production was dramatically reduced in the experimental model of endophthalmitis. Unfortunately, TNFα$^{-/-}$ mice displayed poor retinal function retention, presumably due to increased bacterial load (121), providing rationale for the development of novel and more targeted therapies.

R161H mice which spontaneously developed uveitis or EAU mouse models are devoid of disease phenotypes when raised in germ-free environment or treated with broad-spectrum antibiotics (73, 74). Mechanistic basis to these phenomena has been proven by Horai et al. to be originated from gut microbe-activated T cells (74). Our recent findings of the existence of intraocular microbes imply that intraocular commensals might also contribute to the pathogenesis of uveitis, as germ-free environment and antibiotics theoretically also remove intraocular commensals, although direct evidence for this notion is still lacking. Therapies manipulating commensal microbiome have been emerged as a novel strategy to prime the host immune system to counteract several inflammatory diseases, such as inflammatory bowel disease, graft-vs.-host disease, HIV infection, and psychological-stress-induced inflammation (125–127). This is presumably due to the reason that host microbiota could shape the host immune system to dictate the proinflammatory effects of other proinflammatory stimuli (128). A recent study demonstrated that the combination of remodeling of gut microbiome and microglia inhibition significantly attenuate the progression of EAU after inflammation onset (129). A potential explanation is that antigens from commensals reprogram naïve $CD4^+$ T cells to the regulatory T cells lineage to restrain lymphocyte response (130). Nonetheless, it remains to be determined whether the clinical intervention targeting gut microbiome is efficacious in improving uveitis humans.

CONCLUSION

Commensals are a large source of intrinsic antigens that are continuously sensed by the immune system but typically do not elicit inflammation. Since the discovery of ocular surface microbiota, their interactions with the innate immunity of the ocular surface have been explored by many researchers. Up to date, the intraocular microbiota could be considered a black box. The interior of the eye is highly vascularized and contains miscellaneous types of immune cells or immune mediators. How the intraocular microbiota and intraocular immune environment interplay to modulate inflammatory eye diseases, such as uveitis, remains an open question. Most of the microorganisms that constitute the intraocular microbiome are sparse in number, anaerobic, and extremely difficult to culture. Our laboratory has employed state-of-the-art metagenomic sequencing, combined with cultural technique and micrographical analysis to unveil the mask of intraocular microbiota, which may advance our understanding toward the mechanisms of intraocular inflammation. However, puzzles as to how commensals occupy the inside of the eye, whether the intestinal microbiota contribute to or modulate the intraocular commensals, and how intraocular commensals regulate the innate and adaptive ocular immune responses await to be answered. This process is most likely involved roles of TLRs, APCs, MHCs, and many inflammatory mediators. Further delineation of the commensal types that altered in ocular inflammatory diseases, and clarification of the question that whether the commensals as a whole or specific commensal epitopes are mainly responsible for disease progression are of significant importance to expand our knowledge of the ocular immune system and intraocular inflammation.

AUTHOR CONTRIBUTIONS

JL and LW wrote the manuscript. SY prepared the figures. All authors contributed to the article and approved the submitted version.

REFERENCES

1. McDermott AM. Antimicrobial compounds in tears. *Exp Eye Res* (2013) 117:53–61. doi: 10.1016/j.exer.2013.07.014
2. Graham JE, Moore JE, Jiru X, Moore JE, Goodall EA, Dooley JS, et al. Ocular pathogen or commensal: a PCR-based study of surface bacterial flora in normal and dry eyes. *Invest Ophthalmol Vis Sci* (2007) 48(12):5616–23. doi: 10.1167/iovs.07-0588
3. Willcox MD. Characterization of the normal microbiota of the ocular surface. *Exp Eye Res* (2013) 117:99–105. doi: 10.1016/j.exer.2013.06.003
4. Miller D, Iovieno A. The role of microbial flora on the ocular surface. *Curr Opin Allergy Clin Immunol* (2009) 9(5):466–70. doi: 10.1097/ACI.0b013e3283303e1b
5. Ueta M. Innate immunity of the ocular surface and ocular surface inflammatory disorders. *Cornea* (2008) 27(Suppl 1):S31–40. doi: 10.1097/ICO.0b013e31817f2a7f
6. Owens CD, Stoessel K. Surgical site infections: epidemiology, microbiology and prevention. *J Hosp Infect* (2008) 70(Suppl 2):3–10. doi: 10.1016/S0195-6701(08)60017-1
7. Cristina ML, Sartini M, Schinca E, Ottria G, Spagnolo AM. Operating room environment and surgical site infections in arthroplasty procedures. *J Prev Med Hyg* (2016) 57(3):E142–E8.
8. Rahmani S, Eliott D. Postoperative Endophthalmitis: A Review of Risk Factors, Prophylaxis, Incidence, Microbiology, Treatment, and Outcomes. *Semin Ophthalmol* (2018) 33(1):95–101. doi: 10.1080/08820538.2017.1353826
9. Damgaard C, Magnussen K, Enevold C, Nilsson M, Tolker-Nielsen T, Holmstrup P, et al. Viable bacteria associated with red blood cells and plasma in freshly drawn blood donations. *PloS One* (2015) 10(3):e0120826. doi: 10.1371/journal.pone.0120826
10. Potgieter M, Bester J, Kell DB, Pretorius E. The dormant blood microbiome in chronic, inflammatory diseases. *FEMS Microbiol Rev* (2015) 39(4):567–91. doi: 10.1093/femsre/fuv013
11. Paisse S, Valle C, Servant F, Courtney M, Burcelin R, Amar J, et al. Comprehensive description of blood microbiome from healthy donors assessed by 16S targeted metagenomic sequencing. *Transfusion* (2016) 56 (5):1138–47. doi: 10.1111/trf.13477
12. Schierwagen R, Alvarez-Silva C, Madsen MSA, Kolbe CC, Meyer C, Thomas D, et al. Circulating microbiome in blood of different circulatory compartments. *Gut* (2019) 68(3):578–80. doi: 10.1136/gutjnl-2018-316227
13. Sorrentino FS, Matteini S, Bonifazzi C, Sebastiani A, Parmeggiani F. Diabetic retinopathy and endothelin system: microangiopathy versus endothelial dysfunction. *Eye (Lond)* (2018) 32(7):1157–63. doi: 10.1038/s41433-018-0032-4
14. Beli E, Yan Y, Moldovan L, Vieira CP, Gao R, Duan Y, et al. Restructuring of the Gut Microbiome by Intermittent Fasting Prevents Retinopathy and Prolongs Survival in db/db Mice. *Diabetes* (2018) 67(9):1867–79. doi: 10.2337/db18-0158

15. Sinclair SH, Schwartz SS. Diabetic Retinopathy-An Underdiagnosed and Undertreated Inflammatory, Neuro-Vascular Complication of Diabetes. *Front Endocrinol (Lausanne)* (2019) 10:843. doi: 10.3389/fendo.2019.00843
16. Camelo S, Castellanos J, Lafage M, Lafon M. Rabies virus ocular disease: T-cell-dependent protection is under the control of signaling by the p55 tumor necrosis factor alpha receptor, p55TNFR. *J Virol* (2001) 75(7):3427–34. doi: 10.1128/JVI.75.7.3427-3434.2001
17. Egger SF, Buxbaum A, Georgopoulos M, Scholda C, Vecsei VP, Huber-Spitzy V, et al. Bacterial growth in human vitreous humor. *Exp Eye Res* (1997) 65(6):791–5. doi: 10.1006/exer.1997.0385
18. Metchnikoff E. On aqueous humour, micro-organisms and immunity. *J Pathol Bacteriol* (1892) 1:13–20.
19. Goto H, Usui Y, Umazume A, Uchida K, Eishi Y. Propionibacterium acnes as a possible pathogen of granuloma in patients with ocular sarcoidosis. *Br J Ophthalmol* (2017) 101(11):1510–3. doi: 10.1136/bjophthalmol-2016-309248
20. Nagata K, Eishi Y, Uchida K, Yoneda K, Hatanaka H, Yasuhara T, et al. Immunohistochemical Detection of Propionibacterium acnes in the Retinal Granulomas in Patients with Ocular Sarcoidosis. *Sci Rep* (2017) 7(1):15226. doi: 10.1038/s41598-017-15710-0
21. Hori Y, Maeda N, Sakamoto M, Koh S, Inoue T, Tano Y. Bacteriologic profile of the conjunctiva in the patients with dry eye. *Am J Ophthalmol* (2008) 146(5):729–34. doi: 10.1016/j.ajo.2008.06.003
22. Fernandez-Rubio ME, Rebolledo-Lara L, Martinez-Garcia M, Alarcon-Tomas M, Cortes-Valdes C. The conjunctival bacterial pattern of diabetics undergoing cataract surgery. *Eye (Lond)* (2010) 24(5):825–34. doi: 10.1038/eye.2009.218
23. Schabereiter-Gurtner C, Maca S, Rolleke S, Nigl K, Lukas J, Hirschl A, et al. 16S rDNA-based identification of bacteria from conjunctival swabs by PCR and DGGE fingerprinting. *Invest Ophthalmol Vis Sci* (2001) 42(6):1164–71.
24. Ozkan J, Nielsen S, Diez-Vives C, Coroneo M, Thomas T, Willcox M. Temporal Stability and Composition of the Ocular Surface Microbiome. *Sci Rep* (2017) 7(1):9880. doi: 10.1038/s41598-017-10494-9
25. Schloss PD, Handelsman J. Status of the microbial census. *Microbiol Mol Biol Rev* (2004) 68(4):686–91. doi: 10.1128/MMBR.68.4.686-691.2004
26. Moeller CT, Branco BC, Yu MC, Farah ME, Santos MA, Hofling-Lima AL. Evaluation of normal ocular bacterial flora with two different culture media. *Can J Ophthalmol* (2005) 40(4):448–53. doi: 10.1139/i05-014
27. Clarridge JE3. Impact of 16S rRNA gene sequence analysis for identification of bacteria on clinical microbiology and infectious diseases. *Clin Microbiol Rev* (2004) 17(4):840–62. doi: 10.1128/CMR.17.4.840-862.2004
28. Rausch P, Ruhlemann M, Hermes BM, Doms S, Dagan T, Dierking K, et al. Comparative analysis of amplicon and metagenomic sequencing methods reveals key features in the evolution of animal metaorganisms. *Microbiome* (2019) 7(1):133. doi: 10.1186/s40168-019-0743-1
29. Dong Q, Brulc JM, Iovieno A, Bates B, Garoutte A, Miller D, et al. Diversity of bacteria at healthy human conjunctiva. *Invest Ophthalmol Vis Sci* (2011) 52(8):5408–13. doi: 10.1167/iovs.10-6939
30. Zhou Y, Holland MJ, Makalo P, Joof H, Roberts CH, Mabey DC, et al. The conjunctival microbiome in health and trachomatous disease: a case control study. *Genome Med* (2014) 6(11):99. doi: 10.1186/s13073-014-0099-x
31. Huang Y, Yang B, Li W. Defining the normal core microbiome of conjunctival microbial communities. *Clin Microbiol Infect* (2016) 22 (7):643 e7– e12. doi: 10.1016/j.cmi.2016.04.008
32. Doan T, Akileswaran L, Andersen D, Johnson B, Ko N, Shrestha A, et al. Paucibacterial Microbiome and Resident DNA Virome of the Healthy Conjunctiva. *Invest Ophthalmol Vis Sci* (2016) 57(13):5116–26. doi: 10.1167/iovs.16-19803
33. Wen X, Miao L, Deng Y, Bible PW, Hu X, Zou Y, et al. The Influence of Age and Sex on Ocular Surface Microbiota in Healthy Adults. *Invest Ophthalmol Vis Sci* (2017) 58(14):6030–7. doi: 10.1167/iovs.17-22957
34. Li Z, Gong Y, Chen S, Li S, Zhang Y, Zhong H, et al. Comparative portrayal of ocular surface microbe with and without dry eye. *J Microbiol* (2019) 57 (11):1025–32. doi: 10.1007/s12275-019-9127-2
35. Suzuki T, Sutani T, Nakai H, Shirahige K, Kinoshita S. The Microbiome of the Meibum and Ocular Surface in Healthy Subjects. *Invest Ophthalmol Vis Sci* (2020) 61(2):18. doi: 10.1167/iovs.61.2.18
36. Kelly BJ, Gross R, Bittinger K, Sherrill-Mix S, Lewis JD, Collman RG, et al. Power and sample-size estimation for microbiome studies using pairwise distances and PERMANOVA. *Bioinformatics* (2015) 31(15):2461–8. doi: 10.1093/bioinformatics/btv183
37. Tedeschi S, Negosanti L, Sgarzani R, Trapani F, Pignanelli S, Battilana M, et al. Superficial swab versus deep-tissue biopsy for the microbiological diagnosis of local infection in advanced-stage pressure ulcers of spinal-cord-injured patients: a prospective study. *Clin Microbiol Infect* (2017) 23 (12):943–7. doi: 10.1016/j.cmi.2017.04.015
38. Prast-Nielsen S, Tobin AM, Adamzik K, Powles A, Hugerth LW, Sweeney C, et al. Investigation of the skin microbiome: swabs vs. biopsies. *Br J Dermatol* (2019) 181(3):572–9. doi: 10.1111/bjd.17691
39. Glassing A, Dowd SE, Galandiuk S, Davis B, Chiodini RJ. Inherent bacterial DNA contamination of extraction and sequencing reagents may affect interpretation of microbiota in low bacterial biomass samples. *Gut Pathog* (2016) 8:24. doi: 10.1186/s13099-016-0103-7
40. Knight R, Vrbanac A, Taylor BC, Aksenov A, Callewaert C, Debelius J, et al. Best practices for analysing microbiomes. *Nat Rev Microbiol* (2018) 16 (7):410–22. doi: 10.1038/s41579-018-0029-9
41. Lu LJ, Liu J. Human Microbiota and Ophthalmic Disease. *Yale J Biol Med* (2016) 89(3):325–30.
42. Zhang Y, Liu ZR, Chen H, Fan YC, Duo J, Zheng H, et al. Comparison on conjunctival sac bacterial flora of the seniors with dry eye in Ganzi autonomous prefecture. *Int J Ophthalmol* (2013) 6(4):452–7. doi: 10.3980/j.issn.2222-3959.2013.04.08
43. Dong X, Wang Y, Wang W, Lin P, Huang Y. Composition and Diversity of Bacterial Community on the Ocular Surface of Patients With Meibomian Gland Dysfunction. *Invest Ophthalmol Vis Sci* (2019) 60(14):4774–83. doi: 10.1167/iovs.19-27719
44. Soh Qin R, Tong Hak Tien L. Healthcare delivery in meibomian gland dysfunction and blepharitis. *Ocul Surf* (2019) 17(2):176–8. doi: 10.1016/j.jtos.2018.11.007
45. Markoulli M, Flanagan J, Tummanapalli SS, Wu J, Willcox M. The impact of diabetes on corneal nerve morphology and ocular surface integrity. *Ocul Surf* (2018) 16(1):45–57. doi: 10.1016/j.jtos.2017.10.006
46. Li S, Yi G, Peng H, Li Z, Chen S, Zhong H, et al. How Ocular Surface Microbiota Debuts in Type 2 Diabetes Mellitus. *Front Cell Infect Microbiol* (2019) 9:202. doi: 10.3389/fcimb.2019.00202
47. Shivaji S. We are not alone: a case for the human microbiome in extra intestinal diseases. *Gut Pathog* (2017) 9:13. doi: 10.1186/s13099-017-0163-3
48. Thomason CA, Leon A, Kirkpatrick LT, Belden LK, Hawley DM. Eye of the Finch: characterization of the ocular microbiome of house finches in relation to mycoplasmal conjunctivitis. *Environ Microbiol* (2017) 19(4):1439–49. doi: 10.1111/1462-2920.13625
49. Consolandi C, Turroni S, Emmi G, Severgnini M, Fiori J, Peano C, et al. Behcet's syndrome patients exhibit specific microbiome signature. *Autoimmun Rev* (2015) 14(4):269–76. doi: 10.1016/j.autrev.2014.11.009
50. Terzulli M, Contreras-Ruiz L, Kugadas A, Masli S, Gadjeva M. TSP-1 Deficiency Alters Ocular Microbiota: Implications for Sjogren's Syndrome Pathogenesis. *J Ocul Pharmacol Ther* (2015) 31(7):413–8. doi: 10.1089/jop.2015.0017
51. de Paiva CS, Jones DB, Stern ME, Bian F, Moore QL, Corbiere S, et al. Altered Mucosal Microbiome Diversity and Disease Severity in Sjogren Syndrome. *Sci Rep* (2016) 6:23561. doi: 10.1038/srep23561
52. Tsigalou C, Stavropoulou E, Bezirtzoglou E. Current Insights in Microbiome Shifts in Sjogren's Syndrome and Possible Therapeutic Interventions. *Front Immunol* (2018) 9:1106. doi: 10.3389/fimmu.2018.01106
53. Zaheer M, Wang C, Bian F, Yu Z, Hernandez H, de Souza RG, et al. Protective role of commensal bacteria in Sjogren Syndrome. *J Autoimmun* (2018) 93:45–56. doi: 10.1016/j.jaut.2018.06.004
54. Callegan MC, Gilmore MS, Gregory M, Ramadan RT, Wiskur BJ, Moyer AL, et al. Bacterial endophthalmitis: therapeutic challenges and host-pathogen interactions. *Prog Retin Eye Res* (2007) 26(2):189–203. doi: 10.1016/j.preteyeres.2006.12.001
55. Streilein JW. Ocular immune privilege: therapeutic opportunities from an experiment of nature. *Nat Rev Immunol* (2003) 3(11):879–89. doi: 10.1038/nri1224
56. Stein-Streilein J. Immune regulation and the eye. *Trends Immunol* (2008) 29 (11):548–54. doi: 10.1016/j.it.2008.08.002
57. Cone RE, Pais R. Anterior Chamber-Associated Immune Deviation (ACAID): An Acute Response to Ocular Insult Protects from Future Immune-Mediated Damage? *Ophthalmol Eye Dis* (2009) 1:33–40. doi: 10.4137/oed.s2858

58. Yiu G, Chung SH, Mollhoff IN, Nguyen UT, Thomasy SM, Yoo J, et al. Suprachoroidal and Subretinal Injections of AAV Using Transscleral Microneedles for Retinal Gene Delivery in Nonhuman Primates. *Mol Ther Methods Clin Dev* (2020) 16:179–91. doi: 10.1016/j.omtm.2020.01.002
59. Anand V, Chirmule N, Fersh M, Maguire AM, Bennett J. Additional transduction events after subretinal readministration of recombinant adeno-associated virus. *Hum Gene Ther* (2000) 11(3):449–57. doi: 10.1089/10430340050015914
60. Engelbert M, Gilmore MS. Fas ligand but not complement is critical for control of experimental Staphylococcus aureus Endophthalmitis. *Invest Ophthalmol Vis Sci* (2005) 46(7):2479–86. doi: 10.1167/iovs.04-1139
61. Maeda Y, Takeda K. Role of Gut Microbiota in Rheumatoid Arthritis. *J Clin Med* (2017) 6(6):60. doi: 10.3390/jcm6060060
62. Maeda Y, Takeda K. Host-microbiota interactions in rheumatoid arthritis. *Exp Mol Med* (2019) 51(12):1–6. doi: 10.1038/s12276-019-0283-6
63. Cekanaviciute E, Yoo BB, Runia TF, Debelius JW, Singh S, Nelson CA, et al. Gut bacteria from multiple sclerosis patients modulate human T cells and exacerbate symptoms in mouse models. *Proc Natl Acad Sci U S A* (2017) 114 (40):10713–8. doi: 10.1073/pnas.1711235114
64. Gulden E, Wong FS, Wen L. The gut microbiota and Type 1 Diabetes. *Clin Immunol* (2015) 159(2):143–53. doi: 10.1016/j.clim.2015.05.013
65. Zheng P, Li Z, Zhou Z. Gut microbiome in type 1 diabetes: A comprehensive review. *Diabetes Metab Res Rev* (2018) 34(7):e3043. doi: 10.1002/dmrr.3043
66. Matsuoka K, Kanai T. The gut microbiota and inflammatory bowel disease. *Semin Immunopathol* (2015) 37(1):47–55. doi: 10.1007/s00281-014-0454-4
67. Kostic AD, Xavier RJ, Gevers D. The microbiome in inflammatory bowel disease: current status and the future ahead. *Gastroenterology* (2014) 146 (6):1489–99. doi: 10.1053/j.gastro.2014.02.009
68. Rosenbaum JT, Asquith M. The microbiome and HLA-B27-associated acute anterior uveitis. *Nat Rev Rheumatol* (2018) 14(12):704–13. doi: 10.1038/s41584-018-0097-2
69. Huang X, Ye Z, Cao Q, Su G, Wang Q, Deng J, et al. Gut Microbiota Composition and Fecal Metabolic Phenotype in Patients With Acute Anterior Uveitis. *Invest Ophthalmol Vis Sci* (2018) 59(3):1523–31. doi: 10.1167/iovs.17-22677
70. Lin P, Bach M, Asquith M, Lee AY, Akileswaran L, Stauffer P, et al. HLA-B27 and human beta2-microglobulin affect the gut microbiota of transgenic rats. *PloS One* (2014) 9(8):e105684. doi: 10.1371/journal.pone.0105684
71. Ye Z, Zhang N, Wu C, Zhang X, Wang Q, Huang X, et al. A metagenomic study of the gut microbiome in Behcet's disease. *Microbiome* (2018) 6 (1):135. doi: 10.1186/s40168-018-0520-6
72. Janowitz C, Nakamura YK, Metea C, Gligor A, Yu W, Karstens L, et al. Disruption of Intestinal Homeostasis and Intestinal Microbiota During Experimental Autoimmune Uveitis. *Invest Ophthalmol Vis Sci* (2019) 60 (1):420–9. doi: 10.1167/iovs.18-24813
73. Heissigerova J, Seidler Stangova P, Klimova A, Svozilkova P, Hrncir T, Stepankova R, et al. The Microbiota Determines Susceptibility to Experimental Autoimmune Uveoretinitis. *J Immunol Res* (2016) 2016:5065703. doi: 10.1155/2016/5065703
74. Horai R, Zarate-Blades CR, Dillenburg-Pilla P, Chen J, Kielczewski JL, Silver PB, et al. Microbiota-Dependent Activation of an Autoreactive T Cell Receptor Provokes Autoimmunity in an Immunologically Privileged Site. *Immunity* (2015) 43(2):343–53. doi: 10.1016/j.immuni.2015.07.014
75. Nakamura YK, Metea C, Karstens L, Asquith M, Gruner H, Moscibrocki C, et al. Gut Microbial Alterations Associated With Protection From Autoimmune Uveitis. *Invest Ophthalmol Vis Sci* (2016) 57(8):3747–58. doi: 10.1167/iovs.16-19733
76. Fritsche LG, Igl W, Bailey JN, Grassmann F, Sengupta S, Bragg-Gresham JL, et al. A large genome-wide association study of age-related macular degeneration highlights contributions of rare and common variants. *Nat Genet* (2016) 48(2):134–43. doi: 10.1038/ng.3448
77. Fritsche LG, Chen W, Schu M, Yaspan BL, Yu Y, Thorleifsson G, et al. Seven new loci associated with age-related macular degeneration. *Nat Genet* (2013) 45(4):433–99e1–2. doi: 10.1038/ng.2578
78. Warwick A, Lotery A. Genetics and genetic testing for age-related macular degeneration. *Eye (Lond)* (2018) 32(5):849–57. doi: 10.1038/eye.2017.245
79. Wen X, Hu X, Miao L, Ge X, Deng Y, Bible PW, et al. Epigenetics, microbiota, and intraocular inflammation: New paradigms of immune regulation in the eye. *Prog Retin Eye Res* (2018) 64:84–95. doi: 10.1016/j.preteyeres.2018.01.001
80. Zinkernagel MS, Zysset-Burri DC, Keller I, Berger LE, Leichtle AB, Largiader CR, et al. Association of the Intestinal Microbiome with the Development of Neovascular Age-Related Macular Degeneration. *Sci Rep* (2017) 7:40826. doi: 10.1038/srep40826
81. Rullo J, Far PM, Quinn M, Sharma N, Bae S, Irrcher I, et al. Local oral and nasal microbiome diversity in age-related macular degeneration. *Sci Rep* (2020) 10(1):3862. doi: 10.1038/s41598-020-60674-3
82. Ho EXP, Cheung CMG, Sim S, Chu CW, Wilm A, Lin CB, et al. Human pharyngeal microbiota in age-related macular degeneration. *PloS One* (2018) 13(8):e0201768. doi: 10.1371/journal.pone.0201768
83. Rowan S, Jiang S, Korem T, Szymanski J, Chang ML, Szelog J, et al. Involvement of a gut-retina axis in protection against dietary glycemia-induced age-related macular degeneration. *Proc Natl Acad Sci U S A* (2017) 114(22):E4472–81. doi: 10.1073/pnas.1702302114
84. Uchiki T, Weikel KA, Jiao W, Shang F, Caceres A, Pawlak D, et al. Glycation-altered proteolysis as a pathobiologic mechanism that links dietary glycemic index, aging, and age-related disease (in nondiabetics). *Aging Cell* (2012) 11 (1):1–13. doi: 10.1111/j.1474-9726.2011.00752.x
85. Andriessen EM, Wilson AM, Mawambo G, Dejda A, Miloudi K, Sennlaub F, et al. Gut microbiota influences pathological angiogenesis in obesity-driven choroidal neovascularization. *EMBO Mol Med* (2016) 8(12):1366–79. doi: 10.15252/emmm.201606531
86. Astafurov K, Elhawy E, Ren L, Dong CQ, Igboin C, Hyman L, et al. Oral microbiome link to neurodegeneration in glaucoma. *PloS One* (2014) 9(9): e104416. doi: 10.1371/journal.pone.0104416
87. Libby RT, Anderson MG, Pang IH, Robinson ZH, Savinova OV, Cosma IM, et al. Inherited glaucoma in DBA/2J mice: pertinent disease features for studying the neurodegeneration. *Vis Neurosci* (2005) 22(5):637–48. doi: 10.1017/S0952523805225130
88. Chen H, Cho KS, Vu THK, Shen CH, Kaur M, Chen G, et al. Commensal microflora-induced T cell responses mediate progressive neurodegeneration in glaucoma. *Nat Commun* (2018) 9(1):3209. doi: 10.1038/s41467-018-05681-9
89. Gong H, Zhang S, Li Q, Zuo C, Gao X, Zheng B, et al. Gut microbiota compositional profile and serum metabolic phenotype in patients with primary open-angle glaucoma. *Exp Eye Res* (2020) 191:107921. doi: 10.1016/j.exer.2020.107921
90. Botos I, Segal DM, Davies DR. The structural biology of Toll-like receptors. *Structure* (2011) 19(4):447–59. doi: 10.1016/j.str.2011.02.004
91. Chang JH, McCluskey PJ, Wakefield D. Recent advances in Toll-like receptors and anterior uveitis. *Clin Exp Ophthalmol* (2012) 40(8):821–8. doi: 10.1111/j.1442-9071.2012.02797.x
92. Kawai T, Akira S. Toll-like receptors and their crosstalk with other innate receptors in infection and immunity. *Immunity* (2011) 34(5):637–50. doi: 10.1016/j.immuni.2011.05.006
93. Liu X, Wang C, Ye Z, Kijlstra A, Yang P. Higher expression of Toll-like receptors 2, 3, 4, and 8 in ocular Behcet's disease. *Invest Ophthalmol Vis Sci* (2013) 54(9):6012–7. doi: 10.1167/iovs.13-12159
94. Fang J, Chen L, Tang J, Hou S, Liao D, Ye Z, et al. Association Between Copy Number Variations of TLR7 and Ocular Behcet's Disease in a Chinese Han Population. *Invest Ophthalmol Vis Sci* (2015) 56(3):1517–23. doi: 10.1167/iovs.14-15030
95. Jiang Y, Wang H, Yu H, Li L, Xu D, Hou S, et al. Two Genetic Variations in the IRF8 region are associated with Behcet's disease in Han Chinese. *Sci Rep* (2016) 6:19651. doi: 10.1038/srep19651
96. Chang JH, Hampartzoumian T, Everett B, Lloyd A, McCluskey PJ, Wakefield D. Changes in Toll-like receptor (TLR)-2 and TLR4 expression and function but not polymorphisms are associated with acute anterior uveitis. *Invest Ophthalmol Vis Sci* (2007) 48(4):1711–7. doi: 10.1167/iovs.06-0807
97. Triantafilou M, Manukyan M, Mackie A, Morath S, Hartung T, Heine H, et al. Lipoteichoic acid and toll-like receptor 2 internalization and targeting to the Golgi are lipid raft-dependent. *J Biol Chem* (2004) 279(39):40882–9. doi: 10.1074/jbc.M400466200
98. Nomura F, Akashi S, Sakao Y, Sato S, Kawai T, Matsumoto M, et al. Cutting edge: endotoxin tolerance in mouse peritoneal macrophages correlates with down-regulation of surface toll-like receptor 4 expression. *J Immunol* (2000) 164(7):3476–9. doi: 10.4049/jimmunol.164.7.3476
99. Rosenbaum JT, McDevitt HO, Guss RB, Egbert PR. Endotoxin-induced uveitis in rats as a model for human disease. *Nature* (1980) 286(5773):611–3. doi: 10.1038/286611a0

100. Allensworth JJ, Planck SR, Rosenbaum JT, Rosenzweig HL. Investigation of the differential potentials of TLR agonists to elicit uveitis in mice. *J Leukoc Biol* (2011) 90(6):1159–66. doi: 10.1189/jlb.0511249
101. Fang J, Fang D, Silver PB, Wen F, Li B, Ren X, et al. The role of TLR2, TRL3, TRL4, and TRL9 signaling in the pathogenesis of autoimmune disease in a retinal autoimmunity model. *Invest Ophthalmol Vis Sci* (2010) 51(6):3092–9. doi: 10.1167/iovs.09-4754
102. Chang JH, McCluskey PJ, Wakefield D. Toll-like receptors in ocular immunity and the immunopathogenesis of inflammatory eye disease. *Br J Ophthalmol* (2006) 90(1):103–8. doi: 10.1136/bjo.2005.072686
103. Wakefield D, Gray P, Chang J, Di Girolamo N, McCluskey P. The role of PAMPs and DAMPs in the pathogenesis of acute and recurrent anterior uveitis. *Br J Ophthalmol* (2010) 94(3):271–4. doi: 10.1136/bjo.2008.146753
104. Chang JH, McCluskey P, Wakefield D. Expression of toll-like receptor 4 and its associated lipopolysaccharide receptor complex by resident antigen-presenting cells in the human uvea. *Invest Ophthalmol Vis Sci* (2004) 45 (6):1871–8. doi: 10.1167/iovs.03-1113
105. Brito BE, Zamora DO, Bonnah RA, Pan Y, Planck SR, Rosenbaum JT. Toll-like receptor 4 and CD14 expression in human ciliary body and TLR-4 in human iris endothelial cells. *Exp Eye Res* (2004) 79(2):203–8. doi: 10.1016/j.exer.2004.03.012
106. Liversidge J, McKay D, Mullen G, Forrester JV. Retinal pigment epithelial cells modulate lymphocyte function at the blood-retina barrier by autocrine PGE2 and membrane-bound mechanisms. *Cell Immunol* (1993) 149(2):315–30. doi: 10.1006/cimm.1993.1158
107. Mai K, Chui JJ, Di Girolamo N, McCluskey PJ, Wakefield D. Role of toll-like receptors in human iris pigment epithelial cells and their response to pathogen-associated molecular patterns. *J Inflammation (Lond)* (2014) 11:20. doi: 10.1186/1476-9255-11-20
108. Dodge IL, Carr MW, Cernadas M, Brenner MB. IL-6 production by pulmonary dendritic cells impedes Th1 immune responses. *J Immunol* (2003) 170(9):4457–64. doi: 10.4049/jimmunol.170.9.4457
109. Gregerson DS, Heuss ND, Lew KL, McPherson SW, Ferrington DA. Interaction of retinal pigmented epithelial cells and CD4 T cells leads to T-cell anergy. *Invest Ophthalmol Vis Sci* (2007) 48(10):4654–63. doi: 10.1167/iovs.07-0286
110. Hsu SM, Mathew R, Taylor AW, Stein-Streilein J. Ex-vivo tolerogenic F4/80 (+) antigen-presenting cells (APC) induce efferent CD8(+) regulatory T cell-dependent suppression of experimental autoimmune uveitis. *Clin Exp Immunol* (2014) 176(1):37–48. doi: 10.1111/cei.12243
111. Wieczorek M, Abualrous ET, Sticht J, Alvaro-Benito M, Stolzenberg S, Noe F, et al. Major Histocompatibility Complex (MHC) Class I and MHC Class II Proteins: Conformational Plasticity in Antigen Presentation. *Front Immunol* (2017) 8:292. doi: 10.3389/fimmu.2017.00292
112. Gill T, Asquith M, Brooks SR, Rosenbaum JT, Colbert RA. Effects of HLA-B27 on Gut Microbiota in Experimental Spondyloarthritis Implicate an Ecological Model of Dysbiosis. *Arthritis Rheumatol* (2018) 70(4):555–65. doi: 10.1002/art.40405
113. Baggia S, Lyons JL, Angell E, Barkhuizen A, Han YB, Planck SR, et al. A novel model of bacterially-induced acute anterior uveitis in rats and the lack of effect from HLA-B27 expression. *J Invest Med* (1997) 45(5):295–301.
114. Rosenbaum JT, Lin P, Asquith M. Does the Microbiome Cause B27-related Acute Anterior Uveitis? *Ocul Immunol Inflamm* (2016) 24(4):440–4. doi: 10.3109/09273948.2016.1142574
115. Misiuk-Hojlo M, Miedzybrodzki R, Grzybowski A, Lugowski C, Niedziela T, Turno-Krecicka A, et al. Elevated levels of anti-endotoxin antibodies in patients with bilateral idiopathic acute anterior uveitis. *Acta Ophthalmol* (2011) 89(3):e283–8. doi: 10.1111/j.1755-3768.2010.01969.x
116. Curnow SJ, Murray PI. Inflammatory mediators of uveitis: cytokines and chemokines. *Curr Opin Ophthalmol* (2006) 17(6):532–7. doi: 10.1097/ICU.0b013e32801094b5
117. Mirshahi A, Hoehn R, Lorenz K, Kramann C, Baatz H. Anti-tumor necrosis factor alpha for retinal diseases: current knowledge and future concepts. *J Ophthalmic Vis Res* (2012) 7(1):39–44.
118. Bazzoni F, Beutler B. The tumor necrosis factor ligand and receptor families. *N Engl J Med* (1996) 334(26):1717–25. doi: 10.1056/NEJM199606273342607
119. Cid MC, Kleinman HK, Grant DS, Schnaper HW, Fauci AS, Hoffman GS. Estradiol enhances leukocyte binding to tumor necrosis factor (TNF)-stimulated endothelial cells via an increase in TNF-induced adhesion molecules E-selectin, intercellular adhesion molecule type 1, and vascular cell adhesion molecule type 1. *J Clin Invest* (1994) 93(1):17–25. doi: 10.1172/JCI116941
120. Deshmukh D, Chakrabarti M, Jayasudha R, Hasnat Ali M, Tyagi M, Sharma S, et al. Elevated cytokine levels in vitreous as biomarkers of disease severity in infectious endophthalmitis. *PloS One* (2018) 13(10):e0205292. doi: 10.1371/journal.pone.0205292
121. Ramadan RT, Moyer AL, Callegan MC. A role for tumor necrosis factor-alpha in experimental Bacillus cereus endophthalmitis pathogenesis. *Invest Ophthalmol Vis Sci* (2008) 49(10):4482–9. doi: 10.1167/iovs.08-2085
122. Parkunan SM, Randall CB, Astley RA, Furtado GC, Lira SA, Callegan MC. CXCL1, but not IL-6, significantly impacts intraocular inflammation during infection. *J Leukoc Biol* (2016) 100(5):1125–34. doi: 10.1189/jlb.3A0416-173R
123. Jabs DA. Immunosuppression for the Uveitides. *Ophthalmology* (2018) 125 (2):193–202. doi: 10.1016/j.ophtha.2017.08.007
124. Pleyer U, Pohlmann D, Kardes E, Poddubnyy D, Rademacher J. Emerging drugs for the treatment of noninfectious uveitis. *Expert Opin Emerg Drugs* (2019) 24(3):173–90. doi: 10.1080/14728214.2019.1663823
125. Ouyang J, Isnard S, Lin J, Fombuena B, Peng X, Nair Parvathy S, et al. Treating From the Inside Out: Relevance of Fecal Microbiota Transplantation to Counteract Gut Damage in GVHD and HIV Infection. *Front Med (Lausanne)* (2020) 7:421. doi: 10.3389/fmed.2020.00421
126. Mishima Y, Sartor RB. Manipulating resident microbiota to enhance regulatory immune function to treat inflammatory bowel diseases. *J Gastroenterol* (2020) 55(1):4–14. doi: 10.1007/s00535-019-01618-1
127. Xu C, Lee SK, Zhang D, Frenette PS. The Gut Microbiome Regulates Psychological-Stress-Induced Inflammation. *Immunity* (2020) 53(2):417–28 e4. doi: 10.1016/j.immuni.2020.06.025
128. Suriguga S, Luangmonkong T, Mutsaers HAM, Groothuis GMM, Olinga P. Host microbiota dictates the proinflammatory impact of LPS in the murine liver. *Toxicol In Vitro* (2020) 67:104920. doi: 10.1016/j.tiv.2020.104920
129. Zhou J, Yang J, Dai M, Lin D, Zhang R, Liu H, et al. A combination of inhibiting microglia activity and remodeling gut microenvironment suppresses the development and progression of experimental autoimmune uveitis. *Biochem Pharmacol* (2020) 180:114108. doi: 10.1016/j.bcp.2020.114108
130. Kuczma MP, Szurek EA, Cebula A, Chassaing B, Jung YJ, Kang SM, et al. Commensal epitopes drive differentiation of colonic Tregs. *Sci Adv* (2020) 6 (16):eaaz3186. doi: 10.1126/sciadv.aaz3186

20

CFH I62V as a Putative Genetic Marker for Posner-Schlossman Syndrome

Ming Ming Yang[1], *Hong Yan Sun*[1], *Ting Meng*[1], *Shan Hu Qiu*[2], *Qi Qiao Zeng*[1], *Tsz Kin Ng*[3,4], *Li Jiang*[1], *Ting Ming Deng*[1], *Ai Neng Zeng*[1], *Jun Wang*[2*] *and Xiao Ling Luo*[1*]

[1] *Department of Ophthalmology, Shenzhen People's Hospital, The Second Clinical Medical College of Jinan University & The First Affiliated Hospital of Southern University of Science and Technology, Shenzhen, China,* [2] *Department of Endocrinology, Shenzhen People's Hospital, The Second Clinical Medical College of Jinan University & The First Affiliated Hospital of Southern University of Science and Technology, Shenzhen, China,* [3] *Joint Shantou International Eye Center of Shantou University and The Chinese University of Hong Kong, Shantou, China,* [4] *Department of Ophthalmology and Visual Sciences, The Chinese University of Hong Kong, Hong Kong, China*

***Correspondence:**
Jun Wang
wangjun4622@163.com
Xiao Ling Luo
lxl2603@vip.sina.com

Objective: Posner-Schlossman syndrome (PSS), also known as glaucomatocyclitic crisis, is an ocular condition characterized by recurrent attacks of anterior uveitis and raised intraocular pressure. Previous studies by our team and others have identified the genetic association of complement pathway genes with uveitis and glaucoma. This study aimed to investigate the complement genes in PSS patients with the view of elucidating the genetic background of the disease.

Methods: A total of 331 subjects (56 PSS patients and 275 controls) were recruited for this study. We selected 27 variants in six complement pathway genes (*SERPING1*, *C2*, *CFB*, *CFH*, *C3*, and *C5*) and detected them using TaqMan single nucleotide polymorphism (SNP) Genotyping Assays. Univariate SNP association analysis, haplotype-based association analysis, gene-gene interaction analysis among complement genes, and genotype-phenotype correlation analysis were performed.

Results: Among the 27 variants of six complement pathway genes, the functional variant I62V (rs800292) at the *CFH* gene was found to be significantly associated with PSS; there was a significant increase in the frequency of A allele and AA homozygosity in PSS patients than in controls ($P = 1.79 \times 10^{-4}$; odds ratio (OR) 2.18, 95% CI: 1.44–3.29; $P = 4.65 \times 10^{-4}$; OR 3.66, 95% CI: 1.70–7.85, respectively). The additive effect of *CFH*-rs800292 and *SERPING1*-rs3824988 was identified with an OR of 12.50 (95% CI: 2.16–72.28). Genotype-phenotype analysis indicated that the rs800292 AA genotype was associated with a higher intraocular pressure and higher frequency of recurrence. Unlike a high proportion of human leukocyte antigen (HLA)-B27 positivity in anterior uveitis, only 3 in 56 (5.36%) PSS patients were HLA-B27 positive. In addition, one haplotype block (GC) in the *SERPING1* gene showed a nominal association with PSS with an increased risk of 2.04 ($P = 0.01$; 95% CI: 1.18–3.53), but the *P*-value could not withstand the Bonferroni correction ($P_{corr} > 0.05$).

Conclusion: This study revealed a genetic association of a *CFH* variant with PSS as well as its clinical parameters, implying that the alternative complement pathway might play an important role in the pathogenesis of PSS. Further studies to enrich the understanding of the genetic background of PSS and the role of the complement system in ocular inflammation are warranted.

Keywords: uveitis, posner-schlossman syndrome (PSS), complement system, genes, single nucleotide polymorphisms, complement factor H

INTRODUCTION

Posner-Schlossman syndrome (PSS), also known as glaucomatocyclitic crisis, is an ocular condition that presents with recurrent anterior uveitis and acutely with markedly elevated intraocular pressure (IOP). It is often classified as secondary inflammatory glaucoma (1, 2). The main clinical manifestations of PSS are elevated IOP and blurred vision, with a tendency to affect patients between 20 and 50 years of age. Long-term recurrent PSS patients are at a high risk of developing permanent complications, such as optic nerve atrophy and loss of vision (2).

The exact pathogenesis of PSS is largely unknown, and previous studies have suggested that genetic susceptibility, infection, and autoimmune drive may contribute to the disease (1, 3, 4). Multiple genetic loci in human leukocyte antigen (*HLA*) have been identified to be associated with PSS in Japanese and Chinese populations, such as *HLA-Ia, HLA-II, HLA-Bw54, HLA-E,* and *HLA-G.* These recent genetic studies have not only helped shed light on the pathogenesis of the disease, but also have suggested that they share common etiologies with other hypertensive uveitic conditions (5–8). To date, however, no specific gene other than *HLA* has been found to directly cause PSS.

The complement system, a key innate immune defense system, plays an important role in modulating various immune and inflammatory responses. In our previous studies, we intensively studied the genetic profiles of complement pathway genes in uveitis, including complement factor H (*CFH*), complement factor B (*CFB*), complement component 2 (*C2*), complement component 3 (*C3*), complement component 5 (*C5*), and complement component 1 inhibitor gene (*SERPING1*) (9–17). Moreover, recent studies have implicated complement cascades in glaucomatous neurodegeneration. IOP also modulates the immune system by inducing several complement components such as *CFH*, *C3*, *C1q*, and *C1r* (18, 19).

In view of the above findings and considering that PSS shared the characteristics of both anterior uveitis and glaucoma, the primary aim of this study was to investigate the genetic associations of 27 variants in complement pathway genes in PSS patients. Our secondary aim was to further identify any associations between these genes and specific phenotypes to understand the genetic background of this disease.

Abbreviations: PSS, Posner-Schlossman syndrome; IOP, intraocular pressure; *HLA*, human leukocyte antigen; *CFH*, complement factor H; *CFB*, complement factor B; *C2*, complement component 2; *C3*, complement component 3; *C5*, complement component 5; *SERPING1*, complement component 1 inhibitor gene; KP, keratic precipitates; SNPs, single nucleotide polymorphisms; OR, odds ratio; CI, confidence interval; *C1*, complement component 1.

MATERIALS AND METHODS

Study Participants

All study subjects were enrolled at the Chinese University of Hong Kong Eye Center and Shenzhen Peoples' Hospital. Informed consent was obtained from each study participant, and the study protocol was in accordance with the ethical guidelines of the Declaration of Helsinki. The study was approved by the Medical Ethics Committee of the Chinese University of Hong Kong Eye Center and the Clinical Research Ethics Committee of Shenzhen Peoples' Hospital.

Fifty-six PSS patients were recruited for this study. The diagnosis of PSS was based on the following clinical features: repeated episodes of unilateral moderate to high elevation of IOP with blurred vision, mild anterior chamber inflammation and mutton-fat-like keratic precipitates (KPs), open anterior chamber angles under high IOP, and no obvious posterior synechiae of the iris (20). For each patient, the clinical course of ocular inflammation was documented, including visual acuity, slit-lamp biomicroscopy, IOP, age at onset, clinical features (KPs, posterior synechiae, and anterior chamber cells), laterality, frequency of recurrence, and complications of PSS. A total of 275 individuals without any systemic immune-related disorders and major eye diseases except senile cataract were recruited as control subjects. All subjects underwent full clinical examination and basic ophthalmic investigations.

Selection and Genotyping of Single Nucleotide Polymorphisms

Twenty-seven single nucleotide polymorphisms (SNPs) in six genes/loci in the complement pathway were selected in the present study, including rs17030, rs344555, rs2241393, rs2241392, rs428453, rs11672613, rs2230205, and rs2250656 in *C3*; rs3020644, rs9332739, rs4151667, rs1048709, rs17201431, rs537160, and rs2072633 in the *C2/CFB* locus; rs1005511 and rs3824988 in *SERPING1*; rs12237774, rs2269066, rs17611, rs1548782, rs10985126, and rs1017119 in *C5*; and rs3753394, rs800292, and rs1065489 in *CFH*. Genomic DNA was extracted from peripheral blood using the QIAamp Blood Kit (Qiagen; Hilden, Germany). The 27 SNPs were assessed using TaqMan genotyping assays (Applied Biosystems, Foster City, CA, USA) in a Roche LightCycler 480 real-time polymerase chain reaction System (Roche Diagnostics, Basel, Switzerland), according to the manufacturer's instructions. The HLA-B27 allele was detected using nested polymerase chain reaction as described by Konno et al. (21).

Statistical Analysis

The Hardy-Weinberg equilibrium of each SNP in the controls was assessed using the χ^2 test in PLINK (V.1.07, available in the public domain at http://pngu.mgh.harvard.edu/~purcell/plink/). Allelic and genotypic frequencies between cases and controls were compared using the χ^2 test or Fisher's exact test. Dominant and recessive models were applied to investigate the disease association with regard to the minor allele, and the odds ratio (OR) and 95% confidence intervals (CI) were calculated. Logistic regression analysis was applied to adjust for the association of these SNPs with age and sex. IOP, age at onset, anterior chamber cells, and frequency of recurrence were analyzed by the *t*-test or Mann–Whitney *U* test, whereas the presence of posterior synechiae and KPs were analyzed by χ^2 test or Fisher's exact test. Moreover, stratified analysis based on the clinical manifestations was also performed. Pairwise linkage disequilibrium between polymorphisms and expectation-maximization algorithm-based haplotype association analyses were performed using Haploview (ver. 4.2). Furthermore, we applied the W-test for gene-gene interaction analysis. The joint effects of these pairs of SNPs were also analyzed with reference to the individuals with both the non-risk genotypes at the two studied SNPs. In individual association analysis, a $P < 0.05$ was considered statistically significant. The Bonferroni method was used to correct the *P*-values in multiple testing, with a $P < 0.0019$ ($P = 0.05/27$, where 27 was the number of SNPs included in this study) being considered statistically significant.

RESULTS

Clinical Characteristics

The demographic and clinical characteristics of the PSS patients and healthy controls are shown in **Table 1**. This study involved a total of 331 unrelated subjects, including 56 patients with PSS (24 males, 32 females; mean age ± SD: 49.9 ± 14.0 years) and 275 controls (122 males, 153 females; mean age ± SD: 54.3 ± 7.6 years). Among the PSS patients, 53 (94.6%) had increased IOP at first onset, 50 (89.3%) had recurrent episodes of PSS, and the average frequency of recurrence was 6.3±4.9. Forty-two (75.0%) patients had KP signs and only three (5.4%) were HLA-B27 positive.

Association of Complement Genes With PSS

All the selected SNPs conformed to the Hardy-Weinberg equilibrium in the control group. Twenty-seven SNPs in *C3*, *C2/CFB*, *SERPING1*, *C5*, and *CFH* in the complement pathway were genotyped and statistically analyzed in PSS patients and healthy controls. Among the 27 SNPs, rs800292 in *CFB* was significantly associated with PSS ($P = 1.79\times10^{-4}$; OR 2.18, 95% CI: 1.44–3.29), with the minor allele A conferring a 2.18-fold increased risk of PSS (**Table 2**). Meanwhile, genetic association was also identified in the genotypic recessive model; there was a significant increase in the frequency of AA homozygosity in PSS patients than in controls ($P = 4.65\times10^{-4}$; OR 3.66, 95% CI: 1.70–7.85). In addition, a higher frequency of the *SERPING1*/rs3824988 CC genotype and C allele was found in PSS patients than in healthy controls (CC: $P = 0.036$; OR 7.73; C: $P = 0.01$, OR 1.99). A lower frequency of the *C5*/rs1017119 C allele was found in PSS patients ($P = 0.043$; OR 0.47) (**Table 3**). However, these two associations lost significance after adjusting for multiple testing. No significant association was identified for the other 24 SNPs, either in allelic or genotypic models. Gender stratification analysis of rs800292 showed a statistically significant association in female PSS patients ($P = 0.001$; OR 2.60, 95% CI: 1.50–4.51), but not in male patients (**Table 4**).

TABLE 1 | The demographic and clinical features of the PSS cases and controls.

	Total	%
PSS patients		
Age (year, mean ± SD)	49.9 ± 14.0	
Male	24	42.9
Female	32	57.1
Affected eyes		
Right eye	29	51.8
Left eye	25	44.6
Both eyes	2	3.6
IOP >21 mmHg	53	94.6
IOP (mmHg, mean ± SD)	42.8 ± 11.7	
KPs	42	75.0
Recurrent frequency (times, mean ± SD)	6.3 ± 4.9	
Healthy controls		
Age (year, mean ± SD)	54.3 ± 7.6	
Male	122	44.4
Female	153	55.6

PSS, Posner-Schlossman syndrome; IOP, intraocular pressure, the highest IOP of the affected eye; KPs, keratic precipitates.

Comparison of Clinical Parameters in Different Genotypes

Genotype-phenotype correlation analysis was done in terms of multiple clinical features such as IOP, age of onset, number of flares, frequency of recurrence, and the presence of KPs. Considering the significant association of *CFH*-rs800292 with PSS in this study, correlations between specific genotypes and clinical features were evaluated in the PSS patients. We discovered a relationship between rs800292 and IOP level, as well as frequency of recurrence. The mean IOP (49.69 ± 6.58 mmHg) in patients homozygous for the risk allele A at SNP rs800292 was significantly higher than patients with the genotypes AG+GG (40.67 ± 12.14 mmHg; $P = 0.001$; **Figure 1**). Similarly, patients with genotype AA had a relatively higher frequency of recurrence (9.83 ± 5.25 times) than those with G carriers (6.11 ± 4.81 times; $P = 0.026$; **Figure 2**). Associations with other clinical features were not observed.

Gene-Gene Interaction and Joint-Effect Analysis

We applied the W-test for pairwise gene-gene interaction analysis and identified a significant interaction of one pair: *CFH*-rs800292 with *SERPING1*-rs3824988. Joint-effect analysis was conducted

TABLE 2 | Allelic association of genetic variants with PSS.

No.	Gene/Locus	Variants	Minor allele	PSS($n = 56$)	Control($n = 275$)	*P*-values	OR (95% CI)
1	*C3*	rs17030	G	0.420	0.415	0.92	1.02 (0.07–1.54)
2		rs344555	A	0.312	0.251	0.18	1.35 (0.87–2.12)
3		rs2241393	G	0.312	0.344	0.53	1.15 (0.74–1.78)
4		rs2241392	G	0.330	0.313	0.71	1.08 (0.70–1.67)
5		rs428453	C	0.170	0.162	0.84	1.06 (0.62–1.82)
6		rs11672613	G	0.455	0.427	0.58	1.12 (0.75–1.69)
7		rs2230205	A	0.464	0.424	0.43	1.18 (0.78–1.77)
8		rs2250656	G	0.232	0.236	0.92	1.02 (0.63–1.66)
9	*C2-CFB*	rs3020644	A	0.429	0.484	0.29	1.25 (0.83–1.88)
10		rs9332739	C	0.009	0.027	0.49*	2.94 (0.39–22.53)
11		rs4151667	A	0.018	0.029	0.75*	1.65 (0.37–7.27)
12		rs1048709	A	0.317	0.280	0.44	1.20 (0.76–1.88)
13		rs17201431	C	0	0.020	0.23*	1.02 (1.01–1.03)
14		rs537160	A	0.491	0.484	0.89	1.03 (0.69–1.55)
15		rs4151657	C	0.277	0.251	0.57	1.14 (0.72–1.80)
16		rs2072633	G	0.393	0.435	0.42	1.19 (0.78–1.80)
17	*C1INH*	rs1005511	G	0.295	0.227	0.13	1.42 (0.90–2.23)
18		rs3824988	C	0.188	0.104	0.01	2.00 (1.15–3.45)
19	*C5*	rs12237774	T	0.152	0.198	0.25	1.38 (0.79–2.41)
20		rs2269066	C	0.170	0.218	0.25	1.37 (0.80–2.33)
21		rs17611	G	0.357	0.411	0.29	1.26 (0.82–1.92)
22		rs1548782	T	0.214	0.204	0.80	1.07 (0.65–1.75)
23		rs10985126	C	0.188	0.244	0.20	1.40 (0.84–2.33)
24		rs1017119	C	0.071	0.142	0.04	2.15 (1.01–4.58)
25	*CFH*	rs3753394	C	0.491	0.400	0.08	1.45 (0.95–2.19)
26		rs800292	A	0.491	0.307	1.79×10^{-4}	2.18 (1.44–3.29)
27		rs1065489	T	0.482	0.442	0.15	1.35 (0.89–2.05)

*PSS, Posner-Schlossman syndrome; C3, component 3; C2, component 2; CFB, complement factor B; SERPING1, component 1 inhibitor gene; C5, component 5; CFH, complement factor H; CI, confidence interval; OR, odds ratio; *Fisher exact test.*

TABLE 3 | Genotypic association of rs3824988, rs1017119, and rs800292 in PSS patients and healthy controls.

SNP	Genotype/Allele	PSS		Controls		*P*-value	OR	95% CI
		n	%	*n*	%			
rs3824988	CC	3	5.4	2	0.7	0.046	1.90	1.01–3.57
SERPING1	CT	15	26.8	53	19.3	0.036*	7.73	1.26–47.36
	TT	38	67.9	220	80.0			
	C	21	18.8	57	10.4	0.012	1.99	1.15–3.45
rs1017119	CC	0	0.0	5	1.8	0.052	0.46	0.21–1.02
C5	CT	8	14.3	68	24.7	0.594*	1.02	1.00–1.04
	TT	48	85.7	202	73.5			
	C	8	0.9	78	14.2	0.043	0.47	0.22–0.99
rs800292	AA	13	23.2	21	7.6	0.003	2.61	1.36–5.00
CFH	AG	29	51.8	127	46.2	4.65×10^{-4}	3.66	1.70–7.85
	GG	14	25.0	127	46.2			
	A	55	49.1	169	30.7	1.79×10^{-4}	2.18	1.44–3.29

*PSS, Posner-Schlossman syndrome; SERPING1, component 1 inhibitor gene; C5, component 5; CFH, complement factor H; CI, confidence interval; OR, odds ratio; *Fisher exact test.*

TABLE 4 | Polymorphisms of *CFH*-rs800292 in PSS patients and healthy controls stratified by gender.

SNP	Genotype/Allele	PSS		Controls		*P*-value	OR	95% CI
		n	%	*n*	%			
Male	AA	4	16.7	10	6.5	0.085	2.47	0.86–7.04
	AG	15	62.5	64	41.8	0.248*	2.24	0.64–7.85
	GG	5	20.8	48	31.4			
	A	23	47.9	84	34.4	0.076	1.75	0.94–3.27
Female	AA	9	28.1	11	9.0	0.015	2.73	1.19–6.28
	AG	14	43.8	63	51.6	0.002*	5.05	1.89–13.53
	GG	9	28.1	79	64.8			
	A	32	50.0	85	27.8	0.001	2.60	1.50–4.51

*PSS, Posner-Schlossman syndrome; CFH, complement factor H; CI, confidence interval; OR, odds ratio; *Fisher exact test.*

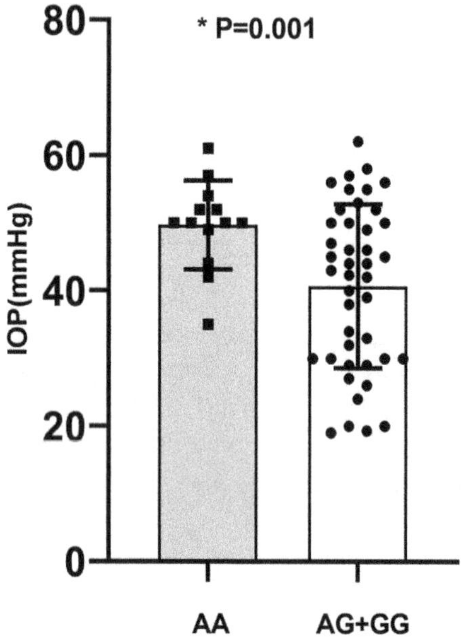

FIGURE 1 | The average of IOP in PSS patients according to genotype of rs800292. AA: 49.69 ± 6.58; AG+GG: 40.67 ± 12.14 (mmHg). *statistical significance.

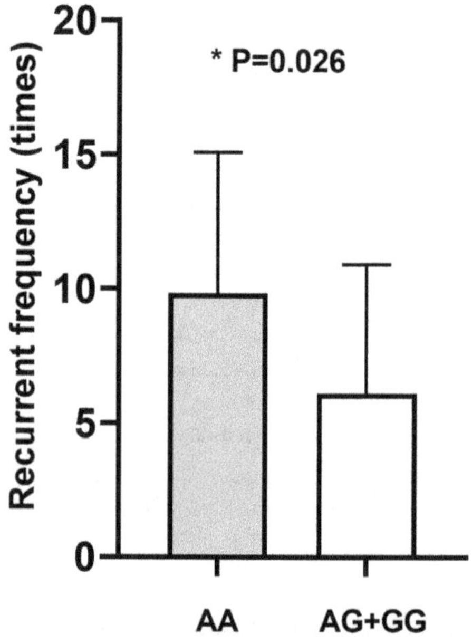

FIGURE 2 | The average disease recurrent frequency of PSS according to genotype. AA: 9.83 ± 5.25; AG+GG: 6.11 ± 4.81 (times). *statistical significance.

to estimate the ORs of PSS for each possible combination of genotypes from these two loci, with the homozygous non-risk genotypes as reference. A joint disease OR of 12.50 in individuals with the rs800292 AA genotype and rs3824988 risk allele (C) carriers was observed than in the baseline non-risk genotypes, with the calculated 95% CI in a wide range from 2.16 to 72.28 ($P = 0.012$; **Table 5**; **Figure 3**)

Linkage Disequilibrium and Haplotype Association Analysis

Pairwise linkage disequilibrium analysis was performed for all six selected genes in the complement pathway using these 27 SNPs, and five haplotype blocks were detected. Block 1 involved SNPs rs17030 and rs344555 at *C3*; Block 2 involved SNPs rs428453 and rs11672613 at *C3*; Block 3 involved SNPs rs1048709, rs537160, rs4151667, and rs2072633 at the *C2/CFB* locus; Block 4 involved SNPs rs1005511 and rs3824988 at *SERPING1*; and Block 5 involved SNPs rs17611 and rs1548782 at *C5* (**Figure 4**). A risk haplotype, GC, defined by block 4 was identified. It conferred a 2.04-fold increased risk of PSS, but the statistical significance did not remain after multiple corrections ($P = 0.01$; permutation $P = 0.24$; **Table 6**).

DISCUSSION

In this study, we identified the functional variant rs800292 (I62V) at *CFH* involved in the complement system to be significantly associated with PSS ($P = 1.79 \times 10^{-4}$), conferring a 2.18-fold

TABLE 5 | Interaction analysis between *CFH*-rs800292 and *SERPING1*-rs3824988.

a. Genotype distribution	***CFH*-rs800292**					
SERPING1-rs3824988	**Controls (*n* = 275)**			**PSS (*n* = 56)**		
	GG	**AG**	**AA**	**GG**	**AG**	**AA**
TT	100 (36.3)	102 (37.1)	18 (6.5)	8 (14.3)	20 (35.7)	10 (17.9)
CT+CC	27 (9.8)	25 (9.1)	3 (1.1)	6 (10.7)	9 (16.1)	3 (5.4)

b. Joint odds ratios and 95% confidence interval	***CFH*-rs800292**		
***SERPING1*-rs3824988**	**GG**	**AG**	**AA**
TT	1.00 (Ref)	2.45 (1.03–5.82)	1.06 (0.40–2.79)
CT+CC	2.78 (0.89–8.69)	4.50 (1.58–12.84)	12.50 (2.16–72.28)

PSS, Posner-Schlossman syndrome; SERPING1, component 1 inhibitor gene; CFH, complement factor H.

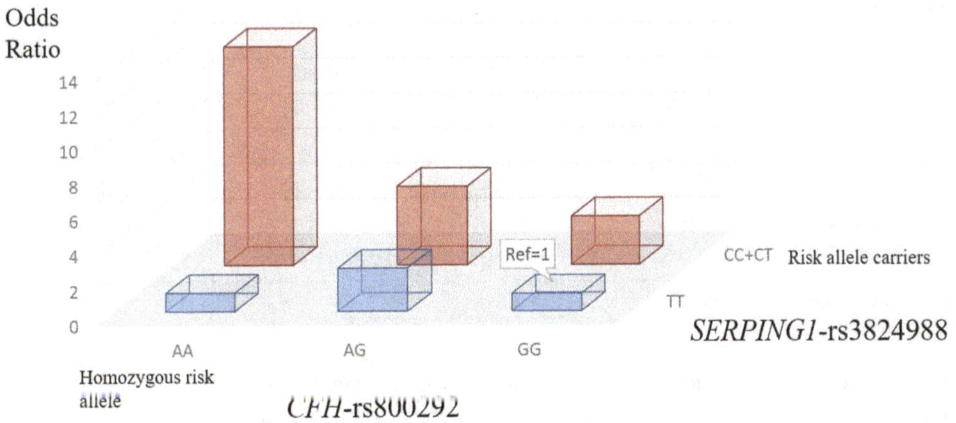

FIGURE 3 | Two-locus (*CFH* and *SERPING1*) genotype-specific PSS risk.

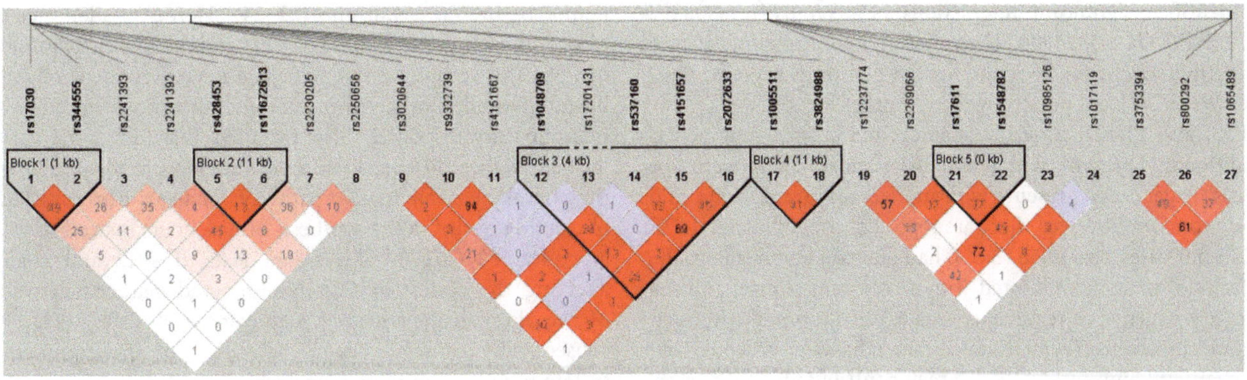

FIGURE 4 | Pairwise LD among 27 SNPs in complement genes across complement system. The haplotype block was defined by the confidence interval method implemented in the Haploview software. The LD (r^2) between any two SNPs is listed in the cross cells.

TABLE 6 | Haplotype analysis of complement pathway genes in PSS patients and healthy controls.

Haplotype	Frequency	Frequency		*P*	*Chi square*	Odds ratio 95% CI
		PSS	Controls			
Block 1 (rs17030, rs344555)						
AG	0.585	0.580	0.585	0.921	0.010	-
GA	0.261	0.312	0.251	0.176	1.829	-
GG	0.154	0.107	0.164	0.131	2.278	-
Block 2 (rs428453, rs11672613)						
GG	0.430	0.455	0.424	0.551	0.356	-
GA	0.407	0.375	0.414	0.450	0.570	-
CA	0.161	0.169	0.159	0.785	0.074	-
Block 3 (rs1048709, rs537160, rs4151657, rs2072633)						
AATA	0.279	0.309	0.273	0.437	0.605	-
GGCG	0.255	0.277	0.251	0.567	0.328	-
GATA	0.204	0.181	0.208	0.520	0.415	-
GGTG	0.165	0.115	0.175	0.117	2.456	-
GGTA	0.089	0.116	0.084	0.273	1.202	-
Block 4 (rs1005511, rs3824988)						
AT	0.760	0.705	0.771	0.138	2.197	-
GT	0.123	0.107	0.126	0.592	0.287	-
GC	0.116	0.187	0.102	0.010	6.639	2.04 (1.18–3.53)
Block 5 (rs17611, rs1548782)						
AA	0.596	0.643	0.587	0.274	1.199	-
GT	0.204	0.214	0.201	0.763	0.091	-
GA	0.198	0.143	0.209	0.109	2.576	-

PSS, Posner-Schlossman syndrome; CI, confidence interval.

increase in risk of PSS. Such an association was also found in the genotypic dominant and recessive models. In particular, rs800292 showed a significant association with the IOP level and frequency of recurrence ($P = 0.001$ and 0.026, respectively). Patients with the risk genotype AA had a higher IOP level and higher frequency of recurrence, indicating an association with severity of inflammation and disease prognosis. Furthermore, we identified significant interactions between *CFH* rs800292 and *SERPING1* rs3824988. These findings confirmed *CFH* as a susceptibility gene for PSS, and for the first time, revealed *CFH* rs800292 (I62V) as a putative genetic marker for PSS.

PSS, also known as glaucomatocyclitic crisis, is an ocular condition that presents with markedly elevated IOP and anterior uveitis. It generally presents with unilateral blurred vision and eye discomfort; however, there are reported cases of bilateral PSS (2). In our cases, two in 56 (3.6%) had bilateral involvement, the majority of patients presented with a recurrent course, and the average frequency of recurrence was 6.3 ± 4.9 times. Although the exact mechanism remains uncertain, it has been accepted that infection and autoimmune drive may contribute to the disease. In addition, identification of the HLA locus in PSS implies a role for genetic variants of immune regulation in PSS pathogenesis (5, 7, 8). However, no specific genes other than HLA were identified to be significantly associated with PSS.

Our previous studies have made significant advancements in depicting the genetic profiles of complement pathway genes in uveitis, and *CFH* has been identified to be significantly associated with anterior uveitis as well as intermediate and posterior uveitis entities (13, 14, 16). Furthermore, *CFH* gene polymorphisms are also associated with multiple inflammatory diseases, such as age-related macular degeneration, diabetic retinopathy, and atypical hemolytic-uremic syndrome (22–24). Here, we identified the association between rs800292 at *CFH* and the clinical parameters of PSS. The complement system is a key component of innate immunity and is involved in modulating various immune and inflammatory responses. SNP rs800292 is a functional variant located in the *CFH* gene which is a major soluble inhibitor of the complement alternative pathway. Changes in the rs800292 nucleotide results in the synthesis of isoleucine instead of valine at codon 62 (I62V). This might lead to structural changes affecting the ability of C3b binding and reduced activation of the alternative pathway C3-convertase (C3bBb) (25). This subsequently causes excessive activation of the complement system to induce immunologic disorders.

We identified genotype-phenotype correlations between *CFH* rs800292 (I62V) and PSS. The functional variant conferred a higher risk for elevated IOP ($P = 0.001$) and higher frequency of recurrence ($P = 0.026$). Clinically, patients with higher IOP and more recurrent episodes have more visual complications and are at risk of developing permanent complications such as optic nerve atrophy and loss of vision (26). Therefore, rs800292 identified in this study might be a useful genetic biomarker for the prediction of severe courses and may provide guidance for the frequency of follow-up.

Furthermore, the female-specific association and SNP-gender interaction between rs800292 and PSS suggested that additional risk factors may be required for *CFH* to exert its effect on the pathogenesis of PSS. Gender differences in inflammation susceptibility have been found in previous studies by our team and others (13, 14, 27). The di?erence in susceptibility to microbial infection between males and females may be partially explained by the di?erence in sex hormones, or likely through an epistatic function (28). However, the exact mechanism is still elusive, and further validation in a larger cohort of PSS is warranted.

Considering the biological relevance of these genes in the complement cascade, we performed pairwise gene-gene interaction analysis and identified significant interactions of one particular pair: *CFH*-rs800292 with *SERPING1*-rs3824988. CFH and *SERPING1* proteins are key regulators of the alternative and classical complement pathways respectively, the protein encoded by *SERPING1* regulates complement component 1 (*C1*) by inhibiting the proteolytic activity of its subcomponents C1r and C1s (29). *SERPING1* has been shown to be associated with age-related macular degeneration and multiple immune-mediated diseases; *SERPING1* mRNA is also expressed in both the retina and the retinal pigment epithelium-choroid layers of human donor eyes (30). In addition, a risk haplotype, GC, defined by *SERPING1* SNPs rs3824988 and rs1005511 was identified, although the statistical significance did not remain after multiple corrections. Our findings provide additional evidence for the involvement of the complement system, especially the upstream cascade, in relation to PSS. Unfortunately, the functions of these genes and proteins in PSS are yet to be elucidated.

Several limitations of our study need to be discussed. First, the relatively small sample size may lower the statistical power and may generate a type II error in our statistical analysis. To reduce the likelihood of such errors, we have increased the number of healthy controls. Second, although we analyzed 27 tag-SNPs to capture the majority of common genetic variations of the complement cascade, they may not sufficiently reflect the genetic impact of the complement system on PSS, as some identified functional SNPs conferring susceptibility to immune-related diseases were not investigated in this study because of lower minor allele frequency. Last but not least, the exact biological function of these genes/loci has not yet been reported. Therefore, further investigations of more regions in the complement cascade using a larger cohort and in other ethnic groups could help to consolidate our findings. In addition, a comprehensive evaluation of the "hot" region, especially the alternative pathway, by extensive sequencing to uncover unknown variations is worthwhile.

In summary, we have identified the association of *CFH* functional variant rs800292 (I62V) with PSS and its clinical parameters, providing new evidence to support *CFH* as a susceptibility gene for PSS. This insight would help to understand the genetic background of PSS and help in the early detection of manifestations of the disease.

ETHICS STATEMENT

The studies involving human participants were reviewed and approved by the Medical Ethics Committee of the Chinese University of Hong Kong and the Clinical Research Ethics Committee of Shenzhen Peoples' Hospital. The patients/participants provided their written informed consent to participate in this study.

AUTHOR CONTRIBUTIONS

MY, JW, and XL designed the experiments. HS, TM, AZ, TD, QZ, and LJ performed the experiments. MY, SQ, and JW performed the analysis and wrote the paper. TN and XL revised the paper. All authors contributed to the editing of the paper and to scientific discussions.

ACKNOWLEDGMENTS

We express our greatest gratitude to all the participants in this study.

REFERENCES

1. Megaw R, Agarwal PK. Posner-Schlossman syndrome. *Surv Ophthalmol.* (2017) 62:277–85. doi: 10.1016/j.survophthal.2016.12.005
2. Shazly TA, Aljajeh M, Latina MA. Posner-Schlossman glaucomatocyclitic crisis. *Semin Ophthalmol.* (2011) 26:282–4. doi: 10.3109/08820538.2011.605821
3. Chan NS, Chee SP, Caspers L, Bodaghi B. Clinical features of CMV-associated anterior uveitis. *Ocul Immunol Inflamm.* (2018) 26:107–15. doi: 10.1080/09273948.2017.1394471
4. Hedayatfar A, Chee SP. Posner-Schlossman syndrome associated with cytomegalovirus infection: a case series from a non-endemic area. *Int Ophthalmol.* (2014) 34:1123–9. doi: 10.1007/s10792-014-9928-6
5. Hirose S, Ohno S, Matsuda H. HLA-Bw54 and glaucomatocyclitic crisis. *Arch Ophthalmol.* (1985) 103:1837–9. doi: 10.1001/archopht.1985.01050120071023
6. Huang X, Xu Y, Chen W, Zhu T, He L, Wang S, et al. The genetic contribution of HLA-E*01:03 and HLA-E*01:03-G*01:01 to Posner-Schlossman syndrome in southern Chinese. *Ann Transl Med.* (2019) 7:749. doi: 10.21037/atm.2019.11.70
7. Zhao J, Huang XS, Peng SM, Mei SY, Xu YP. A novel HLA-G allele, HLA-G*01:01:01:07, was identified in a Chinese patient with Posner-Schlossman syndrome. *HLA.* (2017) 90:136–40. doi: 10.1111/tan.13058
8. Zhao J, Zhu T, Chen W, Fan BJ, He L, Yang B, et al. Human leukocyte antigens-b and -c loci associated with posner-schlossman syndrome in a southern chinese population. *PLoS ONE.* (2015) 10:e0132179. doi: 10.1371/journal.pone.0132179
9. Wang QF, Huang XF, Zheng ZL, Dai ML, Cai WJ, Yang MM, et al. Association of CD59 and CFH polymorphisms with acute anterior uveitis in Chinese population. *Eye (Lond).* (2016) 30:1452–7. doi: 10.1038/eye.2016.146
10. Wang Y, Huang XF, Yang MM, Cai WJ, Zheng MQ, Mao G, et al. CFI-rs7356506 is a genetic protective factor for acute anterior uveitis in Chinese patients. *Br J Ophthalmol.* (2014) 98:1592–6. doi: 10.1136/bjophthalmol-2014-305296
11. Yang M, Fan JJ, Wang J, Zhao Y, Teng Y, Liu P. Association of the C2-CFB locus with non-infectious uveitis, specifically

predisposed to Vogt-Koyanagi-Harada disease. *Immunol Res.* (2016) 64:610–8. doi: 10.1007/s12026-015-8762-x
12. Yang MM, Lai TY, Luk FO, Pang CP. The roles of genetic factors in uveitis and their clinical significance. *Retina.* (2014) 34:1–11. doi: 10.1097/IAE.0b013e31829f7415
13. Yang MM, Lai TY, Tam PO, Chiang SW, Chan CK, Luk FO, et al. CFH 184G as a genetic risk marker for anterior uveitis in Chinese females. *Mol Vis.* (2011) 17:2655–64.
14. Yang MM, Lai TY, Tam PO, Chiang SW, Chan CK, Luk FO, et al. Complement factor H and interleukin gene polymorphisms in patients with non-infectious intermediate and posterior uveitis. *Mol Vis.* (2012) 18:1865–72. doi: 10.1246/bcsj.46.2869
15. Yang MM, Lai TY, Tam PO, Chiang SW, Ng TK, Liu K, et al. Association of C2 and CFB polymorphisms with anterior uveitis. *Invest Ophthalmol Vis Sci.* (2012) 53:4969–74. doi: 10.1167/iovs.12-9478
16. Yang MM, Lai TY, Tam PO, Chiang SW, Ng TK, Rong SS, et al. Association of CFH and SERPING1 polymorphisms with anterior uveitis. *Br J Ophthalmol.* (2013) 97:1475–80. doi: 10.1136/bjophthalmol-2013-303679
17. Yang MM, Wang J, Dong L, Kong J, Teng Y, Liu P, et al. Lack of association of C3 gene with uveitis: additional insights into the genetic profile of uveitis regarding complement pathway genes. *Sci Rep.* (2017) 7:879. doi: 10.1038/s41598-017-00833-1
18. Ren L, Danias J. A role for complement in glaucoma? *Adv Exp Med Biol.* (2010) 703:95–104. doi: 10.1007/978-1-4419-5635-4_7
19. Rosen AM, Stevens B. The role of the classical complement cascade in synapse loss during development and glaucoma. *Adv Exp Med Biol.* (2010) 703:75–93. doi: 10.1007/978-1-4419-5635-4_6
20. Jiang JH, Zhang SD, Dai ML, Yang JY, Xie YQ, Hu C, et al. Posner-Schlossman syndrome in Wenzhou, China: a retrospective review study. *Br J Ophthalmol.* (2017) 101:1638–42. doi: 10.1136/bjophthalmol-2016-309863
21. Konno Y, Numaga J, Tsuchiya N, Ogawa A, Islam SM, Mochizuki M, et al. HLA-B27 subtypes and HLA class II alleles in Japanese patients with anterior uveitis. *Invest Ophthalmol Vis Sci.* (1999) 40:1838–44.
22. Bernabeu-Herrero ME, Jimenez-Alcazar M, Anter J, Pinto S, Sanchez Chinchilla D, Garrido S, et al. Complement factor H, FHR-3 and FHR-1 variants associate in an extended haplotype conferring increased risk of atypical hemolytic uremic syndrome. *Mol Immunol.* (2015) 67(2 Pt B):276–86. doi: 10.1016/j.molimm.2015.06.021
23. Lu F, Liu S, Hao Q, Liu L, Zhang J, Chen X, et al. Association between complement factor c2/c3/cfb/cfh polymorphisms and age-related macular degeneration: a meta-analysis. *Genet Test Mol Biomarkers.* (2018) 22:526–40. doi: 10.1089/gtmb.2018.0110
24. Wang J, Yang MM, Li YB, Liu GD, Teng Y, Liu XM. Association of CFH and CFB gene polymorphisms with retinopathy in type 2 diabetic patients. *Mediators Inflamm.* (2013) 2013:748435. doi: 10.1155/2013/748435
25. Jha P, Bora PS, Bora NS. The role of complement system in ocular diseases including uveitis and macular degeneration. *Mol Immunol.* (2007) 44:3901–8. doi: 10.1016/j.molimm.2007.06.145
26. Lippert J, Falgiani M, Ganti L. Posner-Schlossman Syndrome. *Cureus.* (2020) 12:e6584. doi: 10.7759/cureus.6584
27. Aigner C, Gaggl M, Kain R, Prohaszka Z, Garam N, Csuka D, et al. Sex differences in clinical presentation and outcomes among patients with complement-gene-variant-mediated thrombotic microangiopathy. *J Clin Med.* (2020) 9:964. doi: 10.3390/jcm9040964
28. Scotland RS, Stables MJ, Madalli S, Watson P, Gilroy DW. Sex differences in resident immune cell phenotype underlie more efficient acute inflammatory responses in female mice. *Blood.* (2011) 118:5918–27. doi: 10.1182/blood-2011-03-340281
29. Davis AE III, Whitehead AS, Harrison RA, Dauphinais A, Bruns GA, Cicardi M, et al. Human inhibitor of the first component of complement, C1: characterization of cDNA clones and localization of the gene to chromosome 11. *Proc Natl Acad Sci USA.* (1986) 83:3161–5. doi: 10.1073/pnas.83.10.3161
30. Ennis S, Jomary C, Mullins R, Cree A, Chen X, Macleod A, et al. Association between the SERPING1 gene and age-related macular degeneration: a two-stage case-control study. *Lancet.* (2008) 372:1828–34. doi: 10.1016/S0140-6736(08)61348-3

Permissions

All chapters in this book were first published by Frontiers; hereby published with permission under the Creative Commons Attribution License or equivalent. Every chapter published in this book has been scrutinized by our experts. Their significance has been extensively debated. The topics covered herein carry significant findings which will fuel the growth of the discipline. They may even be implemented as practical applications or may be referred to as a beginning point for another development.

The contributors of this book come from diverse backgrounds, making this book a truly international effort. This book will bring forth new frontiers with its revolutionizing research information and detailed analysis of the nascent developments around the world.

We would like to thank all the contributing authors for lending their expertise to make the book truly unique. They have played a crucial role in the development of this book. Without their invaluable contributions this book wouldn't have been possible. They have made vital efforts to compile up to date information on the varied aspects of this subject to make this book a valuable addition to the collection of many professionals and students.

This book was conceptualized with the vision of imparting up-to-date information and advanced data in this field. To ensure the same, a matchless editorial board was set up. Every individual on the board went through rigorous rounds of assessment to prove their worth. After which they invested a large part of their time researching and compiling the most relevant data for our readers.

The editorial board has been involved in producing this book since its inception. They have spent rigorous hours researching and exploring the diverse topics which have resulted in the successful publishing of this book. They have passed on their knowledge of decades through this book. To expedite this challenging task, the publisher supported the team at every step. A small team of assistant editors was also appointed to further simplify the editing procedure and attain best results for the readers.

Apart from the editorial board, the designing team has also invested a significant amount of their time in understanding the subject and creating the most relevant covers. They scrutinized every image to scout for the most suitable representation of the subject and create an appropriate cover for the book.

The publishing team has been an ardent support to the editorial, designing and production team. Their endless efforts to recruit the best for this project, has resulted in the accomplishment of this book. They are a veteran in the field of academics and their pool of knowledge is as vast as their experience in printing. Their expertise and guidance has proved useful at every step. Their uncompromising quality standards have made this book an exceptional effort. Their encouragement from time to time has been an inspiration for everyone.

The publisher and the editorial board hope that this book will prove to be a valuable piece of knowledge for researchers, students, practitioners and scholars across the globe.

List of Contributors

S. M. Shamsul Islam and Hasan M. Sayeed
Department of Biomedical Science, School of Medicine, Ajou University, Suwon, South Korea

Hye-Myung Ryu
Department of Microbiology, Ajou University School of Medicine, Suwon, South Korea

Seonghyang Sohn
Department of Biomedical Science, School of Medicine, Ajou University, Suwon, South Korea
Department of Microbiology, Ajou University School of Medicine, Suwon, South Korea

Sahar A. Alhakeem
Molecular Immunology Section, Laboratory of Immunology, National Eye Institute (NEI), National Institutes of Health, Bethesda, MD, United States
Department of Biomedical Sciences, College of Health Sciences, University of Wisconsin- Milwaukee, Milwaukee, WI, United States

Charles E. Egwuagu and Evaristus C. Mbanefo
Molecular Immunology Section, Laboratory of Immunology, National Eye Institute (NEI), National Institutes of Health, Bethesda, MD, United States

Claudia Barfüßer, Carmen Wiedemann, Anne L. C. Hoffmann, Sieglinde Hirmer and Cornelia A. Deeg
Chair of Physiology, Department of Veterinary Sciences, Ludwig-Maximilians-Universität (LMU) Munich, Martinsried, Germany

Jing Xu, Guannan Su, Xinyue Huang, Rui Chang, Zhijun Chen, Zi Ye and Qingfeng Cao
The First Affiliated Hospital of Chongqing Medical University, Chongqing Branch of National Clinical Research Center for Ocular Diseases, Chongqing, China

Peizeng Yang
The First Affiliated Hospital of Chongqing Medical University, Chongqing Key Lab of Ophthalmology, Chongqing Eye Institute, Chongqing Branch of National Clinical Research Center for Ocular Diseases, Chongqing, China

Aize Kijlstra
University Eye Clinic Maastricht, Maastricht, Netherlands

Roxane L. Degroote
Chair of Physiology, Department of Veterinary Sciences, LMU Munich, Munich, Germany

MinHee K. Ko and Deming Sun
Doheny Eye Institute and Department of Ophthalmology, David Geffen School of Medicine at UCLA, Los Angeles, CA, United States

Hui Shao
Department of Ophthalmology and Visual Sciences, Kentucky Lions Eye Center, University of Louisville, Louisville, KY, United States

Henry J. Kaplan
Department of Ophthalmology, Saint Louis University (SLU) Eye Institute, SLU School of Medicine, Saint Louis, MO, United States

Han Jiang, Min Wu, Hangyu Liu, Zhu Song, Qiangqiang Wang, Junwei Zhang and Junyan Han
Department of Immunology, School of Basic Medicine, Tongji Medical College, Huazhong University of Science and Technology, Wuhan, China

Zhaohui Li, Jianhua Wu, Jing Yuan, Mengyao Han, Tao Xu, Junwen He, Chengfeng Yu and Sha Pan
Retinal and Vitreous Diseases Department of Wuhan Aier Eye Hospital, Wuhan University, Wuhan, China

Long Yu, Haihong Zeng, Yafei Huang and Shen Qu
Department of Pathogen Biology, School of Basic Medicine, Tongji Medical College, Huazhong University of Science and Technology, Wuhan, China

Ying Zhang and Shan Wang
Ophthalmic Imaging Department of Wuhan Aier Eye Hospital, Wuhan University, Wuhan, China

Li Zhou
Cataract Department of Wuhan Aier Eye Hospital, Wuhan University, Wuhan, China

Jessica Matas, Victor Llorenç, Maria Teresa Sainz de la Maza, Marc Figueras-Roca, Marina Mesquida, Alfredo Adán and Blanca Molins
Group of Ocular Inflammation, Institut d'Investigacions Biomèdiques Agustí Pi i Sunyer (IDIBAPS), Hospital Clínic de Barcelona, Barcelona, Spain

Alex Fonollosa, Joseba Artaraz and Barbara Berasategui
Department of Ophthalmology, BioCruces Health Research Institute, Hospital Cruces, University of the Basque Country, Baracaldo, Spain

David Díaz-Valle
Ophthalmology Department and Health Research Institute (IdISSC), Hospital Clinic of San Carlos, Madrid, Spain

Cristina Esquinas
Valle Hebron Research Institute, Autonomous University of Barcelona, Barcelona, Spain

Minghang Pei
Department of Ophthalmology, The First Affiliated Hospital of Zhengzhou University, Zhengzhou, China

Xinshu Liu
Department of Ophthalmology, The Fourth People's Hospital of Shenyang, Shenyang, China

Chan Zhao, Fei Gao, Yi Qu, Anyi Liang, Junyan Xiao and Meifen Zhang
Department of Ophthalmology, Peking Union Medical College Hospital, Chinese Academy of Medical Sciences and Peking Union Medical College, Beijing, China

Jonas J. W. Kuiper and Wouter J. Venema
Department of Ophthalmology, University Medical Center Utrecht, University of Utrecht, Utrecht, Netherlands
Center for Translational Immunology, University Medical Center Utrecht, University of Utrecht, Utrecht, Netherlands

Denis Wakefield
Faculty of Medicine, University of NSW Sydney, Kensington, NSW, Australia
NSW Health Pathology and South Eastern Sydney, LHD, Sydney, NSW, Australia

Daniel Clarke
Department of Medicine, South Eastern Sydney, LHD, Sydney, NSW, Australia

Peter McCluskey
Save Sight Institute, The University of Sydney, Sydney, NSW, Australia
Discipline of Clinical Ophthalmology and Eye Health, Faculty of Medicine and Health, The University of Sydney, Sydney, NSW, Australia

Gerhild Wildner and Maria Diedrichs-Möhring
Section of Immunobiology, Department of Ophthalmology, University Hospital, LMU Munich, München, Germany

Lydia J. Bradley, Amy Ward, Madeleine C. Y. Hsue and Lindsay B. Nicholson
School of Cellular and Molecular Medicine, University of Bristol, Bristol, United Kingdom

Jian Liu and David A. Copland
Academic Unit of Ophthalmology, Translational Health Sciences, University of Bristol, Bristol, United Kingdom

Andrew D. Dick
School of Cellular and Molecular Medicine, University of Bristol, Bristol, United Kingdom
Academic Unit of Ophthalmology, Translational Health Sciences, University of Bristol, Bristol, United Kingdom
University College London, Institute of Ophthalmology, London, United Kingdom

Feargal J. Ryan
Precision Medicine Theme, South Australian Health & Medical Research Institute, Adelaide, SA, Australia

Jillian M. Carr, Yuefang Ma, Liam M. Ashander, Genevieve F. Oliver, G. Bracho Granado, Abby C. Dawson, Michael Z. Michael and Binoy Appukuttan
Flinders University College of Medicine and Public Health, Bedford Park, SA, Australia

David J. Lynn and Justine R. Smith
Precision Medicine Theme, South Australian Health & Medical Research Institute, Adelaide, SA, Australia
Flinders University College of Medicine and Public Health, Bedford Park, SA, Australia

João M. Furtado and Milena Simoes
Ophthalmology Division, Ribeirão Preto Medical School, University of São Paulo, Ribeirão Preto, Brazil

Christine Mölzer, Heather M. Wilson and John V. Forrester
Institute of Medical Sciences, University of Aberdeen, Aberdeen, United Kingdom

Jarmila Heissigerova
Department of Ophthalmology, First Faculty of Medicine, Charles University and General University Hospital in Prague, Prague, Czechia

Lucia Kuffova
Institute of Medical Sciences, University of Aberdeen, Aberdeen, United Kingdom
Eye Clinic, Aberdeen Royal Infirmary, Aberdeen, United Kingdom

Tong Zhang and Xiaofeng Hou
Shenzhen Eye Institute, Shenzhen Eye Hospital, Jinan University, Shenzhen, China

Xiaosheng Huang, Xinhua Liu, Zonghui Yan, Kun Zeng, Danyao Nie, Shaoyi Mei, Tianhui Zhu, Shiming Peng and Liangnan Sun
Shenzhen Eye Institute, Shenzhen Eye Hospital, Jinan University, Shenzhen, China
School of Ophthalmology, Optometry, Shenzhen Eye Hospital, Shenzhen University, Shenzhen, China

Jiamin Cai and Ye Ye
School of Ophthalmology, Optometry, Shenzhen Eye Hospital, Shenzhen University, Shenzhen, China

Jun Zhao
Department of Ophthalmology, Shenzhen People's Hospital (The Second Clinical Medical College, Jinan University; The First Affiliated Hospital, Southern University of Science and Technology), Shenzhen, China

Nafeesa Mehmood, Liying Low and Graham R. Wallace
Institute of Inflammation and Ageing, College of Medical and Dental Sciences, University of Birmingham, Birmingham, United Kingdom

Masaki Takeuchi and Nobuhisa Mizuki
Department of Ophthalmology and Visual Science, Yokohama City University Graduate School of Medicine, Yokohama, Japan

Shigeaki Ohno
Department of Ophthalmology, Faculty of Medicine and Graduate School of Medicine, Hokkaido University, Sapporo, Japan

Jing Jing Li, Sanjun Yi and Lai Wei
State Key Laboratory of Ophthalmology, Zhongshan Ophthalmic Center, Sun Yat-sen University, Guangzhou, China

Ming Ming Yang, Hong Yan Sun, Ting Meng, Qi Qiao Zeng, Li Jiang, Ting Ming Deng, Ai Neng Zeng and Xiao Ling Luo
Department of Ophthalmology, Shenzhen People's Hospital, The Second Clinical Medical College of Jinan University & The First Affiliated Hospital of Southern University of Science and Technology, Shenzhen, China

Shan Hu Qiu and Jun Wang
Department of Endocrinology, Shenzhen People's Hospital, The Second Clinical Medical College of Jinan University & The First Affiliated Hospital of Southern University of Science and Technology, Shenzhen, China

Tsz Kin Ng
Joint Shantou International Eye Center of Shantou University and The Chinese University of Hong Kong, Shantou, China
Department of Ophthalmology and Visual Sciences, The Chinese University of Hong Kong, Hong Kong, China

Index

L

M

N

O

P

R

S

T

U

V

Z

www.ingramcontent.com/pod-product-compliance
Lightning Source LLC
LaVergne TN
LVHW082213200926
848484LV00008B/2246